Brain Dynamics Series

Induced Rhythms in the Brain

Brain Dynamics Series

Induced Rhythms in the Brain

Edited by
E. Başar
T.H. Bullock

Preface by V.B. Mountcastle

With 93 figures, some in color

Birkhäuser
Boston · Basel · Berlin

Erol Başar
Institute of Physiology
Medical University Lübeck
Ratzeburger Allee 160
D-2400 Lübeck 1
GERMANY

Theodore H. Bullock
Department of Neurosciences, 0201
University of California, San Diego
La Jolla, CA 92093
USA

Library of Congress Cataloging-in-Publication Data
Induced rhythms in the brain / edited by E. Başar, T.H. Bullock;
preface by V.B. Mountcastle.
p. cm. — (Brain dynamics series)
Includes bibliographical references and index.
ISBN 0-8176-3537-8 (alk. paper). — ISBN 3-7643-3537-8 (alk.
paper)
1. Visual cortex. 2. Electroencephalography. 3. Visual evoked
response. I. Başar, Erol. II. Bullock, Theodore Holmes.
III. Series.
[DNLM: 1. Brain—physiology. 2. Evoked Potentials.
3. Periodicity. WL 300 I42]
QP383.12.I53 1991
612.8′2—dc20
DNLM/DLC
for Library of Congress 92-7081
CIP

Printed on acid-free paper.

ISBN 0-8176-3537-8
ISBN 3-7643-3537-8

Typeset by Asco Trade Typesetting Ltd., Hong Kong.
Printed and bound by Quinn-Woodbine, Woodbine, New Jersey
Printed in U.S.A.

9 8 7 6 5 4 3 2 1

Brain Dynamics

Series Editors:

Erol Başar (Editor in Chief), Medical University of Lübeck
W.J. Freeman, University of California, Berkeley
W.-D. Heiss, Max-Planck-Institut für Neurologische Forschung
D. Lehmann, University Hospital, Zürich
F.H. Lopes da Silva, University of Amsterdam
E.-J. Speckmann, University of Münster

Books in the Series:

Dynamics of Sensory and Cognitive Processing by the Brain
E. Başar, editor
ISBN 0-387-16994-6

Brain Dynamics: Progress and Perspectives
E. Başar and T.H. Bullock, editors
ISBN 0-387-50867-8

Chaos in Brain Function
E. Başar, editor
ISBN 0-387-52329-4

Induced Rhythms in the Brain
E. Başar and T.H. Bullock, editors
ISBN 0-8176-3537-8

Forthcoming:

Slow Potential Changes in the Brain
W. Haschke, E.-J. Speckmann, and A. Roitbak, editors
ISBN 0-8176-3583-1

Publisher's Note

With this volume, the publication of the *Brain Dynamics Series* is being transferred from Springer-Verlag Heidelberg to Birkhäuser Boston.

The aim of this Series continues to be the publication of monographs and multi-authored subject collections in interdisciplinary neuroscience research, clinical as well as basic, with emphasis on "brain dynamics", the complex interactions of the ever-changing states of the brain's machinery.

The transfer of the Series (of which most of the Editors are European) to Birkhäuser Boston will further reaffirm the importance of international cooperation in research on the brain, and help strengthen the neuroscience publication bridge between scientists in Europe and in the United States.

Books in the *Brain Dynamics Series* will include the following subject areas:

EEG, MEG, evoked and event-related brain responses
Neural populations and neural networks
Neuropathology and brain function
Model epilepsies
Brain imaging
Dynamics of neural populations at the cellular level
Comparative neurophysiology
Chaotic dynamics in brain function
Cognitive functions of the brain

Contents

Cortical Rhythms, Ongoing (EEG) and Induced (ERPs)

Thalamic Oscillations

Contributors

W. Ross Adey
Pettis Memorial Veteran's Hospital
Loma Linda, California, USA

L. F. Abbott
Brandeis University
Waltham, Massachusetts, USA

Martin Arndt
Institut für Angewandte Physik und Biophysik
Philipps-Universität Marburg
Marburg, Germany

Erol Başar
Institut für Physiologie
Medizinische Universität Lübeck
Lübeck, Germany

Canan Başar-Eroglu
Institut für Physiologie
Medizinische Universität Lübeck
Lübeck, Germany

Roman Bauer
Institut für Angewandte Physik und Biophysik
Philipps-Universität Marburg
Marburg, Germany

Michael Brosch
Institut für Angewandte Physik und Biophysik
Philipps-Universität Marburg
Marburg, Germany

Theodore H. Bullock
Department of Neurosciences 0201
University of California, San Diego
La Jolla, California, USA

György Buzsáki
Center for Molecular and Behavioral Neuroscience
Rutgers University
Newark, New Jersey, USA

Roberto Curró Dossi
Université Laval
Faculté de Médécine
Cité Universitaire
Québec, Canada

Peter Dicke
Institut für Angewandte Physik und Biophysik
Philipps-Universität Marburg
Marburg, Germany

Reinhard Eckhorn
Institut für Angewandte Physik und Biophysik
Philipps-Universität Marburg
Marburg, Germany

Gerald M. Edelman
The Neurosciences Institute of the Neurosciences Research Program
New York, New York, USA

Andreas K. Engel
Neurophysiologische Abteilung
Max-Planck-Institut für Hirnforschung
Frankfurt, Germany

Walter J. Freeman
Department of Molecular & Cell Biology
Division of Neurobiology
University of California
Berkeley, California, USA

Robert Galambos
University of California at San Diego
School of Medicine
La Jolla, California, USA

Albert Goldbeter
Faculté des Sciences
Université Libre de Bruxelles
Bruxelles, Belgium

Charles M. Gray
The Salk Institute for Biological Studies
San Diego, California, USA

H. Haken
Institut für Theoretische Physik und Synergetik
Universität Stuttgart
Stuttgart, Germany

Scott L. Hooper
Department of Biology
Brandeis University
Waltham, Massachusetts, USA

Thomas B. Kepler
Department of Physiology and Biophysics
Mt. Sinai Medical School
New York, New York, USA
and
Center for Neurobiology and Behavior
College of Physicians and Surgeons of Columbia University
New York, New York, USA

Wolfgang Klimesch
Department of Physiological Psychology
Institute of Psychology
University of Salzburg
Salzburg, Austria

Peter König
Neurophysiologische Abteilung
Max-Planck-Institut für Hirnforschung
Frankfurt, Germany

Rodolfo R. Llinás
Department of Physiology & Biophysics
NYU Medical Center
New York, New York, USA

Fernando Lopes da Silva
Department of Experimental Zoology
University of Amsterdam
Amsterdam, The Netherlands

William W. Lytton
Computational Neurobiology Laboratory
Howard Hughes Medical Institute
The Salk Institute for Biological Studies
La Jolla, California, USA

George R. Mangun
Department of Psychiatry and Program in Cognitive Neuroscience
Dartmouth Medical School
Hanover, New Hampshire, USA

Eve Marder
Department of Biology
Brandeis University
Waltham, Massachusetts, USA

Keld B. Mikkelsen
Laboratory of Physics I
Technical University of Denmark
Lyngby, Denmark

Vernon B. Mountcastle
Philip Bard Labs of Neurophysiology
Johns Hopkins University School of Medicine
Baltimore, Maryland, USA

Denis Paré
Université Laval
Faculté de Medecine
Cité Universitaire
Québec, Canada

Ralph Parnefjord
Institut für Physiologie
Medizinische Universität Lübeck
Lübeck, Germany

Hellmuth Petsche
Institut für Neurophysiologie-Hirnforschung
Universität Wien
Wien, Austria

Gert Pfurtscheller
Department of Medical Informatics
Institute of Biomedical Engineering
Graz University of Technology
Graz, Austria

Elke Rahn
Institut für Physiologie
Medizinische Universität Lübeck
Lübeck, Germany

Peter Rappelsberger
Institut für Neurophysiologie-Hirnforschung
Universität Wien
Wien, Austria

Herbert Reitboeck
Institut für Angewandte Physik und Biophysik
Philipps-Universität Marburg
Marburg, Germany

Urs Ribary
Department of Physiology and Biophysics
NYU Medical Center
New York, New York, USA

Knud Saermark
Laboratory of Physics I
Technical University of Denmark
Lyngby, Denmark

Wageda Salem
Institut für Angewandte Physik und Biophysik
Philipps-Universität Marburg
Marburg, Germany

Thomas Schanze
Institut für Angewandte Physik und Biophysik
Philipps-Universität Marburg
Marburg, Germany

Martin Schürmann
Institut für Physiologie
Medizinische Universität Lübeck
Lübeck, Germany

Terrence J. Sejnowski
Computational Neurobiology Laboratory
Howard Hughes Medical Institute
The Salk Institute for Biological Studies
La Jolla, California, USA

Wolf Singer
Neurophysiologische Abteilung
Max-Planck-Institut für Hirnforschung
Frankfurt, Germany

Olaf Sporns
The Neurosciences Institute of the Neurosciences Research Program
New York, New York, USA

Mircea Steriade
Université Laval
Faculté de Médécine
Cité Universitaire
Québec, Canada

Felix Strumwasser
Marine Biological Laboratory
Woods Hole, Massachusetts, USA

Giulio Tononi
The Neurosciences Institute of the Neurosciences Research Program
New York, New York, USA

This book derives in part from a work session organized and chaired by Professors Başar and Bullock and hosted by the Neurosciences Institute of the Neurosciences Research Program, Rockefeller University, April 9–11, 1990. The support of this organization is gratefully acknowledged.

Preface

It is easy to imagine the excitement that pervaded the neurological world in the late 1920's and early 1930's when Berger's first descriptions of the electroencephalogram appeared. Berger was not the first to discover that changes in electric potential can be recorded from the surface of the head, but it was he who first systematized the method, and it was he who first proposed that explanatory correlations might be found between the electroencephalogram, brain processes, and behavioral states. An explosion of activity quickly followed: studies were made of the brain waves in virtually every conceivable behavioral state, ranging from normal human subjects to those with major psychoses or with epilepsy, to state changes such as the sleep-wakefulness transition. There evolved from this the discipline of Clinical Electroencephalography which rapidly took a valued place in clinical neurology and neurosurgery. Moreover, use of the method in experimental animals led to a further understanding of such state changes as attention–inattention, arousal, and sleep and wakefulness. The evoked potential method, derived from electroencephalography, was used in neurophysiological research to construct precise maps of the projection of sensory systems upon the neocortex. These maps still form the initial guides to studies of the cortical mechanisms in sensation and perception. The use of the event-related potential paradigm has proved useful in studies of the brain mechanisms of some cognitive functions of the brain.

The use of electroencephalography in the study of basic brain mechanisms reached a peak in the 1940–50's; thereafter such studies plateaued and ceased to be attractive to most experimental neuroscientists. I believe this was due to the growing conviction that while slow wave events recorded from the surface of the head or the brain itself might reflect some aspects of behavioral states, their study had, in spite of herculean efforts, revealed little of brain mechanisms. The central questions became as follows. Are slow wave events passive epiphenomena in the sense that they reflect summed potential changes caused by the net ionic current flow through the extracellular space of the brain, currents produced by cellular events of several types? Indeed, the net current flow at any moment might very well be produced by any of a variety of patterns of actions in the populations of neurons contributing to it. *Or*, contrarily, are at least some slow wave events active agents of signal transmission within and between neuronal populations? The first proposition came to dominate main-stream thinking in neuroscience for several decades.

Rather suddenly, however, a paradigm change is upon us, for the proposition that slow wave events are active agents for signal transmission now stands as a testable hypothesis with some evidence to support it. Such a radical change has not occurred by chance. It is due to the development of new theories and concepts, new methods of data collection and analysis, and more importantly to skillful studies over a long period of time by investigators like Freeman, Bullock, Petsche, Başar and Galambos, followed now by a host of others. Many of these individuals have contributed to the present volume. All neuroscientists are indebted to them for opening—for re-opening—this old and now once again new window through which to observe the workings of the brain.

This book deals with a particular class of slow wave events—the induced rhythms. Bullock emphasizes in a masterly introduction that induced brain rhythms have been studied for a long time and were frequently surmised by earlier investigators to be related to higher order brain functions. He defines them as a widespread, heterogeneous class of oscillations that includes a rhythm not present in the stimulus—an oscillation caused or modulated by stimuli or state changes that do not directly drive the successive cycles of the slow wave rhythm; thus they differ from both spontaneous and driven oscillations. Interest in these phenomena was stimulated anew in the decades of the 1960's and 1970's by the seminal studies of Walter Freeman and his colleagues on the olfactory system. Study of induced rhythms has now been extended to include many neural systems in many species, in a number of different behavioral states. The general proposition driving the field is that the stimulus induced slow wave oscillations are related to / are signs of / generate or are generated by / are representations of / those higher-order neural operations intercalated between initial central sensory processing and such complex brain functions as perception, or the willing and execution of movement patterns, or storage in memory—in short, those functions whose study makes up a large part of what is now called by the inclusive term of Cognitive Neuroscience. Currently, the most actively investigated and potentially illuminating derivative hypothesis is that the oscillations induced by sensory stimuli in spatially separate parts of a cortical sensory area, or in different cortical areas or other brain regions constitute, *when coherent*, a mechanism for binding together neural activities evoked by parts of complex stimuli into correlated activity in distributed neural ensembles. When that activity is coherent it is thought to be important in generating the neural basis of holistic perceptions like pattern recognition; when incoherent it is not. How far this idea will lead is uncertain, but all will recognize its heuristic value.

The chapters in this book are written by active investigators who provide here a cross section of the state of knowledge in the field. Different ones of these scientists hold different views concerning the active agent/passive epiphenomenon question described above. Regardless of the outcome of that debate, the studies described in this book provide a mass of new information about the function of the brain, function viewed from a different perspective than that of presently received opinion. It is thus of great interest and importance for all neuroscientists.

Vernon B. Mountcastle

Philip Bard Laboratories of Neurophysiology
Johns Hopkins University School of Medicine

Introduction to Induced Rhythms: A Widespread, Heterogeneous Class of Oscillations

THEODORE H. BULLOCK

Adrian (1950) introduced the term "induced waves" for oscillations caused by odor stimuli in the olfactory bulb of cats, rabbits, and hedgehogs, distinguishing these events from intrinsic, spontaneous waves. Recent findings on the coherence of oscillations among and between small sets of neurons in the visual cortex, upon stimulation with moving stripes or gratings, have attracted wide notice (see chapters in this volume by Gray et al. and Eckhorn et al.). Particularly intriguing is the coherence between widely separated sets when stimulated by one long bar and its absence when the bar is separated into two, moving in the same direction and orientation out of phase. Our attention having thus been called to the class of responses that includes a rhythm not present in the stimulus, the question arises where else such phenomena have been seen and whether they reflect a common mechanism or a common role in the brain. The aim of this chapter is to survey previous information as background for the rest of the book, which brings together the new information.

Definitions and Examples

Induced rhythms are here defined as oscillations caused or modulated by stimuli or state changes that do not directly drive successive cycles. They form a category distinct from **spontaneous** and from **driven oscillations**. We cannot omit the word modulated since it is unreasonable to confine ourselves to systems that have no ongoing background rhythms or to require proof that the induced rhythm is something quite new. "Directly drive" must be understood to embrace not only 1:1 driving but cases of frequency doubling or frequency entraining events; hence this exclusion has the potential for transitional or intermediate cases. Since some term was needed for the category of oscillations triggered or altered by events, the word "induced" has been chosen to distinguish it from the long established category of **evoked rhythms**. It would avoid confusion if authors would use evoked rhythms for those driven or entrained by rhythmic stimuli, as in "steady state" responses to 40 Hz stimuli. Thus, one might say the evoked potential to a moving bar includes or is followed by an induced rhythm. A few authors have used the terms **endogenous** and **exogenous** rhythms. These are not so heuristic since endogeny, as it refers to self-paced rather than self-started, must include both the ongoing, spontaneous, and the triggered induced oscillations.

Many familiar phenomena belong under the rubric of induced rhythms including ringing a bell and changing the pitch of a flute by placing a finger on a hole. In biology, the wing beat of a fly is an induced rhythm in the *muscle* since it is myogenic and depends on the properties of the oscillating muscle whereas the flight muscle of a locust or butterfly is driven 1:1 by motor neurons and the term induced would apply to the *neuronal* rhythm. The synchronized cell divisions of the fertilized egg and the rhythmic secretion of hormones by endocrine glands triggered by adequate stimuli (see Strumwasser, this volume) are other examples. The change in heart beat with a frightening sight and the change in breathing rate with a change in supply or demand of oxygen are examples. Subclasses can be recognized on various grounds, for example those that last a short time, like a damped bell ringing and those that persist during sustained states, like the pitch of the flute. This volume deals with rhythms that arise in the brain and with some others, from peripheral and model systems and even some that are not induced but are driven, when they are considered to illuminate the cluster of problems relevant to induced rhythms. These problems run the gamut of levels, from subcellular to cognitive.

A word of warning belongs here, near the definitions. Empirical research that undertakes to detect rhythms presents classical yet often overlooked problems, particularly in the presence of wide-band activity of similar magnitude, in short samples ("spindles"), or where the rhythm damps out or is not highly regular or not well time locked to the triggering event. Cole (1957) and Enright (1965, 1989) have shown pitfalls that "find" spurious rhythms. A common technique in neurophysiology is to band-pass the time series to reduce "noise" in other bands. Figure 1 shows the danger of "seeing" bursts of gamma band (approx. 40 Hz) activity in a stochastic or pseudorandom time series as a result, even when the filter is nearly two octaves wide, especially when the activity suddenly increases or a single large pulse occurs. Seeing peaks in power spectra without adequate statistical tests or demonstration of repeatability is another kind of danger; Enright shows several forms of artifacts.

Induced rhythms as a category of brain oscillations have hardly been recognized hitherto but many examples belonging in this category have been reported. We now believe they hold promise for revealing some fundamental mechanisms of integration. The present survey of the literature, without pretending to completeness, finds *evidence for the proposition that induced rhythms do not form a homogeneous class but are diverse in many ways, including mechanism and significance.* This assertion is worth scrutiny, however, to see whether the similarities go deeper, and possibly some common mechanisms or properties are widespread (Bullock, 1956, 1961, 1962, 1965). If it does prove appropriate to conclude that the category of induced brain rhythms is not homogeneous, the underlying mechanisms are likely to be many and the opportunities for new research multiple. This background, it is hoped, will serve to tie together the chapters that follow and to emphasize the need to view a variety before erecting types or subclasses.

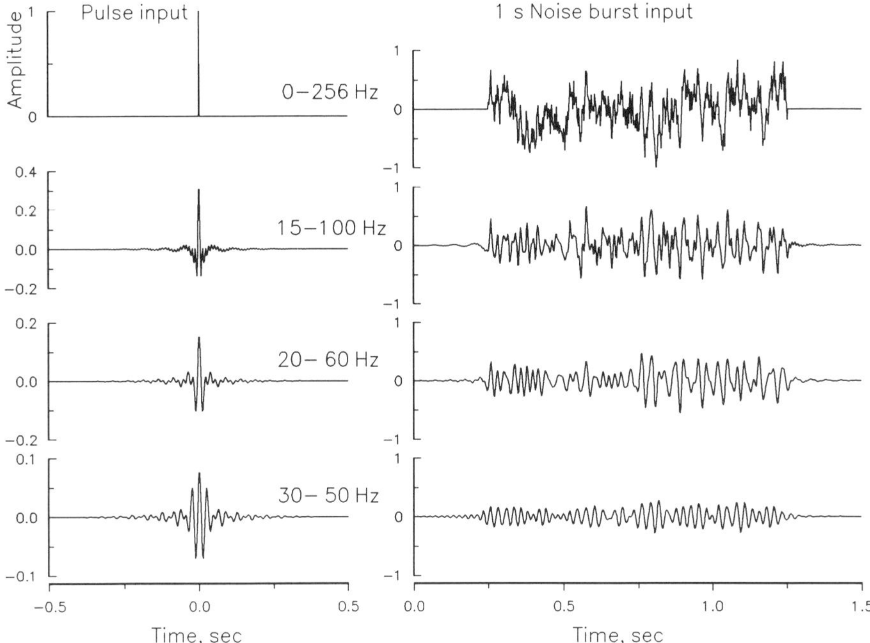

Figure 1. Artificial test data through band-pass filters. **Left:** Impulse functions from input of a single point. Gains are successively higher from top to bottom. **Right:** Input is a sudden burst of "noise," a pseudo random time series, starting with whiteness–equal energy at all frequencies, modified to simulate EEG by reducing high frequency power through a 6-dB/octave, 15 Hz low-pass filter. All gains are equal. Note that even the 20- to 60-Hz filter makes a single event or a burst of pink noise look like a burst of gamma band spindles.

The references selected are chosen from a longer bibliography, which itself cannot pretend to be a complete list of induced rhythms in the brain but represents an extensive sample. I pass over many rhythms, such as the respiratory and endocrine examples, in order to lift up somewhat less familiar cases that might offer advantages for new studies. A few general reviews and books with material relevant to the theme are included (Freeman, 1975, 1985; Başar, 1980, 1988; Başar et al., 1983; Başar, 1988; Freeman and Skarda, 1985; Lopes da Silva, 1987; Başar and Bullock, 1989; Bullock, 1989; Sheer, 1989).

Early Examples, from the Retina

The oldest study I will cite is Fröhlich's (1913) on the general physiology of sense organs. He describes 30- to 90-Hz rhythms in isolated octopus eyes during illumination and 20- to 45-Hz waves after light OFF, and attributes them to the retina. These oscillations change frequency with light intensity and temperature. They are labile and require the preparation to be in very good condition. Having no amplifier, his string galvanometer had to be of sufficiently high resistance not to short circuit the EMF, and critically strung to be aperiodic, yet sufficiently sensitive. A proper history of our topic would go much farther back. Even if we confine ourselves to observation of electrically recorded fluctuations, a good many authors, some cited by Fröhlich, had already described oscillations in muscle and in sensory nerves under steady stimuli in gastropods, elasmobranchs, frogs, and mammals.

The next to be cited, skipping over years that saw many relevant studies, is Adrian and Matthews (1928), on the isolated eye of the eel (*Conger*), whose whole optic nerve was touched by gross electrodes. The usual "rapid and irregular succession of action currents" gave way to a rhythmic succession of large waves under certain conditions, especially illumination of a large part of the retina. More commonly seen during the light, rhythmic waves were also seen after light OFF, in both cases after a long latency. The usual frequency range was 5 to 15 Hz, depending on the light intensity and duration. Adrian and Matthews's main conclusion was that the waves can be attributed to synaptic interactions leading to synchronized waxing and waning of impulse discharge. Later authors added observations on other species and properties of these induced retinal rhythms (Granit, 1941, 1963; Steinberg, 1966; Wachtmeister and Dowling, 1978; Mastronarde, 1989; Maffei and Galli-Resta, 1990; Kergoat and Lovasik, 1990; Lestienne et al., 1990; Bullock et al., 1991). Typically, certain combinations of stimulus conditions are more conducive to the particular form of induced activity described, but no general statement can be made covering the various manifestations; they are unlikely to represent the same physiological event in these different preparations. The induced rhythms in the retina due to omitted stimuli in a train, recently found by Bullock et al. (1991), are briefly described below.

Abandoning a chronological sequence, it is not self-evident which possible basis for grouping is most heuristic. Certainly a lumping by frequency would make strange bedfellows. The following rubrics do not altogether prevent odd proximities either.

Sense Organs

Sense organs other than retinal also show induced rhythms. To generate oscillations in sensory structures it is not necessary to have the complex circuitry of the retina. Tuberous electroreceptors in electric fish, which resemble octavolateralis receptors in that they have an innervated secondary sense cell like a hair cell, give a damped oscillation of a characteristic frequency in response to a pulse or a step stimulus (Zakon and Meyer, 1983). A stretch receptor, such as that in crayfish or in the mammalian muscle spindle, shows an induced rhythm whose frequency is a function of the mechanical step and which, in different kinds of organs, is more tonic or more rapidly adapting. The mechanism of the oscillation in the crayfish stretch receptor is perhaps one of the **most fully analyzed examples of induced rhythms** in neurons, extending to patch-clamp data on single-channel openings and closings (Erxleben, 1989; Morris, 1990).

Isolated Axons

Isolated axons vary in response to brief pulse or step stimuli from essentially no oscillation or a few damped cycles to rhythmic discharge riding on subthreshold oscillatory local potentials lasting up to dozens of cycles, according to the type of fiber (Arvanitaki et al., 1936; Arvanitaki, 1938, 1939a, 1939b; Hodgkin, 1948; Wright and Adelman, 1954; Tasaki and Terakawa, 1982). It will not be surprising if these examples have basically the same mechanism as stretch receptors.

Ganglia

Ganglia in invertebrates and in the peripheral nervous system of vertebrates have been found on occasion to respond rhythmically to nonrhythmic input. Early studies of the effects of polarizing ganglia were among the first uses of the giant neurons of the gastropod mollusc, *Aplysia* (Arvanitaki and Cardot, 1941; Arvanitaki and Chalazonitis, 1955, 1961). Optic lobes of insects were studied in a brief flurry of interest, when it was discovered that they can, under certain conditions difficult to define, generate large 20- to 30-Hz rhythms of compound field potentials for a second or more after the onset of light (Jahn and Wulff, 1942; Crescitelli and Jahn, 1942; Bernhard, 1942). In recent literature lobster stomatogastric ganglia have been shown to modulate their spontaneous rhythm with suitable input (Ayers and Selverston, 1979) and some suggestions of mechanisms are available (Hartline et al., 1988; Hartline, 1989; Kepler et al., 1990). An insect motor control model (Altman and Kien, 1989) as well as gastropod intrinsic rhythms can also be modulated (Arshavsky et al., 1988a, 1988b; Gelperin, 1989; Gelperin and Tank, 1990; Kleinfeld et al., 1990). Autonomic ganglia of mammals may offer material for study of oscillations to transient inputs (Horn and Dodd, 1983). These preparations, especially the well studied, few-celled crustacean peripheral ganglia, make it clear how difficult it can be to decide whether a rhythm should be attributed to pacemaker cells that others follow, with modifications, or to the whole array of cells or to some essential subset acting in a circuit with particular time constants and interaction strengths. This question may seem elementary but can be refractory (Selverston, 1980; Robertson and Moulins, 1981) even with favorable conditions for intracellular recording and for eliminating single, chosen cells from the circuit—partly because of the ability of the system to regulate.

The Vertebrate Brain Stem

The vertebrate brain stem, from the midbrain caudally, has various examples of induced rhythms, each facultative and labile. The tectum sometimes oscillates to certain light pulses or steps (Konishi, 1960; O'Benar, 1976; Bullock et al., 1990a). Cerebellar cells can sometimes be triggered to oscillate (Lee and Bullock, 1990). Synchronized oscillations in the primary nucleus of the sensory pathway from electroreceptors in the medulla as well as in the tectum of rays after 10 ms electric pulse stimuli in the water are described below. Neurons of the inferior olive (Llinás and Yarom, 1986), substantia nigra (Fujimura and Matsuda, 1989), and other nuclei (Llinás, 1988) show autogenous oscillation modulated by various impinging influences, especially calcium channel blockers. This set of cases is surely diverse in mechanism as well as in dynamic properties.

The Olfactory Bulb

The olfactory bulb and associated structures are well known substrates for oscillations brought on by physiological odor stimuli (Adrian 1942, 1950; Freeman, 1968, 1972, 1975, 1978, 1979a, 1979b, 1979c, 1981, 1988; Freeman and Schneider, 1982; Viana di Prisco and Freeman, 1985; Gray et al., 1986; Gray and Skinner, 1988; Boejinga and Lopes da Silva, 1989a, 1989b). A number of authors have modeled the bulb, the pyriform cortex, and their oscillatory processing (Freeman, 1975, 1979a, 1979b, 1979c, 1987; Haberly and Bower, 1989; Li and Hopfield, 1989; Wilson and Bower, 1989). Even in this relatively well studied phenomenon it is not at all clear whether we have to do with a single, common physiological process or whether more than one alternative or sequential mechanism may be involved in inducing the rhythms.

Subcortical Structures

Subcortical structures including the **thalamus** and the **hippocampus** have frequently been observed to oscillate in response to stimuli. Chang (1950) was one of the first to analyze the repetitive discharges in the corticothalamic "reverberating circuit." Others who reported repetitive or oscillatory firing in various nuclei of the thalamus include Galambos et al. (medial geniculate; 1952), Bishop et al. (lateral geniculate; 1953), Jahnsen and Llinás (slices of thalamus; 1984a, 1984b), Lenz et al. (humans with central pain; 1989), and

Leresche et al. (thalamocortical cells; 1990). After acoustic or other stimuli hippocampal field potentials can show a few cycles or more at approximately 40 Hz (Başar, 1980; Başar et al., this volume). Hippocampal cells burst synchronously in sustained rhythms or spindles under certain conditions, *in vivo* as well as in slices (Jeffreys and Haas, 1982; Miles et al., 1988). These properties have been modeled (Traub et al., 1987a, 1987b, 1989). Septal cell synchronized bursting in response to sensory stimuli or activity such as walking in rats or to administration of certain drugs initiates the much studied theta rhythm or RSA (Sainsbury, 1985; Lopes da Silva, this volume) that spreads widely through the limbic and related structures.

The Central Visual System

The central visual system provides a number of examples, probably not to be reduced to one or two phenomena, but basically disparate in mechanism, as well as in triggering conditions and cell substrates. The classical alpha rhythm has sometimes been considered an example, induced by closing the eyes or, as Adrian emphasized, by simply shifting attention to sounds. Başar (this volume) quotes Grey Walter on the variety of kinds of alpha band responses—some sensitive to opening and closing the eyes, some not, some driven by flicker, some not, some influenced by mental activity, some not. More commonly alpha activity is considered exemplary of spontaneous rhythms since it occurs in the absence of visual and other arousing stimulation. Bishop (1933, 1935) observed some suggestions of cyclic changes already at subcortical levels as well as in the cortex (Bartley and Bishop, 1933; Bishop and O'Leary, 1936, 1938; Bishop and Clare, 1952; Clare and Bishop, 1956). Brazier (1960) showed bursts of alphalike activity after light ON and Lansing and Barlow (1972) found the time-locked average evoked burst after a flash is quite distinct from the envelope of alpha blocking and return, although they are roughly parallel; the larger the background alpha, the larger was the evoked burst, contrary to Başar's (1980) usual case. Chatrian et al. (1960) reported a fast rhythm in human visual cortex under steady illumination. Pöppel and Logothetis (1986) also described cellular oscillations in the human brain. A number of workers have described different forms of periodic responses to brief stimuli in the visual cortex of cats, monkeys, and other species; these are much in need of comparison and reconciliation especially with the following group of reports (Grüsser and Grüsser-Cornehls, 1962; Doty and Kimura, 1963; Hughes, 1964; Regan, 1968; Sturr and Shansky, 1971; Abdullaev et al., 1977; Whittaker and Siegfried, 1983; Friedlander, 1983).

Freeman and van Dijk (1987) found stable spatial patterns of activity in the monkey visual cortex during sustained, conditioned checkerboard stimulation, with irregular bursts having multiple power peaks in the 20- to 40-Hz range; in selected time intervals there was coherence among several electrodes. Something special was happening at the time of visual stimulation, provided it had been conditioned, but it was not as simple as an oscillation. It must have been another form of activity than the next described.

New properties and perhaps new forms of oscillation were uncovered in the striate cortex of anesthetized cats, triggered by moving stripes in the preferred orientation, by two laboratories in recent years (Gray and Singer, 1987a, 1987b; 1989; Eckhorn and Reitboek, 1988; Eckhorn et al., 1988a, 1988b, 1989a, 1989b, 1990; Lohmann et al., 1988; Gray et al., 1990a, 1990b, 1991; Engel et al., 1990 see the chapters by Gray et al. and by Eckhorn et al. in this volume). It remains to be learned whether some of the previously reported oscillatory responses are parts of these column-specific rhythms. The papers just cited not only describe the properties of oscillations but also propose an important role (see further below, under Roles of induced rhythms) in information processing.

Other studies that may have a bearing on the relation of these oscillations to visual evoked potentials and spatiotemporal receptive field organization are those of Ducati et al. (1988), Seiple and Holopigian (1989), Lestienne et al. (1990), and Dinse et al. (1991).

Other Cortical Areas

Other cortical areas have also yielded various hints and signs of induced rhythms, under such a variety of conditions that identifying them with a common mechanism, manifestation, or even stimulus is not yet possible. We can go back at least to Loomis et al. (1938), who recorded from the scalp in humans and described a "K complex" after acoustic stimuli during sleep: after a long latency negative and then positive swing a series of 8- to 14-Hz oscillations lasts for a second or more. Bremer (1949) illustrated rhythmic afterpotentials, like damped oscillations, after a single nerve shock recording in the frog spinal cord and after an acoustic click recording in the cat cortex and sometimes in the medial geniculate, most conspicuous in the strychninized state. Among the stimulus conditions that have elicited rhythms of a wide range of frequencies are nasal respiration (frog and turtle, Servít and Strejčková, 1976), acoustic stimuli (Schreiner and Joris, 1986), somatosensory stimuli (manual manipulation of textures; Ahissar and Vaadia, 1990), discrimination tasks (Simpson et al., 1977), attention (Rougeul et al., 1979; Montaron et al., 1982) and epilepsy (Traub and Wong, 1982). State changes that modulate the steady 40-Hz click-driven evoked potentials have been demonstrated (Galambos and Makeig, 1988; Makeig and Galambos, 1989).

Several studies aim to unravel mechanisms (Llinás, 1988; White et al., 1989; Silva et al., 1991) and the influence of agents such as anesthetics (Madler and Pöppel, 1987, Pöppel and Logothetis, 1986). Bressler (1990) discusses the possible role of gamma rhythms (approx. 40 Hz) as a cortical information carrier.

Theoretical and Other Studies

Theoretical and other studies bearing on induced rhythms include a few general works (Haken, 1977; Başar, 1980, 1983a, 1983b; Başar et al., 1983; Malsburg, 1981, 1985; Abraham and Shaw, 1982; Rapp, 1987; Lopes da Silva, 1987; Freeman, 1988) and some modeling studies (Malsburg and Schneider, 1986; Rotterdam et al., 1982; Freeman, 1987; Sporns et al., 1989; Reeke et al., 1990; Lee and Chay, 1990). Some studies of real systems that are not neural are nevertheless so germane they must be cited (Moran and Goldbeter, 1985; Goldbeter and Moran, 1988; Goldbeter, 1988; Li and Goldbeter, 1989).

An interesting area of experiment and theory is that lying on and over the arbitrary boundary of our definition of induced rhythms, namely, studies of interactions of more or less rhythmic ongoing activity with more or less rhythmic input (Altschuler et al., 1990; Barrio and Buño, 1990a, 1990b; Lee and Chay, 1990; Adey, this volume).

Induced rhythms can either be quite time-locked to the triggering event by having a consistent latency and frequency or frequency modulation, or they can be poorly or not at all time-locked when these independently variable parameters are not consistent in successive trials. The rhythms, like all biological rhythms, can be more or less regular or periodic. Exceptional instances are rather precisely periodic, with a very small standard deviation of the periods (e.g., high frequency electric fish), but more commonly there is a considerable or even quite large fluctuation of periods. It is not yet known whether in the cases of large fluctuation of periods a pattern of consistent frequency modulation occurs each time the "rhythm" is induced by its adequate stimulus or only a stochastic or possibly a chaotic sequence.

The now substantial literature on *dynamical analysis and chaos* in brain activity, usually confined to the ongoing electroencephalogram (EEG) without discrete stimuli, is not discussed in this chapter but in the epilogue of Başar. Induced rhythms are typically not precise limit cycles but are only relatively periodic, at best. Dynamical analysis might well reveal significant features not otherwise appreciated.

There is, no doubt, a significant chapter yet to be written on the *natural history* of induced rhythms, as well as of the spontaneous rhythms. Such an account will, among other things, be concerned with the departures from perfect periodicity, whether they are stochastic or chaotic, and whether they might be systematic or even patterned modulation of the period. Too little is yet known to see a broad picture.

Besides the temporal aspect of a more adequate characterization, the *spatial aspect* must surely be important, particularly in the millimeter or smaller domain, as opposed to the usual EEG spatial resolution of centimeters. The findings of Singer et al. and Eckhorn et al. (see their chapters) clearly show this, since high correlation of the oscillations can be absent between neighboring electrode loci equivalent to columns having different preferred orientations, and present between columns having the same orientation preference. We have shown (Bullock and McClune, 1989) that the coherence between cortical surface electrodes in the ongoing micro-EEG in rat, rabbit, and human (Bullock et al., 1990b) typically declines from high to negligible values in a few millimeters for all frequencies (1–70 Hz), except for single frequencies in the special cases of strong alpha and theta activity. In the 1989 study it was found that *intracortical* electrodes are commonly much less coherent than surface loci. Microstructure of the dynamical characteristics in space is a frontier still poorly explored. Such exploration is currently limited by the poor time resolution of the methods for characterizing nonspike activity that changes significantly in fractions of a second; we have to integrate over many seconds (i.e., blur the temporal fine structure) in order to use the powerful methods for spatial analysis.

Roles of Induced Rhythms

Propositions that brain rhythms play a role in information processing go back at least to Bremer and Titeca (1940), Bremer (1941, 1944, 1949, 1953, 1958), Gerard (1941), and Bullock (1945) but became much more explicit with Freeman (1975). Quite distinct types of speculation about role have been put forward by Freeman and by others, for example Madler and Pöppel (1987) and Lopes da Silva (this volume). Sheer (1989) associates the gamma band rhythms (approx. 40 Hz) with focused arousal and cognitive performance, a proposal that overlaps but may be subtly different from those just referenced. The papers by Gray, Singer, and coworkers and those by Eckhorn and coworkers cited above propose still different kinds of meaning (see their chapters). All these ideas are inherently difficult to test, even if they were made specific in terms of the mechanism by which the oscillations might exert the hypothesized influence. Nevertheless, speculation need not be premature if it is heuristic in suggesting do-able experiments—as is certainly the case in both of these groups of papers.

New Experiments from This Laboratory

Bullock et al. (1991) found highly labile oscillations of many cycles at 15 to 25 Hz (15°C) in the tectum and traced them to an origin in the retina in elasmobranchs and teleosts after the main visual evoked potential to single flashes or after the OFF of a long light (at least 500 ms). Bullock et al. (1990a) found similar oscillations after omitting flashes from a long conditioning train (at least 2 flashes per second for tens of cycles or many seconds) (Fig. 2A). The rhythmic waves facultatively follow a more dependable initial complex; the whole sequence was named the omitted stimulus potential (OSP). The notable feature of the OSP is the nearly fixed latency after the due-time of the first omitted stimulus. As though the retina "expected" the missing flash, it emits an OSP on schedule, approximately 80 ms after the missing stimulus was due (see Galambos, this volume, for "emitted potentials" equivalent to OSPs). An explanation seems reasonable in terms of an accumulated inhibition with a decay time specific to each conditioning frequency, leading to the OSP as a postinhibitory rebound. The induced rhythm is very labile in amplitude but fixed in frequency for a given preparation and temperature, not influenced by interstimulus interval, intensity, or train duration, except in the number of cycles of oscillation, which can be more than 20. Originating in the retina and large in the tectum, the induced rhythm is small or not visible in the telencephalon, whereas a late, slow wave OSP is conspicuous. The complex circuitry of the retina is not necessary since similar OSPs and induced rhythms, of approximately 7 Hz for >1 s and also of approximately 55 Hz for up to 0.15 s have recently been found (Fig. 2B, C) in a somatosensory (electrosensory) cranial nerve nucleus in the medulla of rays after trains of physiological stimuli—feeble electric pulses in the bath at >2 Hz (Bullock and Hofmann, 1991). Whereas OSPs are also found in the midbrain and forebrain, the rhythmic component is reduced or lost in the telencephalon.

Chapters of This Book

The chapters that follow represent a variety of approaches and treatments. According to one logic, they may be grouped in the following sequence. First are updated accounts of the recently analyzed example of *oscillations in the striate cortex* upon stimulation with moving stripes in the preferred orientation. In the chapter by **Gray et al.**, new measures of the fine temporal structure are reported in cross-correlations of the single unit spike activity with local field potentials from electrodes 5 mm and more apart, showing the high degree of dynamic variability of the duration of synchrony, as well as its phase and frequency. The chapter by **Eckhorn, Schanze et al.** reiterates strongly a somewhat similar hypothesis of a causal meaning of the stimulus-specific synchronous oscillations in the binding or linking problem: those combinations of neurons should be synchronized that code relevant combinations of visual features linked in the stimulus to define it as one object. They report new experiments with sudden movements and slow retinal image shifts during fixation, showing suppression of background oscillations followed by synchronized oscillation of wide (35–80 Hz) frequency range. They also refer to models that behave like the brain, dealt with more fully in the later chapter by Eckhorn, Dicke, et al.

A number of contributors then deal with descriptive information about the correlates of induced *cortical rhythms, both ongoing* (*EEG*) *and evoked* (*ERPs*), in humans and in laboratory mammals. **Lopes da Silva** analyzes the rhythmic

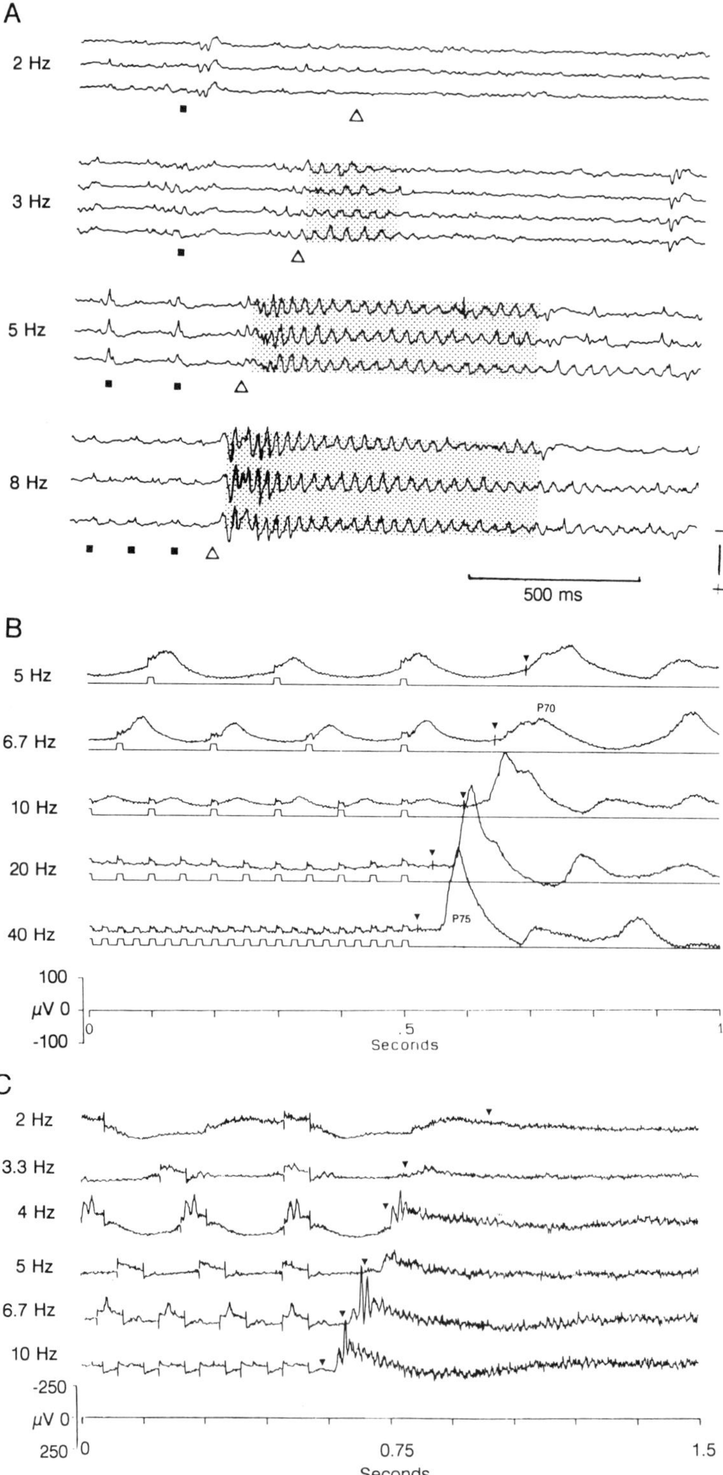
A
2 Hz
3 Hz
5 Hz
8 Hz
500 ms
B
5 Hz
6.7 Hz
P70
10 Hz
20 Hz
40 Hz
P75
100
μV 0
-100
0
.5
1
Seconds
C
2 Hz
3.3 Hz
4 Hz
5 Hz
6.7 Hz
10 Hz
-250
μV 0
250
0
0.75
1.5
Seconds

slow activity (RSA; theta waves) of the limbic cortex, emphasizing the problem of its meaning but also considering its origin and even providing a model, concluding that it is more a network rhythm than due to intrinsic neuronal oscillations **Petsche and Rappelsberger** reexamine human scalp EEGs using probability mapping of power and coherence of five frequency bands before and during lasting mental tasks, such as mental arithmetic, listening to music or to speech, reading, mental cube rotation, and playing chess. By comparing groups of individuals they found significant differences between tasks, between trained and untrained subjects, and between the sexes, even in the resting state. **Pfurtscheller and Klimesch** examine the event-related synchronization and desynchronization of alpha and beta band scalp EEG in humans during cognitive tasks and find that occipital alpha activity can be attenuated at the same time that central beta activity is enhanced. They relate the two states to relatively active versus inhibited or "idling" cortex and propose that alpha desynchronization is a prerequisite for gamma (40-Hz) synchronization.

Saermark et al. present new results of seven-channel *magnetoencephalographic* (*MEG*) comparison of auditory evoked responses with ongoing, spontaneous activity in subjects with pronounced alpha power, finding that stimuli induce time-locked oscillations close to the frequency of the dominant spontaneous rhythm (10 Hz). Furthermore, if each is regarded as arising from a single equivalent dipole there is a close positional relationship between the generators of the evoked and the ongoing alpha. **Llinás and Ribary** present new results with the seven-channel MEG, having placed the seven-sensor probe of a few centimeters' diameter successively over five different parts of the head, from frontal to occipital and temporal. Stimulating with tone bursts they call particular attention to a global gamma (approx. 40 Hz)-induced

◀ **Figure 2.** Omitted stimulus potentials (OSPs) from an elasmobranch, *Platyrhinoidis*. Records are lined up by the time of the last stimulus. First omitted stimuli indicated by triangles. Wide-band recording of the ends of long (10 s) conditioning trains of stimuli; single sweeps. **A:** Visual OSPs from the tectum; light flashes at the frequencies indicated on the left; only the last one to three flashes (*black square symbols*) of the conditioning trains are shown. Note the OSP (*shaded area*) with initial deflections followed by a labile oscillation at ca.25 Hz. (Reproduced with permission from Bullock et al., 1990a.) **B:** Electrosensory OSPs from the midbrain (mesencephalic lateral nucleus); stimulus trains of 10 ms electric pulses, 55 μV/cm, in the bath, at the frequencies shown. Note the large initial "on schedule" P70–P75 = positive peak 70–75 ms after the due-time of the first omitted stimulus (*triangles*) to this lateral line (somatosensory) modality, followed by approximately 5 Hz facultative oscillations which in repeated trials come and go. **C:** The same, from the medulla (dorsal electrosensory nucleus); 10 s train of 60 ms electric pulses. No OSP can be discerned at 2 or 3.3 Hz and only a slightly enhanced slow wave plus some disinhibited irregular activity, like EEG, at 4 Hz. At 6.7 and 10 Hz the pronounced OSP includes large fast oscillations (ca. 50 Hz) which damp down quickly into the background micro-EEG. Slow oscillations like those in B are not evident. (B and C reproduced with permission from Bullock and Hofmann, 1991.)

rhythm and especially its apparent sweep over the cortex in a systematic sequence. They propose an important role for the global gamma in cognitive processing.

Başar et al. report examples of induced rhythms in the theta, alpha, and gamma bands. They emphasize the working hypothesis that these evoked responses are stimulus-induced synchronizations and enhancements of the spontaneous EEG (Başar, 1980).

Predictions are made or called for in the next three chapters. **Freeman** predicts, from studies of the simpler three-layered paleocortex, especially using the concepts of nonlinear dynamical analysis, what will be found in forthcoming applications of these methods to the six-layered neocortex. Among other things, he anticipates that neocortical oscillations in field potentials and in cell firing will be shown to be due to feedback between excitatory and inhibitory neurons, not by coupling of oscillatory cells (Eeckman and Freeman, 1990). He specifies the time constants, the curve that relates dendritic current and spike firing probability, spatial patterns of amplitude modulation of carrier frequencies >25 Hz, and other properties not yet measured. **Galambos** contrasts the human scalp-recorded gamma band activity with the Gray and Singer and the Eckhorn, Schanze et al. gamma band activity from the anesthetized cat, pointing out basic differences as well as the impossibility, at present, of anticipating what activity would be seen from the scalp of the awake cat under the same conditions as the human recordings or from the microelectrode in the human cortex during moving stripe stimuli. **Mangun** points out that the visual evoked potentials in humans (P1-N1-P2-N2) form a brief series of waves of approximately 10 Hz, and raises the question whether the successive deflections are individual "components" (i.e., distinct populations sequentially activated or rhythmic oscillations of one set of neurons). He concludes for the former from current source density analyses and scalp topographic mapping. This surprising result, he suggests, dictates that similar analyses are needed for other induced "rhythms."

A group of chapters deals largely with *thalamic oscillations.* **Buzsáki** proposes that the high voltage spindles of 2 to 12 Hz in the rat are an emergent property of the network between the relay nuclei and the nucleus reticularis, despite the lack of rhythmic firing of relay cells and the lack of endogenous pacemaker neurons in either nuclear group. The frequency of network oscillation is attributed to an interplay between two major classes of voltage-dependent conductances of thalamocortical cells: low-threshold calcium and high-threshold *N*-methyl-D-aspartate (NMDA) channels. A major role of such oscillatory behavior is seen in several kinds of mood disorders. **Steriade et al.** distinguish two main types of thalamic oscillations, of which the first, the slow (<14 Hz) oscillations, are subdivided into spindles (7–14 Hz) and delta waves (0.5–4 Hz). The spindles are timed by inhibitory reticularis input to thalamocortical cells, whereas the delta waves are regarded as endogenous. The second type are fast (25–45 Hz) oscillations, some of which are apparently intrinsic cellular proclivities, unmasked by depolarization, and some are driven by synaptic input, presumably network-timed. **Llinás** draws on intracellular recording studies *in vitro* as well as *in vivo* and concludes that the 40-Hz rhythms seen in the cortex involve the circuitry of a cortico-thalamo-cortical resonant loop but also depend on cellular properties in the thalamic cells that support the 40-Hz resonance. Together these mechanisms underline the intrinsic organization of the central nervous system (CNS) that sculpts the temporal features of its output, as opposed to a fundamentally reflexive view.

Cellular and subcellular mechanisms based on invertebrate examples and other "simpler" systems constitute the next four chapters. Invertebrates may appear to be relatively neglected, although not from lack of appreciation of the majority of the animal kingdom by the editors! The fact is that signs and measures of induced rhythms in assemblies of cells have been little studied in these animals. The information available, apart from some slow wave findings (cited above under Ganglia), is almost confined to the rhythms of single units and small circuits, represented in two chapters. **Marder et al.** explore the behavior of mathematical models simulating the lobster stomatogastric ganglion or other networks consisting of bursting pacemaker neurons and non-bursting neurons electrically coupled to the former. They find that such networks can produce outputs quite different from the properties of the driving oscillators. **Strumwasser** reviews the data on cellular processes underlying three long period rhythms independent of cell–cell interactions: cell division cycles (ca. 30 min), pulsatile neuroendocrine secretion (approx. 1 hr), and circadian (24 hr) cycles. Mechanisms are known in some cases in terms of a few proteins that interact through phosphorylation, dephosphorylation, and selective proteolysis to generate the cyclic time base. Diversity is evident even in these examples, since some appear to require both the transcriptional and translational machinery whereas in others the latter is sufficient. Of special interest is the fact that the frequency of pulsatile secretion of a particular hormonal pathway is important for the optimal target tissue response, as has been occasionally suggested for so-called tuned synapses. **Goldbeter** compares neuronal oscillations with those studied in unicellular models such as *Dictyostelium* amoebae measured by biochemical concentrations or activity. Noting a number of similarities as well as differences, he highlights a common function, the frequency encoding of pulsatile signals in intercellular communication. **Adey** considers preparations from a variety of sources that offer singularly advantageous opportunities or challenges to investigate fundamental mechanisms, not only of the purest kind of induced rhythms but also responses to imposed rhythms, including unfamiliar forms of stimuli—a veritable treasure chest of phenomena demanding innovative technical approaches.

Chapters concerned primarily with *theory and models* come last. Several of the preceding chapters included consideration of theory and models (Eckhorn et al., Lopes da Silva, Freeman, Buzsáki, Marder, Goldbeter). **Lytton and Sejnowski** use three levels of small network models of neurons with many kinds of channels to experiment with the consequences of the long-known rebound from inhibition as a paradoxical driving mechanism and to show

how even a small number of inhibitory neurons can rapidly phase-lock a local neural population or two remote, connected populations such as the induced rhythms in separate columns of visual cortex (Gray et al., this volume). If this mechanism applies to the actual case, it reduces the problem of how the population is synchronized to how the small set of inhibitory cells are synchronized. **Tononi et al.** offer a series of models that generate induced rhythms much like those found in the striate cortex, as described in the chapters by Gray et al. and Eckhorn, Schanze et al. In another chapter **Eckhorn, Dicke et al.** test one- and two-layered models and show that the latter, with enough inhibition and suitable time constants, oscillates much like the induced rhythms of the visual cortex. The models of Tononi et al. and those of Eckhorn, Dicke et al. are far from identical; they raise the question of what to conclude from modeling when various permutations of partly realistic properties can imitate some aspects of the living system to a first approximation. **Haken** discusses the general principles of synergetics that appear relevant to the understanding of induced rhythms.

Başar provides an epilogue highlighting basic issues of the principles underlying higher order neural processing, many of which have been with us for long but can be seen now in a new perspective. Recognizing four bands of induced rhythms, from the delta to the gamma bands, he asks how the brain integrates oscillations of neurons, what underlies its excitability, how oscillation and resonance are partly independent of each other, as well as of synchrony and coherence. He calls attention to some of the new tools that may accelerate progress or break new paths toward insights.

Summary

Induced rhythms are special and unusual although widespread phenomena, requiring particular conditions in each situation where they have been found. We define this class of phenomena as oscillations caused or modulated by stimuli that do not directly drive successive cycles. Hence, they are a class of endogenous rhythms distinguished from purely spontaneous and from entrained (driven) rhythms. Induced rhythms have been recorded in many places, preparations, and conditions, from invertebrates and vertebrates, from peripheral and central neurons, and from spinal to cortical levels. The greater number and variety of reports from higher cortical levels of mammals may or may not be significant; it may be a sampling artifact or it may reflect a greater tendency to induced rhythms in more advanced neural tissue.

Diversity also seems to apply to the mechanisms, although these are principally unknown in most cases. Isolated axons, receptors, or neuron somata possess a degree of iteration, in response to membrane depolarization, characteristic for that type of unit and level of depolarization, from a few cycles per second or less up to more than 100 Hz. Some receptors oscillate after a pulse or step stimulus at a characteristic frequency of many hundreds of Hertz. Some rhythms are triggered by an impinging event or state, perhaps a particular transmitter. Some "ring" for a number of cycles and cease as though damped. Some appear to be circuit rhythms, dependent on the connectivity and the circuit time constants. A major variable is the degree of coherence between the oscillations in separate populations of cells; this can be high when the eliciting visual stimulus is unitary or low when visibly separate objects are the stimuli, suggesting a role in "binding" images together that share signs of belonging to one object. A similar range of coherence values is known for the ongoing micro-EEG, which may show long range high values or values that decline rapidly in a few millimeters of cortex, tangentially, fractions of a millimeter radially; in these cases a role for the coherence is more difficult to demonstrate. Rhythms may be more or less regular and vary from a few Hz up to at least 80 Hz. Some spontaneous oscillations of 1 kHz and more, in electric fish central pacemakers, are characteristically modulated by ethologically significant stimuli, making these examples of induced rhythms.

Systematic study of this class of oscillations has barely begun. It is too early to tell whether there will be a few distinct subclasses, or many, or a continuum graded by properties or by mechanisms. The citations to literature, going back many decades, represent an incomplete collection of earlier studies. The collection of newer studies in this book samples a wide range of cases and approaches, both empirical and theoretical.

References

Abdullaev GB, Gadzhieva NA, Rzaeva NM, Alekperova SA, Kambarli EI, Dimitrenko AI, Gasanova SA (1977): Oscillatory potentials in the structurcs of visual system. *Fiziol Zh SSSR* 12: 1653–1661

Abraham RH, Shaw CD (1982): *Dynamics—The Geometry of Behavior*. Santa Cruz: Aerial Press

Adrian ED (1942): Olfactory reactions in the brain of the hedgehog. *J Physiol* 100: 459–473

Adrian ED (1950): The electrical activity of the mammalian olfactory bulb. *Electroencephalogr Clin Neurophysiol* 2: 377–387

Adrian ED, Matthews R (1928): The action of light on the eye. Part III. The interaction of retinal neurones. *J Physiol* 65: 273–298

Ahissar E, Vaadia E (1990): Oscillatory activity of single units in a somatosensory cortex of an awake monkey and their possible role in texture analysis. *Proc Natl Acad Sci USA* 87: 8935–8939.

Altman JS, Kien J (1989): New models for motor control. *Neural Computation* 1: 173–183

Altschuler E, Garfinkel A, Segundo JP, Stiber M, Wang GH (1990): Pacemaker neurons: periodic and aperiodic responses to periodic PSPs. *Biophys J* 57: 193a

Arshavsky YuI, Deliagina TG, Meizerov ES, Orlovsky GN, Panchin YuV (1988a):

Control of feeding movements in the freshwater snail *Planorbis corneus*. I. Rhythmical neurons of buccal ganglia. *Exp Brain Res* 70:310–322

Arshavsky YuI, Deliagina TG, Orlovsky GN, Panchin YuV (1988b): Control of feeding movements in the freshwater snail *Planorbis corneus*. III. Organization of the feeding rhythm generator. *Exp Brain Res* 70:332–341

Arvanitaki A (1938): *Les variations graduées de la polarisation des systèmes excitables.* Thesis, Univ. Lyons, Paris: Hermann et cie

Arvanitaki A (1939a): Recherche sur la réponse oscillatoire locale de l'axone géant isolé de *Sepia*. *Arch Int Physiol* 49:209–256

Arvanitaki A (1939b): Contributions à l'étude analytique de la réponse électrique oscillatoire locale de l'axone isolé de *Sepia*. *C R Soc Biol* (*Paris*) 131:1117–1120

Arvanitaki A, Cardot H (1941): Réponses rhytmiques ganglionnaires, graduées en fonction de la polarisation appliquée. Lois des latences et des fréquences. *C R Soc Biol* (*Paris*) 135:1211–1216

Arvanitaki A, Chalazonitis N (1955): Les potentiels bioélectriques endocytaires du neurone géant d'*Aplysia* en activité autorhytmique. *C R Acad Sci* (*Paris*) 240:349–351

Arvanitaki A, Chalazonitis N (1961): Excitatory and inhibitory processes initiated by light and infrared radiations in single identifiable nerve cells (giant ganglion cells of *Aplysia*). In: *Nervous Inhibition*, Florey E, ed. Oxford: Pergamon Press.

Arvanitaki A, Fessard A, Kruta V (1936): Mode répétitif de la réponse électrique des nerfs visceraux et étoilés chez *Sepia officinalis*. *C R Soc Biol* (*Paris*) 122:1203–1204

Ayers JL Jr, Selverston AI (1979): Monosynaptic entrainment of an endogenous pacemaker network: a cellular mechanism for von Holst's magnet effect. *J Comp Physiol* 129:5–17

Barrio LC, Buño W (1990a): Dynamic analysis of sensory-inhibitory interactions in crayfish stretch receptor neurons. *J Neurophysiol* 63:1508–1519

Barrio LC, Buño W (1990b): Temporal correlations in sensory-synaptic interactions: example in crayfish stretch receptors. *J Neurophysiol* 63:1520–1527

Bartley SH, Bishop GH (1933): The cortical response to stimulation of the optic nerve in the rabbit. *Am J Physiol* 103:159–172

Başar E (1980): *EEG–Brain Dynamics*. Amsterdam: Elsevier

Başar E (1983a): Toward a physical approach to integrative physiology. I. Brain dynamics and physical causality. *Am J Physiol* 245:R510–R533

Başar E (1983b): EEG and synergetics of neural populations. In: *Synergetics of the Brain*, Başar E, Flohr H, Haken H, Mandell AJ, eds. Berlin: Springer–Verlag, pp 183–200

Başar E (1988): EEG-dynamics and evoked potentials in sensory and cognitive processing by the brain. In: *Sensory and Cognitive Processing by the Brain*, Başar E, ed. Berlin: Springer–Verlag, pp 30–55

Başar E, Bullock TH (1989): *Brain Dynamics: Progress and Perspectives*. Berlin: Springer–Verlag

Başar E, Flohr H, Haken H, Mandell AJ (1983): *Synergetics of the Brain*. Berlin: Springer–Verlag

Bernhard CG (1942): Isolation of retinal and optic ganglion response in the eye of Dytiscus. *J Neurophysiol* 5:32

Bishop GH (1933): Cyclic changes in excitability of the optic pathway of the rabbit. *Am J Physiol* 103:213–224

Bishop GH (1935): Electrical responses accompanying activity of the optic pathway. *Arch Ophthamol* 14:992–1019

Bishop GH, Clare MH (1952): Relations between specifically evoked and "spontaneous" activity of optic cortex. *Electroencephalogr Clin Neurophysiol* 4:321–330

Bishop GH, O'Leary J (1936): Components of the electrical response of the optic cortex of the rabbit. *Am J Physiol* 117:292–308

Bishop GH, O'Leary J (1938): Potential records from the optic cortex of the cat. *J Neurophysiol* I:391–404

Bishop PO, Jeremy D, McLeod JG (1953): Phenomenon of repetitive firing in lateral geniculate of cat. *J Neurophysiol* 16:437–447

Boeijinga PH, Lopes da Silva FH (1989a): A new method to estimate time delays between EEG signals applied to beta activity of the olfactory cortical areas. *Electroencephalogr Clin Neurophysiol* 73:198–205

Boeijinga PH, Lopes da Silva FH (1989b): Modulations of EEG activity in the entorhinal cortex and forebrain olfactory areas during odour sampling. *Brain Res* 478: 257–268

Brazier MAB (1960): Long-persisting electrical traces in the brain of man and their possible relationship to higher nervous activity. In: *The Moscow Colloquium on Electroencephalography of Higher Nervous Activity*, Jasper HH, Smirnov GD, eds. Montreal: The EEG Journal, pp 347–358

Bremer F (1941): La synchronisation neuronique. Sa signification physiopathologique et son mécanisme. *Schweiz Med Wochenschr* 12:570

Bremer F (1944): L'activité "spontanée" des centres nerveux. *Bull Acad R Med Belg* 9:148–173

Bremer F (1949): Considérations sur l'origine et la nature des "ondes" cérébrales. *Electroencephalogr Clin Neurophysiol* 1:177–193

Bremer F (1953): *Some Problems in Neurophysiology*. London: London University Press

Bremer F (1958): Cerebral and cerebellar potentials. *Physiol Rev* 38:357–388

Bremer F, Titeca I (1940): L'activité electrique de l'écorce cérébrale. In: *Traité de Physiologie normale et pathologique*, Tome XII. Paris: Masson

Bressler SL (1990): The gamma wave: a cortical information carrier? *Trends Neurosci* 13:161–162

Bullock TH (1945): Problems in the comparative study of brain waves. *Yale J Biol Med* 17:657–679

Bullock TH (1956): The trigger concept in biology. In: *Physiological Triggers and Discontinuous Rate Processes*, Bullock TH, ed. London: American Physiological Society, pp 1–8

Bullock TH (1961): The origins of patterned nervous discharge. *Behaviour* 17:48–59

Bullock TH (1962): Integration and rhythmicity in neural systems. *Am Zool* 2:97–104

Bullock TH (1965): Mechanisms of integration. In: *Structure and Function in the Nervous Systems of Invertebrates*, New York: WH Freeman and Co, pp 253–351

Bullock TH (1989): The micro-EEG represents varied degrees of cooperativity among wide-band generators: spatial and temporal microstructure of field potentials. In: *Brain Dynamics: Progress and Perspectives*, Başar E, Bullock TH, eds. Berlin: Springer–Verlag, pp 5–12

Bullock TH, Hofmann MH (1991): The neurobiology of expectation: interval-specific event related potentials to omitted stimuli in the electrosensory pathway in elasmobranchs (unpublished data)

Bullock TH, McClune MC (1989): Lateral coherence of the electrocorticogram: a new measure of brain synchrony. *Electroencephalogr Clin Neurophysiol* 73:479–498

Bullock TH, Hofmann MH, Nahm FK, New JG, Prechtl JC (1990a): Event-related potentials in the retina and optic tectum of fish. *J Neurophysiol* 64:903–914

Bullock TH, Iragui VJ, Alksne JF (1990b): Electrocorticogram coherence and correlation of amplitude modulation between electrodes both decline in millimeters in human as well as in rabbit brains. *Soc Neurosci Abstr* 16:1241

Bullock TH, Hofmann MH, New JG, Nahm FK (1991): Dynamic properties of visual evoked potentials in the tectum of cartilaginous and bony fishes, with neuroethological implications. *J Exp Zool Suppl* 5:142–155

Chang H-t (1950): The repetitive discharges of corticothalamic reverberating circuit. *J Neurophysiol* 13:235–257

Chatrian GE, Bickford RG, Uihlein A (1960): Depth electrographic study of a fast rhythm evoked from the human calcarine region by steady illumination. *Electroencephalogr Clin Neurophysiol* 12:167–176

Clare MH, Bishop GH (1956): Potential wave mechanisms in cat cortex. *Electroencephalogr Clin Neurophysiol* 8:583–602

Cole LC (1957): Biological clock in the unicorn. *Science* 125:874–876

Crescitelli F, Jahn TL (1942): Oscillatory electrical activity from the insect compound eye. *J Cell Comp Physiol* 19:47–66

Dinse HR, Krüger K, Best J (1991): Temporal aspects of cortical information processing cortical architecture, oscillations and non-separability of spatio-temporal receptive field organization. In: *Neuronal Cooperativity—Models and Experiments*, Kruger J, ed. Freiburg: Springer–Verlag (in press)

Doty RW, Kimura DS (1963): Oscillatory potentials in the visual system of cats and monkeys. *J Physiol* 168:205–218

Ducati A, Fava E, Motti EDF (1988): Neuronal generators of the visual evoked potentials: intracerebral recording in awake humans. *Electroencephalogr Clin Neurophysiol* 71:89–99

Eckhorn R, Reitboeck HJ (1988): Assessment of cooperative firing in groups of neurons: special concepts for multiunit recordings from the visual system. In: *Dynamics of Sensory and Cognitive Processing by the Brain*, Başar E, ed. Berlin: Springer–Verlag, pp 219–227

Eckhorn R, Bauer R, Brosch M, Jordan W, Kruse W, Munk M (1988a): Functionally related modules of cat visual cortex show stimulus-evoked coherent oscillations: a multiple electrode study. *Invest Ophthalmol Vis Sci* 29:331

Eckhorn R, Bauer R, Brosch M, Jordan W, Kruse W, Munk M, Reitboeck HJ (1988b): Are form- and motion-aspects linked in visual cortex by stimulus-evoked resonances? In: Workshop: *Visual Processing of Form and Motion*, Vol. P7. Tubingen, West Germany: European Brain and Behavior Society

Eckhorn R, Bauer R, Reitboeck HJ (1989a): Discontinuities in visual cortex and possible functional implications: relating cortical structure and function with multielectrode/correlation techniques. In: *Brain Dynamics: Progress and Perspectives*, Başar E, Bullock TH, eds. Berlin: Springer–Verlag, pp 267–278

Eckhorn R, Reitboeck HJ, Arndt M, Dicke P (1989b): Feature linking via stimulus—evoked oscillations: experimental results from cat visual cortex and functional implications from a network model. In: *Neural Networks, Abstr. Vol., Conference on Neural Networks, Washington 1989*

Eckhorn R, Reitboeck HJ, Arndt M, Dicke P (1990): Feature linking via synchronization among distributed assemblies: simulations of results from cat visual cortex. *Neural Computation* 2:293–307

Eeckman FH, Freeman WJ (1990): Correlations between unit firing and EEG in the rat olfactory system. *Brain Res* 528:238–244

Engel AK, König P, Gray CM, Singer W (1990): Stimulus-dependent neuronal oscillations in cat visual cortex: inter-columnar interaction as determined by cross-correlation analysis. *Eur J Neurosci* 20:588–606

Engel AK, König P, Kreiter AK, Gray CM, Singer W (1991): Temporal coding by coherent oscillations as a potential solution to the binding problem: physiological evidence. In *Nonlinear Dynamics and Neuronal Networks*, Schuster HG, ed. Weinheim: VCH Verlagsgesellschaft, pp 3–25

Enright JT (1965): The search for rhythmicity in biological time series. *J Theor Biol* 8:426–468

Enright JT (1989): The parallactic view, statistical testing, and circular reasoning. *J Biol Rhythms* 4:295–304

Erxleben C (1989): Stretch-activated current through single ion channels in the abdominal stretch receptor organ of the crayfish. *J Gen Physiol* 94:1071–1083

Freeman WJ (1968): Relations between unit activity and evoked potentials in prepyriform cortex of cats. *J Neurophysiol* 31:337–348

Freeman WJ (1972): Measurement of oscillatory responses to electrical stimulation in olfactory bulb of cat. *J Neurophysiol* 35:762–779

Freeman WJ (1975): *Mass Action in the Nervous System.* New York: Academic Press

Freeman WJ (1978): Spatial properties of an EEG event in the olfactory bulb and cortex. *Electroencephalogr Clin Neurophysiol* 44:586–605

Freeman WJ (1979a): Nonlinear gain mediating cortical stimulus-response relations. *Biol Cybern* 33:237–247

Freeman WJ (1979b): Nonlinear dynamics of paleocortex manifested in the olfactory EEG. *Biol Cybern* 35:21–37

Freeman WJ (1979c): EEG analysis gives model of neuronal template-matching mechanism for sensory search with olfactory bulb. *Biol Cybern* 35:221–234

Freeman WJ (1981): A physiological hypothesis of perception. *Perspect Biol Med* 561–592

Freeman WJ (1985): Techniques used in the search for the physiological basis for the EEG. In: *Handbook of Electroencephalography and Clinical Neurophysiology*, Vol. 3A, Part 2. Gevins A, Remond A, eds. Amsterdam: Elsevier.

Freeman WJ (1987): Simulation of chaotic EEG patterns with a dynamic model of the olfactory system. *Biol Cybern* 56:139–150

Freeman WJ (1988): A watershed in the study of nonlinear neural dynamics. In: *Dynamics of Sensory and Cognitive Processing by the Brain*, Başar E, ed. Heidelberg: Springer–Verlag, pp 378–380

Freeman WJ, Schneider W (1982): Changes in spatial patterns of rabbit olfactory EEG with conditioning to odors. *Psychophysiology* 19:44–56

Freeman WJ, Skarda CA (1985): Spatial EEG patterns, non-linear dynamics and perception: the neo- Sherringtonian view. *Brain Res Rev* 10:147–175

Freeman WJ, van Dijk BW (1987): Spatial patterns of visual cortical fast EEG during conditioned reflex in a rhesus monkey. *Brain Res* 422:267–276

Friedlander MJ (1983): The visual prosencephalon of teleosts. In: *Fish Neurobiology, Vol. 2: Higher Brain Areas and Functions*, Davis RE, Northcutt RG, eds. Ann Arbor: University of Michigan Press, pp 91–115

Fröhlich FW (1913): Beiträge zur allgemeinen Physiologie der Sinnesorgane. *Z Sinnesphysiol* 48:28–164

Fujimura K, Matsuda Y (1989): Autogenous oscillatory potentials in neurons of the guinea pig substantia nigra pars compacta in vitro. *Neurosci Lett* 104:53–57

Galambos R, Makeig S (1988): Dynamic changes in steady-state responses. In: *Dynamics of Sensory and Cognitive Processing by the Brain*, Başar E, ed. Berlin: Springer-Verlag, pp 103–122

Galambos R, Rose JE, Bromiley RB, Hughes JR (1952): Microelectrode studies on medial geniculate body of cat. II. Response to clicks. *J Neurophysiol* 15:359–380

Gelperin A (1989): Neurons and networks for learning about odors. In: *Perspectives in Neural Systems and Behavior*, Carew TJ, Kelley D, eds. New York: Alan R. Liss, Inc, pp 121–136

Gelperin A, Tank DW (1990): Odor-modulated collective network oscillations of olfactory interneurons in a terrestrial mollusc (personal communication)

Gerard R (1941): The interaction of neurones. *Ohio Acad Sci* 41:160–172

Goldbeter A (1988): Periodic signaling as an optimal mode of intercellular communication. *Int Union Physiol Sci/Am Physiol Soc* 3:103–105

Goldbeter A, Moran F (1988): Dynamics of a biochemical system with multiple oscillatory domains as a clue for multiple modes of neuronal oscillations. *Eur Biophys J* 15:277–287

Granit R (1941): Rotation of activity and spontaneous rhythms in the retina. *Acta Physiol Scand* 1:370–379

Granit R (1963): *Sensory Mechanisms of the Retina*. New York: Hafner Publishing Co. (reprinted from 1947)

Gray CM, Singer W (1987a): Stimulus-dependent neuronal oscillations in the cat visual cortex area 17. *Neuroscience* 22 (Suppl.): 1301P

Gray CM, Singer W (1987b): Stimulus specific neuronal oscillations in the cat visual cortex: a cortical functional unit. *Soc Neurosci Abstr* # 404.3

Gray CM, Singer W (1989): Stimulus-specific neuronal oscillations in orientation columns of cat visual cortex. *Proc Natl Acad Sci USA* 86:1698–1702

Gray CM, Skinner JE (1988): Centrifugal regulation of neuronal activity in the olfactory bulb of the waking rabbit as revealed by reversible cryogenic blockade. *Brain Res* 69:378–386

Gray CM, Freeman WJ, Skinner JE (1986): Chemical dependencies of learning in the rabbit olfactory bulb: acquisition of the transient spatial pattern change depends on norepinephrine. *Behav Neurosci* 100:585–596

Gray CM, König P, Engel AK, Singer W (1989): Oscillatory responses in cat visual cortex exhibit inter-columnar synchronization which reflects global stimulus properties. *Nature (Lond)* 338:334–337

Gray CM, Engel AK, König P, Singer W (1990a): Stimulus-dependent neuronal oscillations in cat visual cortex: receptive field properties and feature dependence. *Eur J Neurosci* 20:607–619

Gray CM, Engel AK, König P, Singer W (1991): Temporal properties of synchronous oscillatory neuronal interactions in cat striate cortex. In: *Nonlinear Dynamics and Neuronal Networks*, Schuster HG, ed. Weinheim: VCH Verlagsgesellschaft, pp 27–55

Gray CM, König P, Engel AK, Singer W (1990b): Synchronization of oscillatory responses in visual cortex: a plausible mechanism for scene segmentation. In: *Pro-*

ceedings of Conference on: Synergetics of the Brain, June 1989. Bavaria: Schloss Elman.
Grüsser O-J, Grüsser-Cornehls U (1962): Periodische Aktivierungsphasen visueller Neurone nach kurzen Lichtreizen verschiedener Dauer. *Pflügers Arch* 275:291–311
Haberly LB, Bower JM (1989) Olfactory cortex: model circuit for study of associative memory? *Trends Neurosci.* 12:258–264
Haken H (1977): *Synergetics. an Introduction.* Heidelberg: Springer–Verlag
Hartline DK (1989): Simulation of restricted neural networks with reprogrammable neurons. *IEEE Trans Circuits and Systems* 36:653–660
Hartline DK:, Russell DF, Raper JA, Graubard K (1988): Special cellular and synaptic mechanisms in motor pattern generation. *Comp Biochem Physiol* 91C:115–131
Hodgkin AL (1948): The local electric changes associated with repetitive action in a non-medullated axon. *J Physiol* 107:165–181
Horn JP, Dodd J (1983): Inhibitory cholinergic synapses in autonomic ganglia. *Trends Neurosci* 6:180–184
Hughes JR (1964): Responses from the visual cortex of unanesthetized monkeys. *Int Rev Neurobiol* 7:99–152
Jahn TL, Wulff VJ (1942): Allocation of electrical responses from the compound eye of grasshoppers. *J Gen Physiol* 26:75–88
Jahnsen H, Llinás R (1984a): Electrophysiological properties of guinea-pig thalamic neurones: an in vitro study. *J Physiol (Lond)* 349:205–226
Jahnsen H, Llinás R (1984b): Ionic basis for the electroresponsiveness and oscillatory properties of guinea-pig thalamic neurones *In vitro*. *J Physiol (Lond)* 349:227–247
Jefferys JGR, Haas HL (1982): Synchronized bursting of CA1 hippocampal pyramidal cells in the absence of synaptic transmission. *Nature* 300:448–450
Kepler TB, Marder E, Abbott LF (1990): The effect of electrical coupling on the frequency of model neuronal oscillators. *Science* 248:83–85
Kergoat H, Lovasik JV (1990): The effects of altered retinal vascular perfusion pressure on the white flash scotopic ERG and oscillatory potentials in man. *Electroencephalogr Clin Neurophysiol* 75:306–322
Kleinfeld D, Raccuia-Behling FR, Chiel HJ (1990): Circuits constructed from identified *Aplysia* neurons exhibit multiple patterns of persistent activity. *Biophys J* 57: 697–715
Konishi J (1960): Electric response of visual center in fish, especially to colored light flash. *Jpn J Physiol* 10:13–27
Lansing RW, Barlow JS (1972): Rhythmic after-activity to flashes in relation to the background alpha which precedes and follows the flash stimuli. *Electroencephalogr Clin Neurophysiol* 32:149–160
Lee LT, Bullock TH (1990): Cerebellar units show several types of long-lasting posttetanic responses to telencephalic stimulation in catfish. *Brain Behav Evol* 35:291–301
Lee YS, Chay TR (1990): Electrical bursting in excitable cell model: a step toward understanding the neural network mechanisms. *Biophys J* 57:130a
Lenz FA, Kwan HC, Dostrovsky JO, Tasker RR (1989): Characteristics of the bursting pattern of action potentials that occurs in the thalamus of patients with central pain. *Brain Res* 496:357–360
Leresche N, Jassik-Gerschenfeld D, Haby M, Soltesz I, Crunelli V (1990): Pacemaker-like and other types of spontaneous membrane potential oscillations of thalamocortical cells. *Neurosci Lett* 113:72–77

Lestienne R, Gary-Bobo E, Przybyslawski J, Saillour P, Imbert M (1990): Temporal correlations in modulated evoked responses in the visual cortical cells of the cat. *Biol Cybern* 62:425–440

Li Y-X, Goldbeter A (1989): Frequency specificity in intercellular communication. *Biophys J* 55:125–145

Li Z, Hopfield JJ (1989): Modeling the olfactory bulb and its neural oscillatory processings. *Biol Cybern* 61:379–392

Llinás R (1988): The intrinsic electrophysiological properties of mammalian neurons: insights into central nervous system function. *Science* 242:1654–1664

Llinás R, Yarom Y (1986): Oscillatory properties of guinea-pig inferior olivary neurones and their pharmacological modulation: an *in vitro* study. *J Physiol (Lond)* 376:163–182

Lohmann H, Eckhorn R, Reitboeck HJ (1988): Visual receptive fields of local intracortical potentials. *J Neurosci Methods* 25:29–44

Loomis AL, Harvey EN, Hobart GA III (1938): Distribution of disturbance-patterns in the human electroencephalogram, with special reference to sleep. *J Neurophysiol* 1:413–430

Lopes da Silva F (1987): Dynamics of EEGs as signals of neuronal populations: models and theoretical considerations. In: *Electroencephalography: Basic Principles, Clinical Applications and Related Fields*, Niedermeyer E, Lopes da Silva F, eds. Baltimore–Munich: Urban and Schwarzenberg, pp 15–28

Madler C, Pöppel E (1987): Auditory evoked potentials indicate the loss of neuronal oscillations during general anaesthesia. *Naturwissenschaften* 74:S.42

Maffei L, Galli-Resta L (1990): Correlation in the discharges of neighboring rat retinal ganglion cells during prenatal life. *Proc Natl Acad Sci USA* 87:2861–2864

Makeig S, Galambos R (1989): The 40-Hz band evoked response lasts 150 msec and increases in size at slow rates. *Soc Neurosci Abstr* 15:113

Malsburg C von der (1981): *The correlation theory of the brain.* Goettingen, Germany: Internal Report, Max-Planck-Institut for Biophysical Chemistry

Malsburg C von der (1985): Nervous structure with dynamical links. *Ber Bunsen-ges Phys Chem* 89:703–710

Malsburg C von der, Schneider W (1986): A neural cocktail-party processor. *Biol Cybern* 54:29–40

Mastronarde DN (1989): Correlated firing of retinal ganglion cells. *Trends Neurosci* 12:75–80

Miles R, Traub RD, Wong RKS (1988): Spread of synchronous firing in longitudinal slices from the CA3 region of the hippocampus. *J Neurophysiol* 60:1481–1496

Montaron M-P, Bouyer J-J, Rougeul A, Buser P (1982): Ventral mesencephalic tegmentum (VMT) controls electrocortical beta rhythms and associated attentive behaviour in the cat. *Behav Brain Res* 6:129–145

Moran F, Goldbeter A (1985): Excitability with multiple thresholds. A new mode of dynamic behavior analyzed in a regulated biochemical system. *Biophys Chem* 23:71–77

Morris C (1990): Mechanosensitive ion channels. *J Membr Biol* 113:93–107

O'Benar JD (1976): Electrophysiology of neural units in goldfish optic tectum. *Brain Res Bull* 1:529–541

Pöppel E, Logothetis N (1986): Neuronal oscillations in the human brain. *Naturwissenschaften* 73:267–268

Rapp PE (1987): Why are so many biological systems periodic? *Prog Neurobiol* 29: 261–273

Reeke GN Jr, Finkel LH, Sporns O, Edelman GM (1990): Synthetic neural modeling: a multilevel approach to the analysis of brain complexity. In: *Signal and Sense: Local and Global Order in Perceptual Maps*, Edelman GM, Gall WE, Cowan WM, eds. New York: Wiley-Liss, pp 607–707

Regan D (1968): A high frequency mechanism which underlies visual evoked potentials. *Electroencephalogr Clin Neurophysiol* 25:231–237

Robertson RM, Moulins M (1981): Firing between two spike thresholds: implications for oscillating lobster interneurons. *Science* 214:941–943

Rotterdam A van, Lopes da Silva FH, van den Endee J, Viergever MA, Hermans AJ (1982): A model of the spatial-temporal characteristics of the Alpha rhythm. *Bull Math Biol* 44:283–305

Rougeul A, Bouyer JJ, Dedet L, Debray O (1979): Fast somato-parietal rhythms during combined focal attention and immobility in baboon and squirrel monkey. *Electroencephalogr Clin Neurophysiol* 46:310–319

Sainsbury RS (1985): Type 2 theta in the guinea pig and the cat. In: *Electrical Activity of the Archicortex*, Buzsáki G, Vanderwolf CH, eds. Budapest: Akademiai Kiado, pp 11–22

Schreiner CE, Joris PX (1986): Intrinsic oscillations in the primary auditory cortex of cats. *Proc XXX Cong Int Union of Physiol Sci*, p. 81

Seiple W, Holopigian K (1989): An examination of VEP phase. *Electroencephalogr Clin Neurophysiol* 73:520–531

Selverston AI (1980): Are central pattern generators understandable? *Behav Brain Sci* 3:535–571

Servít Z, Strejčková A (1976): Influence of nasal respiration upon normal EEG and epileptic electrographic activities in frog and turtle. *Electroencephalogr Clin Neurophysiol* 25:109–114

Sheer DE (1989): Sensory and cognitive 40-Hz event-related potentials: behavioral correlates, brain function, and clinical application. In: *Brain Dynamics: Progress and Perspectives*, Başar E, Bullock TH, eds. Berlin: Springer–Verlag, pp 339–374

Silva LR, Amitai Y, Connors BW (1991): Intrinsic oscillations of neocortex generated by layer 5 pyramidal neurons. *Science* 251:432–435

Simpson R, Vaughan HG Jr, Ritter W (1977): The scalp topography of potentials in auditory and visual discrimination tasks. *Electroencephalogr Clin Neurophysiol* 42: 528–535

Sporns O, Gally JA, Reeke GN Jr, Edelman GM (1989): Reentrant signaling among simulated neuronal groups leads to coherence in their oscillatory activity. *Proc Natl Acad Sci USA* 86:7265–7269

Steinberg RH (1966): Oscillatory activity in the optic tract of cat and light adaptation. *J Neurophysiol* 29:139–156

Sturr JF, Shansky MS (1971): Cortical and subcortical responses to flicker in cats. *Exp Neurol* 33:279–290

Tasaki I, Terakawa S (1982): Oscillatory miniature responses in the squid giant axon: origin of rhythmical activities in the nerve membrane. In: *Cellular Pacemakers*, vol. 1, Carpenter D, ed. New York: John Wiley and Sons, Inc, pp 163–186

Traub RD, Wong RKS (1982): Cellular mechanism of neuronal synchronization in epilepsy. *Science* 216:745–747

Traub RD, Miles R, Wong RKS (1987a): Models of synchronized hippocampal bursts in the presence of inhibition. I. Single population events. *J Neurophysiol* 58:739–751

Traub RD, Miles R, Wong RKS, Schulman LS, Schneiderman JH (1987b): Models of synchronized hippocampal bursts in the presence of inhibition. II. Ongoing spontaneous population events. J Neurophysiol 58:752-764

Traub RD, Miles R, Wong RKS (1989): Model of the origin of rhythmic population oscillations in the hippocampal slice. *Science* 243:1319–1325

Viana Di Prisco G, Freeman WJ (1985): Odor-related bulbar EEG spatial pattern analysis during appetitive conditioning in rabbits. *Behav Neurosci* 99:964–978

Wachtmeister L, Dowling JE (1978): The oscillatory potentials of the mudpuppy retina. *Invest Ophthalmol Visual Sci* 17:1176–1188

White G, Lovinger DM, Weight FF (1989): Transient low-threshold Ca^{2+} current triggers burst firing through an afterpolarizing potential in an adult mammalian neuron. *Proc Natl Acad Sci USA* 86:6802–6806

Whittaker SG, Siegfried JB (1983): Origin of wavelets in the visual evoked potential. *Electroencephalogr Clin Neurophysiol* 55:91–101

Wilson MA, Bower JM (1989): The stimulation of large- scale neural networks. In: *Methods in Neuronal Modeling: From Synapses to Networks*, Koch C, Segev I, eds. Cambridge, MA: MIT Press, pp 291–333

Wright EB, Adelman WJ (1954): Accommodation in three single motor axons of the crayfish claw. *J Cell Comp Physiol* 43:119–132

Zakon HH, Meyer JH (1983): Plasticity of electroreceptor tuning in the weakly electric fish, *Sternopygus dariensis*. *J Comp Physiol* 153:477–487

Oscillations in the Striate Cortex

Mechanisms Underlying the Generation of Neuronal Oscillations in Cat Visual Cortex

CHARLES M. GRAY, ANDREAS K. ENGEL, PETER KÖNIG, and WOLF SINGER

Place an electrode on the surface or in the depth of nearly any neuronal structure in the brain of either vertebrates or invertebrates. Record the fluctuations of voltage produced by the flow of current, and what you are likely to observe is an irregular sequence of rhythmic changes of potential having a multitude of frequencies (Bullock and Başar, 1988). If your electrode happens to be within one of many structures responsive to sensory stimuli, the presentation of a stimulus will in many cases evoke a sustained rhythmic fluctuation of potential outlasting the stimulus. This propensity for neural structures to generate oscillatory waves of activity has come to be termed an "induced rhythm". It is a general property of sensory as well as many other neuronal networks that is expressed during periods of activation. In this chapter we describe some of our recent observations of induced rhythms in the mammalian visual cortex and discuss the evidence for several neuronal mechanisms thought to underlie their generation.

One of the most striking examples of sensory-induced rhythms in the brain was originally described by Adrian (1942, 1950). Adrian placed electrodes in the olfactory bulbs of anesthetized hedgehogs, cats, and rabbits and recorded the activity of individual olfactory neurons as well as the macroscopic local field potential. He then stimulated the olfactory receptor sheet with an odorant mixture that evoked a brisk neuronal response at short latency. Associated with this response he observed a pronounced rhythmic wave of activity in the field potential recording that occurred at roughly the same latency and outlasted the presence of the stimulus. This oscillatory response, having a frequency of 30 to 60 Hz, he termed the "induced wave" (Adrian, 1950). Subsequently, a wide array of investigations revealed this phenomenon to be a general property of olfactory cortical structures. Induced waves were observed in the olfactory bulb and pyriform cortex of a variety of mammalian species (Bressler and Freeman, 1980; Freeman, 1975). They were seen in amphibia and fish as well as humans (Hughes et al., 1969; Libet and Gerard, 1939; Thommesen, 1978).

Induced high-frequency rhythms were later found to be prominent in many areas of the human brain (Chatrian et al., 1960; Perez-Borja et al., 1961; Sem-Jacobsen et al.,1956). Further investigations revealed the presence of induced waves in the somatosensory and visual modalities of cats and monkeys and from the scalp in humans (Hubel and Wiesel, 1965; Bauer and Jones, 1976; Sheer, 1976; Rougeul et al., 1979; Galambos et al., 1981; Bouyer et al., 1981).

The rhythmic activity was found to range in frequency from 20 to 60 Hz, could be evoked under a variety of stimulus conditions, and was most apparent when the subjects were engaged in a behavioral task.

The widespread distribution of these neuronal oscillations, their stimulus specificity, and dependence on behavioral state led to a number of predictions regarding their function (Freeman, 1981). Among these postulates, a specific functional role for rhythmic neuronal activity in the neocortex was proposed by Malsburg (1981, 1986). He predicted that by selectively synchronizing the rhythmic activity of neurons responding to features in an image a sensory scene could be unambiguously segmented into its component objects. For example, response synchronization could be used to bind together the elementary features of a spoken word in a noisy environment or to identify the features belonging to a visual object in a complex scene (Milner, 1974).

Experimental evidence for the synchronization of rhythmic activity was abundantly available from investigations in the olfactory system (Freeman, 1975, 1978; Freeman and Schneider, 1982). When recorded at multiple locations in the olfactory bulb or pyriform cortex, the induced waves were found to synchronize with little or no phase lag. These synchronous interactions were transient (i.e., 100–200 ms in duration) and were later found to be stimulus specific (Bressler, 1988; Vianna Di Prisco and Freeman, 1985). Moreover, when recorded in both the bulb and cortex, at loci separated by as much as 1 cm, the induced rhythms were found to be synchronous (Bressler, 1987). Such transient, stimulus-specific and synchronous-rhythmic interactions clearly constituted a close parallel to the type postulated by Malsburg.

Induced Waves in Visual Cortex (The Visual Sniff)

Persuaded by Malsburg's theoretical predictions and the experimental findings of Freeman and his colleagues, we investigated the temporal structure of neuronal responses in cat striate cortex. Initially, we searched for oscillatory responses in the visual cortex by recording multiunit activity (MUA) and the local field potential (LFP) from single electrodes in awake behaving kittens. In a number of our recordings we observed a clear stimulus-dependent oscillation of both the neuronal firing probability and the LFP during the presentation of a slowly drifting square wave grating at the optimal orientation (Gray and Singer, 1987a, 1987b). Correlation and frequency analysis revealed that the two signals were tightly correlated and had a frequency distribution of approximately 40 to 60 Hz. These induced waves were strikingly similar to those observed in the olfactory system, thereby conjuring up the notion of a "visual sniff."

In two subsequent studies utilizing multiunit recordings (Gray et al., 1989; Gray and Singer, 1989), we found that a large fraction of neurons (66% and 47%, respectively) in areas 17 and 18 engage in oscillatory activity in a frequency range of 40 to 60 Hz when activated with optimally oriented light stimuli. This neuronal activity was associated with a high-amplitude oscillatory LFP signal of the same frequency (Gray and Singer, 1989). In those recordings where the spike train was periodic, the action potentials typically occurred during the peak negativity of the LFP oscillation (Fig. 1). Analysis of the autocorrelation histograms of the spike trains and the frequency spectra of the LFPs revealed that the two signals were, on the average, of the same frequency. Spike-triggered averaging of the LFP demonstrated that the two signals were closely correlated in time.

In order to determine if such oscillatory responses were the result of a rhythmic afferent input we also made recordings of single-unit and multiunit activity as well as the LFP signal in the lateral geniculate nucleus (LGN) of the cat (Gray and Singer, 1989). Under conditions in which we observed robust oscillatory responses in cortex we found no evidence for stimulus-dependent oscillatory responses in the frequency range of 20 to 70 Hz in the LGN. It must be pointed out, however, that ganglion cells in the retina of a variety of species have long been known to exhibit oscillatory responses (Adrian and Matthews, 1928; Laufer and Verzeano, 1967; Ariel et al., 1983). And a number of investigators have reported finding 30- to 70-Hz oscillatory activity in a small percentage of the cells in the LGN (Arnett, 1975; Ghose and Freeman, 1990; Munemori et al., 1984).

Taken together, the results of these experiments demonstrated that units close enough to be recorded with a single electrode, if responsive to the same stimulus, show a synchronization of their respective oscillatory responses. The close correlation of the unit activity with the LFP suggests that the LFP signal results from the combined, correlated activity of a population of neurons firing in synchrony. The mechanisms for generation of the oscillations appear to be largely intracortical since we did not find rhythmic activity in a similar frequency range in the LGN. We cannot exclude the likely possibility, however, that rhythmic afferent input from the LGN may contribute to the generation of oscillatory responses in the cortex. This possibility could be tested by performing cross-correlation measurements between simultaneously recorded LGN and cortical oscillatory responses.

Laminar Distribution of the LFP

These results prompted a number of further experiments. Among these we sought to determine the spatial distribution of the coherently active population of cells and the extent to which cells in different layers of the cortex respond in synchrony. To achieve this we first utilized a 16-channel, multielectrode array to record the laminar distribution of LFP responses in cortex. These linear arrays of electrodes were advanced perpendicular to the surface of the cortex in order to sample the activity of neurons in a single cortical

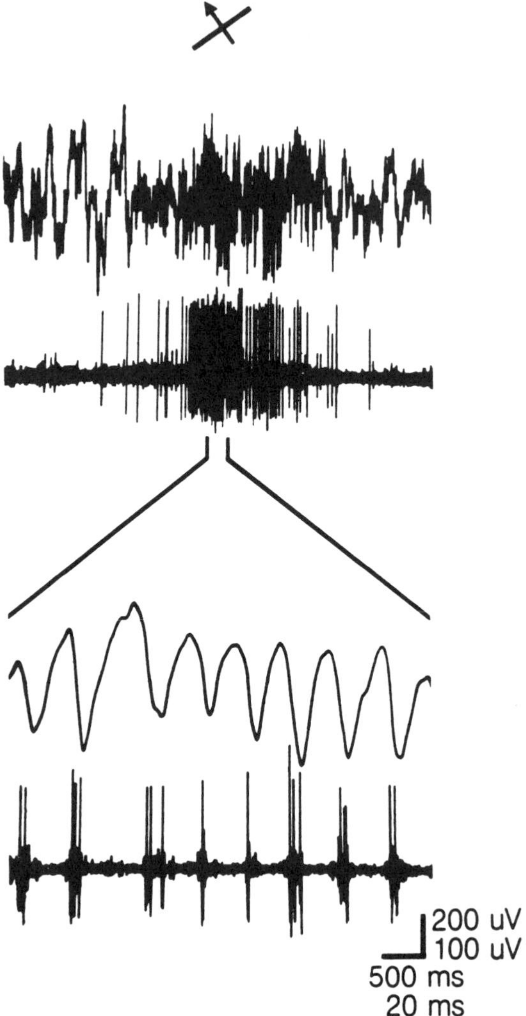

Figure 1. Local field potential (LFP) and multiunit activity (MUA) responses recorded from area 17 in an adult cat to the presentation of an optimally oriented light bar moving across the receptive field of the recorded neurons. The upper (slow time scale) and lower (fast time scale) plots show oscilloscope traces of the LFP (*upper trace* in each plot) and MUA (*lower trace* in each plot) recorded during a single trial illustrating the response to the preferred direction of stimulus movement. Reprinted from Gray et al. (1989): the Proceedings of the National Academy of Sciences, 86:1698–1702.

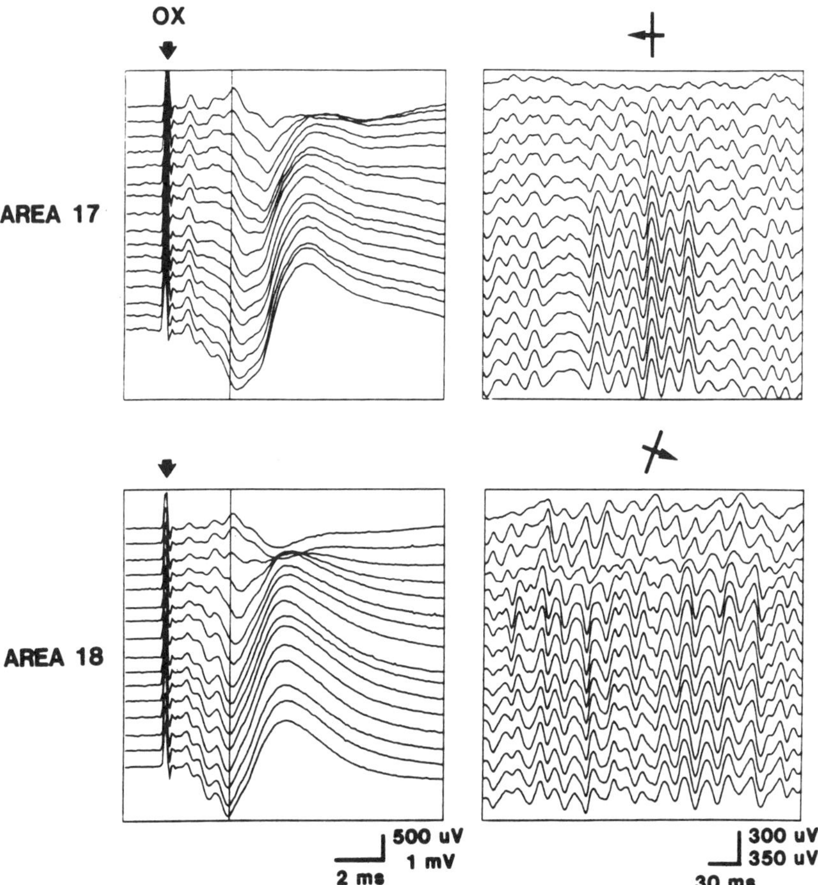

Figure 2. Synchronization of oscillatory LFP responses across the cortical layers in areas 17 and 18. The panels show parallel recordings from 16 electrodes implanted perpendicular to the cortical surface. The interelectrode distance is 150 μm. The left column shows responses evoked by electrical stimulation of the optic chiasm. The right column displays the responses evoked by stimulation of the receptive fields using a moving light bar.

column from the surface to the white matter. Measurements were carried out separately for areas 17 and 18. We also implanted stimulating electrodes into the optic chiasm in order to compare the visual responses with those evoked by electrical stimulation. The results obtained from a typical experiment are shown in Figure 2. Stimulation of the optic chiasm evoked a characteristic spatiotemporal distribution of potential in both areas 17 and 18 (Mitzdorf and Singer, 1980). In contrast, the presentation of a moving light bar across the receptive field mapped for the LFP activity evoked a well resolved oscillatory response in areas 17 and 18 that was highly synchronized throughout all the layers of the cortex. In area 18, prominent phase gradients in the LFP typically occurred in the upper cortical layers, a result previously noted for area 18 (Mitzdorf and Singer, 1980). In area 17, these sharp phase gradients were largely absent.

The results of these measurements further supported our contention that the oscillatory responses reflect activity in a coherently active population of cells. Nevertheless, for several reasons it seems likely that the generation of LFP responses does not involve all cells within an orientation column, but rather a subpopulation. First, we found many instances in which the multiunit responses showed no evidence of rhythmic activity (Gray et al., 1989; Gray and Singer, 1989). Second, consideration of the mechanisms underlying the electrogenesis of field potentials (Freeman, 1975; Mitzdorf, 1985) suggest that relatively few pyramidal cells, having vertically oriented dendrites spanning multiple layers (Martin, 1984), if synchronously active, could easily generate the distribution of potential seen in our laminar analysis of the LFP. For these reasons we conducted a further set of experiments designed to examine the temporal properties of single cells with respect to their laminar position and receptive field types (Gray et al., 1990).

Receptive Field Properties

We examined the receptive field dependence of oscillatory responses in 133 single cells. In general, we found a clear difference in the temporal pattern of firing between simple and complex cells. The vast majority of simple cells showed little or no evidence of oscillatory activity in response to their preferred stimulus. The firing pattern of these cells, as revealed by the autocorrelation histogram, typically showed a refractory period of 2 to 5 ms followed by a relatively flat distribution. This indicated that the range of interspike intervals showed broad variation with no clear evidence of periodicity. Only 12% of the simple cells recorded showed evidence of an oscillatory firing pattern (Gray et al., 1990).

In contrast to the typical temporal behavior of simple cells, a large fraction of the complex cells (42%) exhibited an oscillatory firing pattern. This propensity for rhythmic firing was much more pronounced in the standard than in the special complex cells (Gray et al., 1990). The oscillatory firing pattern consisted of bursts of two to five spikes in which the interburst intervals ranged from 15 to 30 ms. An example of an oscillatory standard complex cell is shown in Figure 3.

Although in our sample more than 50% of the standard complex cells showed evidence of oscillatory behavior, there were many clear and unambiguous examples of standard complex as well as other cells that did not oscillate. In these cases, the cells often fired at rates as high as 200 Hz but showed no tendency for bursting. Spikes usually occurred in isolation, having a refractory period of 3 to 8 ms. The distribution of interspike intervals was

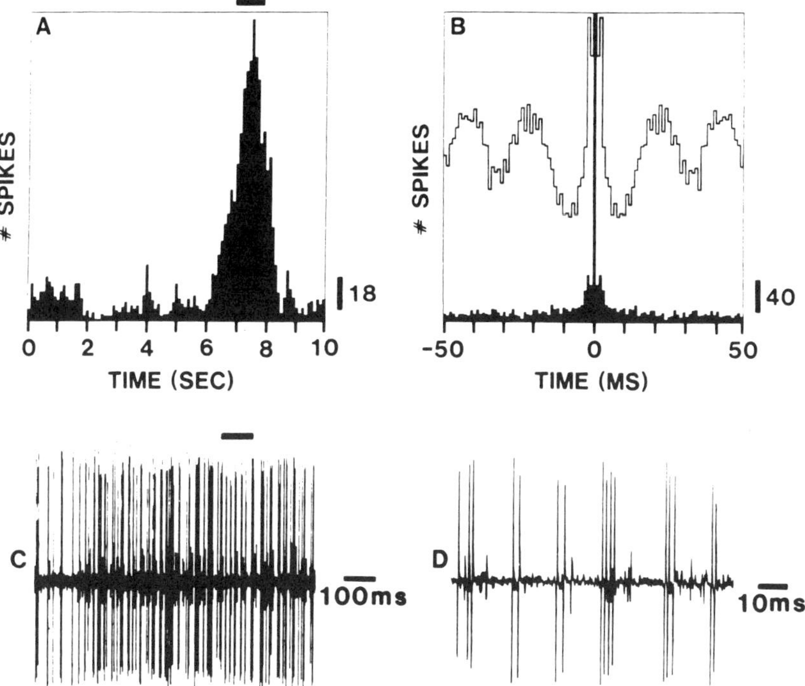

Figure 3. The firing pattern of an oscillatory standard-complex cell. **A:** Post–stimulus–time histogram of the neuronal spike train recorded over 10 trials. The response is selective for the second direction of stimulus movement. **B:** Autocorrelation histograms. Filled and unfilled bars display the correlograms computed for the first and second direction of stimulus movement, respectively. **C:** Plot of the spike train recorded during a single presentation to the second direction of stimulus movement. **D:** High resolution plot of the same data shown in C. Reprinted by permission of Oxford University Press, *European Journal of Neuroscience* 1990; 2:607–619.

randomly distributed, yielding a flat autocorrelogram over a range of intervals extending to 60 ms.

Finally, reconstruction of the laminar position of cells exhibiting oscillatory responses revealed them to be located in all layers, but sparsely distributed in layer 4 (Gray et al., 1990). These findings thus confirmed our results on the laminar distribution of the oscillatory LFP responses.

These results clearly demonstrate a high degree of heterogeneity in the firing patterns of different cell types in cat striate cortex. Moreover, they raise the likely possibility that intrinsic membrane properties contribute to shaping the temporal character of these firing patterns. A number of experimental as well as theoretical studies have demonstrated that rhythmic patterned firing is controlled in part by a combination of intrinsic membrane conductances (Agmon and Connors, 1989; Berman et al., 1989; Llinas, 1988; McCormick et al., 1985; Schwindt et al., 1988).

Response Variability

In search for mechanisms that contribute to the generation of the induced wave in visual cortex, we considered the possibility that the rhythmic response could be phase-locked to the visual stimulus. The movement of a visual stimulus might be expected to generate a sequence of repetitive firing in a cortical neuron as a result of sequential activation of excitatory and inhibitory subregions in the neuron's receptive field. If such a mechanism were present, one would expect to find a close temporal relation between the stimulus presentation and the phase of the induced wave.

To test this idea we examined oscillatory unit responses to both moving and stationary stimuli (Gray et al., 1990). We selected 12 recordings of both single and multiunit activity in which the autocorrelation histogram exhibited a pronounced oscillatory modulation. The temporal firing patterns of these cells were such that stimulus-evoked oscillations could be easily seen in the raw spike trains. In each of the 12 recordings the oscillatory responses were not synchronized across trials (Fig. 4). We observed a complete lack of oscillatory modulation in the trial-shuffled auto-correlograms and the exact onset and duration of the responses varied from trial to trial. These findings were confirmed by computing the autocorrelogram on each trial and comparing the distributions across trials. This approach revealed that the modulation amplitude and the frequency of the oscillatory responses also varied from trial to trial.

These results also held if we activated the cells with stationary stimuli flashed on and off within their receptive fields. We found a high degree of temporal variability for the onset of an oscillatory response to a stationary stimulus. The trial-shuffled autocorrelogram revealed no synchronization of the oscillations across trials and thus no precise phase-locking to the stimulus onset.

Combined with our previous observations (Engel et al., 1990; Gray and Singer, 1989), these data demonstrate that oscillatory responses exhibit a high degree of dynamic variability. The amplitude, frequency, and phase of the activity fluctuates over time. The onset of the oscillations is variable and bears no fixed relation to the stimulus. This evidence argues against the possibility that the rhythmic responses and their synchronous interactions reflect a temporal coupling to the visual stimulus.

Recurrent Inhibitory Interactions Underlying Oscillatory Responses

In addition to specialized conductance mechanisms capable of generating rhythmic burst firing, it is highly probable that network interactions also play an important role in the generation of this behavior. In particular, it seems likely that inhibitory feedback mechanisms contribute to the oscillatory firing

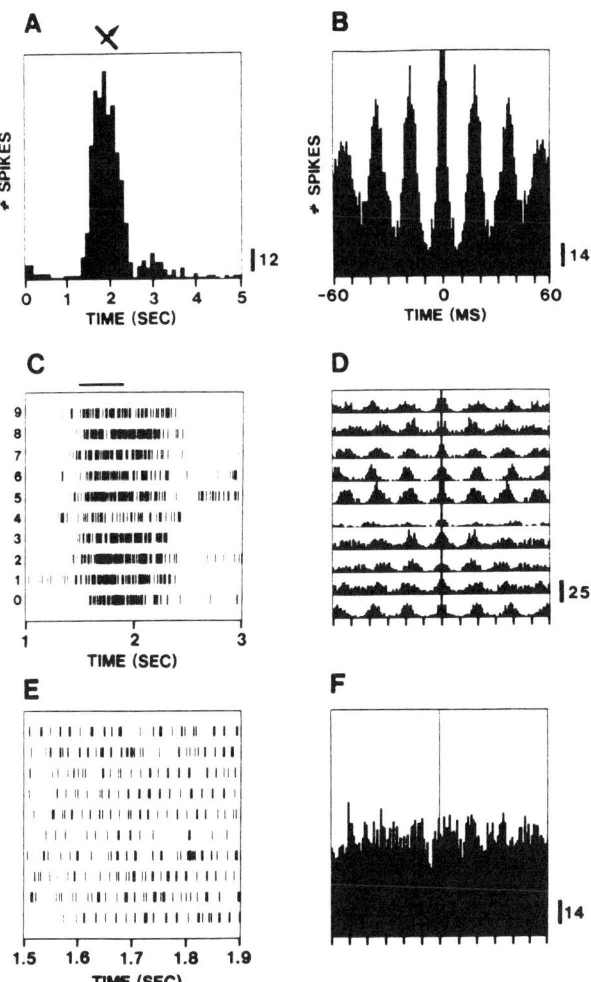

Figure 4. The onset latency, frequency, amplitude, and temporal phase of oscillatory responses are not time-locked to the stimulus presentation. **A:** Post–stimulus-time histogram of a multiunit recording computed from the response to the preferred direction of stimulus movement. **B:** Autocorrelation histogram computed from the same spike train data shown in A. **C:** Raw spike trains displayed for each of the 10 trials recorded between the second and third seconds of the stimulus presentation. **D:** Autocorrelation histograms computed from the spike trains recorded during each of the 10 stimulus presentations. **E:** High-resolution display of the spike trains recorded on each of the 10 trials shown in C. The epoch chosen for display is indicated by the time axis as well as the dark bar overlying the plot in C. **F:** Recomputation of the autocorrelogram after shuffling the trial sequence by one stimulus period. Reprinted by permission of Oxford University Press, *European Journal of Neuroscience* 1990; 2: 607–619.

patterns observed. This assumption results from the consideration of oscillations in the olfactory system.

In olfactory structures, and particularly in the bulb, recurrent inhibition onto excitatory neurons is thought to be responsible for the generation of the induced wave (Freeman, 1975). These findings have led to a set of specific predictions for the mechanism underlying the generation of neocortical induced waves: first, oscillatory responses should coexist in both excitatory and inhibitory neurons at the same frequency; second, the rhythmic activity in the two populations should be correlated; third, owing to their position in the negative feedback circuit, the inhibitory interneurons should exhibit a one-quarter cycle phase lag relative to the excitatory population. Such predictions appear plausible since local circuit inhibitory interneurons exist in abundance in the neocortex (Lund et al., 1979; Martin, 1984). However, it is likely that many forms of inhibition may coexist in the cortical network and such specific interactions may occur in only a subpopulation of inhibitory interneurons. Demonstration of such interactions is further complicated by the difficulties associated with recording from identified inhibitory cells. Thus, one may be largely limited to indirect sources of evidence.

We searched for such evidence and Figure 5 shows one particularly good example. A wide-band signal (1Hz–10kHz) was recorded from a single electrode implanted into area 17. From this signal we were able to detect the presence of two cells of differing amplitude as well as the LFP through the use of analog filtering and window discriminators. The two cells had receptive fields of similar size and location and they had similar orientation preferences. By using a single light bar at the optimal orientation and velocity we were able to activate both cells and evoke an oscillatory response in the LFP. A brief epoch of the response is shown in Figure 5A. The LFP can be easily discerned by the regular fluctuations of the baseline at roughly 45 Hz. The spike trains of the two neurons can also be seen. One is of greater amplitude than the other and they show different phase relations with the LFP. The activity of the large unit (cell 1) appears to coincide with the peak negativity of the LFP whereas the smaller cell (cell 2) shows a slight lag and fires most often during the rising phase of the LFP.

After separating the two cells using a window discriminator, we computed their post–stimulus-time histograms (PSTH) (Fig. 5B). Cell 1 is direction selective, whereas cell 2 shows no direction preference. In the null direction cell 1 even appears to be inhibited. We then computed the auto- and cross-correlation histograms for the two cells (Fig. 5C). These measurements revealed that cell 1 fired rhythmically at roughly 45 Hz whereas cell 2 showed only a weak indication of oscillatory activity at the same frequency. The cross-correlation between the two cells, however, revealed a clear peak at a phase difference of -5 ms. Since cell 2 was the reference cell this finding indicated that cell 1 was firing, on the average, 5 ms before cell 2. Given that the latency of the secondary peak in the autocorrelogram of cell 1 occurred at 22 ms, the phase difference between the two cells was, on the average, 82°, a value quite close to a one-quarter cycle phase difference.

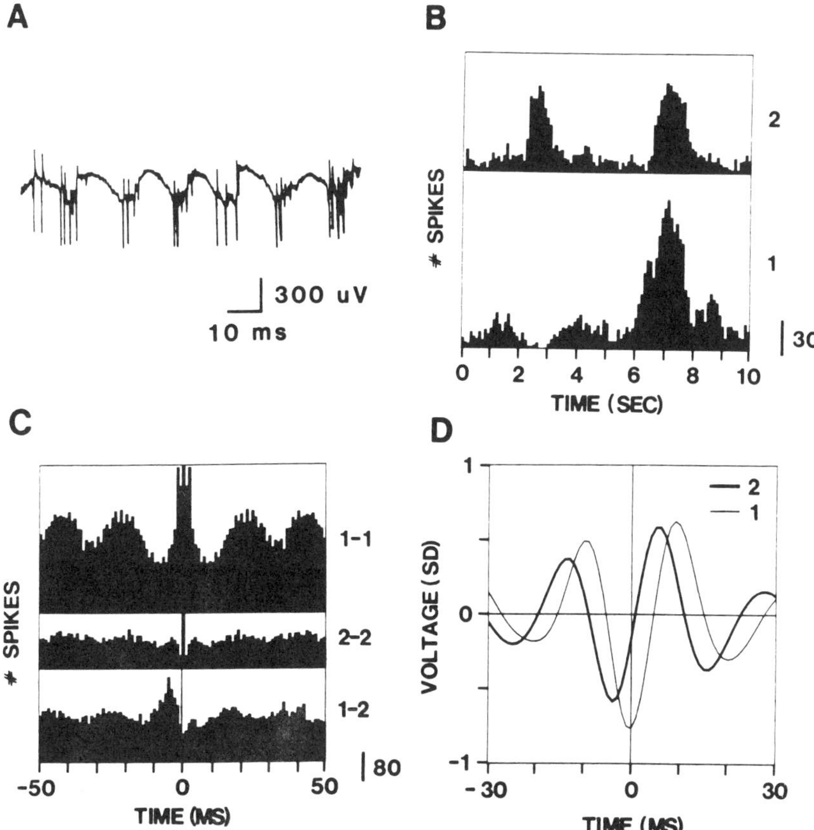

Figure 5. Two cells recorded from the same electrode in area 17 exhibit a one-quarter cycle phase difference during an oscillatory response. **A:** Oscilloscope trace of a brief epoch of data sampled during the peak of an oscillatory response to the preferred stimulus. The responses of the two cells were separated by means of a window discriminator after removing the low frequency components, i.e., the LFP, by band-pass filtering. **B:** Post–stimulus-time histograms of the spike trains of each of the two neurons displayed in A. The high amplitude unit is defined as cell 1 and the low-amplitude unit as cell 2. **C:** Auto (1–1, 2–2) and cross-correlation (1–2) histograms of the spike trains for cells 1 and 2 shown in A and B during the second direction of stimulus movement. **D:** Spike triggered average of the LFP signal with cell 1 (*thin line*) and cell 2 (*thick line*).

These findings were further confirmed by computing the spike-triggered average of the LFP for each of the two cells (Fig. 5D). On average, cell 1 fired during the peak negativity of the LFP (thin line). Cell 2, on the other hand, fired at a latency of 5 ms after the peak negativity of the LFP (thick line), again demonstrating a nearly one-quarter cycle phase lag.

Although the evidence is indirect, if one assumes for the sake of argument that cell 2 is an inhibitory interneuron reciprocally coupled to cell 1, then this experiment provides evidence for a recurrent negative feedback model underlying the generation of rhythmic activity. Such an interaction, when modeled in a network of excitatory and inhibitory neurons, can easily generate oscillatory activity, the frequency being dependent on the transmission delays between excitation and inhibition (Freeman, 1975, 1979; Sporns et al., 1989; Wilson and Cowan, 1972).

These findings, combined with those described above, suggest that recurrent inhibition as well as specific membrane conductances in a subpopulation of neurons contribute to the generation of induced waves in the visual cortex. At this stage it is not possible to determine if either mechanism in isolation is sufficient to generate neuronal oscillations. It is likely, however, that both mechanisms acting in synergy would be the most effective solution. In fact, recent evidence from *in vitro* studies supports this notion. Llinas et al (1991) have demonstrated the existence of a subpopulation of nonspiny stellate neurons in layer 4 of the frontal cortex which, when activated by subthreshold current injection, exhibit membrane potential oscillations at or near 40 Hz. These findings suggest that when sufficiently activated, a cortical network containing these neurons would automatically shift into a resonant state of rhythmic activity, the frequency being determined by the time constants of the membrane conductances. If such conductance mechanisms were present in the basket cells of layer 4 in the visual cortex, their widespread distribution of synaptic contacts (Martin, 1984) could place them in a key position to regulate the generation and coordination of coherent oscillations in a local population of cells.

Modulation of Oscillatory Responses

Among the factors regulating the occurrence and properties of rhythmic activity in the brain, behavioral state has a profound influence. In general, lower frequency rhythms (1–12 Hz) occur most often in states of habituation, drowsiness or sleep, and anesthesia. In contrast, rhythms of higher frequency in the beta and gamma range (15–80 Hz) are often associated with attentive states and behavioral arousal (Bouyer et al., 1981; Raether et al.,1989; Rougeul et al., 1979; Sheer, 1976). In the olfactory system 40- to 80-Hz activity is strongly influenced by behavioral state (Freeman, 1962, 1975). This facilitory effect of arousal is thought to depend in part on ascending modulatory influences arising in several midbrain and brain stem nuclei. Among these structures, the mesencephalic reticular formation (MRF) has long been thought to play a key role in regulating arousal states in the brain (Moruzzi and Magoun, 1949; Singer, 1979). Moreover, it has been demonstrated that conditioning stimulation of the MRF strongly augments the amplitude of neuronal responses in visual cortex (Singer, 1979) as well as the amplitude and coherence of oscillatory responses in the olfactory bulb and cortex (Arduini and Moruzzi, 1953) in a manner similar to that observed during arousal reactions (Freeman, 1962).

For these reasons, we considered it likely that MRF stimulation would also influence oscillatory responses recorded in the striate cortex. To test this idea we implanted stimulating electrodes in the MRF of anesthetized cats and recorded LFP and multiunit responses in the striate cortex to visual stimulation with and without conditioning stimulation of the MRF. Figure 6 illustrates a typical result from these experiments. In the absence of visual and/or MRF stimulation we observed little or no neuronal activity and only low frequency fluctuations in the LFP. MRF stimulation delivered alone produced no detectable change in this pattern of activity. The presentation of a drifting square wave grating at the optimal orientation evoked a neuronal response associated with well resolved, but irregular, oscillations in the LFP.

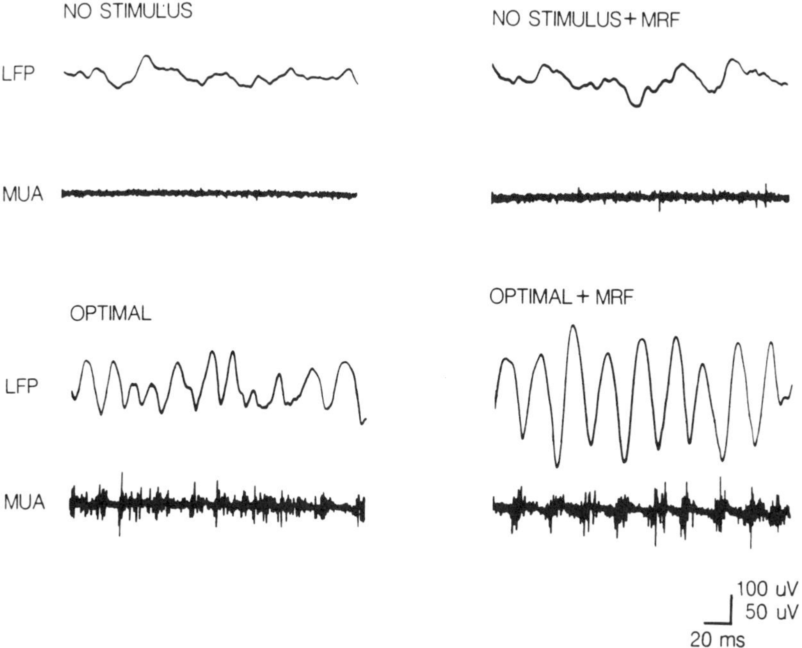

Figure 6. The amplitude and regularity of oscillatory responses in area 17 are enhanced by conditioning stimulation of the mesencephalic reticular formation. Each quadrant of the figure shows a pair of oscilloscope traces displaying a brief epoch of LFP and MUA signals recorded from a single electrode. The plots in the upper left show the signals recorded during spontaneous activity. The upper right traces show the activity recorded immediately following (100 ms) a train of electrical pulses to the MRF. The lower left traces show the activity recorded during the peak of a visual response to an optimally oriented drifting square wave grating. The lower right traces illustrate the changes observed in both signals when the same visual stimulus is presented 100 ms following a train of pulses to the MRF.

However, when applied in conjunction with a visual stimulus, MRF activation resulted in an increase in the amplitude and coherence of both the LFP and multiunit responses.

These findings demonstrate that the widely distributed afferent inputs to the visual cortex arising in the MRF are not reponsible for the generation of oscillatory responses. Rather, it appears that the MRF can exert a powerful modulatory influence on both the amplitude and temporal properties of the neuronal oscillations. This facilitory effect may provide a powerful control mechanism to regulate response synchronization under specific conditions of visual stimulation.

Summary

Our measurements of single-unit, multiunit, and local field potential responses in the striate cortex of the cat have revealed a number of properties of visual cortical-induced rhythms. We find that they occur in a large fraction of cells, most often having standard complex receptive field properties. The rhythmic activity, seen in both single-unit responses as well as the LFP, is distributed throughout all the layers of the cortex. Single-unit measurements indicate, however, that the neuronal oscillations are much less prominent in layer 4. Despite earlier reports to the contrary, similar measurements in the lateral geniculate nucleus revealed no evidence of induced rhythms in the same frequency range under stimulus conditions that resulted in robust oscillatory responses in cortex. Analysis of the variability of visual cortical oscillatory responses suggest that their generation cannot be explained by a sequential activation of excitatory and inhibitory subunits in their receptive fields. Rather, the evidence suggests that the oscillatory responses are generated intracortically Finally, extraretinal input from the MRF appears to play no role in the generation of oscillatory responses in the cortex. This input, however, is strongly facilitory and may serve to regulate synchronous interactions as a function of behavioral state.

We propose that two mechanisms acting together constitute the most likely explanation for the generation of 40- to 60-Hz induced waves in the visual cortex. First, the synaptic coupling between excitatory neurons and inhibitory interneurons is expected to generate rhythmic activity when excitation is imposed on the network from external and/or intrinsic sources. The frequency of oscillation will depend on the time delays inherent in this negative feedback loop. Second, intrinsic membrane properties, distributed in both excitatory and inhibitory neurons, are likely to contribute to the generation of burst firing and to the regulation of the interburst interval underlying rhythmic firing (Baxter and Byrne 1991). The absence of oscillatory responses in a significant fraction of cells suggests, however, that these mechanisms may be differentially distributed within the cortex.

References

Adrian ED (1942): Olfactory reactions in the brain of the hedgehog. *J. Physiol* 100: 459–473

Adrian ED (1950): The electrical activity of the mammalian olfactory bulb. *Electroenceph Clin Neurophysiol* 2:377–388.

Adrian ED, Matthews R (1928): The action of light on the eye. Part III. The interaction of retinal neurons. *J. Physiol* 65:273–298

Agmon A, Connors BW (1989): Repetitive burst-firing neurons in the deep layers of mouse somatosensory cortex. *Neurosci Lett* 99:137–141

Arduini A, Moruzzi G (1953): Olfactory arousal reactions in the "cerveau isole" cat. *Electroencephalogr Clin Neurophysiol* 2:243–250

Ariel M, Daw NW, Rader RK (1983): Rhythmicity in rabbit retinal ganglion cell responses. *Vision Res* 23(12):1485–1493

Arnett DW (1975): Correlation analysis of units recorded in the cat dorsal lateral geniculate nucleus. *Exp Brain Res* 24:111–130

Bauer RH, Jones CN (1976): Feedback training of 36–44 Hz EEG activity in the visual cortex and hippocampus of cats: evidence for sensory and motor involvement. *Psychol Behav* 17:885–890

Baxter DA, Byrne JH (1991): Ionic conductance mechanisms contributing to the electrophysiological properties of neurons. *Current Opinion in Neurobiology* 1:105–112.

Berman NJ, Bush PC, Douglas RJ (1989): Adaptation and bursting in neocortical neurons may be controlled by a single fast potassium conductance. *Q J Exp Physiol* 74:223–226

Bouyer JJ, Montaron MF, Rougeul A (1981): Fast fronto-parietal rhythms during combined focused attentive behavior and immobility in cat: cortical and thalamic localizations. *Electroencephalogr Clin Neurophysiol* 51:244–252

Bressler SL (1987): Relation of olfactory bulb and cortex: I Spatial variation of bulbocortical interdependence. *Brain Res* 409:285–293

Bressler SL (1988): Changes in electrical activity of rabbit olfactory bulb and cortex to conditioned odor stimulation. *Behav Neurosci* 102(5):740–747

Bressler SL, Freeman WJ (1980): Frequency analysis of olfactory system EEG in cat, rabbit and rat. *Electroencephalogr Clin Neurophysiol* 50:19–24

Bullock T, Başar E (1988): Comparison of ongoing compound field potentials in the brains of invertebrates and vertebrates. *Brain Res Rev* 13:57–75

Chatrian GE, Bickford RG, Uilein A (1960): Depth electrographic study of a fast rhythm evoked from the human calcarine region by steady illumination. *Electroencephalogr Clin Neurophysiol* 12:167–176

Engel AK, König P, Gray CM, and Singer W (1990): Stimulus-dependent neuronal oscillations in cat visual cortex: inter-columnar interaction as determined by cross-correlation analysis. *Eur J Neurosci* 2:588–606

Freeman WJ (1962): Changes in prepyriform evoked potential with food deprivation and consumption. *Exper Neurol* 6:12–29

Freeman WJ (1975): *Mass Action in the Nervous System.* New York: Academic Press

Freeman WJ (1978): Spatial properties of an EEG event in the olfactory bulb and cortex. *Electroencephalogr Clin Neurophysiol* 44:586–605

Freeman WJ (1979): Nonlinear dynamics of paleocortex manifested in the olfactory EEG. *Biol Cybern* 35:21–34

Freeman WJ (1981): A physiological hypothesis of perception. In: *Perspectives in Biology and Medicine*. Chicago: University of Chicago, pp 561–592

Freeman WJ, Schneider W (1982): Changes in spatial patterns of rabbit olfactory EEG with conditioning to odors. *Psychophysiology* 19(1):44–56

Galambos R, Makeig S, Talmachoff P (1981): A 40-Hz auditory potential recorded from the human scalp. *Proc Natl Acad Sci* 78:2643–2647

Ghose GM, Freeman RD, (1990): Origins of oscillatory activity in the cat's visual cortex. *Soc Neurosci Abst* 16:523.4

Gray C, Engel AK, König P, Singer W (1990): stimulus-dependent neuronal oscillations in cat visual cortex: receptive field properties and feature dependence. *Eur J Neurosci* 2:607–619

Gray C, König P, Engel AK, Singer W (1989): Oscillatory responses in cat visual cortex exhibit inter-columnar synchronization which reflects global stimulus properties. *Nature* 338:334–337

Gray C, Singer W (1987a): Stimulus-dependent neuronal oscillations in the cat visual cortex area 17. *Neuroscience* 22 (Suppl):S434

Gray C, Singer W (1987b): Stimulus-specific neuronal oscillations in the cat visual cortex: a cortical functional unit. *Soc Neurosci Abst* 13:404.3

Gray C, Singer W (1989): Stimulus-specific neuronal oscillations in orientation columns of cat visual cortex. *Proc Natl Acad Sci USA* 86:1698–1702

Hubel DH, Wiesel TN (1965): Receptive fields and functional architecture in two nonstriate visual areas (18 and 19) of the cat. *J Neurophysiol* 28:229–289

Hughes JR, Hendrix DE, Wetzel NS, Johnston JW (1969): Correlations between electrophysiological activity from the human olfactory bulb and the subjective response to odoriferous stimuli. In: *Olfaction and Taste III*, Pfaffman C, ed. New York: Rockefeller

Laufer M, Verzeano M (1967): Periodic activity in the visual system of the cat. *Vision Res.* 7:215–229

Libet B, Gerard RW (1939): Control of the potential rhythm of the isolated frog brain. *J Neurophysiol* 2:153–169

LLinas RR (1988): The intrinsic electrophysiological properties of mammalian neurons: insights into central nervous system function. *Science* 242:1654–1664

Llinas RR, Grace AA, Yarom Y (1991): In vitro neurons in mammalian cortical layer 4 exhibit intrinsic oscillatory activity in the 10- to 50-Hz frequency range. *Proc Natl Acad Sci.* 88:897–901

Lund JS, Henry GH, MacQueen CL, Harvey AR, (1979): Anatomical organization of the primary visual cortex (area 17) of the cat: A comparison with area 17 of the macaque monkey. *J Comp Neurol* 184:599–618

Malsburg C von der (1981) The correlation theory of brain function. Internal Report, Max-Planck-Institute for Biophysical Chemistry, Goettingen, West Germany

Malsburg C von der (1986): Am I thinking assemblies? In: *Brain Theory*, Palm G, Aertsen A, eds. Berlin: Springer–Verlag

Martin KAC (1984), Neuronal circuits in cat striate cortex. In: *Cerebral Cortex vol. 2, Functional Properties of Cortical Cells*, Jones EG, Peters A, eds. New York: Plenum Press

McCormick DA, Connors BW, Lighthall JW, Prince DA (1985): Comparative electrophysiology of pyramidal and sparsely spiny stellate neurons of the neocortex. *J Neurophysiol* 54(4):782–806

Milner P (1974): A model for visual shape recognition. *Psychol Rev* 8(6):521–535

Mitzdorf U (1985) Current source-density method and application in cat cerebral cortex: investigation of evoked potentials and EEG phenomena. *Physiol Rev* 65(1): 37–100

Mitzdorf U, Singer W (1980): Monocular activation of visual cortex in normal and monocularly deprived cats: an analysis of evoked potentials. *J Physiol* 304:203–220

Moruzzi G, Magoun HW (1949): Brain stem reticular formation and activation of the EEG. *Electroencephalogr Clin Neurophysiol* 1:455–473

Munemori J, Hara K, Kimura M, Sato R (1984): Statistical features of impulse trains in cat's lateral geniculate neurons. *Biol Cybern* 50:167–172

Perez-Borja C, Tyce FA, McDonald C, Uihlein A (1961): Depth electrographic studies of a focal fast response to sensory stimulation in the human *Electroencephalogr Clin Neurophysiol* 13:695–702

Raether A, Gray CM, Singer W (1989): Intercolumnar interactions of oscillatory neuronal responses in the visual cortex of alert cats. *Eur Neurosci Assoc Abst* 72.5

Rougeul A, Bouyer JJ, Dedet L, Debray O (1979): Fast somato-parietal rhythms during combined focal attention and immobility in baboon and squirrel monkey. *Electroencephalogr Clin Neurophysiol* 46:310–319

Schwindt PC, Spain WJ, Foehring RC, Stafstrom CE, Chubb MC, Crill WE (1988): Multiple potassium conductances and their functions in neurons from cat sensorimotor cortex in vitro. *J Neurophysiol* 59(2):424–449

Sem-Jacobsen CW, Petersen MC, Dodge HW, Lazarte JA, Holman CB (1956): Electroencephalographic rhythms from the depths of the parietal, occipital and temporal lobes in man. *Electroencephalogr Clin Neurophysiol.* 8:263–278

Sheer DE, (1976): Focused arousal and 40-Hz EEG. In: *The Neuropsychology of Learning Disorders*, Knights RM, Bakker DJ, eds., Baltimore: University Park Press, pp 71–78

Singer W (1979): Central-core control of visual cortex functions. In: The *Neurosciences Fourth Study Program*, Schmitt FO, Worden FG, Cambridge, MA: eds. MIT Press, pp 1093–1109

Sporns O, Gally JA, Reeke GN, Edelman GM (1989) Reentrant signaling among simulated neuronal groups leads to coherency in their oscillatory activity. *Proc Natl Acad Sci* 86:7265–7269

Thommesen G. (1978) The spatial distribution of odor-induced potentials in the olfactory bulb of char and trout (*Salmonidae*). *Acta Physiol Scand* 102:205–217

Vianna Di Prisco G, Freeman WJ (1985): Odor-related bulbar EEG spatial pattern analysis during appetitive conditioning in rabbits. *Behav Neurosci* 99(5):964–978

Wilson HR, Cowan JD (1972): Excitatory and inhibitory interactions in localized populations of model neurons. *Biophys J* 12:1–24

Stimulus-Specific Synchronizations in Cat Visual Cortex: Multiple Microelectrode and Correlation Studies from Several Cortical Areas

REINHARD ECKHORN, THOMAS SCHANZE, MICHAEL BROSCH, WAGEDA SALEM, ROMAN BAUER

Neural Synchronization: A Flexible Mechanism for Feature Linking?

It might be imagined that the recently observed synchronizations among neurons of cat visual cortex are epiphenomena or side products of cellular properties with no causal significance for visual signal processing. Our working hypothesis, on the contrary, assumes that synchronization of neural activities forms the basis of a flexible mechanism for feature linking in sensory systems. Specified for the visual system, the hypothesis states that the receptive field properties of visual neurons in different parts ol the visual system can be linked into a perceptual whole by synchronizing the activities of those neurons that are activated by a coherent visual stimulus. We further assume that synchronization among the activities in distributed neural assemblies is internally enhanced or even generated via a specific linking (association) network that connects corresponding and noncorresponding locations of the cortical representations of visual space. Endogenous generations of synchronized states would be necessary in cases where the degree of direct (exogenous) stimulus-evoked synchronization is not sufficient in order to fulfill the demands for feature binding Linking networks are assumed to have connections and coupling strengths that follow rules of "perceptual coherence and plausibility" (for example, neurons that have neighboring receptive fields and that represent similar visual features by their RFs will have relatively strong linking connections compared with neurons having large inter-RF distance and different RF properties). This means that those combinations of neurons should be favored for synchronizing their activities via the linking network that code relevant and often occurring combinations of visual features.

This chapter gives a brief review of results on stimulus-induced synchronizations at 35 to 80 Hz in the visual cortex of lightly anesthetized cats. This is followed by a presentation of new data about signal properties of oscillatory events and on how and when they are generated, synchronized, desynchronized, and inhibited under stimulus control. For this we analyzed dynamic interactions among stimulus-locked responses (as evoked by sudden stimulus movements) and synchronized oscillatory cortical activities (as induced during fixation periods with slow retinal image shifts). We found that synchronized stimulus-locked responses first suppress ongoing oscillations and that after a period of inhibition oscillatory synchronizations occur with enhanced probability. The succession from synchronized to desynchronized states and vice versa is discussed in the context of the "linking-by-synchronization hypothesis" for visual situations like sudden object displacements and saccade/fixation sequences. A condensed version of our experimental findings in cat visual cortex was tested by us in computer simulations that mimicked a variety of our neurophysiological findings on stimulus-related synchronizations and that supports our coding hypothesis (see Eckhorn et al., *in press a*).

Linking of Local Visual Features into Coherent Visual Percepts

Stimuli comprising coherent features are integrated by our sensory systems into perceptual entities, even if the features are dispersed among different sensory modalities. We can perceive a sensory object as a perceptual whole even if various aspects of the object are occluded, obscured by the background, or are not present at all. The visual system can easily detect coherencies in an object's local stimulus features and is able to link, intensify, and isolate them. These capabilities of grouping, mutual facilitation, and figure/ground separation require highly flexible neural mechanisms for self-organization that are able to construct reliable and unique percepts out of ambiguous sensory signals. The perceptual capabilities of sensory systems for flexible region definition and feature linking have been studied extensively by psychophysical methods, but the underlying neuronal mechanisms are still largely unknown.

Visual Coding: Invariant and Flexible Principles

The neural mechanisms underlying perception are mainly not known. Some basic principles of "neural coding" are, however, discovered that probably play a role in sensory perception. In this respect, the visual system is studied most intensively among the sensory modalities. Here the concept of *receptive fields* (RFs) reveals highly specific *local coding properties* of single visual neurons that are the physical basis of local feature representations. The visual structures, including retina, lateral geniculate body, and visual cortical areas, form two-dimensional retinotopically organized "maps" of RFs. Each map has specific processing properties that rely on the prominent RF properties of that area. In cats as many as 15 such retinotopically arranged cortical maps have been found in each of the two hemispheres, and in primates this number is even higher.

RF properties and their retinotopic arrangements in "feature maps" form the basis of relatively invariant coding mechanisms that can serve as frame of reference between the outer world and visual perception. Even though visual processing is relatively well understood on this level of invariable coding, the necessary flexible mechanisms of feature linking and integration are unknown. Flexible mechanisms are needed, because otherwise an unlimited number of connections would be necessary if all the occurring "sensory situations" would each be coded by "hard-wired" subsystems specified for the particular sensory situation. Flexibly acting linking connections might be realized anatomically among feature detectors via the reciprocal "association" fiber systems that were found to project within and between visual cortical areas to targets far outside the representations of classical receptive fields. Such linking requires special types of connections between neural assemblies that can mutually facilitate and synchronize their activities without deteriorating their local RF properties (Eckhorn et al., 1988c; Eckhorn et al., in accompanying chapter 21) and that probably evolve from absence or primitive states in lower vertebrates and invertebrates to greater elaboration in mammals.

Analyses of Global Visual Processing Requires Recordings From Sufficiently Large Numbers of Neurons

We assume in our working hypothesis that dynamic ensemble coding is used for the representation of global visual relations: synchronization of stimulus-related activities serves to define visual objects and their perceptual continuity (Damasio, 1989a, 1989b; Eckhorn, 1991; Eckhorn et al., 1988a, 1988b, 1988c, 1989a, 1990a, 1990b, 1991 in press c 1991). To prove this statement, we should record the synchronized signal components from as many neurons as possible that are involved in the processing of a certain visual situation. It is, *a priori*, not clear which types of local "mass activities" are relevant for the study of global cortical sensory coding and on what temporal scale (how precise) "synchrony" is expected in order to support feature linking. In addition, we have to cope with the available techniques for recording and data analysis and the neural structures that will be investigated.

In recordings from the primary areas of cat visual cortex we can take advantage of the special local structures known as "patches," columns, layers, and so forth. The local cortical compartments are formed by groups of neurons that have common receptive field properties (local assemblies). (Eckhorn, 1991; Eckhorn et al., 1989a, 1989b; Gilbert and Wiesel, 1983; Hubel and Wiesel, 1962; Mountcastle, 1978) Neurons in local cortical assemblies, therefore, generally respond "in concert" to appropriate common stimuli, which means that their activities are nearly "synchronized." Synchronization in this context means a correlation delay range of about 20 ms, but not a precision of single spike coincidences. An estimate of the average synchronized response components of such a local assembly can be obtained by extracellular recordings of local neural mass activities. This is possible because extracellular neural signals superimpose linearly in extracellular space: synchronized components add up to high amplitudes whereas statistically independent signals average out. Parallel multiple electrode recordings of extracellular mass activities and single neuron spike trains, therefore, can give us valuable insights into the dynamic interactions among specified single neurons and local assemblies and also between different local assemblies (Eckhorn, 1991).

We developed multiple electrode techniques that are appropriate for simultaneous recordings from several areas of sensory cortex (Reitboeck, 1983a, 1983b; Reitboeck et al., 1981). From each of the (individually drivable) fiber microelectrodes we record in parallel single cell and local mass signals (Eckhorn, 1991; Eckhorn et al., 1988c); that is: local extracellular slow wave field potentials (LFPs; 13–120 Hz), which comprise an estimate of the average dendritic and somatic postsynaptic membrane potentials near the electrode tip (the "synchronized mass input signals" of a local assembly) 2) multiple unit activities (MUA; 1–10 kHz), comprising the "average mass output" of a local assembly near the electrode tip, and 3) single unit activity (SUA), that is, the output signals of single neurons (Fig. 1). The separation of the signals is made by combinations of band-pass filtering (LFPs, MUA, SUA), by envelope demodulation (MUA), and by amplitude window discriminators (SUA) (Eckhorn, 1991; Eckhorn et al., 1988c).

A Short Review of Stimulus-Induced Oscillations in Cat Visual Cortex

Gray and Singer (1987a) found in kitten visual cortex area 17 that *signal oscillations of 40 to 65 Hz* can be induced in local neural assemblies by specific visual stimulation. (We will call these oscillatory events "γ-spindles" because their frequencies are in the electroencephalogram's γ-range and because they are limited in duration to 50 to 500 ms). These authors first observed the oscillations as a local phenomenon restricted to single cortical columns and they proposed the oscillations to play a role for the stabilization between pre- and postsynaptic structures in the developing visual cortex (Gray and Singer, 1987a). They also already mentioned that the "local oscillator may provide a good model of the cortical columnar functional unit" (Gray and Singer, 1987b).

The above findings led us to the proposal that stimulus-induced γ-spindles might occur synchronized in separated cortical assemblies and that they could serve to define global visual relations (Eckhorn et al., 1988a, 1988b, 1988c). We could, indeed, discover correlated stimulus-specific γ-spindles (35–80Hz) in spatially separate cortical positions with our Marburg multiple-electrode technique (Reitboeck, 1983a, 1983b; Reitboeck et al., 1981): lateral synchronizations among neighboring cortical hypercolumns of the same visual area (both in A17 and A18) as well as synchronizations between different cortical areas (A17 and A18) were found (Eckhorn et al., 1988a, 1988b, 1988c). Recently, we could show that appropriate global stimuli induce stimulus-specific synchronizations among three cortical areas (A17, 18, 19). Our finding

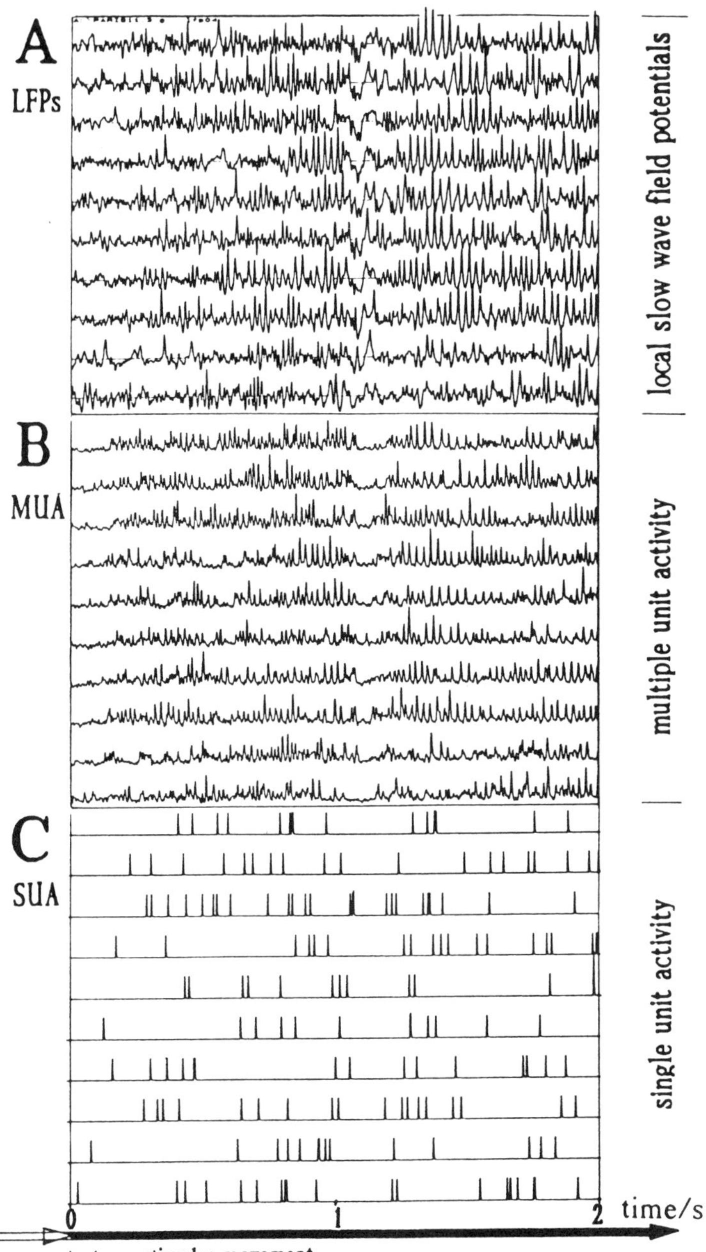

Figure 1. Three types of cortical signals, recorded simultaneously with the same microelectrode. Responses to 10 identical consecutive stimulus repetitions. **A:** Local field potentials (LFPs; 13–120 Hz). **B:** Multiple unit activities [MUA; derived by filtering (1–10 kHz) and subsequent envelope demodulation (0–120Hz)]. **C:** Single unit spike activity (SUA). Stimulus: grating of 0.25 cycl/°, moving at $v = 4.5°/s$. Black trace below indicates the duration of the stimulus movement. A 10 μs whole-field flash was applied at about the middle of the traces. (Note the 200-ms post–flash depressions of LFP high-frequency components and of MUA and single unit spike discharges).

of stimulus-specific synchronizations of γ-spindles between cortical columns in the same visual area (A17, A18) with similar orientation specificities was confirmed by the group of W. Singer who found correlated γ-rhythms at distances up to several millimeters (Gray et al., 1989; Ts'o et al., 1986); recently this group reported synchronizations of γ-rhythms between cortical areas A17 and the visual area PMLS, (Engel et al., 1990).

If the "linking" hypothesis is correct, (in the postero-medial lateral sulcus) such synchronizations should also be present between the different hemispheres of the same cortical area, because parts of the same visual object that activate different hemispheres should also be linked. Interhemispheric correlations of stimulus-induced γ-spindles could, indeed, also be proved for cat A17 (Engel et al., 1990), and it is shown for simultaneous inter-hemispheric synchronizations of A17 and A18 from experiments in our laboratory (Fig. 11).

Stimulus-response characteristics of γ-spindles (LFPs and MUA) were found to have specific correlations with classical single cell receptive field properties (Eckhorn et al., 1988a, 1988b, 1988c, 1989a; Gray et al., 1989; Gray and Singer, 1987a, 1987b). This means that the generation of γ-spindles can specifically be correlated with tuning properties of local cell assemblies, including RF position, ocularity, binocular disparity, orientation, contrast, movement direction, and velocity of contrast borders and textures (Eckhorn, 1991, Eckhorn et al., 1988a, 1988b, 1988c, 1989a).

We have been using *correlation profiles* to illustrate the spatial distributions of stimulus-induced correlation of γ-spindles in the horizontal direction, which comprise correlations between functional cortical columns (Eckhorn, 1991; Eckhorn et al., 1988c, 1991). Such profiles depend on the type of stimulation: different stimulus movement directions, for example, reveal coupling maxima between different cortical columns (Fig. 2). In Figure 2A the stimulus moved in the preferred direction of the neurons near electrodes 2, 3, and 7 whereas in Figure 2B the perpendicular direction was preferred by neurons near electrodes 5 and 6. It can be seen that γ-activities of cell groups with similar orientation/direction specificities are more strongly correlated (electrodes 3 and 7) than in neighboring cell groups with different orientation/direction properties (about orthogonal; electrodes 3, 4, and 5).

We discovered also stimulus-induced LFP and MUA γ-spindles that occurred correlated in different cortical areas (Eckhorn, 1991; Eckhorn et al., 1988a, 1988b, 1988c, 1989a, 1990b, 1991, in press b, c). The degree of interareal correlations at positions with RF overlap were as high as intra-areal correlations in about 1 mm lateral recording distance (up to 70% linearly correlated LFP amplitudes; e.g., between two patches of the same prefered stimulus orientation). With "appropriate stimulation" (see below), significant correlations of LFP spindles were present in almost all cortical positions where RFs overlapped (corresponding positions of visual representations), whereas significant correlations between MUA spindles where found only in "patchy" subareas of the RF overlap regions. RF properties at patches with interareal

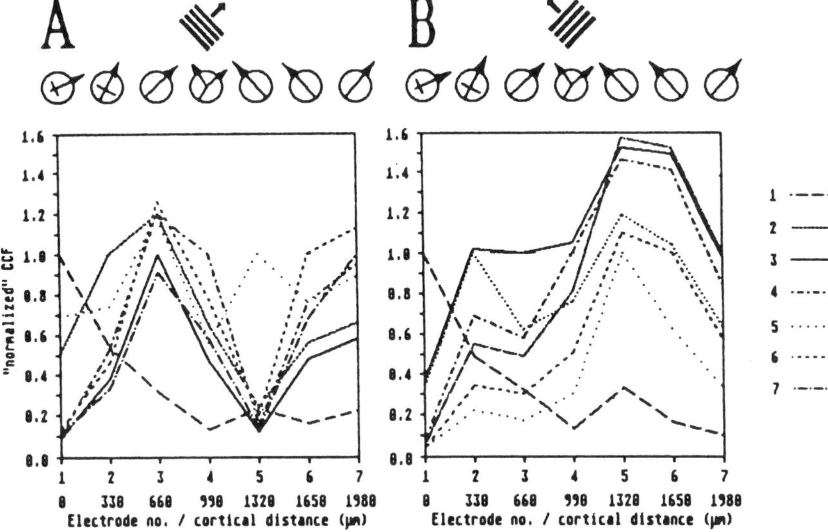

Figure 2. Spatial profiles of stimulus-specific gamma-spindle correlations within and between orientation columns of the same cortical area (A17). Simultaneous recordings of LFPs from layers II/III with a linear array of seven microelectrodes. Stimulus parameters: as in Fig. 2.1 (orthogonal movement directions, as indicated above). RFs of neighboring recording positions overlapped. *Ordinates*: peak amplitudes of normalized cross-correlograms were plotted over cortical distance (normalization to RMS values during stimulus pause). Different profiles were obtained by taking signals from each electrode as reference for cross-correlations with those on the remaining electrodes. Orientation/direction specificities of single neurons at each recording position are indicated above. Reprinted with permission of Springer–Verlag from Eckhorn R (1991): Stimulus-evoked synchronizations in the visual cortex: Linking of local features into global figures? In: *Neural Cooperativity*, Krüger, ed. New York: Springer–Verlag.

synchronizations, including ocularity, orientation, movement direction, and velocity preferences, could be considerably different in the different visual cortex areas. However, correlated γ-spindles could only be induced in those positions with RF overlap, where the cells (in both areas) could be activated by the same stimulus. (Simultaneous activation is a general requirement for the occurrence of synchronized γ-spindles.) This means that sufficient "coding overlap" (in RF properties) is required in order for a stimulus to induce correlated γ-spindles in separated cortical assemblies. The latter statement holds also for nonoverlapping RF positions, as we found: γ-spindles (MUA and LFP) that are correlated in the two visual areas were observed in those positions where the RF properties have one of their RF properties in common (for example, a directional preference for stimulus motion in a range $< \pm 15°$).

Two States of Visual Cortical Processing With Synchronized Activities

Stimulus-locked (non-oscillatory) and stimulus-induced (oscillatory) synchronizations

In natural vision, short stimulus shifts are often followed by phases with more stationary retinal images, for example during saccade-fixation sequences or when a visual object suddenly moves and stops again. We partly mimicked such visual situations in our cat experiments by applying sequences of stationary or slowly drifting stimuli that were superimposed by sudden larger stimulus displacements. Two types of stimulus-related synchronized activations were observed under such conditions: 1) "primary" stimulus-locked responses occur synchronized with precisely timed poststimulus delays, and 2) stimulus-induced γ-spindle synchronizations often followed such stimulus-locked responses (Eckhorn, 1991; Eckhorn et al., 1988c, 1991 in press c).

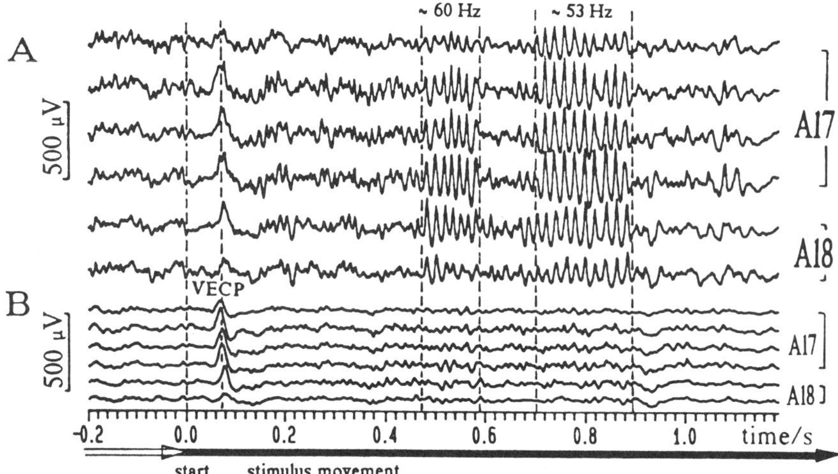

Figure 3. Two types of stimulus-related synchronizations of LFPs in two cortical areas: stimulus-locked local field potentials, and stimulus-induced γ-spindles. **A:** Single-sweep LFP-responses (band-pass: 13–120 Hz). **B:** Averages of 18 LFP responses to identical stimuli. Note that the oscillatory components (480–900 ms poststimulus) are average out, while averaging pronounces the primary evoked potentials (VECPs, at $t = 50–120$ ms). *Binocular stimulation*: drifting grating; 0.7 cycles/° swept at 4°/s; movement starts at $t = 0$ and continues for 3.4 s. Simultaneous recordings with linear array of seven microelectrodes from layers II/III; the RFs of A17 and A18 neurons overlapped partially. Reprinted with permission of Elsevier from Eckhorn R (1990a): Feature linking across cortical maps via synchronization. In: *Proceedings Intern Conf. Parallel Processing in Neural Systems and Computers*, Eckmiller R, ed. Amsterdam: Elsevier.

Both types of stimulus-specific synchronizations can be identified to contribute to the local postsynaptic mass activities (LFPs) shown in Figure 3. Signal components due to stimulus-locked synchronization are contained in the averaged visually evoked cortical potentials (VECPs) (Fig. 3B). VECPs are revealed by stimulus-locked averaging, whereas the rhythmic γ-spindle components generally are averaged out by this procedure. Figure 3 also shows that oscillations do not persist throughout visual stimulation. Instead, we found that oscillatory events of 35 to 80 Hz occur as γ-spindles with durations of about 50 to 700 ms that are separated by irregular pauses with more stochastic activity of lower amplitudes and less coherence. Post stimulus latencies of γ-spindles were found to be significantly longer than the latencies of the VECPs. More details of γ-spindle properties are given in the next sections and elsewhere (Eckhorn et al., 1988c, 1991 in press c).

Properties of γ-spindles under different stimulus conditions

Quantitative and selective estimates of oscillatory synchronizations were derived with a computer algorithm for automatic γ-spindle detection that proved to have high sensitivity as well as high temporal resolution (Eckhorn et al. 1991, in press c; Schanze et al., 1990).

Some typical statistical parameters of LFP γ-spindles are listed in Table 1. Table 1A shows that during *stimulation with a drifting grating* (1Aa), the γ-spindle parameters were of considerably higher magnitude than during

Table 1. Oscillation spindle statistics of LFP recordings from two cortex areas under different stimulations

	a				b		
		drifting	—	Stimulus	—	stationary	
	A18	A18★A17	A17		A18	A18★A17	A17
A Amplitude/μV	28 ± 6.4	29 ± 6.8	31 ± 7.8		11 ± 0.9	12 ± 1.3	15 ± 2.2
Duration/ms	125 ± 93	138 ± 110	119 ± 94		78 ± 31	81 ± 40	81 ± 41
Frequency/Hz	60 ± 11	60 ± 9.7	60 ± 10		53 ± 13	54 ± 12	55 ± 14
Probability	0.72	0.74	0.72		0.23	0.17	0.24
				two superimposed stimulus jerks			
B Amplitude/μV	23 ± 5.6	25 ± 6.1	27 ± 7.6		21 ± 5.5	23 ± 5.9	27 ± 9.1
Duration/ms	88 ± 53	93 ± 60	89 ± 54		104 ± 57	115 ± 68	119 ± 83
Frequency/Hz	68 ± 15	68 ± 15	67 ± 14		57 ± 11	59 ± 9.1	60 ± 9.0
Probability	0.48	0.48	0.53		0.66	0.70	0.81

A18: Recording from visual cortex area 18. **A17:** Recording from area 17. **A18★A17:** Values of "correlation spindles," calculated from the simultaneously recorded A17 and A18 data. Stimulation: **A:** whole-field grating of 0.25 cycl/deg, **a:** drifting at $v = 8.5°/s$ in "preferred" direction, or **b:** remaining stationary. **B:** stimulation as in *a*, with two additional stimulus jerks of half a spatial cycle of the grating; one jerk in, the other against the stimulus drifting direction (interjerk interval: 750 ms). Amplitudes are half peak-to-peak values. For more details of the spindle-search algorithm see text. RFs in the two A17 and A18 recording positions: adjacent, nonoverlapping, same preferences of orientations and stimulus movement directions. Reprinted with permission of Plenum Press from Eckhorn R, Schanze T (in press): Possible neural mechanisms of feature linking in the visual system: stimulus-locked and stimulus-induced synchronizations. In: *Self-Organized, Emerging Properties and Learning*, Babloyantz A, ed. New York: Plenum Press.

stimulation with the stationary grating (1Ab): we found a factor of 2.3 for amplitudes, 1.6 for durations, 1.1 for frequencies, and 3.4 for probabilities of γ-spindle occurrence in this typical example. These and most other results described in this chapter were obtained under light anesthetic conditions in semi-chronically prepared cats. Light anesthesia was maintained during recording sessions with nitrous-oxide/oxygen (70/30%). Some data were recorded while anesthesia was maintained with small amounts of continuously infused ketamine (1–2 mg/kg h), while the cat was ventilated with room air. Both types of anesthesia were supplemented by inhalation of 0.1–0.3% Fluothane if heart rate or other changes indicated a demand for that. With ketamine anesthesia stimulus-response properties of cortical cells were noticeably more brisk and "spontaneous" activities were slightly higher compared with nitrous oxide/oxygen, but occurrence rates and amplitudes of stimulus-induced γ-spindles were similar in both conditions.

Part B of Table 1 shows γ-spindle parameters that were obtained under the same conditions as in Table 1A, except that the grating stimulus made two sudden jerks. These jerks were either superimposed on the constant velocity drift (1Ba) or they were given in isolation (1Bb). *Jerks* in a slowly drifting grating considerably affected the generation of γ-spindles: superimposed jerks led, in this example, to a reduction of average spindle amplitudes (17%) and spindle durations (41%), to an increase in average spindle oscillation frequency (13%), and to a lower oscillation probability (46%).

When the *jerks* were applied to the stationary grating we found a remarkable effect (Fig. 4): after a short stimulus-locked burst and an inhibitory pause, γ-spindles were generated over several hundred milliseconds. The spindles' amplitudes and durations were slightly smaller under these conditions, while oscillation frequencies and probabilities did not change significantly compared with the values obtained with drifting stimuli. The possible significance of these findings for feature linking in natural vision will be discussed below.

Interactions between stimulus-locked responses and stimulus-induced oscillations in the visual cortex

Stimulus-locked responses of sufficient strength show a typical temporal course in slow wave VECPs (Başar, 1980, 1983, 1988; Bullock, 1988; Mitzdorf, 1985, 1987). In the following two sections we describe how the primary stimulus-locked response, the succeeding "silent" phase, and the last phase of increased excitability affect the generation of stimulus-induced γ-spindles. In the third section possible implications of these interactions for feature integration during saccade and fixation periods are discussed.

Delayed oscillatory state after fast stimulus transients. Efficient "jerk" stimuli (short and fast movements) (Fig. 4) or flashes (Fig. 1) generally evoke a short, precisely timed primary response peak in the cortical mass activities, and also in many single neurons (standard deviation of LFP response delays is typi-

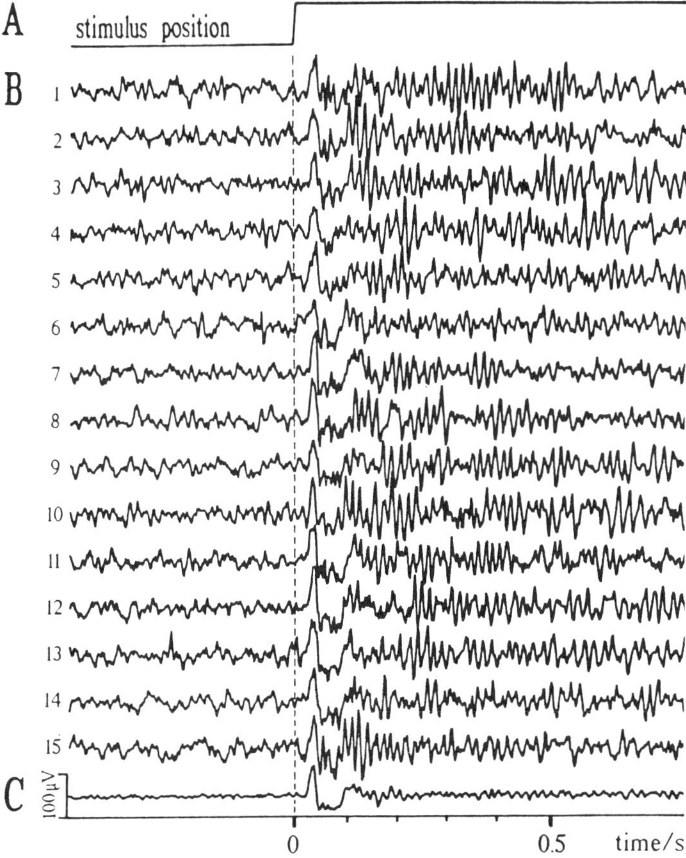

Figure 4. Jerk-induced oscillatory LFPs in visual cortex (A18). **A:** At $t = 0$ the previously stationary grating (same as in Table 1) jerks by half a spatial cycle; orientation and jerk direction correspond with the preferences of the neurons at the recording position in visual cortex area 18. **B:** 15 consecutively recorded LFP epochs from the same electrode in response to identical jerk stimuli (upward is negative). **C:** Stimulus-locked ensemble average of LFP epochs in A. Amplitudes in B and C are calibrated to the same scale. Note the high amplitude oscillation spindles after the primary "jerk potential" in B and the suppression of oscillatory components in C due to stimulus-locked averaging. Reprinted with permission of Plenum Press from Eckhorn R (1991): Possible neural mechanisms of feature linking in the visual system: stimulus-locked and stimulus-induced synchronizations. In: *Self-Organized, Emerging Properties and Learning*, Babloyantz, ed. New York: Plenum Press.

cally a few milliseconds). This response peak is followed by a silent phase (50–150 ms) and by a long period of moderate activation (200–700 ms), during which γ-spindles occur with enhanced probabilities. The primary response is obviously due to direct input from lateral geniculate afferents that activate a considerable number of cortical neurons for a short period. The inhibitory phase partly might be due to a discharge pause in the geniculate input, but it is probably influenced more by intra cortical inhibition (Creutzfeld et al., 1966). During the inhibitory phase the LFP components of higher frequencies and nearly all spike discharges (MUA) are suppressed; they "recover" gradually toward the end of the silent period (Figs. 1, 4).

In the subsequent long postinhibitory activation phase γ-spindles of considerable amplitudes were found to be generated. In the example shown, they appeared 90 $\pm$ 55 ms after the primary VECP peak (mean $\pm$ standard deviation; $n = 55$ response sweeps; Table 1Bb and Fig. 4). The observed activation is probably a postinhibitory rebound effect during which the spike encoders of the inhibited cortical cells are highly sensitive.

Suppression of stimulus-specific oscillations by stimulus transients. Oscillatory cortical synchronizations induced, for example, by a drifting stimulus, can immediately be suppressed by strong stimulus-locked cortical responses that are evoked, for example, by a flash (Fig. 1) or by a stimulus jerk (Fig. 4). Strong transient stimuli lead to a succession of two prominent response periods: initially, there is a period of complete or partial suppressions of γ-spindles; this is followed by a period where stimulus-induced oscillations occur with reduced amplitudes, lower probabilities, and increased variability and average oscillation frequencies, compared with values during constant velocity stimulation (see Table 1Ba).

Explanations for the transitions between different states of cortical synchronizations. We assume two mechanisms leading to the observed suppression and the reduced occurrence probability of γ-spindles following transient evoked responses. The first is an interruption of γ-spindles by the evoked response that dominates cortical single cell activity patterns; the other is due to intracortical inhibition.

Transient visual activation generates a variety of different spike patterns in individual cortical neurons that are essentially nonrhythmic in the sense of constant cycle periods. We assume that these stimulus-dominated heterogeneous responses have to wear off partly until the relatively weak mutual cortical coupling connections can support a common oscillatory mode. Our neural network simulations revealed that the more similar the discharge patterns in the different stimulated neurons are and the nearer they are to the preferred γ-spindle frequencies, the higher the probability that they will join into a common oscillatory state (see Eckhorn et al., in press a). For the function of the visual system, weak coupling connections are, however, of advantage, because they can provide many different coupling configurations among the same neural elements. It is therefore able to represent a large variety of sensory situations. In contrast, afferent visual feeding connections should be strong in order to provide fast and reliable detection with unexpected and weak visual stimuli.

The second argument why transient responses do not directly initiate synchronized γ spindles in cortical neurons but suppress their occurrence is probably due to intracortical inhibition. Inhibition immediately follows the first excitatory responses and generally lasts longer than 100 ms (depending on the strength of the stimulus transient), which is much longer than the oscillatory period of a typical γ spindle (21 ms) and often longer than a γ-spindle's duration (Table 1).

Relations between synchronized states and natural visual situations

In natural vision, short stimulus shifts are often followed by phases with more stationary retinal images, for example during saccade-fixation sequences or when a visual object suddenly moves and stops again. In both visual situations the primary stimulus-locked responses, that occur synchronized in many cortical neurons, might provide the basis for signaling relatively crudely but rapidly the "when," "where" and some aspects of "what" of the current visual events. The following inhibitory phase may play a role for perceptual suppression during fast retinal image shifts. But more probably, the inhibitory period may provide the previously activated part of the system with a transitory desensitization during which fast and strong stimulus-locked signals can be transmitted with high signal-to-noise ratios and processing speeds, while the internally generated synchronous γ-spindles are largely suppressed (see also our models of these effects in Eckhorn et al., in accompanying chapter 21). Post inhibitory rebound activations that occur after transient stimulations by sudden shifts of an object or after saccades can support sensitive generations and synchronizations of γ-spindles just in those cortical locations where a visual object continues to activate the neurons during the following period of retinal fixation or slow drift. During this state the coupling connections are assumed to be still sensitized by the fast stimulus-locked response components (Eckhorn et al. 1991, in press a, c). Only during periods of fixation or smooth pursuit would there be enough time for γ-spindle generation (21 ms per cycle at 48-Hz spindle frequency; spindle durations up to several hundred milliseconds; Table 1). In temporally critical situations it is therefore of advantage that stimulus-induced oscillatory states are quickly suppressed by sudden stimulus transients.

Sensory systems that are never supplied with well-timed signals from their receptors, like the olfactory system, would always have to use the mechanism of self-generation of repetitive synchronized activities in order to form global temporal association codes (for oscillations in olfactory system see Freeman, 1975; Freeman and Skarda, 1985). The auditory system, on the other hand, is probably more often directly supplied with synchronized activities from its receptors and cortically generated γ-spindles, therefore, might play a less important role.

In summary, we found that stimulus-locked (exogenous/nonoscillatory) and stimulus-induced (endogenous/γ-spindle) synchronization processes are two states that can, in extreme cases, occur only in alternation (as reported above). However, if the stimuli contain only "mild" transients that evoke stimulus-locked responses of only small amplitudes, then both types of synchronizations occur intermingled (as we recently could show).

Synchronizations Between Corresponding and Non-Corresponding Locations of the Visual Representations in Different Cortical Areas

Combined signal correlation and anatomical labeling analysis of cortical A17 and A18 connections

Tracer studies in mammals revealed reciprocal "association" fiber systems between visual cortical areas that massively connect corresponding locations of the visual cortical representations, where the RFs of neurons in both cortical areas overlap. However, there are considerable numbers of fibers that project to non corresponding targets (Bullier et al., 1984, 1988; Eckhorn et al., 1990b; Ferrer et al., 1988; Gilbert, 1985; Gilbert and Wiesel, 1983, 1987; Ts'o et al., 1986). Projections with such "RF mismatch" thus cannot contribute to the classical RF properties.

We investigated where and how the reciprocal association fiber systems between cat visual cortex areas 17, 18, and 19 might play a role in synchronizations among locations with and without RF overlap. For this, projections from A17 to A18 were labeled repeatedly during multiple microelectrode recordings by microinjections of a retrogradely transported tracer (HRP) at a "reference" recording position in A18 (Fig. 5) while we scanned A17 with other electrodes in steps (Ekhorn et al., 1990b).

Retrogradely stained cell bodies appeared in supragranular layers of A17 as patches covering regions with and without RF overlap relative to the A18 injection site. We found correlations between A17-18 MUA oscillations to depend on stimulation type and cell specificities. With our types of stimulation (binocular grating stimuli), A17-18 MUA spindles with high degrees of correlation occurred mainly in "patch positions" (see MUA cross-correlograms in Fig. 5). Correlated A17-18 LFP components were also present at "interpatch" positions. High density patches of labeled neurons in A17 coincided with recording positions where A17 RFs overlapped those of the A18 injection site. At such RF overlap positions significantly correlated A17-18 MUAs and LFPs were induced, even if the cells' preferred orientations and directions were markedly different. Spatially extensive stimuli could induce synchro-

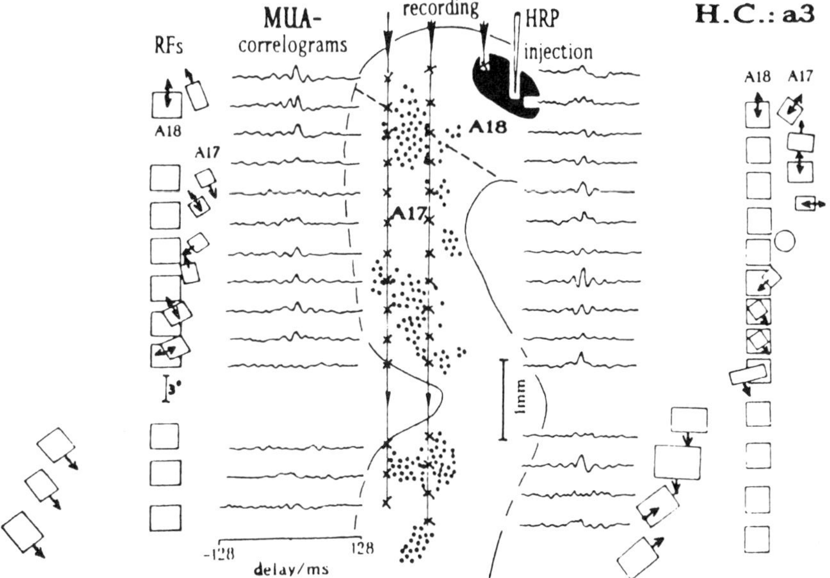

Figure 5. Couplings between cat areas 17 and 18 revealed with signal correlations and labelling of connections by a tracer. **Center:** Frontal section of a cat's visual cortex at Horsley Clark coordinates 3 mm anterior. The retrograde tracer HRP was injected into A18 (*black patch*). Small black dots indicate retrogradely labeled cell bodies (note their clustered distributions). Two microelectrodes were advanced in steps through A17. Mass spike activities (MUA) were recorded while a drifting whole-field grating stimulated the cells in both areas. **Sides:** Cross-correlograms between MUA recorded at the A18 injection site and those A17 positions where the MUA cross-correlograms have been plotted. **Outer sides**: RF-distributions at the A17 recording positions, plotted relative to the reference RF of A18. Simplified "rules," where interareal correlation patches were found, are described in the text. Reprinted with permission of Thieme from Eckhorn (1990): Cooperativity between cat area 17 and 18 revealed with signal correlations and HRP. In: *Brain and Perception*, Elsner N and Roth G, eds. Stuttgart–New York: Thieme.

nized A17-18 MUAs and LFPs even in cortical positions with "mismatch" between RFs of A17 and A18, albeit mostly with less coherence.

Correlations between γ-spindles in A17 and A18

Interareal correlations of stimulus-induced γ-spindles were analyzed in more detail by applying our "spindle detection algorithm" to the short-epoch cross-spectra of recording pairs in two different cortex areas (Eckhorn et al., in press

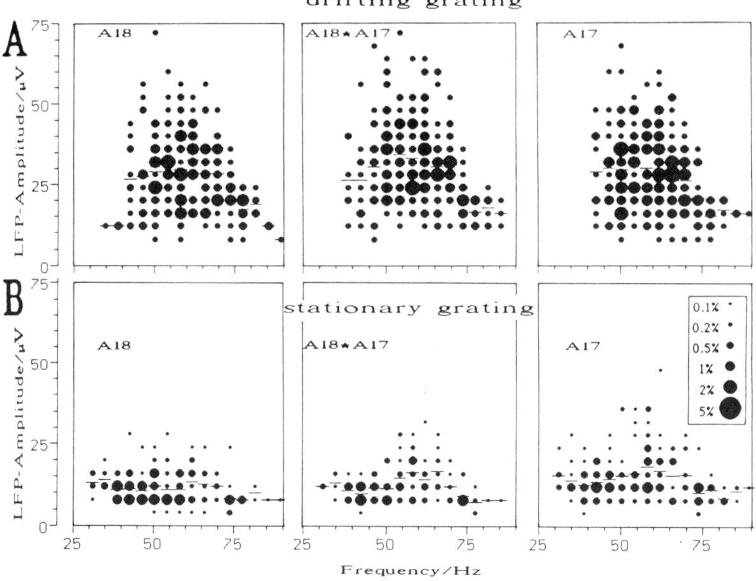

Figure 6. Distributions of occurrence frequencies of LFP gamma-spindle amplitudes versus their oscillation frequencies (single channel and correlation data). Simultaneous LFP recordings from visual cortex areas A17 and A18 (same data as for Table 1.A). Gamma-spindle events in single-channel recordings were isolated from the other remaining signal components by digital filtering (30–90 Hz, Blackman–Harris window) and a "spindle search algorithm" (Eckhorn et al., in press c; Schanze et al., 1990). "Correlation spindles" were searched for by the same algorithm, but instead of original records here short-epoch cross-correlograms (128 ms) were taken for the spindle search procedure. Search for correlation spindles was carried out on temporally overlapping parts in intervals of 32 ms. Dot size indicates relative spindle occurrence frequency, normalized to the data where the stimulus grating remained stationary (calibrations in the insert of the lower right panel). Spindle occurence frequencies are shown for data recorded during stimulation with a drifting grating (**A**) and while the grating remained stationary (**B**). A18 and A17 (*outer panels*) denote that single channel data were analyzed, whereas A18★A17 in the center panels denote that "correlation spindles" of the two channels are shown. Note the wide "spread" in the direction of large oscillation amplitudes and the higher occurrence frequencies of γ-spindles in the data obtained during stimulation (A) compared with those obtained while the grating stimulus remained stationary. Note also that during stationary stimuli low frequency spindles appear that are absent during drift stimulation. Reprinted with permission of Plenum Press from Eckhorn R, Schanze T (in press): Possible neural mechanisms of feature linking in the visual system: stimulus locked and stimulus induced synchronizations. In: *Self-Organization, Emerging Properties and Learning*, Babloyantz A, ed. New York: Plenum Press.

c; Schanze et al., 1990) (analysis details in Fig. 6). Our method enables us to analyze correlations among single γ-spindle events without major deteriorations by other correlated and uncorrelated signal components. As of January 1991 we analyzed data from 55 pairs of A17-18 recordings of LFPs in detail. Our results show that stimulus-induced γ-spindle events occur with high degrees of correlation in the two areas, which indicates that spindle parameters, including times of occurrences, frequencies, phases, and amplitudes, can covary in both areas with a high degree, if the stimulus drives both assemblies simultaneously (Table 1 and Fig. 6 show typical results from 2 of 55 recording pairs). The stimulus-specificity of spindle correlations is often high. In the examples shown relative occurrence frequencies of "correlation spindles" (for explanation see legend of Fig. 6) are larger by a factor of 3.4 and their amplitudes are larger by a factor of 2.4 during specific stimulation compared with no stimulation ("spontaneous" activities). We assume that the observed correlations are either mediated via the interareal association fibers and/or they might be due to a common drive outside of A17 and A18 (not observed). We currently consider interareal synchronization via association fibers to be more probable, as will be discussed below.

Correlation dynamics of γ-spindles from two different cortical areas were evaluated by calculating the spectral coherence of LFPs. In order to obtain reliable estimates for short response epochs, we repeated the stimulus cyclically and calculated an ensemble average of the coherence values of equivalent "time slices" ($n = 12$; each of 250 ms duration; frequency resolution, 2 Hz) of the stimulus cycle. Significance of these short-duration coherence values was estimated by subtracting from them the average coherence values that were calculated from the activities of the interleaved stimulation pauses ($n = 12$; each of 2 s duration). Figure 7 shows a time course of such A17-18 coherence values at the respective γ-spindle frequencies. Shortly after the grating stimulus starts to move ($t = 0$, Fig.7), coherence increases from 0.1 to about 0.6 during the movement and goes down again to low values after the stimulus stops. This example shows (together with other results from our laboratory) that the coupling strength between two visual cortical areas (its "efficacy") is highly "modulated" under stimulus control. More detailed analyses of individual gamma-spindle pairs from two areas revealed that coupling can increase within a single cycle of a γ-oscillation.

Correlations between single-cell and mass activities in two cortical areas

We often found in recording positions with binocularly driven neurons that LFP and MUA γ-spindles could be induced, with high amplitudes and coherence only by appropriate binocular stimuli (Eckhorn, 1991; Eckhorn et al., 1988a, 1988b, 1988c). Such a *dependence on binocular stimulation* also was often present in correlations between single cells and γ oscillations of mass activities in the same and between different cortex areas. Figure 8 shows that

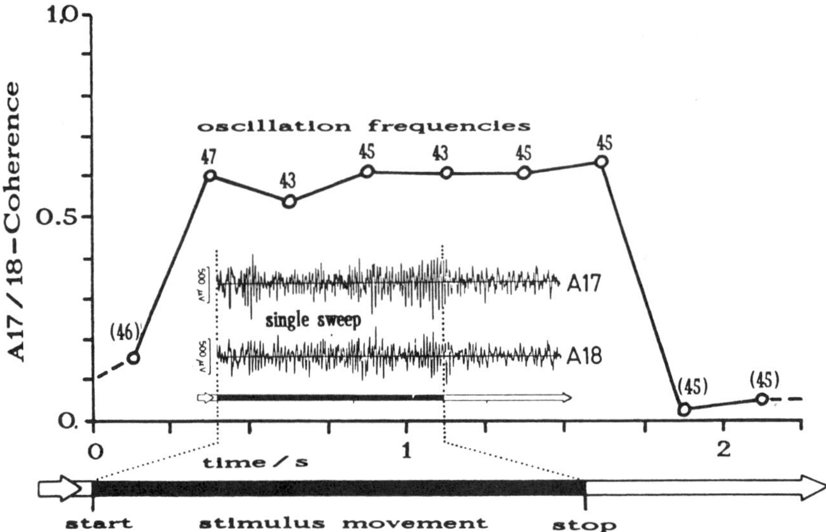

Figure 7. Temporal course of γ-spindle coherence in two different cortex areas in response to a moving stimulus. Coherence values were determined as averages from short-epoch (250 ms) LFP responses to 10 identical stimulus repetitions. Recordings were from A17 and A18 positions with overlapping RFs. A single sweep response pair is shown as insert. More details are in the text. Reprinted with permission of Springer–Verlag from Eckhorn R (1991): Stimulus-evoked synchronizations in the visual cortex: linking of local features into global figures? In: *Neural Cooperativity*, Krüger J, ed. New York: Springer–Verlag.

with monocular stimulation of the dominant eye, single-cell spikes of one area are only loosely coupled with the LFPs in the other area and γ-components are barely visible, although the RFs of the recording positions in both areas overlapped. Such binocularly induced correlations might support processing of global binocular correspondence in order to compute depth from disparity cues. In positions with mainly monocular driven cells, however, γ-spindles of considerable amplitudes could also be induced.

Figure 9 is another example of specific stimulus influences on A17-A18 correlations between γ-spindle mass activities (LFPs and MUA) and single-cell spike trains (SUA). Data from three (of 19) electrodes were selected for this figure. The two A17 recordings (electrodes 3 and 6) have nonoverlapping RFs and perpendicular directional preferences for moving stimuli whereas the A18 recording has an overlapping RF (electrode 13) with one of the A17 positions (electrode 6; a schema of the RFs is plotted in the upper right of Fig. 9).

The correlograms in Figure 9 confirm again our (preliminary) general rules for the dependence of γ-spindle correlations on RF (coding) properties of visual cortical neurons: Correlations between γ-spindles are stronger the nearer the local coding (RF) properties at the recording positions are in "cod-

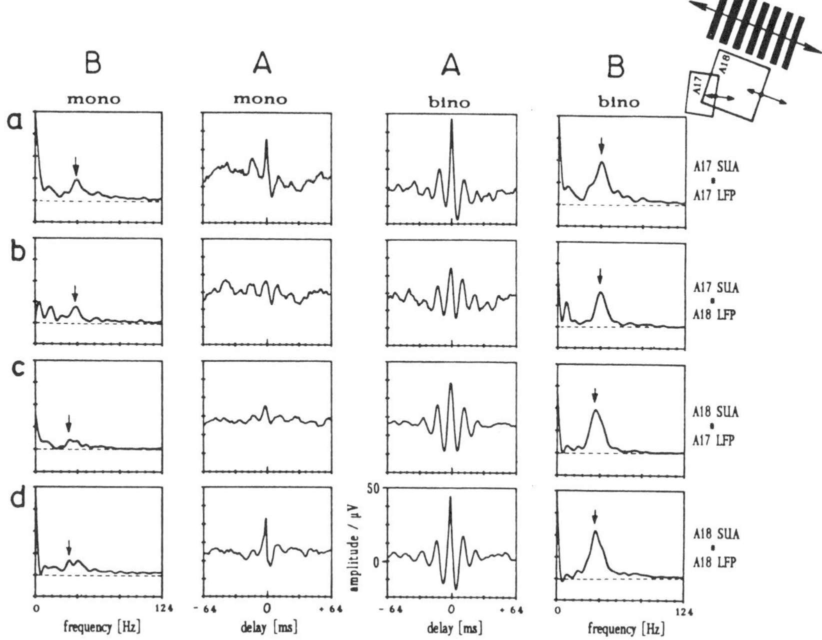

Figure 8. Dependence of γ-spindle correlations in two cortical areas on monocular versus binocular stimulation. **A:** Spike-triggered averages of LFPs, calculated for all combinations of A17 and A18 spikes and LFPs (symbols shown at right side). **B:** Spectral functions calculated by Fourier transformation from the respective spike-triggered averages of A. RFs at the A17 and A18 recording positions slightly overlapped (RF symbols at the upper right). Stimulus: Grating of 0.7 cyc/° moving in and against preferred direction at 8°/s. Note the remarkable degree of γ-spindle correlations due to binocular (bino) compared with monocular (mono) stimulation. The latter was applied to the dominant eye. Reprinted with permission of Springer–Verlag from Eckhorn R (1991): Stimulus-evoked synchromizations in the visual cortex: Linking of local features into global figures? In: *Neural Cooperativity*, Krüger J, ed. New York: Springer–Verlag.

ing space" (i.e., the more similar their RF properties are). A second condition is that a common stimulus has to activate the neurons simultaneously and "gently," which means that it should not evoke major stimulus-locked responses (otherwise γ-spindles are suppressed).

The above-mentioned "correlation rule" can be followed in Figure 9: In both of the shown stimulus directions no correlations were induced between spikes on electrode 6 and MUA and LFPs on electrode 3 (Fig. 9Aa); these positions have no RF properties in common (corresponding to a relatively high distance in RF coding space). Spikes from another cortical area (A18, electrode 13) are, on the other hand, well correlated with γ-spindles on electrode 3 (Fig. 9Ba; right panels). Correlations are only present, however, if the stimulus moves in the direction that is preferred by the neurons in both re-

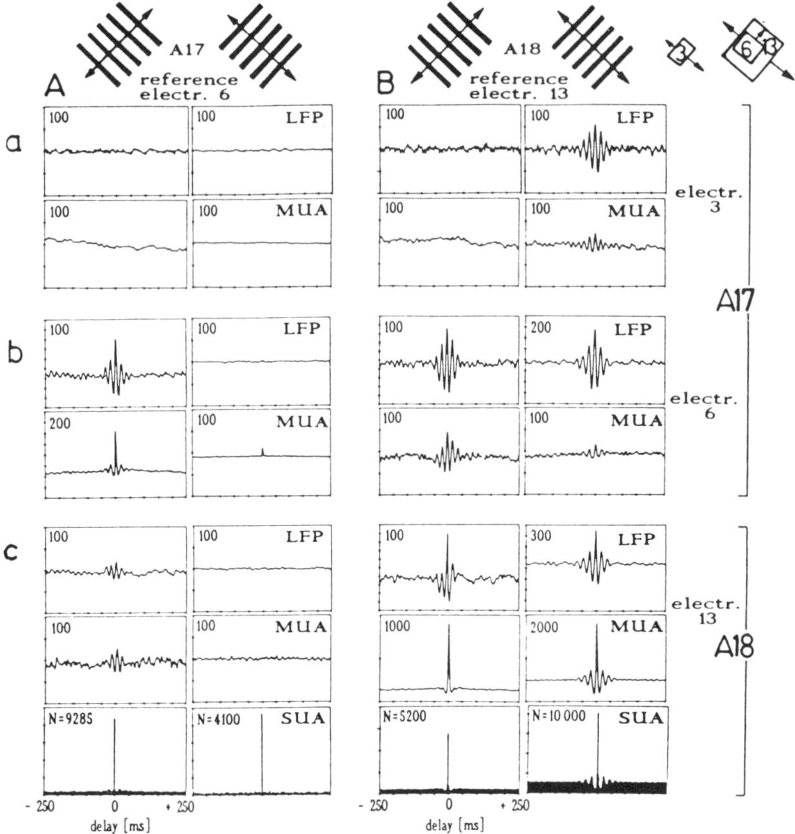

Figure 9. Stimulus-induced correlations between cortex areas 17 and 18 as revealed with cross-correlations between single cell spiketrains and mass activities (LFPs and MUAs). Correlation is revealed by spike-triggered averaging of LFPs and MUAs that were recorded with the same microelectrodes as the spiketrains. Two electrodes were in A17 (electrodes 3 and 6) and one in A18 (electrode 13). **A:** Trigger spikes from electrode 6 in A17. **B:** Trigger spikes from electrode 13 in A18. **a:** LFPs and MUAs from electrode 3. **b:** From electrode 6. **c:** From electrode 13. LFPs and MUAs for averaging were recorded with the same three electrodes (indicated at the right margin). A schema of the RFs and preferred movement directions is shown at the upper right. The lowermost panels show the auto-coincidence histograms of the trigger spiketrains (N = number of trigger spikes). The numbers in the upper left corners of individual correlograms indicate the relative amplitude scales. Stimuli: Grating of 0.7 cyc/° drifting at 8°/s in the directions (sketched above). Note the relations between RF-properties, stimulation and the degree of correlation. (For more details see text.) Modified from Eckhorn R (1991); Stimulus-evoked synchronizations in the visual cortex: linking of local features into global figures? In: *Neural Cooperativity*, Krüger J, ed. New York: Springer–Verlag.

cording positions (these neurons also have nonoverlapping RFs). The other correlograms in Figure 9 are also in support of the "rules" formulated above.

Stimulus-specific synchronizations between three cortical areas

Stimulus-specific synchronizations of γ-spindles between three areas of cat visual cortex were recently discovered by us (Fig. 10) (Eckhorn et al., in press b). The results from three areas generally confirmed earlier findings for A17–A18 and intra-areal correlations of γ-spindles. Our data so far show that stimulus-induced synchronizations of γ-spindles occur when the RFs at a recording position in one area had at least a single coding property in common with those in another area. This means that a common "stimulus object" must activate the neurons in different areas simultaneously, and for internally mediated correlations to occur, the neurons must be coupled by appropriate connections. Figure 10 shows auto- (panels at the diagonal) and cross-spectral (other panels) estimates of simultaneous recordings from A17, A18, and A19 that were specifically "modulated" by changing stimulus conditions. For example, stimulation with a grating that drifts upward in vertical direction (Fig. 10A) induced only small power γ-rhythms on electrodes 1 in A19 and 7 in A17, and the cross-power between electrodes 1 and 7 was correspondingly small. Neurons at both recording positions preferred horizontal stimulus movements, like those applied for Figure 10B. During specific stimulation, here the power of γ-rhythms increased, due to "better stimulation" by a factor of 2.4 on electrode and by 3.4 on electrode 7, while the cross-power increased by a factor of 2.1.

Figure 10 taken alone, however, does not show simple "rules" of stimulus-specific changes in couplings of γ-rhythms between all recording positions, because at three of the seven electrodes oblique movement directions were preferred (electrodes 2, 4, 5), whereas only responses with horizontal and vertical movement directions are shown. Two of these three positions with "oblique preference" (electrodes 4 and 5) were in A18 and they had very broad characteristics for stimulus movement direction. In addition, the spatial frequency and stimulus velocity of the stimulus grating used was in the ranges preferred by A18 neurons (in particular, those at electrode 4). The A18 responses were correspondingly strong, even to horizontal and vertical movements in this case. We made more than 200 recordings simultaneously from three areas (in addition to the seven recordings shown in Fig. 10), and these results confirmed the "linking rules" that we found for A17-18 couplings.

Spindle Synchronizations Between Visual Cortical Hemispheres

According to our linking-by-synchronization hypothesis, one should expect stimulus-induced γ-spindles to occur synchronized in both hemispheres of a cortical area in situations where the same visual object or region extends into

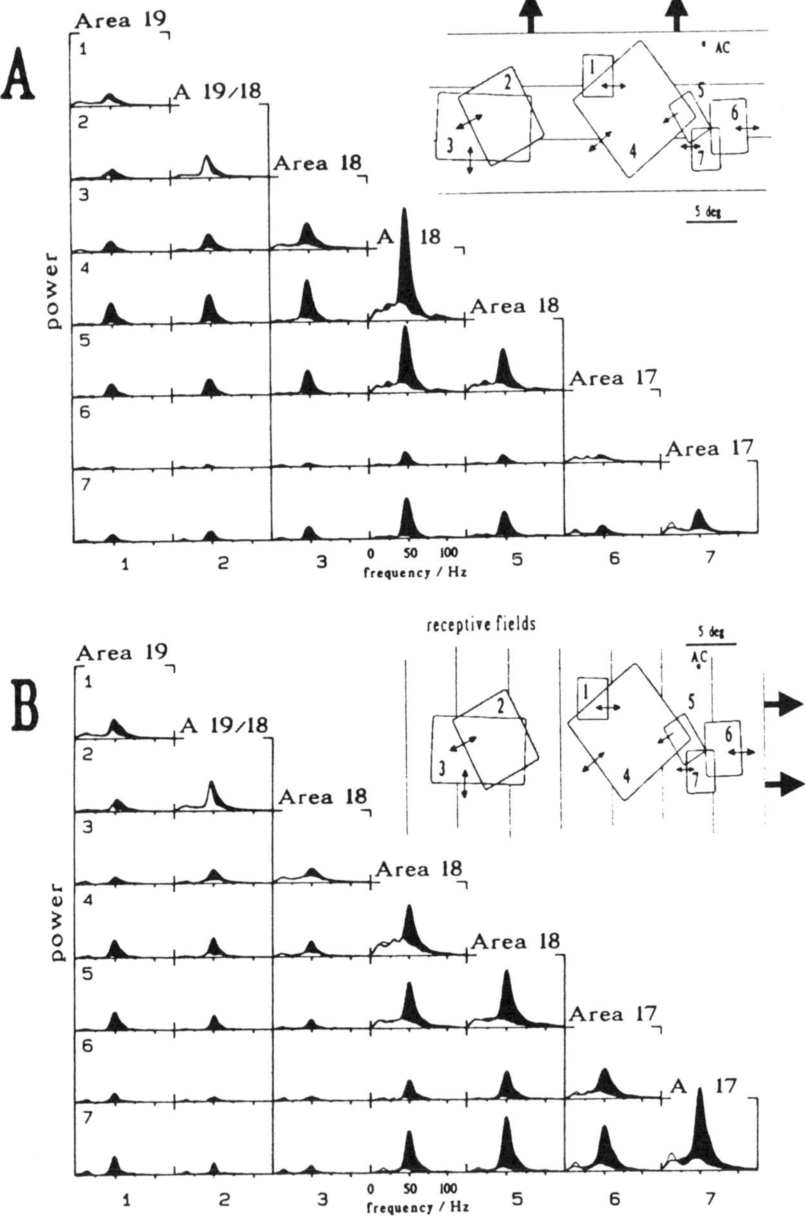

Figure 10. Stimulus-induced correlations among γ-rhythms of three different visual cortex areas (A17, 18, 19). Auto- (*diagonals*) and cross-power spectra (*off-diagonals*) were derived with upward movement of a drifting grating (**A**) and movement to the right (**B**). Black areas indicate the difference between the spectral power derived during the 3.45 s of stimulus movement and those obtained during the 2.45 s interstimulus

both visual half fields. Such synchronized γ-spindles have indeed been found recently (Engel et al., 1990). An example of interhemispheric coupling from our laboratory (A17, 18) is shown in Figure 11. Our preliminary data revealed that interhemispheric correlations are significantly weaker than those found in a single hemisphere. However, similar "rules" seem to hold also for interhemispheric correlations between γ-spindles. With overlapping receptive fields coupling strengths depend less on other preferred stimulus features (in the border region of A17 and A18 where the vertical meridian of the visual field is represented with overlap), whereas at positions with nonoverlapping RFs at least one "strong linking feature" (like stimulus movement direction) should be similar for the neurons in both hemispheres.

How and Where are γ-Spindles Generated and Synchronized?

Possible functional structures on several levels of organization

Little is known about how stimulus-induced γ-spindles are generated and little is known about the connections that lead to their correlated occurrence in remote parts of the visual cortex. In order to prompt more detailed investigations we provide a short overview about possible mechanisms and structures that might be involved. These are guided by clues from neurophysiological observations and from models of stimulus-induced synchronizations that allow one to reduce the huge variety of possibilities to a few probable mechanisms. Different structural levels have to be considered for their involvement in oscillatory synchronizations, including the following:

At the level of *synapses and dendrites*, we expect active bandpass properties in the preferred γ-spindle frequency range of 45 to 65 Hz in those cortical pyramide cells that participate actively in the generation of oscillatory synchronizations ("rhythmically discharging neurons"). We further assume that in (some subclasses of) cortical pyramide cells the apical dendrites are the locations where oscillatory signals are injected, amplified, and possibly also

Figure 10 (*Continued*)
pauses (blank areas below thin curves). Simultaneous recordings of LFPs from layers II/III with a linear array of seven microelectrodes (1 mm interelectrode spacing). Stimulus: Grating, 0.2 cycl/°, drifting at 4°/s in the directions indicated by the arrows in the inserts at the upper rights, where grating and RFs are plotted to the same scale. Numbers in rows and columns of power spectra and on RFs denote the electrodes' numbers. Note the stimulus-specific oscillatory coupling among the different areas, depending on stimulus movement direction and the neurons' preferred stimulus directions (*small arrows* at RF borders; more details in the text). Modified from Eckhorn R, et al. (1991): Stimulus-related facilitation and synchronization among visual cortical areas: Experiments and models. In: *Nonlinear Dynamics and Neural Networks*, Schuster HG, ed. Stuttgart: VNC–Verlag.

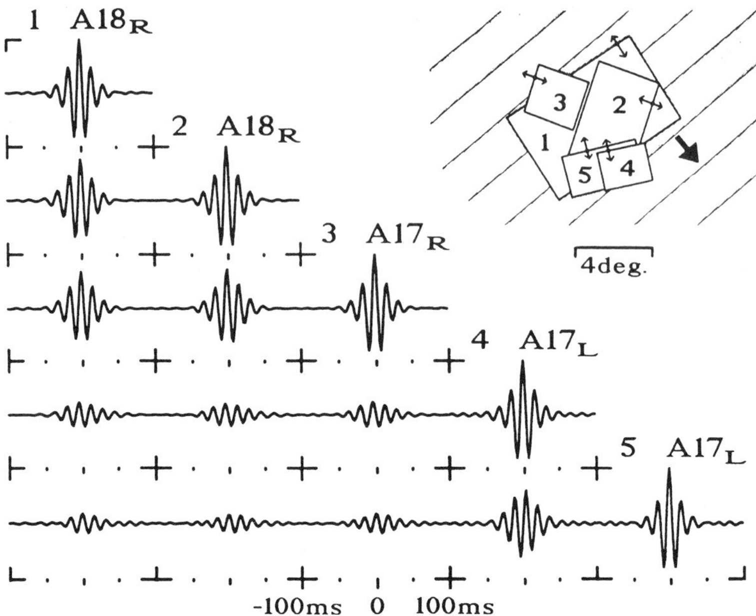

Figure 11. Intra- and interhemispheric correlations between stimulus-induced γ-spindles of cat visual cortex A17 and A18. Normalized auto- (*at diagonal*) and cross-correlograms' (at *off-diagonals*) of LFPs recorded with five microelectrodes in response to 24 stimulus repetitions. Recordings in A17 and A18 of the right (R) and left (L) hemispheres, as indicated on top of the columns of the correlation matrix. The insert at the upper right indicates the stimulus grating and the RFs, drawn to the same scale. Stimulus: grating of 0.25 cyc/° moving at 8.5°/s in the indicated direction (*bold arrow*). Note the high intra-areal correlations (0.6–0.8 between electrodes 1-2-3 and 4-5), compared with the lower interhemispheric coupling (0.1–0.2 between electrodes 1–3 in the right and 4, 5 in the left hemisphere). The interhemispheric correlations are highly significant with the stimulus direction shown (proved with the "shift predictor" method). Application of the same drifting stimulus in perpendicular direction resulted in greatly reduced rhythmic correlations (below significance) between electrodes 1, 4, and 5 because this stimulus direction was also perpendicular to the preferred directions at that recording position.

synchronized with other pyramide cells (see below; while the basal dendrites are assumed to receive mainly the visual feeding signals that establish the receptive field properties).

At the *single neuron* level, oscillatory and synchronizing properties might be due to the combined properties of several processes. The interactions between synaptic, dendritic, and somatic signal transfer properties, together with the spike encoders' dynamic threshold mechanism, can lead to repetitive bursting (at 35–80 Hz) under appropriate sustained drive that does not contain oscillatory components itself (Llinas, 1988). Recently cortical pyramide cells were found that have spike encoders responding with repetitive bursts at

γ-frequencies to intracellular injections of direct currents (e.g., see Chagnac-Amitai and Connors, 1989).

At the level of *local assemblies* (where neurons have similar RF properties), oscillatory synchronization might be accomplished by short synaptic feedback links via local interneurons (e.g., Llinas, 1988) and/or by dendro-dendritic coupling. If coupling via interneurons is essential for the generation of γ-spindles, we would expect phase shifts between the activities of pyramide cells and inhibitory interneurons of 90° to 180 We have no clear experimental indication for such phase shifts yet, possibly as the small neurons contribute little to the recorded mass signals (MUAs and LFPs) because of their high generator impedances. The expected phase shift should, however, be clearly visible in single-cell spike recordings, and especially in intracellular recordings from neurons participating in the oscillatory state.

The possibility of dendro-dendritic coupling was reinforced by the discovery of vertical bundles of closely packed apical dendrites of layer III and larger-V pyramide cells that could support direct dendro-dendritic coupling among the cells, even if oscillatory dendritic potentials are subthreshold (for dendritic bundles in cat cortex see Fleischhauer, 1974).

On the level of *remotely coupled local assemblies*, the "member" neurons are located in the same or in different cortical areas and they differ in their RF properties in at least one aspect (e.g., RF position for neurons in the same area, or movement sensitivity for neurons in different areas). We assume that special association fiber systems with linking synapses provide the mutual couplings that are necessary for oscillatory and nonoscillatory synchronizations (Eckhorn, 1991; Eckhorn et al., 1988c, 1989a, 1989b, 1990a, 1990b, 1991, in press a, c). These networks are assumed to be different, also in the type of their synapses, to the "feeding" connections that are assumed to establish the receptive field properties. Such linking networks were tested by us in computer simulations and the results support our assumptions of two types of connections (see Eckhorn, 1991; Eckhorn et al., in press b).

Are stimulus-induced γ-spindles generated and synchronized in the visual cortex?

We have several reasons for assuming that local groups of few cortical neurons can generate γ-spindles autonomously without the necessity for linking connections with more remote assemblies (in principle, a single neuron would be sufficient for the generation of a rhythmic bursting sequence of action potentials in the γ-range, as is argued by us in Chapter 21). The following arguments are mainly in support of local γ-spindle generation and global synchronization in the cortex, but subcortical involvement cannot be excluded.

1. γ-spindles of high coherence are induced by specific stimuli in those cortical locations where the neurons respond with spike discharges preferentially to that stimulus feature. This means that γ-spindle generation is

specifically related with RF properties of cortical (but not of subcortical) neurons, which is a clue to their cortical origin.

2. Neither we nor other researchers have yet found oscillatory activities in subcortical regions that are correlated with cortical γ-spindles. We repeatedly recorded simultaneously from visual cortex and lateral geniculate nucleus (LGNd) (Eckhorn, 1991) as well as from the superior colliculus without finding significant values of correlated γ-oscillations between cortical and subcortical structures. (Oscillations in the LGNd were not present, although we could record high amplitude spindles simultaneously in the visual cortex.) Our negative observation is supported by recordings in Singer's group; they also did not find γ-oscillations in the LGNd (Gray et al., 1989). However, in an older publication about connectivity of cat LGNd, Arnett (1975) mentioned intrageniculate correlated oscillations in the γ-range, but he did not pay any further attention to this finding. In a recent congress report, Ghose and Freeman reported oscillatory spike activities in cat visual cortex A17 and mentioned that some recordings with a high rhythmic modulation in their spike discharges were afferent geniculate fibers (Ghose and Freeman, 1990). They concluded from this finding that oscillatory activity is of a subcortical, rather than intracortical, origin. However, this finding should be confirmed with direct recordings from LGNd, because cortical fiber recordings are not convincing with respect to the origins of the axons.
3. It is known that extracortical inputs, and especially the (transiently activated) afferent geniculate inputs, evoke stimulus-locked cortical potential distributions with a polarity reversal between upper and lower layers (e.g., Mitzdorf 1985, 1987). Stimulus-induced γ-spindles, in contrast, were found by us not to be phase-locked with stimulus transients and they do not have any larger systematic phase changes across cortical layers (Eckhorn, 1991; Eckhorn et al., 1988a, 1988b, 1988c). In the same vertical penetrations, in which γ-spindles had no polarity reversals, we did find such reversals for the stimulus-locked response components, including the so-called stimulus-locked wavelets that occur in the retina, geniculate, and cortex in response to some global and strong transient stimuli, like whole-field flashes (Başar, 1980, 1983, 1988; Cracco and Cracco, 1978; Mitzdorf, 1987) [in the auditory system stimulus-locked wavelets are in the range of 40 Hz (e.g., Başar, 1980, 1983, 1988; Sheer, 1989) and they are also generated in peripheral parts of the auditory system]. We could show that the rhythmic components of cortical γ-spindles (and the related action potential bursts) are generally not phase-locked with stimulus transients (although their envelopes are), which is directly evident in stimulus-triggered averages where γ-spindles are averaged out (Eckhorn et al., 1988). One has to consider, however, the possibility that γ-spindles are "injected" diffusely across the layers into the cortex via an unknown stimulus-influenced pathway that delivers oscillatory signals with a high temporal jitter relative to stimulus transients.

4. Although we frequently observed phase differences between correlated γ-oscillations of up to 180°, we did not yet find systematic "rules" for such differences (e.g., there was no systematic phase shift with distance parallel to the cortical surfaces). The average phase difference between most recording positions with significant spindle correlations was zero. This finding provides arguments in favor of mutual synchronizations between cortical "γ-spindle generators" but also arguments in favor of a common extracortical source. However, two remote and noncoherent (dissimilar) stimuli can induce uncorrelated γ-spindles in separated cortical positions. This is an argument for a cortical generation against common extracortical source (Gray et al., 1989).
5. Another argument for the cortical origin of γ-spindles is that oscillatory spike activities are precisely confined to the cortical representation of a stimulus. However, subcortical sources also cannot be ruled out by this argument, but the spatial resolution (RF widths) of their γ-spindle generators should equal at least that of A17 cortical RFs. Besides the lateral geniculate body, however, other possible subcortical sources with small RFs are not yet known.

Receptive Fields and Linking Fields: Concepts of Local and Global Visual Coding

In order to bring neuronal mechanisms of stimulus-specific synchronizations into correspondence with perceptual feature linking functions, we introduced the concept of the *linking field (association field)* of a local neural assembly (Eckhorn et al. 1991, in press b, c). The linking field extends the concept of single cells' RFs to neural ensemble coding. We defined the linking field of a local (reference) assembly of visual neurons to be that area in visual space where appropriate global stimuli can initiate synchronization between the activities of the reference assembly and other assemblies (that have their aggregate RFs within the range of the linking field). Linking fields are transiently "constructed" by the constituent neurons as a cooperative process of synchronization, as we assume, according to the properties of their RFs, the present stimulation, and the linking connections.

Linking fields of local assemblies in visual cortex can roughly be estimated from recordings of stimulus-induced LFP oscillations, because LFPs, recorded in a single location, are influenced by synchronized activities from remote assemblies in their amplitudes if these signals are transmitted via axonal connections to the recording location. Such "γ-spindle fields" or "oscillations fields" were recently measured by us (Brosch et al., 1990).

LFP oscillation fields were found to be generally much broader and less stimulus-specific than the classical RFs of the assemblies' neurons (and even much broader than the aggregate RFs of local assemblies). Figure 12 shows an example of estimated oscillation fields of cat A18 assemblies. They were

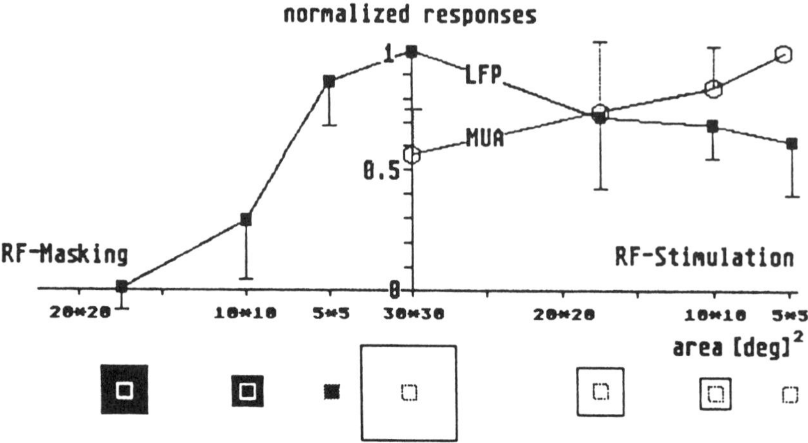

Figure 12. Average "oscillation field" of γ-rhythms induced by varying spatial configurations of a drifting grating. Influences from the classical receptive field (cRF) and the far periphery were estimated from LFPs and MUAs recorded with the same electrode. Stimuli: moving gratings, either in the cRF periphery (by masking the cRF and progressively its surround, shown at the left side of the ordinate) or by stimulating the cRF and additionally the periphery [stepwise increase from cRF size to full field ($30 \times 30°$, shown at the right side of the ordinate)]. Response measures (ordinate): LFP: Average amplitudes of LFP γ-rhythms, normalized to the responses with $30 \times 30°$ grating (LFP: 35–70 Hz; digital filtering with Blackman–Harris window; filled symbols). MUA: Average integrated MUA poststimulus histograms, normalized to the responses with $30 \times 30°$ grating (*open symbols*). Abscissa: stimulus areas were confined by an opaque frame (results at right side of figure) or by an occluder (results at left side). The 5×5 deg square at the center of the indicated stimulus areas denotes the extents of the cRFs. Data from $N = 47$ recordings from upper layers of A18. Note the strong masking effect for oscillatory LFPs by occluding the cRF (*left side*) and the long range contributions to LFP oscillations from the periphery (*right side*) in contrast to the MUA suppression by peripheral stimuli. Reprinted with permission of Thieme from Brosch M, et al. (1990): The spatial distribution of stimuli evoking oscillations of neural responses in the visual cortex of the cat. In: *Brain and Perception*, Elsner N, Roth G, eds. Stuttgart–New York: Thieme.

found to extend to more than 30° by 30° visual angle from the RF of the chosen cortical reference positions, which indicates influences from synchronized locations over many millimeters of cortical distance.

Pair recordings confined to a single visual cortex area and hemisphere revealed that the correlation coefficient of γ-rhythms at any two positions decreases on average down to a value of 0.2 (significance threshold) at 6 mm cortical distance (in A18, anteroposterior direction (Brosch et al., 1991)). We assume that such long-range stimulus-specific synchronizations are mediated by the relatively sparse horizontal intra-areal "association fibers" and by the mutual interareal fibers that connect noncorresponding locations of the visual cortical representation within the same and between different cortical areas (i.e., they connect positions where the RFs do not overlap). The strong shorter range contributions to synchronized γ-components are probably due to the dense intra- and interareal mutual connections that project mainly within the cortical representation range of the assemblies' aggregate RFs (i.e., the RFs overlap partly or totally). Such association connections with "receptive field mismatch" have been known for many years, but their functional roles had remained unclear (Bullier et al., 1984, 1988; Ferrer et al., 1988; Gilbert, 1985; Gilbert and Wiesel, 1983, 1987 Ts'o et al., 1986).

Possible Relations Between Stimulus-Induced Cortical γ-Spindles and 40-Hz Electroencephalogram-Rhythms During Focal Attention

γ-spindles are induced under our experimental conditions with lightly anesthetized cats by (bottom up) visual activations, but under awake attentive conditions also "higher" mental processes, such as focal attention or visualization, may induce (top down) oscillatory states in the visual cortex that might join into a single common synchronized state. Such considerations were already made by Sheer (1989), who reported that 40-Hz rhythms (30–50 Hz) occur in electroencephalogram (EEG) recordings of man, monkey, cat, and rabbit during states of focal attention. Significant 40-Hz amplitudes were recorded *inter alia* at locations above those cortical areas of sensory modalities to which focal attention had been guided (for a review on 40-Hz rhythms during focal attention see Sheer, 1989). 40Hz rhythms are reported to occur mainly during "difficult" tasks, while the rhythms have much less amplitude or are even absent during executions of simple or previously trained tasks. During learning sessions, 40-Hz amplitudes are high at the beginning and they decrease when the task is executed more quickly and more automatically. We would expect a synchronization between stimulus-induced oscillations and 40-Hz EEG rhythms during focal attention. By this means, flexible, transient relations among bottom-up and top-down mechanisms of dynamic visual processing could be established. During a learning process, when the task gradually is executed more quickly, the slow processes of oscillatory synchronizations are expected to be replaced stepwise by the fast processes of stimulus-locked (nonoscillatory) synchronizations.

Summary and Conclusions

We have addressed the following questions in this Chapter: 1). In what visual situations do visual cortical activities become synchronized? 2). Where are stimulus-related synchronizations generated in the visual system and by which neural mechanisms? 3). What are possible roles of stimulus-related synchronized states in visual processing?

We were able to answer these questions in part for stimulus-locked and for γ-spindle (35–80 Hz) synchronizations on the basis of our experiments with lightly anesthetized cats. However, these results have to be confirmed with other mammalian species and especially with awake and behaving animals.

Summarizing, we found that γ-spindles are generated, synchronized, desynchronized, and shut off under stimulus control. Large amplitude LFP and MUA γ-spindles are preferentially generated in visual situations in which no stimulus-locked responses of larger amplitudes are evoked. Optimal stimuli for γ-spindle generation are often slower in movement velocity, they generate "smoother" transients, and they are spatially more extensive than "optimal" stimuli that evoke maximal spike rates. Oscillations do not last throughout continuous stimulations but γ-spindles of variable latencies, frequencies, amplitudes, and durations appear. The phases of γ-spindle oscillations are not phase-locked with physical parameters of the evoking stimulus. Transient stimuli, on the other hand, evoke stimulus-locked cortical responses that can be highly correlated between remote locations. Strong stimulus-locked responses first suppress ongoing γ-spindle activities and, with a delay of about 50 to 200 ms, support a state of enhanced probability of γ-spindle occurrence that can last over several hundred milliseconds. If the stimuli contain only "mild" transients, then small amplitude stimulus-locked synchronized responses and γ-spindles can occur intermingled.

γ-spindle synchronizations can be induced in separate assemblies of the same cortical area (A17, A18, A19), between different cortical areas, and between different hemispheres with stimuli that overlap the RFs and activate the neurons simultaneously.

A general (preliminary) rule can be derived from our results: The coherence of stimulus-induced γ-spindles in separate cortical assemblies depends inversely on the "coding distance" between the assemblies' RF-properties and directly on the degree of overlap between the assemblies' coding properties with the features of a common stimulus. This means that γ-spindles in any two assemblies in the same or in different cortical areas or hemispheres appear correlated if they have (at least to some degree) similar RF properties and if a common stimulus simultaneously activates the assemblies.

Average phase differences between oscillatory activities of the same type (LFPs or MUAs) were typically close to zero (same and different cortex area and hemisphere). The distributions of phase differences between individual γ-spindles generally varied proportionally with their average coupling strengths. Larger average phase differences (up to 180°) were frequently observed, but systematic dependencies with cortical coding properties or distances could not be established.

We present arguments in support of a cortical origin of stimulus-induced γ-spindles: γ-spindles are likely to be generated in local cortical units and they can mutually enhance and synchronize their activities via association fibers with special modulatory linking synapses.

Finally, the results agree with our proposal that mutual enhancement and synchronization of cell activities are general principles of temporal coding within and among sensory systems: *Event-locked synchronizations* may support crude instantaneous preattentive percepts, and *stimulus-induced oscillatory synchronizations* may support more complex, attentive percepts that require iterative interactions among different processing levels and memory.

In a companion chapter in this book we present results of computer simulations of stimulus-related synchronizations that support our concepts of feature linking by explaining a variety of effects observed in cat visual cortex and in visual psychophysics.

Acknowledgments. We thank our colleagues W. Kruse, H. Baumgarten, and A. Obermüller for their help in experiments and data processing, and our technicians W. Lenz, U. Thomas, and J.H. Wagner for their expert experimental support. We also acknowledge the helpful comments on a previous version of the manuscript by Prof. T.H. Bullock. Our project was sponsored by Deutsche Forschungsgemeinschaft (Re 547/2 and Ec 53/4-1) and by Hessisches Kultusministerium (for the doctoral thesis of M.B.).

References

Arnett DW (1975): Correlation analysis of units recorded in the cat dorsal lateral geniculate nucleus. *Exp Brain Res* 24: 111–130

Başar E (1980): *EEG–Brain Dynamics.* Amsterdam–New York–Oxford: Elsevier, North-Holland Biomedical Press

Başar E (1983): Synergetics of neuronal populations. A survey on experiments; In: Synergetics of the Brain, Başar E, Flohr H, H Haken, Mandell A, eds. Berlin–Heidelberg, New York: Springer–Verlag, 183–200

Başar E (1988): EEG—dynamics and evoked potentials in sensory and cognitive processing by the brain. In: *Dynamics of Sensory and Cognitive Processing by the Brain,* Başar E, ed. Heidelberg Springer–Verlag, pp 30–55

Brosch M, Bauer R, Eckhorn R (1990): The spatial distribution of stimuli evoking oscillations of neural responses in the visual cortex of the cat. In: *Brain and Perception,* Elsner N, Roth G, eds. Stuttgart–New York: Thieme, p 236

Brosch M, Bauer R, Eckhorn R (1991): Spatial correlation profiles of stimulus-induced oscillatory activities in cat visual cortex. In: *Synapse–Transmission–Modulation,* Elsner N, Penzlin H, eds. Stuttgurt–New York: Thieme, p 214

Bullier J, Kennedy H, Salinger W (1984): Branching and laminar origin of projections between visual cortical areas in the cat. *J Comp Neurol* 228: 329–341

Bullier J, McCourt ME, Henry GH (1988): Physiological studies on the feedback connection to the striate cortex from cortical areas 18 and 19 of the cat. *Exp Brain Res* 70: 90–98

Bullock TH (1988): Compound potentials of the brain, ongoing and evoked: perspectives from comparative neurology. In: *Dynamics of Sensory and Cognitive Processing by the Brain,* Başar E, ed. Heidelberg Springer–Verlag, pp 3–18

Chagnac-Amitai Y, Connors BW (1989): Horizontal spread of synchronized activity in neocortex and its control by GABA-mediated inhibition. *J Neurophysiol* 62: 1149–1162

Cracco RQ, Cracco JB (1978): Visual evoked potentials in man: early oscillatory potentials. *Electroencephalogr Clin Neurophysiol* 45:731–739

Creutzfeldt OD, Watanabe S, Lux HD (1966): Relation between EEG-phenomena and potentials of single cells. Part I and II. *Electroencephalogr Clin Neurophysiol* 20:1–37

Damasio AR (1989a): The brain binds entities and events by multiregional activation from convergence zones. *Neur Comput* 1:121–129

Damasio AR (1989b): Time-locked multiregional retroactivation: a systems-level proposal for the neural substrates of recall and recognition. *Cognition* 33:25–62

Eckhorn R (1991): Stimulus-evoked synchronizations in the visual cortex: linking of local features into global figures? In: Springer Series in Synergetics, Krüger J, ed. Neuronal Cooperativity Berlin–Heidelberg–Springer–Verlag, pp 184–224

Eckhorn R, Arndt M, Dicke P, Stöcker M, Reitboeck HJ (1992a): Feature linking by stimulus-induced synchronizations of model neurons. In: *Induced Rhythms in the Brain*, Başar E, Bullock TH, eds. Boston: Birkhauser Boston Inc.

Eckhorn R, Bauer R, Brosch M, Jordan W, Kruse W, Munk M (1988a): Functionally related modules of cat visual cortex show stimulus-evoked coherent oscillations: a multiple electrode study. *Invest Ophthalmol Vis Sci* 29:331,12

Eckhorn R, Bauer R, Jordan W, Brosch M, Kruse W, Munk M, Reitboeck HJ (1988b): Are form- and motion-aspects linked in visual cortex by stimulus-evoked resonances? Multiple electrode and cross-correlation analysis in cat visual cortex. EBBS-Workshop on Visual Processing of Form and Motion, Tübingen, Confer. Vol, p 7

Eckhorn R, Bauer R, Jordan W, Brosch M, Kruse W, Munk M, Reitboeck HJ (1988c): Coherent oscillations: a mechanism of feature linking in the visual cortex? Multiple electrode and correlation analysis in the cat. *Biol Cybern* 60:121–130

Eckhorn R, Bauer R, Reitboeck HJ (1989b): Discontinuities in visual cortex and possible functional implications: relating cortical structure and function with multielectrode/correlation techniques. *Springer Series in Brain Dynamics 2*, Başar E, Bullock TH, eds. Berlin–Heidelberg: Springer–Verlag, pp 267–278

Eckhorn R, Brosch M, Salem W, Bauer R (1990b): Cooperativity between cat area 17 and 18 revealed with signal correlations and HRP. In: *Brain and Perception*, Elsner N, Roth G, eds. Stuttgart–New York: Thieme p 237

Eckhorn R, Dicke OP, Kruse W, Reitboeck HJ (1991): Stimulus-related facilitation and synchronization among visual cortical areas: experiments and models. In: *Nonlinear Dynamics and Neural Networks*, Schuster HG, ed. Stuttgart: VCN-Verlag, pp 57–75

Eckhorn R, Reitboeck HJ, Arndt M, Dicke P (1989a): A neural network for feature linking via synchronous activity: results from cat visual cortex and from simulations. In: *Models of Brain Function*, Cotterill, RMJ, ed. Cambridge University Press Cambridge (UK), pp 255–272

Eckhorn R, Reitboeck HJ, Dicke P, Arndt M, Kruse W (1990a): Feature linking across cortical maps via synchronization. In: *Parallel Processing in Neural Systems and Computers*, Eckmiller R, eds. Düsseldorf (FRG), North Holland, Amsterdam New York, pp 101–104

Eckhorn R, Schanze T (in press c): Possible neural mechanisms of feature linking in the visual system: stimulus-locked and stimulus-induced synchronizations. In: *Self-Organization, Emerging Properties and Learning*, Babloyantz A, ed. New York: Plenum Press

Eckhorn R, Schanze T, Reitboeck HJ (1991d): Neural mechanisms of flexible feature linking in sensory systems. In: *Mathematical Approaches to Brain Functioning Diagnostics*, Dvorak I., Holden AV, ed. Proceedings in Nonlinear Science Series, Manchester University Press, Manchester New York pp 407–428

Engel AK, König P, Gray CM, Singer W (1990): Stimulus-dependent neuronal oscillations in cat visual cortex: inter-columnar interaction as determined by cross-correlation analysis. *Eur J Neurosci* 2:588–606

Engel AK, König P, Kreiter AK, Singer W (1990): Inter-areal and inter-hemispheric synchronization of oscillatory responses in cat visual cortex. *Soc Neurosci Abst* 16: p 1269

Ferrer JMR, Price DJ, Blakemore C (1988): The organization of cortico-cortical projections from area 17 to area 18 of the cat's visual cortex. *Proc. R Soc Lond* B 233:77–98

Fleischhauer K (1974): On different patterns of dendritic bundling in the cerebral cortex of the cat. *Z Anat Entwickl Gesch* 143:115–126

Freeman W (1975): *Mass Action in the Nervous System.* New York: Academic Press

Freeman W, Skarda CA (1985): Spatial EEG patterns, non-linear dynamics and perception: the Neo-Sherringtonian view. *Brain Res Rev* 10:147–175

Ghose GM, Freeman RD (1990): Origins of oscillatory activity in the cat's visual cortex. *Soc Neurosci Abst* 16:p 1270

Gilbert CD (1985): Horizontal integrations in the neocortex. *Trends Neurosci* 8:160–165

Gilbert CD, Wiesel TN (1983): Clustered intrinsic connections in cat visual cortex. *J Neurosci* 3:1116–1133

Gilbert CD, Wiesel TN (1987): Relationships between cortico-cortical projections, intrinsic cortical connections and orientation columns in cat primary visual cortex. *Soc Neurosci Abst* 13:5.9

Gray CM, Singer W (1987a): Stimulus-dependent neuronal oscillations in the cat visual cortex area 17. 2nd IBRO-Congress, Neurosci Suppl, p 1301

Gray CM, Singer W (1987b): Stimulus specific neuronal oscillations in the cat visual cortex: a cortical functional unit. *Soc Neurosci Abst* 404.3

Gray CM, König P, Engel AK, Singer W (1989): Oscillatory responses in cat visual cortex exhibit inter-columnar synchronization which reflects global stimulus properties. *Nature* 338:334–337

Hubel DH, Wiesel TN (1962): Receptive fields, binocular interaction, and functional architecture in the cat's visual cortex. *J Physiol* 160:106–154

Llinas RR (1988): The intrinsic electrophysiological properties of mammalian neurons: insights into central nervous system function. *Science* 242:1654–1664

Mitzdorf U (1985): Current source density method and application in cat cerebral cortex: investigation of evoked potentials and EEG phenomena. *Physiol Rev* 65:37–100

Mitzdorf U (1987): Properties of the evoked potential generators: current source-density analysis of visually evoked potentials in the cat cortex. *Int J Neurosci* 33: 33–59

Mountcastle VB (1978): An organizing principle for cerebral function: the unit module and the distributed system. In Edelman GM, Mountcastle VB, eds, *The Mindful Brain*, Cambridge, MA: MIT Press

Nelson JI, Frost BJ (1985): Intracortical facilitation among cooriented, co-axially aligned simple cells in cat striate cortex. *Exp Brain Res* 61:54–61

Nelson JI, Munk MHJ, Bullier J, Eckhorn R (1989): Functional connectivity revealed in and outside of receptive field overlap by 3 cross-correlation techniques. *Soc Neurosci Abst* 15(2): p 1057

Reitboeck HJ (1983a): A 19-channel matrix drive with individually controllable fiber microelectrodes for neurophysiological applications. *IEEE SMC* 13:676–682

Reitboeck HJ (1983b): Fiber microelectrodes for electrophysiological recordings. *J Neurosci Meth* 8:249–262

Reitboeck HJ, Adamczak W, Eckhorn R, Muth P, Thielmann R, Thomas U (1981): Multiple single-unit recording: design and test of a 19-channel micro-manipulator and appropriate fiber electrodes. *Neurosci Lett* 7(Suppl): S148

Schanze T, Eckhorn R, Baumgarten H (1990): Properties of stimulus-induced oscillatory events in cat visual cortex. In: *Brain and Perception*, Elsner N, Roth G, eds. Stuttgart–New York: Thieme p 238

Sheer DE (1989): Sensory and cognitive 40-Hz event-related potentials: behavioral correlates, brain function, and clinical application. In: *Springer Series in Brain Dynamics 2*, Başar E, Bullock TH, eds. Berlin–Heidelberg–New York: Springer-Verlag pp 339–374

Singer W, Gray CM, Engel A, König P (1988): Spatio-temporal distribution of stimulus-specific oscillations in the cat visual cortex II: global interactions. *Soc Neurosci Abst* 14:899

Ts'o DY, Gilbert CD, Wiesel TN (1986): Relationships between horizontal interactions and functional architecture in cat striate cortex as revealed by cross-correlation analysis. *J Neurosci* 6:1160–1170

Zeki S, Shipp S (1988): The functional logic of cortical connections, *Nature* 335: 311–317

Cortical Rhythms, Ongoing (EEG) and Induced (ERPs)

The Rhythmic Slow Activity (Theta) of the Limbic Cortex: An Oscillation in Search of a Function

Fernando Lopes da Silva

The existence of a prominent electroencephalogram (EEG) activity within the theta frequency range (4–7 Hz) in the hippocampus has been one of the most studied rhythmic activities of the mammalian brain. However, in lower mammals the hippocampal EEG has a wider frequency range and may extend from 3 to 4 Hz up to 10 to 12 Hz. Therefore, it has become current practice to name this EEG activity Rhythmic Slow Activity (RSA), in order to avoid the term theta rhythm, which does not cover the entire frequency range within which the hippocampal EEG of lower animals may fall. Several reviews on RSA, particularly in relation to behavior, have appeared (Ishizuka et al., 1990; Komisaruk, 1977; Lopes da Silva and Arnolds, 1978; Robinson, 1980; Vanderwolf and Robinson, 1981). Robinson (1980) discussed in particular the influence of species differences on RSA. In this respect, a controversial point is whether hippocampal RSA occurs also in humans. Single cases have been reported in which hippocampal RSA was observed in man (Giaquinto, 1973), but Halgren et al. (1985) were not able to find RSA in recordings in humans. However, using spectral analysis, Arnolds et al. (1980) were able to demonstrate RSA in the hippocampus of epileptic patients. This RSA presented a dominant low frequency (about 3–4 Hz), which was modulated with behavior in a similar way as in lower mammals. The relative difficulty of demonstrating RSA in the human hippocampus may be related to the decrease in RSA amplitude and regularity in higher primates (Crowne and Radcliffe, 1975).

Here we review those aspects of the current knowledge regarding the mechanisms of generation and the functional significance of RSA since this gives the opportunity to illustrate a number of general points that may be relevant for a better understanding of how cooperative behavior can occur in complex neuronal networks.

RSA can be considered an induced rhythm of the brain since it appears to be elicited by changes in motor activity. Indeed, motor activity is an essential factor in determining the properties of RSA in different species (Lopes da Silva and Kamp, 1969; Vanderwolf, 1969; Sainsbury, 1970; Arnolds et al., 1979a, 1979b, 1979c). The general conditions under which RSA can be induced in the hippocampus were studied using spectral analysis by Leung et al. (1982). These authors distinguished three main features of rat hippocampal EEG in relation to behavior (Fig. 1).

1. The first feature is irregular slow activity (ISA), which is present during awake immobility and slow wave sleep.

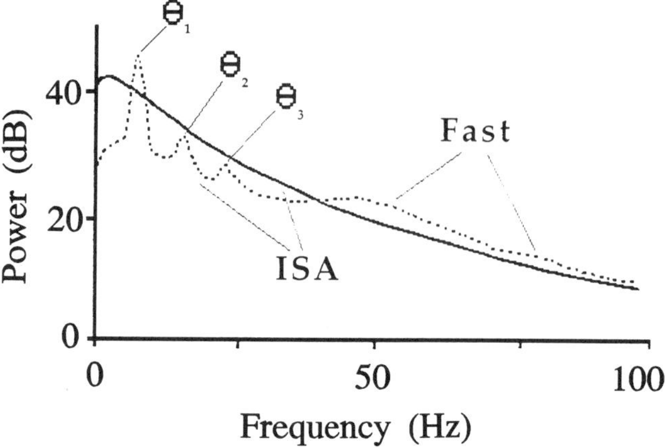

Figure 1. Schematic representation of the power spectra of hippocampal EEG that exhibit the three main features: irregular slow activity (ISA), theta activity drawn with three harmonic components ($\theta_1, \theta_2, \theta_3$), and fast activity. The full line indicates an example of the EEG during awake-immobility, where ISA dominates. The stippled line indicates an example of the EEG as can be recorded during walking. Note that the wideband low frequency components (ISA) decrease in power, whereas the theta and fast frequency components increase as the behavioral state changes from immobility to walking. Adapted from Leung, Wadman, and Lopes da Silva (1982).

2. The second feature is RSA with a narrow band peak in the frequency range of 7 to 8 Hz during voluntary behavior according to Vanderwolf et al. (1978) and sometimes second and third harmonic components (at about 16 and 24 Hz, respectively) as indicated schematically in Fig. 1.
3. The third feature is fast activity of 20 to 70 Hz, which increases in power during voluntary behavior as compared with automatic behavior (Vanderwolf et al., 1978).

Some studies, in which computer spectral analysis was applied, have shown that even during immobility and automatic behavioral acts such as face-washing in rats, small peaks at 5 to 7 Hz occur (Coenen, 1975; Irmis, 1976; Leung et al., 1982; Vanderwolf and Leung, 1983). Spectral analysis of the modulation of the hippocampal EEG in relation to behavior has extensively been carried out by Arnolds et al. (1979a, 1979b, 1979c) in dogs. These studies revealed that statistically significant modulation of the spectral properties of the hippocampal EEG in the sense of increases of amplitude, dominant frequency, and degree of rhythmicity within the RSA frequency band are correlated with the transition from standing to walking, with the increase in speed of a walking animal (Fig. 2), and with head movements. The authors further found significant modulations in the spectral properties of the hippocampal RSA that are related to elementary motor acts such as stepping, respiratory movements, and reflex movements induced by a passive linear acceleration.

Recently, in the monkey also other aspects of the hippocampal EEG were observed to be related to movement (Arezzo et al., 1987). These results taken together support the notion that hippocampal circuits are transiently activated during the preparation of simple voluntary movements.

An especially interesting property of RSA is that this type of EEG activity is characteristic not only of the hippocampus but also of other cortical limbic areas, namely the entorhinal cortex of the temporal lobe and the cingulate cortex. We may state that all limbic cortical areas are capable of displaying RSA, such that the RSA may be considered as an electrophysiological "fingerprint" of the limbic cortex.

Three general questions may be discussed in relation to the specific case of limbic RSA:

1. whether rhythmic activity in a neuronal network depends on intrinsic oscillatory properties of individual neurons or on synaptic interactions at the network level
2. what type of mathematical models can account for the generation of RSA
3. what the functional significance of RSA is in terms of general properties of neuronal networks.

RSA: An intrinsic neuronal property or the result of network (feedback) properties?

It is generally agreed that the RSA of the hippocampus and the other limbic areas is dependent on an intact septal area that acts as a "pacemaker" of the RSA.

The experimental evidence for the notion that the neuronal population of the septal area forms the "pacemaker" of RSA is based on the following findings. Destruction of the medial septum results in the disappearance of the RSA from the hippocampus and other limbic cortical areas (Petsche et al., 1962; Vinogradova et al., 1980). Several investigators using quantitative methods demonstrated that a population of medial septal/diagonal band neurons discharges in phase with the hippocampal RSA (Apostol and Creutzfeldt, 1974; Assaf and Miller, 1978; Gaztelu and Buño, 1982). In the study of Gaztelu and Buño in the rat, about 56% of the total septal population showed a tight phase-locking to the hippocampal RSA. The other septal neurons showed lower degrees of phase-locking and some were nonbursting. The neurons, the activity of which show the highest correlation with the hippocampal RSA, are most densely concentrated within the dorsal part of the vertical limb of the diagonal band and the ventral part of the medial septal nucleus (Assaf and Miller, 1978; Gaztelu and Buno, 1982; Wilson et al., 1976). In the same region, McLennan and Miller (1976) were able to record

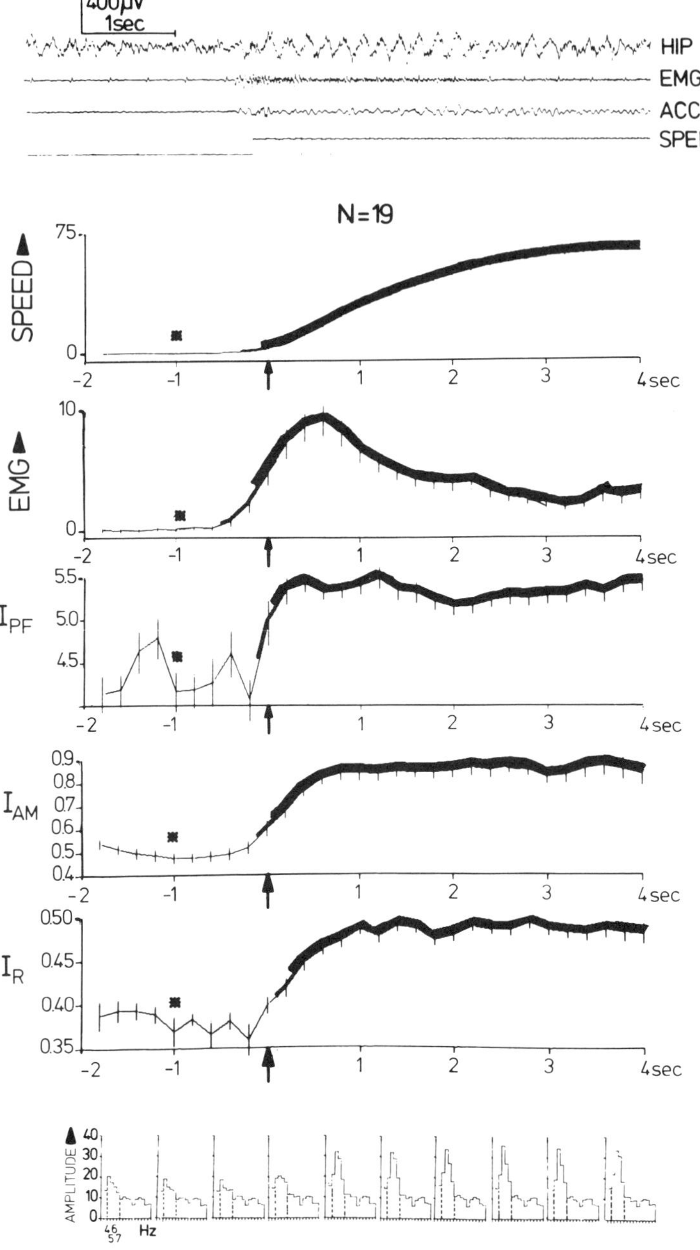

Figure 2. Above: EEG recorded from dorsal hippocampus, along with the EMG of a forepaw muscle, the output of an accelerometer (ACC) indicating wholebody acceleration and a signal indicating the speed of body displacement. **Below:** Curves representing the signals analyzed: speed, rectified and integrated EMG, peak frequency (I_{pF}) of

bursting cells at the frequency of the RSA after fimbria cuts that isolated the medial septum from the hippocampus. However, we should note that the hippocampal neurons need not be considered just as passive followers of the rhythmic septal pacemaker. The local networks may also contribute to the RSA. Indeed, Konopacki et al. (1987b) showed that in hippocampal slices *in vitro*, application of the cholinergic agonist carbachol (50 μM) produced thetalike rhythmical waveforms. This implies that hippocampal networks are capable of producing synchronized rhythmic activity when isolated from septal inputs. The same group of investigators demonstrated that in such a preparation both the CA1 field and the dentate gyrus can independently generate carbachol-induced RSA activity (Konopacki et al., 1987a).

Recently this question was further clarified by an *in vitro* study in hippocampal slices (MacVicar and Tse, 1989). The continuous application of carbachol induced excitation of CA3 pyramidal cells that started as nonrhythmic activity and then changed into quasiperiodic bursts of oscillatory depolarizations. The cholinergic activation was mediated by muscarinic receptors since it was blocked by atropine. Within the local neuronal population, the RSA was synchronous in many CA3 pyramidal neurons. A study of the effect of different agonists and antagonists of the most common, neurotransmitters showed that this type of RSA involves primarily non- *N*-methyl-*D*-aspartate (NMDA) glutamatergic synapses. These authors concluded that recurrent excitation among CA3 pyramidal neurons is necessary for this form of RSA to occur in hippocampal slices but the situation may be different *in vivo*. Indeed, it should be noted that the carbachol-induced RSA corresponds only to one type of RSA occurring in the awake animal, namely that RSA that appears during motionless behavior and REM sleep, but that there are other types of RSA (as those occurring during motor activity) that are not atropine sensitive.

The question of whether cholinergic RSA is mainly determined by intrinsic membrane properties or by synaptic interactions was also examined in the study of MacVicar and Tse (1989). In general it is known that the major

Figure 2 (*Continued*)
hippocampal EEG (in Hz), and the corresponding amplitude (I_{AM}) and peak bandwidth (I_R) in arbitrary units. (Note that a narrow peak, i.e., a small bandwidth, is represented by a large value of I_R: this corresponds to a high degree of rhythmicity.) This registration represents the changes occurring as a dog is displaced in a cart. The speed of the cart is indicated for one trial, on the fourth trace. The arrows indicate the trigger event (start of the displacement in the cart). The results correspond to an average of 19 runs. The values of the means are plotted with the bar through each data point indicating the S.E.M. Where a curve is thickened, there exists a statistically significant difference between that part of the curve and the value indicated by a square asterisk, chosen as a reference (sign test). The thicker the line, the higher the significance ($p < .05$ to $p \ll 0.001$). At the bottom, the series of histograms represents the running spectral analysis of the hippocampal EEG of a number of 200-ms time bins around the trigger event. The placement of the spectra corresponds to the time scale of the curves. Adapted from Arnolds et al. (1979b).

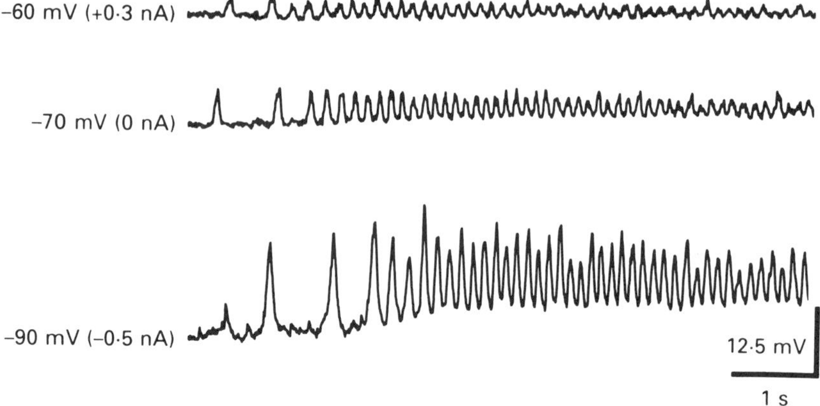

Figure 3. Recording from CA3 pyramidal neuron during carbachol-induced RSA. The membrane potential was altered from an original resting potential of −70 mV by injecting depolarizing or hyperpolarizing current as indicated. Within each burst of RSA, the amplitude of oscillatory depolarizations decreased when membrane potential was progressively depolarized, but the frequency of RSA depolarizations stayed fairly constant from burst to burst. Adapted from MacVicar and Tse (1989).

inward currents carried by Na^+ and Ca^{2+} ions of hippocampal cells are voltage-dependent (Llinás, 1988). MacVicar and Tse (1989) showed that intracellularly recorded carbachol-induced RSA was still present regardless of whether the membrane was deeply hyperpolarized or depolarized, although the amplitude of the oscillations increased or decreased accordingly, just as excitatory (EPSPs) postsynaptic potentials do (Fig. 3). Therefore it can be concluded that hippocampal RSA is not primarily determined by intrinsic membrane conductances; rather, it depends on synaptic interactions.

What Types of Mathematical Models can Account for the Generation of RSA?

Our understanding of both the cellular basis of RSA and the dynamics of the neural networks responsible for its generation have been sharpened by the use of mathematical models combined with physiological observations. These models have not only specific relevance for understanding RSA but they may also be of value for understanding other types of induced or endogenous rhythms of the brain.

Models of the field potentials characteristic of RSA

In order to demonstrate that RSA, recorded at a given cortical site, is indeed locally generated and is not simply the result of volume conduction from another brain site, it is necessary to make a detailed analysis of the local field potential profiles. The demonstration of a dipole field profile, with a phase reversal and zero amplitude at a given cortical layer, in between positive and negative potential poles, allows us to draw the conclusion that the RSA is indeed locally generated.

In the hippocampal formation, a clear dipole field profile of RSA was obtained in the CA1 field with an abrupt phase reversal and null amplitude at the proximal parts of the pyramidal apical dendrites (type I profile of Winson 1976a, 1976b) and an amplitude maximum near the hippocampal fissure under the following experimental circumstances: in freely moving rabbits (Winson, 1976b), urethane-anesthetized rabbits (Bland et al., 1975), curarized rabbits (Artemenko, 1972; Green et al., 1960), and urethane-anesthetized (Green and Rawlins, 1979) or curarized rats (Bland and Whishaw, 1976). However, in freely moving rats (Winson, 1974) a different RSA depth profile was found, the so-called type II profile of Winson (1974). In these cases, there is a gradual phase shift up to 180° in the stratum radiatum of CA1 and an amplitude maximum at the molecular layer of the upper blade of the dentate gyrus. Holsheimer et al. (Feenstra and Holsheimer, 1979; Holsheimer et al., 1979), using spectral analysis methods, found that in urethane-anesthetized rats, besides the phase shift in the stratum radiatum of CA1, a sudden phase reversal in the molecular layer just underneath the granular layer of the dentate gyrus is present.

These findings have been used to obtain a global interpretation of the cellular processes underlying the RSA in the hippocampus. Hippocampal cells were modeled by a linked series of passive membrane compartments representing the soma and the dendritic trees with an active compartment representing the axon hillock. Intracellular, postsynaptic potentials were simulated and the corresponding field potentials were constructed. In this way, Holsheimer et al. (1982) showed that at least some profiles found experimentally (type I of Winson) could be explained by a double dipole activated simultaneously at the CA1 pyramidal and the dentate granular cells with a third RSA source formed by the hilar cells. The type II profile is explained by the model of Leung (1984a), based on that of Buzsàki et al. (1983). This model is suitable to explain also another aspect of the cellular processes that underlie the complex RSA profiles, namely that of their *pharmacological sensitivity*. Vanderwolf (1975) and collaborators (1978, 1983) have shown that in anesthetized rats the RSA is abolished by atropine, whereas in freely moving rats the RSA remains even after large doses of atropine. Accordingly, these authors concluded that there are atropine-resistant and atropine-sensitive RSAs. Recent evidence (Vanderwolf and Baker, 1986) indicates that there are indeed RSA components that are not mediated by cholinergic synapses and that serotonin may be involved in their generation. Leung (1984a, 1984b) demonstrated that the gradual RSA phase shift (type II profile) is related to the relative participation of the atropine-sensitive and the atropine-resistant components. The atropine-sensitive RSA component alone would produce a dipole field with a clear null zone as seen in anesthetized rats. The contribution of the atropine-resistant RSA component is a second dipole that shifts the potential profile to the configuration found in freely moving rats, depending on the relative amplitudes of the two components and the phase lag between them.

The models described above are compatible with different modes of activation of the hippocampal and the dentate cells. In order to establish which model corresponds to the conditions where RSA occurs, *in vivo*, it is important to be able to relate intracellularly recorded membrane potential fluctuations to the extracellular RSA. Nuñez et al. (1987) reported that intracellular RSA activity in identified CA1–CA3 pyramidal cells in rats, curarized and anesthetized with urethane, reflects EPSPs and slow Ca^{2+}-mediated spikes. Moreover, these authors showed that during the RSA most of the CA1 pyramidal cells undergo a depolarization of up to 20 mV above the resting level (Fig. 4). In about 25% of the CA1 cells that were analyzed, the membrane potential

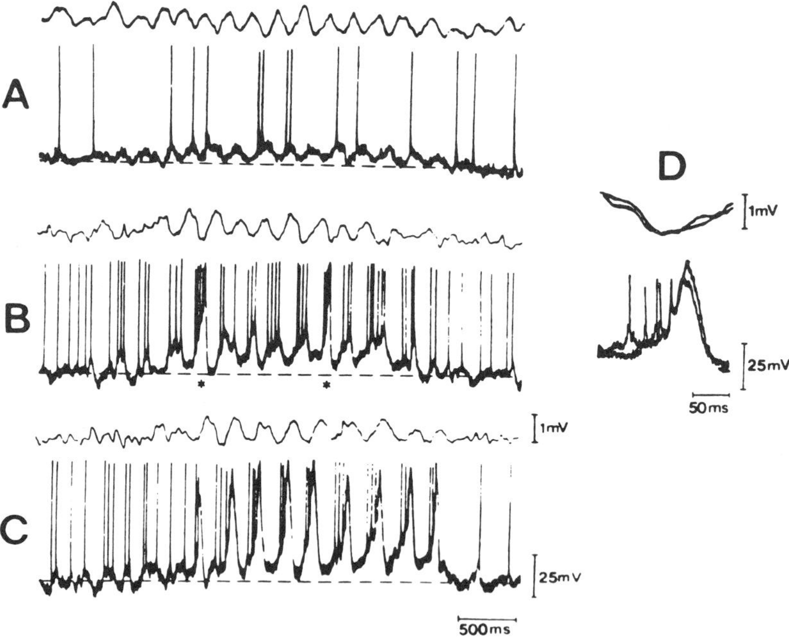

Figure 4. Hippocampal EEG (**upper**) and intracellular (**lower**)in **A**, **B**, and **C** obtained from different CA1 pyramids. With θ, sustained depolarizations above resting level (*broken lines*) are present in all cases. Smooth sine like θ-wave are recorded without (**A**), with occasional (asterisk in **B**), or continously rhythmic (**C**) slow spikes. The expanded time scale records (**D**) show two superimposed EEG θ waves (*upper*) and slow spikes (*lower*). Fast spikes take-off from the rising slopes of slow spikes. Adapted from Nuñez et al. (1987).

oscillated in close relation to the extracellularly recorded RSA. Using small hyperpolarizing pulses, Nuñez et al. (1987) calculated that there is a mean conductance (possibly corresponding mainly to potassium channels) decrease of about 30% during the sustained depolarization. In some CA cells, depolarizing waves were found during the RSA that strongly resembled slow Ca^{2+}-mediated dendritic spikes observed *in vitro*. The injection of depolarizing current pulses decreased the amplitude of the intracellular RSA, whereas hyperpolarizing currents had the opposite effect. According to these data, the hippocampal RSA is correlated with sustained depolarization and periodic transmembrane potential oscillations. This may be caused by cholinergic stimulation, since acetylcholine blocks the hyperpolarizing M current (Halliwell and Adams, 1982) and also blocks the tonic release of gamma-aminobutyric acid GABA from interneurons (Ben-Ari et al., 1981; Hounsgaard, 1978). This would explain the decrease in membrane conductance that has been found. Nuñez et al. (1987) conclude that inhibitory postsynaptic potentials (IPSPs) are not essential in the generation of the RSA.

It is likely that distal dendritic excitation also contributes to RSA (Holsheimer et al., 1982; Leung, 1984a). This may be mediated by a perforant path input. It is important to note that rats with lesions of the entorhinal cortex that received atropine or scopolamine did not show any RSA, despite the fact that the animals continued to walk actively (Vanderwolf and Leung, 1983). Therefore, it may be concluded that atropine-resistant RSA is mediated by the entorhinal cortex. Thus, the question must be raised of how the entorhinal cortex is involved in the generation of this type of RSA. Vanderwolf et al. (1985a, 1985b) showed that atropine-resistant RSA is dependent on a noncholinergic pathway that runs through or arises from the neocortex and the cingulate cortex, and reaches the hippocampus via the entorhinal cortex. It has further been demonstrated that lesions of the lateral hypothalamus abolish atropine-resistant RSA (Whishaw and Kolb, 1979). This noncholinergic pathway may arise from the locus coeruleus (Anden et al., 1966) or from the serotoninergic nuclei (B7, B8, and B9) (Fuxe and Johnsson, 1974). However, there is no experimental evidence that catecholamines play a role in the generation of atropine-resistant RSA. On the contrary, several findings suggest that this may be the case for the serotoninergic fibers (Vanderwolf et al., 1985b). It is becoming clear that RSA is not a uniform phenomenon and that different cellular mechanisms underlie different aspects of the hippocampal rhythmic slow activity.

Models of the dynamic properties of RSA

Here we consider two types of computer models; one consists of a global model that describes the lumped properties of the septohippocampal system (Lopes da Silva et al., 1976), and the other of a network model of the hippocampal CA3 region, which describes the relationship between cellular firing and population rhythmic waves in detail (Traub et al., 1989).

A lumped model of the septohippocampal RSA. The essential properties of RSA of the septohippocampal system can be modeled by means of a neural network consisting of three interconnected populations of neurons, one representing a main type of neuron that receives the external inputs (e.g., a random series of impulses), and the others representing two types of local interneurons responsible for inhibitory and excitatory feedback. There is ample evidence for inhibitory feedback but excitatory feedback has been demonstrated only electrophysiologically but not yet anatomically, at least in the CA3 field (MacVicar and Dudek, 1980; Miles and Wong, 1986; Wong and Traub, 1983).

The interneurons receive not only recurrent collaterals of pyramidal cells, but also afferent fibers directly, by means of which feedforward inhibition may occur. This model includes some of the main intrinsic membrane properties, namely Ca^{2+}-dependent K^+ conductivities. Two main parameters of this model are the time courses of the hyperpolarization and depolarization and the gains of the feedback loops that represent the number of active synapses in these loops. For details see Lopes da Silva et al. (1976). It should be noted that excitatory feedback is necessary to obtain an RSA with the peak frequency and bandwidth encountered *in vivo*. An interesting property of this model is that it shows hysteresis and two main stable oscillatory states: one that corresponds to RSA and another one that corresponds to epileptiform seizure activity. In this respect an interesting feature that the investigations based on the computer simulations have revealed is that the occurrence of epileptiform irregular oscillations depends critically on the presence of the Ca^{2+}-dependent K^+ conductivities. There is a bifurcation point at which the neural network can switch from RSA to epileptiform activity, that depends on the balance between the gains of the excitatory and inhibitory feedback loops. Besides this type of nonlinear dynamic behavior, this model also shows how one important property of RSA can occur, namely that the peak frequency, bandwidth, and amplitude of RSA depends on the intensity of the input reaching the septohippocampal system (Paiva et al., 1976).

From this type of model study, we may obtain some insight into the dynamics of global properties of RSA. In addition, it reveals that the neural networks where RSA occurs also can display epileptiform activity. The latter differs essentially from RSA not only in frequency and amplitude, but also in that RSA is input dependent, whereas epileptiform activity is autonomous. This means that once the system is strongly, albeit briefly, excited it will switch to the irregular oscillations characteristic of an epileptic seizure on condition that the balance between excitatory and inhibitory feedback gains moves in the direction of the former. This type of behavior can be considered as representing a chaotic state of the network. Indeed, it has been shown that during epileptic seizures of the hippocampus the oscillations can be considered as chaotic (Pijn, 1990; Pijn et al., 1991) as those of other brain areas (Babloyantz, 1985). The model study shows also that the threshold to trigger epileptiform oscillations can decrease appreciably just by reducing the gain of the inhibitory feedback by 20%. It is interesting to relate this prediction of the model with the experimental finding that a reduction of a subpopulation of GABAergic interneurons by about 30% is encountered in rats that were submitted to kindling stimuli of the hippocampus and exhibit epilepsy (Kamphuis et al., 1989).

Network model of rhythmic slow activity in the hippocampal CA3. Traub et al. (1989) have simulated the behavior of a population of 9000 pyramidal cells and 900 inhibitory interneurons, forming a network with both excitatory and inhibitory recurrent circuits. This model study permits us to analyze the behavior of the population in terms of individual cells, which cannot be done with the lumped model. In this way it was shown that emergent properties arise in the population that cannot be simply derived from the behavior of the individual cells. For instance, the frequency of the population RSA was systematically higher than the frequency of the bursts of any pyramidal neuron. This study has revealed a number of additional interesting findings: 1) the removal of recurrent excitation led to the disappearance of rhythmic activity, 2) blocking of slow inhibition in the network when cellular excitability was high led to irregular activity instead of RSA; in contrast, when cellular excitability was low the population activity resembled EEG delta activity 3) the pattern of initiation and spatial spread of RSA in the population was studied under many conditions: phase lags between rhythmic bursts as function of distance were observed, but the lag diminished as the cellular excitability increased, and 4) the physical basis for the spatial coherence were the local synaptic connections.

In conclusion, what can we learn from both these types of model studies, with respect to the mechanisms of generation and modulation of RSA? A number of important features of hippocampal RSA have been clarified in this way, and can be summarized as follows:

1. The modulation of RSA peak frequency, amplitude, and bandwidth that occurs *in vivo* as the intensity of motor activity changes can be reproduced in the lumped model just by changing the impulse density of the afferent fibers to the septohippocampal system. In case the input strength becomes very strong, a reduction in RSA occurs in the model and the population activity becomes desynchronized, owing to the activation of the feedforward inhibition with subsequent opening of the inhibitory loop. Similarly, *in vivo*, a very intense motor activity leads to a transition from high frequency RSA to a desynchronized state of the hippocampal EEG.
2. Both the simulations carried out using lumped and network models have demonstrated the critical role that excitatory feedback plays in the generation of RSA of the appropriate frequency and bandwidth.
3. A large amount of synchrony, that is, a high degree of coherence between RSA recorded at different sites with a very small phase lag, depends on the density of the synaptic connectivity and on the degree of cellular excitability, as shown by the simulation using the network model.
4. The network model has shown that transient stimuli induce local evoked

responses that depend on the phase of the ongoing RSA as also found in vivo (Winson and Abzug 1978a, 1978b, Leung, 1980, Rudell et al., 1980, Buzsàki et al., 1981).

5. The rather intriguing experimental finding that most pyramidal cells do not fire at the RSA frequency was clarified using the network model, since the simulation showed that indeed only a small percentage (e.g., 2.8%) of the pyramidal neurons fired bursts in synchrony with the population RSA, whereas a large population of interneurons (e.g., 62%) displayed such synchrony; this is in agreement with the experimental observation that hippocampal interneurons are more likely to behave as theta cells than burst-firing pyramidal neurons.

Functional significance of RSA

It is not simple to assign a functional significance to limbic cortex RSA. Nevertheless, three features of RSA must be put in evidence in this respect.

First, the presence of RSA, at least in the hippocampus, appears to modulate synaptic transmission in the circuits of this brain structure. In this way RSA could serve a "gating function" on the flow of information through the hippocampus.

Second, it is likely that oscillations in hippocampal outputs may facilitate the transmission of information from the hippocampus to target structures, such as the nucleus accumbens (Lopes da Silva et al., 1984) where a pronounced paired-pulse facilitation within the RSA frequency range exists (Boeijinga et al., 1990). In this respect we may suggest that RSA might have a functional role in "matching" the hippocampal output to the circuits of target structures.

Third, the presence of RSA appears to be able to facilitate, or even to induce, long-term potentiation (LTP) in different synaptic circuits of the hippocampus. In this way the presence of RSA may enhance the capacity of these circuits to establish memory traces. Thus, we may suggest that RSA can have a functional role in inducing/enhancing LTP.

In the following we examine these three processes in more detail.

1. A *gating function* of RSA has been suggested in view of the experimental finding that neuronal transmission through the hippocampal circuits depends on the behavioral state of the animal, and thus on the type of hippocampal EEG. Winson and Abzug (1978a, 1978b) have investigated this problem by recording the field potentials evoked by a single electrical pulse to the perforant path in CA1, CA3, and the dentate gyrus under four behavioral states: slow-wave sleep (SWS), rapid eye movement (REM) sleep, "still alert" condition, and during voluntary movements while RSA is present in the hippocampus. A reduced transmission of incoming signals through the CA1 stage of the trisynaptic circuit was observed during all behavioral states except

SWS. A more detailed analysis of these effects (Winson, 1984, 1986) revealed that during "still alert" behavior the attenuation of transmission of the input signals occurs at the first synapse of the trisynaptic circuit at the level of the granule cells of the dentate gyrus, since the population spike recorded in this region is markedly lower in this behavioral state than during SWS. During REM and awake state, both characterized by RSA, the pattern of transmission through the trisynaptic circuit is similar. The population spikes recorded from the granule cell layer are variable from trial to trial and, as a result, the average values fall between those of SWS and those of the "still alert" state. The population spikes in the CA3 field are similarly variable, but in CA1 these spikes are strongly attenuated. Winson (1984, 1986) concluded that during states characterized by RSA some additional mechanism acts at the CA1 level to suppress cell firing. This author interprets the findings in analogy with an electronic logic gate as indicating that the transmission of neural impulses at each synapse of the trisynaptic circuit can be described to result from the open or closed position of a neural gate. For example, during SWS all gates, from the entorhinal cortex to the dentate gyrus, CA3, and CA1, would be in an open state; during RSA, either in the alert state or under REM sleep, the state of the dentate gyrus and CA3 gates would be variable depending on the phase of the rhythmic activity at the time of the arrival of the input (Winson, 1984).

2. The idea that RSA may exert a *matching function* that would enhance the communication between the hippocampus, or other limbic cortical areas, and a target structure, finds support in the finding that the nucleus accumbens, one of the important target structures of the subiculum (Lopes da Silva et al., 1984), presents a marked degree of paired-pulse facilitation at intervals that correspond closely to the main period of hippocampal RSA (Boeijinga et al., 1990) in the rat (i.e., between 100 and 250 ms). Accordingly we may infer from this experimental finding that the transmission of information from the hippocampus (subiculum) through the nucleus accumbens is enhanced when the inputs arive at a frequency corresponding to RSA, in contrast to other frequency ranges. In this way we may state that there is a form of *resonance* at the frequency range of RSA. Considering that the nucleus accumbens constitutes an interface between the hippocampus and the motor circuits of the diencephalon/mesencephalon (ventral pallidum, substantia nigra, superior colliculus, nucleus tegmentalis pedunculopontinus), it may be speculated that in the behavioral condition where RSA is most conspicuous (i.e., during motor activity), it is useful for hippocampal signals to be able to reach those motor circuits in a facilitated way.

3. The suggestion that RSA may have a role in *inducing/enhancing LTP* is based on the observation that there is a preference for LTP to occur in the hippocampal formation if the stimulus is delivered at the frequency range characteristic of RSA. This was recently demonstrated both for synapses of the Schaffer commissural fibers on CA1 neurons in hippocampal slices (Larson and Lynch, 1988; Larson et al., 1986; Rose and Dunwiddie, 1986) and

for synapses of the perforant path fibers on the granular cells of the dentate gyrus *in vivo* (Greenstein et al., 1988; Pavlides et al., 1988). In the CA1 field, LTP induction is optimal when the time interval between stimuli is approximately 200 ms, which corresponds to the frequency band of the spontaneously occurring RSA in the hippocampus. In the dentate gyrus, a significant potentiation of synaptic efficacy, as measured by the field synaptic potential slope and the population spike, can be obtained only when the tetanic pattern consists of a priming pulse followed by a 100-Hz train of six pulses at a 200-ms interval.

It appears that brief high frequency bursts elicit a weak NMDA receptor response that is amplified when the bursts are delivered in a pattern within the frequency range of the RSA. The hypothesis is that the amplification occurs because at this RSA frequency there is a suppression of IPSPs (Larson and Lynch, 1988) and hence a prolongation of the depolarization. This would favor an enhanced influx of Ca^{2+} ions resulting in an amplification of LTP and this implies that during the RSA mode LTP phenomena are facilitated. These findings are compatible with the interpretation that during hippocampal RSA the pyramidal cells are in a state of sustained depolarization (see above).

This property of the hippocampal synapses may be important for a functional role of the hippocampal formation in memory, since this structure appears to act as a sort of holding system that is necessary for the temporary storage of information regarding the temporal order and the spatial context of events (Lopes and Silva et al., 1990; Rawlins, 1985).

Conclusion

The study of the RSA of the limbic cortex permits us to infer the general conclusion that oscillation in neural networks may be not simply a by-product of the activity of neuronal networks, but may have a functional significance in brain functioning, at least in a specific number of cases such as those discussed here. In short, we may state that the RSA type of oscillation may subserve two main types of function: 1) one associated with the frequency of the oscillation as such, and 2) another associated with the state of the neurons induced by the oscillation.

1. The first possibility, that we may call the *frequency-specific role of RSA*, is supported by two experimental observations: that RSA can facilitate the transmission of information between the hippocampus and target structures, such as the nucleus accumbens, and that stimulation at the RSA frequency may induce LTP. With respect to the former mechanism, the presence of RSA may optimize the transmission of signals from the hippocampal formation to output structures at the appropriate time. In fact, signals that would arrive to the nucleus accumbens during a state when RSA is present would tend to be

preferentially transferred to output structures compared to those that would arrive when RSA is absent. In this way, a form of *resonance* between the hippocampal formation and the nucleus accumbens would be established with the optimal level within the RSA frequency range. It would be interesting to explore whether the same time of resonance also occurs with respect to other target structures of different parts of the limbic cortex where RSA predominates. An interesting aspect in this respect is the fact that some motor activities tend to occur in close relationship with hippocampal RSA phase (Arnolds et al., 1979b). With respect to LTP, the main consequence of the presence of RSA would be to facilitate the formation of significant associations between different sets of signals within the limbic cortex subareas themselves, perhaps thus to promote the formation of memory traces.

2. The second possibility that we may call the *gating role of RSA* is supported by the experimental observation that the transmission of signals through the trisynaptic pathway within the hippocampal formation is strongly modulated not only by the presence or absence of RSA but also by the phase of the RSA (Winson and Abzug, 1978a, 1978b; Leung, 1980; Rudell et al., 1980; Buzsàki et al., 1981). Indeed, it has been well documented by Nuñez et al. (1987) that during RSA, CA_1–CA_3 pyramidal cells are in a sustained depolarized state, associated with a conductance decrease. A similar effect can be produced *in vitro* by the application of carbachol (MacVicar and Tse, 1989). These experimental findings lead us to the following generalization: a convenient way to generate a mechanism that operates as a gate within a neuronal network is to bias the membrane potential either in a depolarizing direction, such as during RSA in CA pyramidal neurons, or in a hyperpolarizing direction, such as during sleep spindles in the neurons of the thalamocortical neurons (Lopes da Silvra 1991, Steriade et al., 1990). An interesting observation is that during a burst of oscillatory activity, the mean membrane potential within a neuronal population does not stay clamped at the level of the rest potential, but it may deviate from the latter. This is likely caused by the nonlinear membrane properties of these neurons. In this way, the *state* of the network may change globally during an oscillatory burst. In the case of the CA pyramidal cells, this deviation is in the depolarization direction as shown in Figure 4. Therefore, we put forward the hypothesis that a burst of oscillatory activity in neuronal networks may constitute a mechanism that the nervous system may use to regulate *changes of state* in these networks. Whether such states are accompanied by the release of specific neuromodulators/neuropeptides, as is likely, needs further investigation.

It is interesting to consider this gating function in relation to the functional role of cholinergic systems in the forebrain. An enhancement of the activity of these systems of the brain stem and forebrain causes a number of changes in the oscillatory state of the neural networks of the limbic cortex (i.e., the generation of a given type of RSA), of the thalamus (i.e., the suppression of sleep spindles), and also of the neocortex [i.e., the change of the low frequency type of activity into a state characterized by high frequencies with a wide range of components, as emphasized by Buzsaki and Eidelberg (1983)]. This implies that in this state of enhanced cholinergic activity, the transmission of information in those networks is affected in different ways: the gate is open to allow the flow of specific signals through the thalamus to the cortex, whereas the state of the gate in the trisynaptic pathway that leads from the entorhinal cortex to the hippocampus is changed in a subtle way. In the latter case, the cholinergic state where RSA dominates, impulses arising from the entorhinal cortex are allowed to pass through the two first synapses in the pathway (at the level of the dentate granule cells and at the level of the pyramidal cells of CA3), but in a phased way, according to the frequency of RSA, whereas the synaptic interface to CA1 pyramidal neurons is blocked. In this way, a major shift in the flow of information through a large set of neural pathways can be obtained, a sort of *rerouting of the information*, favoring the flow of "specific sensory" information through the thalamus to the cortex and the flow of "associative" information through the entorhinal cortex to CA3 and from here to target structures of the forebrain, mainly, the septal area (Lopes da Silva et al., 1990) instead of from CA3 to CA1, subiculum, and back to the entorhinal cortex (Witter et al., 1989).

Acknowledgments. I acknowledge the excellent assistance of Cristine Cabi and Ina Huijsen in composing the manuscript and the critical comments of Jan Pieter Pijn and Wytse Wadman.

References

Anden NE, Dahlstrõm K, Fuxe K, Larsson K, Olson L, Ungerstedt U (1966): Ascending monoamine neurons to the telencephalon and diencephalon. *Acta Physiol Scand* 67:313–326

Apostol G, Creutzfeldt OD (1974) Cross correlation between the activity of septal units and hippocampal EEG during arousal. *Brain Res* 67:65–75

Arezzo JC, Tenke CE, Vaughan HG Jr (1987): Movement-related potentials within the hippocampal formation of the monkey. *Brain Res* 401:79–86

Arnolds DEAT, Lopes da Silva FH, Aitink JW, Kamp A (1979a): Hippocampal EEG and behaviour. I. Hippocampal EEG correlates of gross motor behaviour in dog. *Electroencephalogr Clin Neurophysiol* 46:552–570

Arnolds DEAT, Lopes da Silva FH, Aitink JW, Kamp A (1979b): Hippocampal EEG and behaviour. II. Hippocampal EEG correlates of elementary motor acts in dog. *Electroencephalogr Clin Neurophysiol* 46:571–580

Arnolds DEAT, Lopes da Silva FH, Aitink JW, Kamp A (1979c): Hippocampal EEG and behaviour. III. Hippocampal EEG correlates of stimulus response tasks and of sexual behaviour in dog. *Electroencephalogr Clin Neurophysiol* 46:581–591

Arnolds DEAT, Lopes da Silva FH, Aitink JW, Kamp A, Boeijinga P (1980): The spectral properties of hippocampal EEG related to behavior in man. *Electroencephalogr Clin Neurophysiol* 50:324–328

Artemenko DP (1972): Role of hippocampal neurons in theta-wave generation. *Neurophysiology* 4:531–539

Assaf SY, JJ Miller (1978): The role of a raphe serotonin system in the control of septal unit activity and hippocampal desynchronization. *Neuroscience* 3:539–550

Babloyantz A (1985): Evidence of chaotic dynamics of brain activity during the sleep cycle. *Phys Lett (A)* 111:152–156

Ben-Ari Y, Knrjevìc K, Reinhardt W, Ropert N (1981): Intracellular observations on disinhibitory action of acetylcholine in hippocampus. *Neuroscience* 6:2445–2463

Bland BH, Andersen P, Ganes T (1975): Two generators of hippocampal theta activity in rabbits. *Brain Res* 94:199–218

Bland BH, Whishaw IQ (1976): Generators and topography of hippocampal theta (RSA) in the anaesthetized and freely moving rat. *Brain Res* 118:259–280

Boeijinga PH, Pennartz CMA, Lopes da Silva FH (1990): Paired-pulse facilitation in the nucleus accumbens following stimulation of subicular inputs in the rat. *Neuroscience* 35:301–311

Buzsaki, G, Eidelberg (1983) Phase relations of hippocampal projection cells and intereneurons to theta activity in the anesthetized rat. Brain Res. 226:334–339

Buzsàki G, Grastyàn E, Czopf J, Kellènyi L, Prohaska O (1981): Changes in neuronal transmission in the rat hippocampus during behavior. *Brain Res* 225:235–247

Buzsàki G, Leung LW-S, Vanderwolf CH (1983): Cellular bases of hippocampal EEG in the behaving rat. *Brain Res Rev* 6:139–171

Coenen AML (1975): Frequency analysis of rat hippocampal electrical activity. *Physiol Behav* 14:391–394

Crowne DP, Radcliffe D (1975): Some characteristics and functional relations of the electrical activity of the primate hippocampus and hypotheses of hippocampal function. In: *The Hippocampus*, Isaacson RL, Pribam KH, eds. New York: Plenum Press, vol. 2, 185–203

Feenstra BWA, Holsheimer J (1979): Dipole-like neuronal sources of theta rhythm in dorsal hippocampus, dentate gyrus and cingulate cortex of the urethane-anesthetized rat. *Electroencephalogr Clin Neurophysiol* 47:532–538

Fuxe K, Johnsson G (1974): Further mapping of central 5-hydroxytryptamine neurons: studies with the neurotoxic dihydroxytryptamines. *Adv Biochem Psychopharmacol* 10:1–12

Gaztelu JM, Buño W (1982) Septo-hippocampal relationships during EEG theta rhythm. *Electroencephalogr clin Neurophysiol* 54:375–387

Giaquinto S (1973): Sleep recordings from limbic structures in man. *Confin Neurol* 35:285–303

Green JD, Maxwell DS, Schindler WJ, Stumpf C (1960): Rabbit EEG "theta" rhythm: its anatomical source and relation to activity in single neurons. *J Neurophysiol* 23:403–420

Green KF, Rawlins JNP (1979): Hippocampal theta in rats under urethane: generators and phase relations. *Electroencephalogr Clin Neurophysiol* 47:420–429

Greenstein YJ, Pavlides C, Winson J (1988): Long-term potentiation in the dentate gyrus is preferentially induced at theta rhythm periodicity. *Brain Res* 438:331–334

Halgren E, Smith ME, Stapleton JM (1985): Hippocampal field-potentials evoked by repeated v.s. nonrepeated words. In: *Electrical Activity of the Archicortex*, Buszáki G, Vanderwolf CH, eds. Budapest: Akadémiai Kiadó, 67

Halliwell JV, Adams PR (1982): Voltage-clamp analysis of muscarinic excitation in hippocampal neurons. *Brain Res* 250:71–92

Holsheimer J, Boer JJ, Lopes da Silva FH, Van Rotterdam A (1982): The douple dipole model of theta rhythm generation: simulation of laminar field potential profiles in dorsal hippocampus of the rat. *Brain Res* 235:31–50

Holsheimer J, Feenstra BWA, Nijkamp JM (1979): Distribution of field potentials and their relationships during theta and beta activity in the hippocampus and the overlying neocortex of the rat. In: *Origin of Cerebral Field Potentials*, Speckmann EJ, Caspers H, eds. Stuttgart: Thieme, pp 98–114

Hounsgaard J (1978): Presynaptic inhibitory action of acetylcholine in area CA1 of the hippocampus. *Exp Neurol* 62:787–797

Ishizuka N, Weber J, Amaral DG (1990): Organization of intrahippocampal projections originating from CA3 pyramidal cells in the rat. *J Comp Neurol* 295:580–623

Irmis F (1976): Hippocampal rhythmic slow theta activity in relation to certain muscle movements. *Electroencephalogr Clin Neurophysiol* 41:553

Kamphuis W, Huisman E, Wadman WJ, Heizmann CW, Lopes da Silva FH (1989): Kindling induced changes in parvalbumin immunoreactivity in rat hippocampus and its relations to long-term decrease in GABA-immunoreactivity. *Brain Res* 479: 23–34

Komisaruk BR (1977): The role of rhythmical brain activity in sensorimotor integration. In: *Progress in Psychobiology and Physiological Psychobiology*, Sprague JM, Epstein AN, eds. New York Academic Press, vol. 7, pp. 55–90

Konopacki J, Bland BH, MacIver MB, Roth SH (1987a): Cholinergic theta rhythm in transected hippocampal slices: independent CA_1 and dentate generators. *Brain Res* 436:217–222

Konopacki J, MacIver MB, Bland BH, Roth SH (1987b): Carbachol-induced EEG "theta" activity in hippocampal brain slices. *Brain Res* 405:196–198

Larson J, Lynch G (1988): Role of N-methyl-D-aspartate receptors in the induction of synaptic potentiation by burst stimulation patterned after the hippocampal theta rhythm. *Brain Res* 441:111–118

Larson J, Wong D, Lynch G (1986): Patterned stimulation at the theta frequency is optimal for the induction of hippocampal long-term potentiation. *Brain Res* 368: 347–350

Leung L-WS (1980): Behavior-dependent evoked potentials in the hippocampal CA1 region of the rat. I. Correlation with behavior and EEG. *Brain Res* 198:95–117

Leung L-WS (1984a): Model of gradual phase shift of theta rhythm in the rat. *J. Neurophysiol* 52:1051–1065

Leung L-WS (1984b): Pharmacology of theta phase shift in the hippocampal CA_1 region of freely moving rats. *Electroencephalogr Clin Neurophysiol* 58:457–466

Leung L-WS, Lopes da Silva FH, Wadman WJ (1982): Spectral characteristics of the hippocampal EEG in the freely moving rat. *Electroencephalogr Clin Neurophysiol* 54:203–219

Llinás RR (1988): The intrinsic electrophysiological properties of mammalian neurons: insights into central nervous system function. *Science* 242:1654–1664

Lopes da Silvra, F.H. (1991): Neural mechanisms underlying brain waves: from neural membrane to networks, Electroencephalogr Clin Neurophysiol 79:81–93

Lopes da Silva FH, Arnolds DEAT (1978): Physiology of the hippocampus and related structures. *Annu Rev Physiol* 36:291–301

Lopes da Silva FH, Arnolds DEAT, Neijt HC (1984): A functional link between the limbic cortex and ventral striatum: physiology of the subiculum-accumbens pathway. *Exp Brain Res* 55:205–214

Lopes da Silva FH, Kamp A (1969): Hippocampal theta frequency shifts and operant behaviour. *Electroencephalogr Clin Neurophysiol* 26:133–143

Lopes da Silva FH, van Rotterdam A, van Heuden E, Burr W (1976): Models of neuronal populations: The basic mechanisms of rhythmicity. In: *Perspectives in Brain Research*, Corner MA, Swaab DF, eds. Progr Brain Res 45:281–308

Lopes da Silva FH, Witter MP, Boeijinga PH, Lohman AHM (1990): Anatomical organisation and physiology of the limbic cortex. *Physiol Rev* 70:453–511.

MacVicar BA, Dudek FE (1980): Local synaptic circuits in rat hippocampus: interactions between pyramidal cells. *Brain Res* 184:220–223

MacVicar BA, Tse FWY (1989): Local neuronal circuitry underlying cholinergic rhythmical slow activity in CA3 area of rat hippocampal slices. *J. Physiol* 417:197–212

McLennan H, Miller JJ (1976): Frequency-related inhibitory mechanisms controlling rhythmical activity in the septal area. *J Physiol (Lond)* 254:827–841

Miles R, Wong RKS (1986): Excitatory synaptic interactions between CA3 neurons in the guinea-pig hippocampus in vitro. *J Physiol (Lond)* 373:397–418

Nuñez A, Garcia-Austt E, Buño W Jr (1987): Intracellular θ-rhythm generation in identified hippocampal pyramids. *Brain Res* 416:289–300

Paiva T, Lopes da Silva FH, Mollevanger W (1976): Modulating systems of hippocampal EEG. *Electroencephalogr Clin Neurophysiol* 40:470–480

Pavlides C, Greenstein YJ, Goudman M, Winson J (1988): Long-term potentiation in the dentate gyrus is induced preferentially on the positive phase of theta-rhythm. *Brain Res* 439:383–387

Petsche H, Stumpf Ch, Gogolák G (1962): The significance of the rabbit's septum as a relay station between the midbrain and the hippocampus. The contral of hippocampus arousal activity by septum cells. *Electroencephalogr Clin Neurophysiol* 14: 202–211

Pijn JPM (1990): Quantitative evaluation of EEG signals in epilepsy—nonlinear associations, time delays and nonlinear dynamics. Ph.D. Thesis, University of Amsterdam.

Pijn, JP, van Nerveen, J, Noest A, Lopes da Silva FH (1991) Chaos or noise in EEG signals; dependence on state and brain site. *Electroencephalogr Clin Neurophysiol* 79:371–381

Rawlins JNP (1985): Associations across time: the hippocampus as a temporary memory store. *Behav Brain Sci* 8:479–496

Robinson TE (1980): Hippocampal rhythmic slow activity (RSA; theta): A critical analysis of selected studies and discussion of possible species-differences. *Brain Res Rev* 2:69–101

Rose GM, Dunwiddie TV (1986): Induction of hippocampal long-term potentiation using physiologically patterned stimulation. *Neurosci Lett* 69:244–248

Rudell AP, Fox SE, Ranck JB Jr (1980): Hippocampal excitability phase-locked to theta rhythm in waking rats. *Exp Neurol* 68:87–96

Sainsbury RS (1970): Hippocampal activity during natural behaviour in the guinea-pig. *Physiol Behav* 5:317–324

Steriade M, Gloor P, Llinás RR, Lopes da Silva FH, Mesulam M (1990): Basic mechanisms of cerebral rhythmic activities. *Electroencephalogr Clin Neurophysiol* 76:481–508

Traub RD, Miles R, Wong RKS (1989): Model of the origin of rhythmic population oscillations in the hippocampal slice. *Science* 243:1319–1325.

Vanderwolf CH (1969): Hippocampal electrical activity and voluntary movement in the rat. *Electroencephalogr Clin Neurophysiol* 26:407–418

Vanderwolf CH (1975): Neocortical and hippocampal activation in relation to behavior: effects of atropine, eserine, phenothiazines and amphetamine. *J Comp Physiol Psychol* 88:300–323

Vanderwolf CH, Baker GB (1986): Evidence that serotonin mediates noncholinergic neocortical low voltage fast activity, non-cholinergic hippocampal rhytmical slow activity and contributes to intelligent behavior. *Brain Res* 374:342–356

Vanderwolf CH, Kramis R, Robinson TE (1978): Hippocampal electrical activity during waking behaviour and sleep: analyses using centrally acting drugs. In: *Functions of the Septo-Hippocampal System*, Ciba Foundation Symposium 58 (new series). Amsterdam: Excerpta Medica

Vanderwolf CH, Leung L-WS (1983): Hippocampal rhythmical slow activity: a brief history and the effects of entorhinal lesions and phencyclindine. In: *Neurobiology of the Hippocampus*, Seifert W, ed. London: Academic Press, pp 275–302

Vanderwolf CH, Leung L-WS, Cooley RK (1985a): Pathways through the cingulate, neo- and entorhinal cortices mediating atropine-resistant hippocampal rhythmical slow activity. *Brain Res* 347:58–73

Vanderwolf CH, Leung L-WS, Stewart DJ (1985b): Two afferent pathways mediating hippocampal rhythmical slow activity. In: *Electrical Activity of the Archicortex*, Buzsàki G, Vanderwolf CH, eds. Budapest: Akadémiai Kiadó, pp 47–66

Vanderwolf CH, Robinson TE (1981): Reticulo-cortical activity and behavior: A critique of the arousal theory and a new synthesis. *Behav Brain Sci* 4:459–514

Vinogradova OS, Brazhnik ES, Karanov AN, Zhadina SD (1980): Analysis of neuronal activity in rabbit's septum with various conditions of deafferentiation. *Brain Res* 187:354–368

Whishaw IQ, Kolb B (1979): Neocortical and hippocampal EEG in rats during lateral hypothalamic lesion-induced hyperkinesia: relations to behavior and effects of atropine. *Physiol Behav* 22:1107–1113

Wilson CL, Motter BC, Lindsley DB (1976): Influences of hypothalamic stimulation upon septal and hippocampal electrical activity in the cat. *Brain Res* 107:55–68

Winson J (1974): Patterns of hippocampal theta rhythm in the freely moving rat. *Electroencephalogr Clin Neurophysiol* 36:291–301

Winson J (1976a): Hippocampal theta rhythm. I. Depth profiles in the curarized rat. *Brain Res* 103:57–70

Winson J (1976b): Hippocampal theta rhythm. II. Depth profiles in the freely moving rabbit. *Brain Res* 103:71–79

Winson J (1984): Neuronal transmission through the hippocampus: Dependence on behavioural state. In: *Cortical Integration*, Reinoso-Suárez F, Ajmone-Marsan C, eds. New York: Raven Press, p 131

Winson J (1986): Behaviorally dependent neuronal gating in the hippocampus. In: *The Hippocampus*, Isaacson RL, Pribram KH, eds. New York: Plenum Press, vol. 4, pp 77–92

Winson J, Abzug C (1978a): Neuronal transmission through hippocampal pathways dependent on behavior. *J Neurophysiol* 41:716–732

Winson J, Abzug C (1978b): Dependence upon behavior of neuronal transmission from perforant pathway through entorhinal cortex. *Brain Res* 147:422–427

Witter MP, Groenewegen HJ, Lopes da Silva FH, Lohman AHM (1989): Functional organization of the extrinsic and intrinsic circuitry of the parahippocampal region. *Prog Neurobiol* 33:161–253

Wong RKS, Traub RD (1983): Synchronized burst discharge in the disinhibited hippocampal slice. I. Initiation in the CA_2-CA_3 region. *J Neurophysiol* 49:442–458

Is There any Message Hidden in the Human EEG?

HELLMUTH PETSCHE and PETER RAPPELSBERGER

The term "electroencephalogram," or EEG, is ambiguous: it was coined by Hans Berger (1929) who understood by it both the human electrical brain activity as it manifests itself in scalp recordings, and its representation as a potential-time diagram. For activities recorded from the cortex, the proper generator of the EEG, the word "electrocorticogram" was created, a term that did not, however, win much favor; today the term "EEG" is generally used for the designation of electrical brain activity regardless of where and how it is recorded. This also holds true for this chapter.

In contrast to Berger's original ideas, which were virtually aimed at finding ways into the understanding of human thinking, the EEG evolved in a different direction and finally became but an auxiliary laboratory method, mainly in neurology. Particularly epileptology has profited from this method, which developed into a science of its own and greatly contributed to the knowledge of the processes underlying and maintaining epileptic seizures. In the years to come, this evolution of electroencephalography resulted in putting most emphasis on the peculiarities of potential-time diagrams of the electric brain activity of patients (EEG traces) recorded from a few electrodes from the scalp; thus, the EEG was thought of and described chiefly in terms of frequency, amplitude (both estimated by the naked eye) and the shape of so-called graphoelements such as spikes, slow waves, sharp waves, transients and so forth. The spatial aspects of electric brain activity, apart from gross distinctions in location such as occipital, temporal, or frontal were disregarded. For most people working with the EEG, it was merely a useful tool for the examination of a fairly small group of patients. Berger's original endeavor to make use of the EEG for the exploration of mental processes seemed to have pointed into a dead end.

Apart from the host of clinicians who even today regard the EEG under such a narrow viewpoint, there were a few students who, as early as the 1950s and despite the inadequate technological facilities of those days, attempted to consider electric brain activity as a spatiotemporal continuum still hiding its essential secrets, although they were aware of the futility of ever being able to realize such dreams as Pavlov's, who wrote in 1926:

> If one could observe the activity of the brain through the skull, one would see a continuously changing light-spot whisking over the hemispheres and surrounded by darker shadows arrested sometimes here, sometimes there and then again jumping to other regions. In this way the ceaselessly changing function of the consciousness seems to be activated from a central place.

In their attempts to approach a representation of the EEG in a continuous, spatiotemporal way, these few students, mentioned above, made their first steps into topography [a historical review on these attempts is found in Petsche and Shaw, (1972)]. An efficient realization of these efforts, however, could not begin before the past decade when computer technology started opening the doors to EEG mapping methods.

Students of EEG topography wanted to put more weight onto the long disregarded spatial dimension of the EEG without neglecting, however, the time dimension. In this endeavor they soon became intrigued by the observation that even those electrical events that appeared to be synchronous over large regions of the scalp, as for instance the extremely regular 3-Hz spike-and-wave pattern during an absence, displayed phase differences when studied over a more extended time scale. The EEG thus turned out to be far more complex than a mere reflection of its potential-time traces, usually recorded at 3 cm/s in clinical use, would have been assumed to be. Therefore, elucidating the nature of synchrony seemed to be important for the study of epileptic events, because the question of which events may give rise to such a synchronization of electric brain activity seemed to be at the heart of epileptic processes.

Not only seizure patterns but also the background activity at rest are characterized by more or less extended zones of apparently synchronous wave shape. Without synchronization, no EEG would be recordable. It has been shown by Cooper et al. (1965) that cortical areas of several cm^2 must be involved in the same wave pattern to become visible at all on the scalp since the bone and its underlying tissues act as low-pass filters.

Unfortunately, for the study of the processes underlying the generation of the EEG, the human brain is innappropriate because the stratum of EEG "generators," which may be conceived of as perpendicularly arranged dipoles within the cortex, is curved in several planes. For this reason animal studies must be performed when studying EEG generation phenomena. Because of its relatively large and almost ungyrated cortex representing an almost flat generator layer, we chose the rabbit for such studies. The problem of comprehending the electrical continuum of the EEG was approached by using two methods: one was to make use of a multiple semimicroelectrode [16 contacts at 125–150 μm distances on a carrier needle (Prohaska et al., 1979)] for simultaneous recordings from the entire cortical depth; the other was the use of square grids of 4×4 electrodes for cortical surface recordings at distances between 3 and 0.5 mm for the exploration of the behavior of the potential fields during the rise and the course of epileptic seizures (Petsche et al., 1984). Spectral analysis, the most common method for the analysis of the EEG, was used. Since we have been mainly interested in the mutual relationships of electric activities, great emphasis has been put on estimating coherences, a parameter usually disregarded in EEG analysis. This procedure has turned out to be most efficient as it has opened new ways to the understanding of several essential features of the EEG.

Without going into detail about the generation of epileptic patterns and the EEG in general, a few properties of the EEG should be mentioned in this context. First, it should be said that the phenomena recorded from the brain (gross compound field potentials) represent the average of potential differences due to an immense number of currents generated by local de- and hyperpolarizations of neuron and glia cell membranes. These currents flow through the extracellular space and through tissues of different impedance and conductivity. For this reason and until recently the host of neurophysiologists considered field potentials as inappropriate for the study of the current production of the brain and thought of intracellular recordings as the only reliable method. It will be shown that this circumstance does not exclude this neuronal mass activity represented by the EEG from being investigated by appropriate methods which, in effect, have proven to be able to detect not only new aspects of its generation but have even supplied clues to its probable purport.

Volume conduction was usually thought to be the main reason why field potentials were not worth being studied. Nevertheless, this condition turned out to play a far less important part than frequently assumed as may be inferred from the often considerable differences of wave shapes and amplitudes recorded from closely spaced electrodes: in the vertical dimension of the cortex, the wave shapes of spontaneous activity proved to show variations from one layer to the other, particularly in the middle-cortical layers; potential gradients as steep as 4 mV/mm were found here in seizures. The minor role volume conduction also plays in the horizontal dimension has been substantiated by surface recordings: during epileptic events potential gradients of up to 2 mV/mm were seen.

Other observations supporting the minor role of volume conduction even in epileptic activities in which the largest voltages can be seen are as follows: in regularly oscillating EEG activities and in the initial, tonic phase of a seizure, accumulations of synaptic events alternate in the superficial and deeper layers of the cortex; the intracortical spatiotemporal relationships are more irregular and complex in the clonic stage of seizures in which the interactions of regions of maximum current densities demonstrate a highly complex interplay of excitation and inhibition processes between cortex and deeper subcortical structures. Also, during spontaneous activity, the cortex is electrically not uniform but rather behaves as a dipole layer for the basic frequency (Rappelsberger et al., 1982) with many superimposed and less extended dipoles at different depths. It should be mentioned that this high degree of complexity was detected by using current source density analysis (Rappelsberger et al., 1981), a method by which volume conducted phenomena *a priori* are eliminated.

The surface recordings from the grid of 4 $\times$ 4 electrodes served the purpose of comprehending the epicortical behavior of the potential fields during the seizure. When studying these phenomena during a seizure caused by focal cortical application of a small amount of penicillin (5000 IU), the first event to be observed is a localized interictal “spike” from which, after a couple of minutes, a seizure is generated. In the EEG, the beginning of the seizure is characterized by a fast (at about 20 Hz) regular sinusoid activity that, within a few seconds, increases in amplitude and decreases in frequency (the “tonic stage” of the seizure). During this stage the potential fields have turned out to be roughly circular and to cover areas not larger than 3 mm in diameter. Surprisingly, at the onset of the seizure they start circulating with trajectories becoming gradually larger to form a spiral around the penicillin focus. Simultaneously, their amplitudes increase. The time of revolution equals the duration of the waves recorded in the EEG. Later on, the spreading becomes undefinable, saccadic, and more irregular, as does also the wave shape (Petsche 1978; Petsche et al., 1984). At this stage, the potential fields seem to jump to different places without any recognizable rule.

This chapter does not explain this strange behavior; mention should only be made that the immense number of IPSPs, elicited by the heavy focal excitation by penicillin, form both the wall and the bottom of a bowl of inhibition that tries to confine the focal excitation. Only within this bowl of inhibition may the excitatory processes of the seizure develop; since the zone of excitation within the bowl tends to involve adjacent regions (i.e., to spread), it can do this only within this wall, the boundary of the surrounding inhibition, which, however, is gradually overcome by the increasing excitation until finally both the wall and the bottom of the bowl of inhibition break down and the seizure runs rampant.

These observations on pathological EEG patterns led us to the conclusion that the spatiotemporal aspects of the EEG as mass action of the nervous system (Freeman, 1975) might be worth more consideration in the future. Normal activities should also be included in the exploration of the spatiotemporal aspects of the EEG, as our previous studies on the hippocampus–septum system have proven: such an approach demonstrated that the regular 4 to 7/s theta rhythm of the hippocampus is initiated by a neuronal pacemaker (Broca’s nucleus of the diagonal band) in the middle of the septum from where the underlying potential fields spread along the hippocampus in an anterior–posterior direction at speeds of a few meters per second (Petsche and Stumpf, 1960). This was an additional impetus to extend our studies of spatiotemporal aspects of the spontaneous EEG to man.

Two further considerations have supported this idea. The first was that the EEG seems to be an outstanding example of a process fluctuating between chaos and order: even the EEG of a healthy person with its dominant alpha rhythm (between 8 and 12 Hz) presents a mixture of more or less regular and fairly irregular episodes. In epilepsies the range between regular and chaotic activities is even larger; there exist, on the one hand, highly complex activities with bizarre wave shapes at different regions (hypsarrhythmia, an EEG pattern found only in severe deteriorations of brain function in children), and, on the other hand, the already mentioned most regular, machinelike spike-wave pattern during a petit mal seizure.

The second motive for examining the spatiotemporal aspects of the spontaneous EEG in man more closely were experiments by Livanov (1977), who was intrigued by his observations on conditioning experiments in rabbits: when stimulated by flicker light, these animals sometimes reacted with leg movements but sometimes not. It turned out that motor reactions occurred only if the electrical activities of the visual and the motor regions were synchronized. For this reason, Livanov computed the cross-correlation between the activities of these two locations; he found that the light stimulus was more readily transmitted to the cortical motor area when the correlation coefficient was high than when it was low. Synchronization, thus, again proved to have functional significance. Based on these findings, Livanov also examined the human EEG and found that the cross-correlation underwent different changes on different parts of the scalp when the probands were instructed to perform mental tasks.

These observations and our experience on the serviceability of coherence estimates for the understanding of normal and epileptic electrical activities in rabbits prompted us to introduce coherence estimates also in studying the background EEG in man.

The idea that information about thinking may be hidden in the EEG was already suggested by Grey Walter in 1964, when he made conditioning experiments and detected the contingent negative variation or expectancy wave as he also called it: a shift toward negative that arises after a warning stimulus when the subject was suggested to pay attention to another stimulus requiring a response or a decision by him (Walter et al., 1964). In the years to follow the method of obtaining event-related potentials (ERPs) proved to be of great importance for detecting traces of mental processes in the EEG; in this context particular emphasis was paid to the famous P 300, a short positive deviation that could be shown to indicate brain events involved in information processing. But despite the fact that literature on P 300, since its discovery by Sutton et al. in 1965, has literally led to new psychological libraries coming into being, it did not bring essential knowledge to the problem of the EEG's reflection of mental work.

There are several reasons for dissatisfaction with the results evolving from studying P 300 and other ERPs for the elucidation of thinking processes. One is the methodology required by ERP studies: it aims at contriving appropriate psychological paradigms that have to be repeated up to at least 30 times while the superimposed ERPs produced by latency and amplitude changes of P 300 are measured; these are the only data from which often far-reaching conclusions are drawn. For all that the experimenter often forgets that the shape of an ERP is but a minimal aspect of the electrical spatiotemporal continuum that most likely is changed as a whole by the mental task concerned. A further reason for the relative paucity of the results of ERP research are the restrictions imposed by this method: only short-lasting psychological paradigms can be investigated in this way, and, in addition, these paradigms have to be repeated several times, as ERPs arise by the superimposition of many evoked responses and are time-locked to the stimulus. Thus, the paradigms cannot but have more or less laboratory character and mostly are far from the demands daily life makes on the brain. A third reason why probably no far-reaching elucidations on mental processes may be obtained by ERPs is that they are based on reductionistic thinking: it is more than unlikely that any restricted knowledge about fairly primitive thinking processes may contribute at all to the understanding of the thinking processes of daily life.

These thoughts and the conviction of the usefulness of a search for possible temporary changes of the functional connections between brain areas in the course of mental tasks via coherence analysis initiated our own strategy to look for mental processes hidden in the background EEG.

Our method is based on power and coherence analysis of the EEG (Rappelsberger and Petsche, 1988). Its aim is to detect significant changes of these parameters during mental activities with respect to the EEG at rest. Since episodes of at least 1 minute are used for comparison, the duration of the mental task to be studied is not restricted. Even longer lasting mental tasks such as reading, doing mental arithmetic, listening to music, playing chess, and creative thinking may be studied in this manner (Petsche et al., 1986, Petsche 1990). The method has also proved useful to detect EEG differences between psychotic patients and healthy subjects (Pockberger et al., 1985, 1989) as well as to study the influence of drugs on brain activities (Thau et al., 1988). It is based on common-reference recordings (against averaged ear lobe electrodes) from the 19 electrodes of the 10/20 system in order to obtain a survey over the entire skull. Although common-reference recordings have certain disadvantages, they still seem to be the best compromise for use in EEG mapping, particularly if coherence estimates are performed. This was demonstrated by Rappelsberger (1989). Absolute power is computed from each electrode, coherence between adjacent electrodes and electrodes on homologous regions of the two hemispheres. For data reduction the results are compressed to five frequency bands between 4 and 32 Hz. This method permits studies on individuals and on groups of individuals as well as a comparison between individuals and groups of individuals under certain conditions.

Among the results obtained by this procedure, group studies are particularly worth mentioning. Despite the great individual differences of the EEG and of the personal aptitude, it turned out that the probability maps of power and coherence changes obtained by averaging indicate some fundamental thinking strategies becoming evident by virtue of the EEG. This claim first emerged in some findings while listening to music (Petsche et al., 1988a). For 1 minute a quartet by Mozart was presented to 75 students of both sexes, regardless of their interest in music and their musical education, while EEG were recorded. The EEG probability maps, computed with respect to the EEG at rest, exhibited a reduction of alpha power far extended in the left and somewhat more restricted in the right temporal region, an increase of local coherence (between pairs of adjacent electrodes) in the left frontotemporal area in the theta band, and in the right temporo-occipital area in a frequency range between 18 and 24 Hz; furthermore, an increase of the interhemispheric coherence (indicating the degree of functional coupling of the two hemispheres) between the temporo-occipital and the parietal regions was found between 18 and 24 Hz. Such observations hint at the existence of some fundamental thinking strategies involved in the listening of acoustic architectonic structures that can be made visible by the EEG.

When this group of persons was separated according to sex, further characteristic differences were found, the females in general exhibiting more changes while listening to music than males. Incidentally, sex differences have proven to be seen in every mental task studied up to now (Petsche et al., 1988b). When this fairly large group of 75 persons was divided in two parts according to their musical preeducation (at least five years training in any instrument was chosen as criterion) the musically trained group exhibited far more and partially different changes when listening to Mozart than the musically naive.

Listening to spoken language yielded quite different results.

It was instructive to compare also the EEG at rest of these two groups: it too presented us considerable differences. In males, most distinct was a higher degree of local coherence in almost all frequency bands in the right temporo-occipital region; musically trained women differed from untrained ones in the EEG at rest mainly in their stronger functional connectedness of the two hemispheres that concerned the entire frequency spectrum. Common to both sexes were fewer beta activities above 18 Hz in the trained than in the untrained persons.

At first sight it may seem strange for somebody to claim the spontaneous EEG of musically trained persons should differ from the one of the untrained. Musical education as such cannot yet be so important for the brain as to produce a different EEG at rest! However, if one bears in mind the number of abilities that are trained by musical education, this finding loses something of its oddness: musical training on any instrument not only improves manual skill of both hands but also increases the ability to discriminate between sounds and to follow and reconstruct acoustic architectonic structures. Moreover, the sense for both perceiving and performing rhythms is trained. That musical training not only fosters the ability to play an instrument but also contributes to the general training of intellectual abilities was shown by Hassler and Nieschlag (1990).

These findings, however, were not the only ones to suggest that the EEG might contain some information on intellectual abilities. Others came from a study by Rappelsberger et al. (1987), who investigated mental cube rotation in students. Incidentally, in this project the most striking sex differences were found in the theta and beta range with local coherence increased over the posterior parts of the skull. In men, local coherence increased in the theta range in the right posterior quadrant and in the beta range in the left one; in females the contrary happened. This strange observation, however, is not the main reason why the results of this study are dealt with here.

When looking for possible links between the EEG and general traits of intelligence, we posed the question of whether a correlation might exist between the score of ability to rotate cubes mentally and the degree of local coherence change in the EEG while performing this task; indeed, such a correlation could be established in this group of subjects for several electrode positions in the posterior half of the skull. They were positive for males and negative for females ($p < .05$). Moreover, these correlations were found on the opposite hemispheres in the two sexes. Thus, males and females seem to employ almost the opposite strategies while mentally rotating cubes, and, in addition, also have the opposite hemispheres more involved.

This finding also suggests some traits of intelligence to be embodied in the spontaneous electric brain activity. Some support of this claim is supplied by the work of Giannitrapani (1985). A comparison of his findings with ours, however, is not possible as the psychological paradigm and the way of analysis were different.

Our belief that cognitive strategies may be detected in the spontaneous EEG was supported by a variety of other studies concerning mental arithmetic, reading, viewing pictures, and perceiving more or less complex rhythms without music. All these findings encouraged us to look also for possible changes of EEG when investigating higher intellectual abilities such as creative thinking (Petsche et al., 1990). The positive results in this project, however, are too complex to be reported in this short review. Only one example may illustrate the procedure and an outline of the results. In this project the mental task was to imagine, while the EEG was recorded, an abstract concept of the probands' own choice, such as "love," "freedom," "anger," and so forth; moreover, the subjects were requested to attempt to visualize this concept in order to make a sketch of their visualization after the EEG recording on a sheet of paper with colored pencils. The average differences between at rest and task power and coherence values in 21 male and 23 female students were plotted as probability maps as described above. These two groups were homogeneous in terms of age and handedness.

The results are shown in Figure 1. Changes of power caused by this task are largely the same in the two sexes and can probably be interpreted as an arousal phenomenon, whereas coherence changes are distinctly different: as for local coherence, the main differences concern the alpha and theta bands in which females exhibit a decrease of local coherence preponderantly over the right frontal area, and the beta 3 band between 24 and 32 Hz, in which hemispheric differences are seen between the two sexes. Sex differences are also found in interhemispheric coherence: apart from the increase in several locations and frequency bands, females also display decreases of the functional coupling between the two hemispheres.

These characteristics are all the more impressive considering the arbitrarily limited measures of the spatiotemporal pattern—only five bands, limited to upper beta and omitting gamma frequencies, smoothing over many seconds and through the scalp, computing coherence only with nearest neighbors; much more detail can be expected if we used additional dimensions of display.

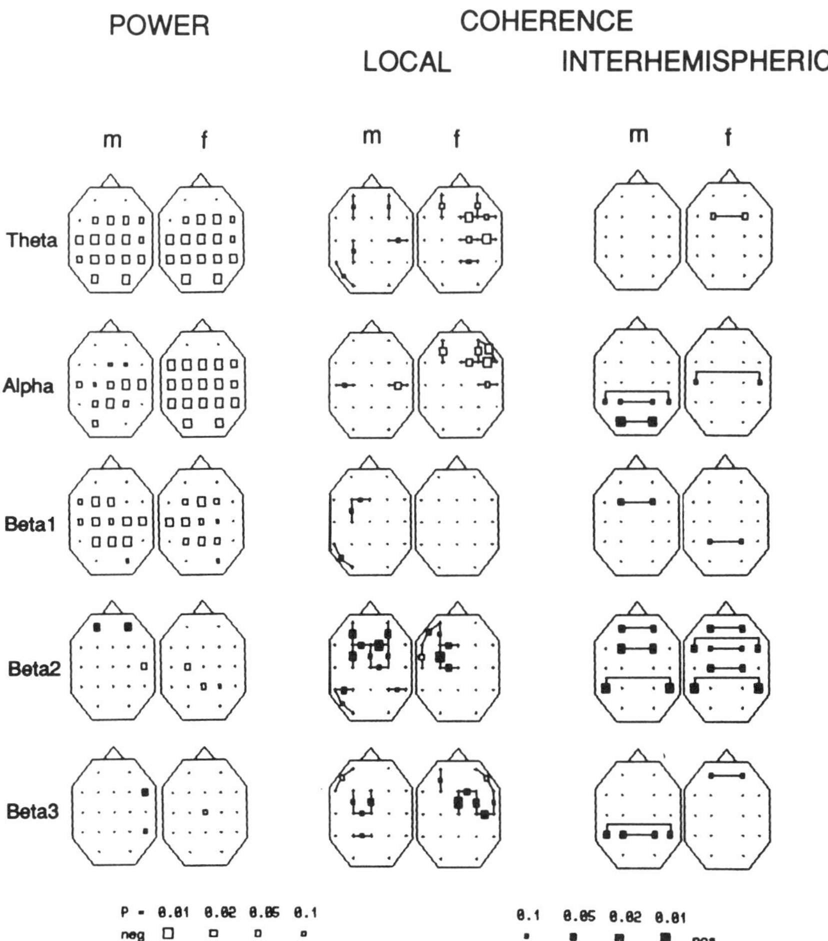

Figure 1. Visualization of an abstract concept. EEG probability maps of the average differences of absolute power and coherence in 21 male (m) and 23 female (f) students. *Black squares*: increase; *white squares*: decrease of the respective parameter. *p* values are given primarily to describe but not to confirm results.

We should rather dedicate the rest of the space to a fairly personal discussion of what we think about the possible significance of these findings.

Both the observations on animals and humans under normal and pathological conditions demonstrate that the gross compound field potentials of the EEG are events laden with information, despite the fact that the EEG recorded from a certain location can all but be clearly defined because it represents the vector sum of very many generators of different nature in the cell membrane. Nevertheless, in animals, a detailed exploration of the EEG has turned out to allow for correlations to the fine structure of the cortex if the distances of the simultaneous multiple recordings were narrowed down to as little as 100 μm. But also in epileptic activities the development of cooperative processes reflected by the EEG has proven to have some functional significance in the competition between excitatory and inhibitory processes. Still more surprising is the observation that the human EEG, recorded from the scalp, despite being blurred and smeared by the different positions of the generators with respect to the recording site and the different tissue layers below the electrodes, also contains information as becomes evident at various locations and in various frequency bands. This information is changed by thinking, as was demonstrated by probability mapping of power and coherence changes during mental processes with respect to the EEG at rest. This conclusion was corroborated by the observation that significant changes of power and coherence were induced if the same mental tasks were performed by fairly large groups of persons. Particularly the changes of coherence, mostly in the beta bands, gave rise to characteristic changes of the probability maps, which may be conceived of as representing sort of electrophysiological reflections of fundamental thinking strategies.

As for the possible meaning of the EEG changes caused by mental tasks, one can only speculate at this stage of knowledge. It seems likely that the greater part of power changes in the alpha and theta range can be related to the level of attentiveness. However, also localized power changes in the beta bands seem to be related to special features of attentiveness as our studies with listening to music have demonstrated (Petsche et al., 1988). Attempts to interpret the coherence changes are more difficult. Livanov's basic idea that an increased territory of synchronization, a hint for a closer functional connection of these two areas, may always be interpreted as an activation of the area in question for mental processes, certainly can not be generalized. In our experience, localized areas of increased as well as of decreased coherence may be interpreted under certain conditions and in certain mental tasks as "hot spots." The physiological meaning of coherence change does not seem to be the same in cortical regions of different functional properties. We have neither an explanation for the frequent observation that coherence changes in the theta and alpha band on the one hand and in the beta bands on the other hand are often contralateral.

Somewhat more easily understood are changes of interhemispheric coherence, which may represent the degree of hemispheric functional connectedness. Nevertheless, further observations, supported by studies with other methods (PET, rCBF), are needed to be able to interpret the greater body of EEG findings during thinking.

A final speculation may be allowed as to a possible functional significance of the human EEG. That it is not mere, meaningless noise could be demonstrated beyond any doubt, as well as that it contains information. But couldn't it also be that it has still additional functions rather than just to preserve traces of thinking?

There is much evidence today to consider the EEG under the aspect of a pseudochaotic event or rather a number of such events that may take on different degrees of order (Babloyantz and Destexhe, 1986; Başar et al., 1989). Besides, there is increasing evidence that pseudochaotic processes underlie the phenomenon of self-organization and, further, that self-organization, as in all living systems, plays an important part in the emerging structures and functions of the brain. In addition, Freeman and Schneider (1982) and Skinner et al. (1989) supplied convincing evidence that the chaotic electric activity produced by the olfactory bulb is obviously an optimum way for the animal to cope with his environment of odors and to recognize new olfactory stimuli as such.

What about the far more complex electrical activity of the neocortex in this respect (see Freeman, this volume)? Admittedly, the function of the olfactory bulb is most simple as compared with the neocortex; this was also the reason why Freeman and his group chose this system for their studies. But if the spontaneous electrical activity actually were involved in optimizing the performance of mental processes by the brain, it is most likely that its tasks would be different according to which regions, whether sensory and motor areas of different hierarchical levels or association or still other areas, are concerned. Under these conditions it would also be easier to realize why the direction of power and coherence changes during mental work would largely depend on the brain regions in which they are observed.

In the ontogenetic development of the brain the top-most stage self-adaptation has attained is thinking, a powerful weapon of the human species in its fight for survival against its perilous environment. Our observations supply several suggestions that the EEG not only hides some traces of thinking but, even more, that it could have a physiological assignment toward the optimization of thinking.

To conclude with the title of a paper by Freeman's group: "How brains make chaos in order to make sense of the world" (Skarda and Freeman, 1987) or with a free translation of a quotation of von Waldeck: "In order to create information, thinking has to be chaotic. Any non-chaotic cognitive process is *malade*: it has got stuck in a circle, again and again returns to the same results and prevents any knowledge. It is the way of fanatics, of fundamentalists in their thinking. Chaotic thinking is only feasible by jumping out of this attractor."

Summary

A look at the history of EEG shows that this method was used mainly as a diagnostic tool in neurology. For this purpose, main emphasis was put on recording potential in the time domain while the spatial domain was largely neglected.

To give equal consideration to both the temporal and the spatial aspects, a micro-EEG method was developed. Its aim was to record from a small cortical volume with a number of electrodes as large as possible, in order to describe its continuous electrical behavior. By doing so in rabbits, both the spontaneous and the seizure EEG turned out to be intricate and conditional on the local cortical structure. When studying the nature of "synchronization" with this method, coherence estimates turned out to be useful.

As there were clues that coherence estimates may give some insight into the degree of the mutual functional connections of cortical regions, this procedure was also tried in humans and studies with probability mapping of power and coherence were performed during a number of mental tasks. Basically, the method consists of examining the differences of these two parameters between task periods of at least 1 minute and the average EEG at rest. Despite the numerous reasons that contribute to the blurring of the EEG when recorded from the scalp, coherence and power values proved to be significantly altered by mental tasks such as silently reading, listening to music and text, mental arithmetic, mental cube rotation, and others. The changes concerned mainly the beta bands, but also the theta and alpha bands were involved. Moreover, distinct sex differences were found in every task. Even the spontaneous EEG proved to be different in groups of subjects who were trained and not trained in a special domain. These findings advocate the idea that the background EEG is not mere noise but rather may serve a certain purpose with respect to mental processes.

Acknowledgment. The authors wish to thank Mrs. Susan Etlinger, Ph.D., for linguistic advice.

References

Babloyantz A, Destexhe A (1986): Low dimensional chaos in an instance of epilepsy. *Proc Natl Acad Sci USA* 83:3513

Başar E, Başar-Eroglu C, Röschke J, Schütt A (1989): The EEG is a quasi-deterministic signal anticipating sensory-cognitive tasks. In: *Brain Dynamics*, Başar E, Bullock TH, eds. Berlin Springer-Verlag.

Berger H (1929): Über das Elektrenkephalogramm des Menschen. *Arch Psychiat* 87: 527–570

Cooper R, Winter AL, Crow HJ, Walter WG (1965): Comparison of subcortical and scalp activity using chronically indwelling electrodes in man. *Electroencephalogr Clin Neurophysiol* 18:217–228

Freeman WJ (1975): *Mass Action in the Nervous System*. New York: Academic Press

Freeman WJ, Schneider WS (1982): Changes in spatial patterns of rabbit olfactory EEG with conditioning to odors. *Psychophysiology* 19:44–56

Giannitrapani D (1985): *The Electrophysiology of Intellectual Functions*. Basel: Karger

Hassler M, Nieschlag (1989): Masculinity femininity. and musical composition. *Arch Psychol* 141:71–84

Livanov MN (1977): *Spatial Organization of Cerebral Processes*. New York: Wiley and Sons

Pavlov JP (1926): *Die höchste Nerventätigkeit (das Verhalten) von Tieren.* Munich: Bergmann

Petsche H (1978): EEG synchronization in seizures. In: *Contemporary Clinical Neurophysiology*, Cobb WA, van Duijn HG, eds. *Electroencephalogr Clin Neurophysiol*, 134 (Suppl): 299–308

Petsche H (1990): EEG und Denken. Z EEG-EMG 21: 207–218

Petsche H, Lindner K, Rappelsberger P, Gruber G (1988a): The EEG—an adequate method to concretize brain processes elicited by music. *Music Percept* 6: 133–159

Petsche H, Lacroix D, Lindner K, Rappelsberger P, Schmidt-Henrich E (1991): Thinking with images or thinking with language: a pilot EEG probability mapping study *Int J Psychophysiol* (in press)

Petsche H, Pockberger H, Rappelsberger P (1984): On the search for the sources of the electroencephalogram. *Neuroscience* 11: 1–27

Petsche H, Pockberger H, Rappelsberger P (1986): EEG topography and mental performance. In: *Topographic Mapping of the Brain.* Duffy F H, ed. Stoneham: Butterworth

Petsche H, Rappelsberger P, Pockberger H (1988b): Sex differences of the on-going EEG: probability mapping at rest and during cognitive tasks. In: *Topographic Brain Mapping of EEG and Evoked Potentials*, Pfurtscheller G, Lopes da Silva F, eds. Berlin Springer-Verlag

Petsche H, Shaw J (1972): EEG Topography. In: *International Handbook of EEG in Clinical Neurophysiology*, 5B, Remond A, ed. Amsterdam: Elsevier

Petsche H, Stumpf C (1960): Topographic and toposcopic study of origin and spread of the regular synchronised arousal pattern in the rabbit. *Electroencephalogr Clin Neurophysiol* 12: 589–600

Pockberger H, Petsche H, Rappelsberger P, Zidek B, Zapotoczky HG (1985): Ongoing EEG in depression: a topographic spectral analytic study. *Electroencephalogr Clin Neurophysiol* 61: 349–358

Pockberger H, Thau K, Lovrek A, Petsche H, Rappelsberger P (1989): Coherence mapping reveals differences in the EEG between psychiatric patients and healthy persons. In: *Topographic Brain Mapping of EEG and Evoked Potentials*, Maurer K, ed. Berlin: Springer-Verlag

Prohaska O, Pacha F, Pfundner P, Petsche H (1979): A 16-fold semimicroelectrode for intracortical recording of field-potentials. *Electroencephalogr Clin Neurophysiol* 47: 629–631

Rappelsberger P (1989): The reference problem and mapping of coherence: a simulation study. *Brain Topography* 2: 63–72.

Rappelsberger P, Krieglsteiner S, Mayerweg M, Petsche H, Pockberger H (1987): Probability mapping of EEG changes: application to spatial imagination studies. *J Clin Monit* 32: 320–322

Rappelsberger P, Petsche H (1988): Probability mapping: power and coherence analyses of cognitive processes. *Brain Mapping* 1: 46–54

Rappelsberger P, Petsche H, Pockberger H (1981): Current source density analysis of simultaneously recorded intracortical field potentials. *Pflüger's Arch* 389: 59–170

Rappelsberger P, Pockberger H, Petsche H (1982): The contribution of the cortical layers to the generation of the EEG: field potential and current source density analysis in the rabbit's visual cortex. *Electroencephalogr Clin Neurophysiol* 53: 255–269

Skarda A, Freeman WJ (1987): How brains make chaos in order to make sense of the world. *Brain Behav Res* 10: 161–195

Skinner JE, Martin JL, Landisman CE, Mommer MM, Fulton K, Mitra M, Burton WD, Saltzberg B (1989): Chaotic attractors in a model of neocortex: dimensionalities of olfactory bulb surface potentials are spatially uniform and event related. In: *Brain Dynamics*, Başar E, Bullock TH, eds. Berlin: Springer–Verlag.

Sutton S, Braren M, Zubin J, John ER (1965): Evoked potential correlates of stimulus uncertainty. *Science* 150:1187–1188

Thau K, Rappelsberger P, Lovrek A, Petsche H, Simhandl C, Topitz A (1988): Effect of Lithium on the EEG of healthy males and females: a probability mapping study. *Neuropsychobiology* 20:158–163

Waldeck, Rvon (1990) Formeln für das Tohuwabohu. *Kursbuch* 98:1–16

Walter WG, Cooper R, Aldridge VJ, McCallam WC, Winter AL (1964): Contingent negative variation: an electric sign of sensori-motor association and expectancy in the human brain. *Nature* 203:380–384

Event-Related Synchronization and Desynchronization of Alpha and Beta Waves in a Cognitive Task

GERT PFURTSCHELLER and WOLFGANG KLIMESCH

Together with the discovery of alpha waves in human scalp electroencephalograms (EEG) by Berger (1930), blocking was reported in response to a light stimulation. Triggered by the pioneering research of Berger, other groups focused on blocking or desynchronization of alpha and beta waves after visual afferences as well as after somatosensory stimulation or movement (Jasper and Andrews 1938; Jasper and Penfield 1949; Gastaut et al., 1952; Chatrian et al., 1959). Besides these findings of alpha or beta wave attenuation after sensory stimulation or with voluntary movement, there were also reports of an enhancement of alpha band activity as a response to visual stimulation (Morrell, 1966; Creutzfeldt et al., 1969) and tactile stimulation (Kreitman and Shaw, 1965).

Sensory stimulation affects not only the spontaneous EEG within the alpha and beta bands but can also evoke 40-Hz oscillations in the visual cortex (Eckhorn et al., 1988; Gray et al., 1989) or fast somatoparietal rhythms over the posterior parietal cortex (Rougeul et al., 1979).

The terms "event-related desynchronization," or ERD, and "event-related synchronization," or ERS, are used in this chapter to describe the ability of neural structures to generate more or less coherent oscillating potentials. ERD describes the attenuation or blocking and ERS (actually the negative ERD) is the enhancement of oscillating potentials within the alpha and beta bands. The ERD (ERS) can be quantified by measuring the power decrease or increase in event-related EEG trials. Time-dependent quantification of the ERD in the alpha and beta bands was first reported by Pfurtscheller and Aranibar (1977) and Pfurtscheller (1981).

The ERD is a topographically localized phenomenon of short duration (phasic) and not identical with the diffuse and tonic EEG desynchronization reported by Moruzzi and Magoun (1949) after reticular formation stimulation resulting in a "flat" EEG spectrum. ERD was reported during visual stimulation (Aranibar and Pfurtscheller, 1978), voluntary movement (Pfurtscheller and Aranibar, 1979, Pfurtscheller and Berghold, 1989), and cognitive activity (Sergeant et al., 1987; Pfurtscheller and Klimesch, 1989; Klimesch et al., 1990a).

Reports about rhythmic activity within the alpha band differentiate between alpha waves and alpha spindles (Lopes da Silva et al., 1973b). Alpha spindles are transient phenomena dominant over the anterior brain regions and are characteristic of the transitional period between waking and sleeping. Alpha waves can be long-lasting and are dominant over the posterior region in the awake state during rest. Andersen and Andersson's (1968) publication on alpha rhythms concentrates on the generation of alpha spindles. A paper recently published by Steriade and Llinas (1988) is also based on the genesis of spindle oscillations. They found that the major factors accounting for the appearance of spindle oscillation are the involvement of reticular thalamic neurons within the thalamocortical system. The alpha waves could be explained as a result of the filter properties of neural networks when submitted to random input (Lopes da Silva, 1973a). A modulation of these "alpha filters" can result in a more synchronized or desynchronized pattern.

In this chapter we focus not on the neural substrate of alpha waves and alpha spindles, but only report some examples of synchronized and desynchronized alpha and beta rhythms during different processing states of the brain.

Data Acquisition Processing and Topographical Display

A modified "electro-cap" with either 29 or 30 electrodes was used for EEG recording. Of these electrodes, more than half were placed according to the international 10–20 system, while the others were assigned to additional points in between (Fig. 1). The EEG was amplified with a 30-channel amplifier system (frequency response 1.5–30 Hz) and sampled by a PDP 11/73 computer. The EEG data were sampled at a rate of 64/s, using stimulus-synchronous epochs of some seconds, with 2 or 4 s (dependent on the type of experiment) before the stimulus. The individual trials were displayed on-line on a monitor

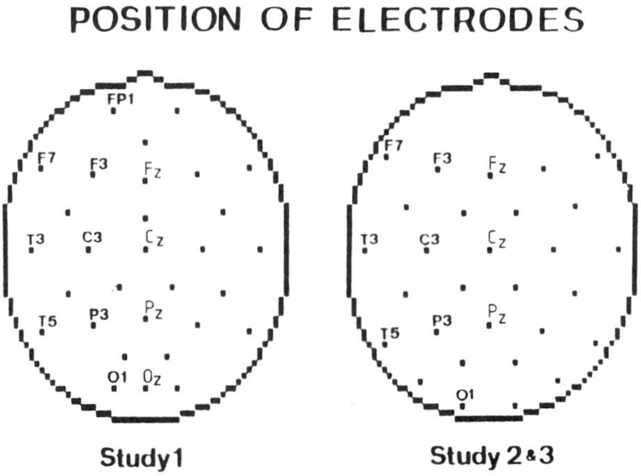

POSITION OF ELECTRODES

Study 1 Study 2 & 3

Figure 1. Position of electrodes used in the three studies. The electrode scheme used in studies 2 and 3 was also used for the movement experiment.

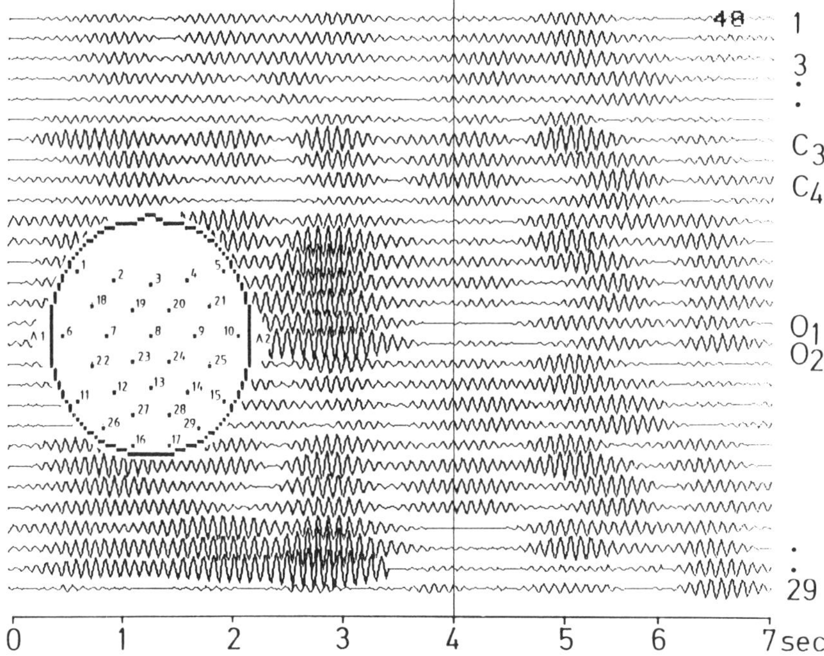

Figure 2. EEG data from one trial (epoch 7 s, filtered in the 10–12-Hz band).

for artifact control and stored on an optical disk. The EEG trials were processed according to the method described elsewhere (Pfurtscheller et al., 1988). After digital band pass filtering, squaring of the samples and averaging over all trials, band power values were obtained. In order to reduce the variance, eight consecutive power values were averaged and, in this manner, power values were obtained at intervals of 125 ms for each channel. The first second of each trial was chosen as a reference interval and the percentage alpha power decrease (or increase), as a measure of the ERD (or ERS) (Pfurtscheller and Aranibar, 1979), was calculated for each 125-ms time interval. A four-nearest-neighbor interpolation algorithm (Buchsbaum et al., 1982) was chosen to compute ERD maps from 30 channels at intervals of 125 ms.

An example of one trial of band-pass filtered (10–12 Hz) EEG data is given in Figure 2. It can be seen that, during visual stimulation, occipital alpha waves were blocked, whereas central mu waves were not affected.

Examples of Grand Average ERD Maps

The data displayed in Figure 3 are grand average maps from three studies performed between 1985 and 1988 (study I: 1985, study II: 1987, study III: 1988). In study I (Pfurtscheller and Klimesch, 1989) words were presented on a computer-controlled video terminal with an exposure time of 250 ms. In the first part of the experiment (reading task) the subjects were instructed to read each word silently. Forty-eight words denoting animals or tools were presented consecutively and a warning signal appeared 1 s before word presentation. After the reading task, a recognition task was performed in which the same set of 48 words served as targets and a different, but semantically related, set of 48 words was used as a distraction. The subjects' task was to distinguish between words already presented in the reading task and words that had not been presented before. The verbal response was either "old" or "new."

In another experiment (study II), subjects had to perform first a reading and then a judgment task (Klimesch et al., 1988, 1990a). Here, a slightly different electrode array (see Fig. 1) was implemented. In these tasks, 48 words and 48 numbers (with two digits each) were used. Study III was a replication of study II with a slight modification: three different, randomly mixed interstimulus intervals between the warning and semantic stimulus were used instead of a fixed time period (Klimesch et al., 1990b).

A common finding in all three studies was an occipital localized decrease of alpha power in the reading and recognition tasks. A significant new observation was a strictly localized alpha power enhancement over both central regions focused at the electrodes C_3 and C_4. This alpha power enhancement was dominant when no verbal response was required; in other words, it occurred primarily in the reading task and less often in the recognition task.

The statistical results (Wilcoxon text for paired differences) of groups II and III (study I had different electrode positions) for two time intervals (375–500 and 500–625 ms) and different electrode positions are summarized in Table 1. The alpha power, for example, was increased by 41.5% ($SE = \pm 12.24, p < 0.01$) at electrode C_4 (at time 500–625 ms poststimulation) and decreased by 30.9% ($SE = \pm 10.02, p < 0.01$) at electrode TPO_2 (at time 500–625 ms).

The major results of these three studies, which were performed in different years and with different groups of subjects, can be summarized as follows:

Synchronization (ERS) and desynchronization (ERD) of alpha frequency components can be observed within the same time interval on different locations on the scalp.

Desynchronization during a reading task is dominant over the posterior region. The magnitude and area of ERD depend on, besides other factors, the frequency band (upper or lower alpha band) chosen and the type of task (reading or recognition) performed (Klimesch et al., 1988, 1990a; Pfurtscheller and Klimesch, 1989).

Synchronization of alpha frequency components, or ERS, defined as an increase of alpha power, was found mainly during the reading task and was strictly localized to the central electrodes C_3 and C_4 overlying the sensorimotor cortex. The ERS pattern showed a high degree of bilateral symmetry and was dominant in the upper alpha band.

It is of interest to note that the enhancement of central localized alpha band rhythms found in the three independent studies is inversely related to the

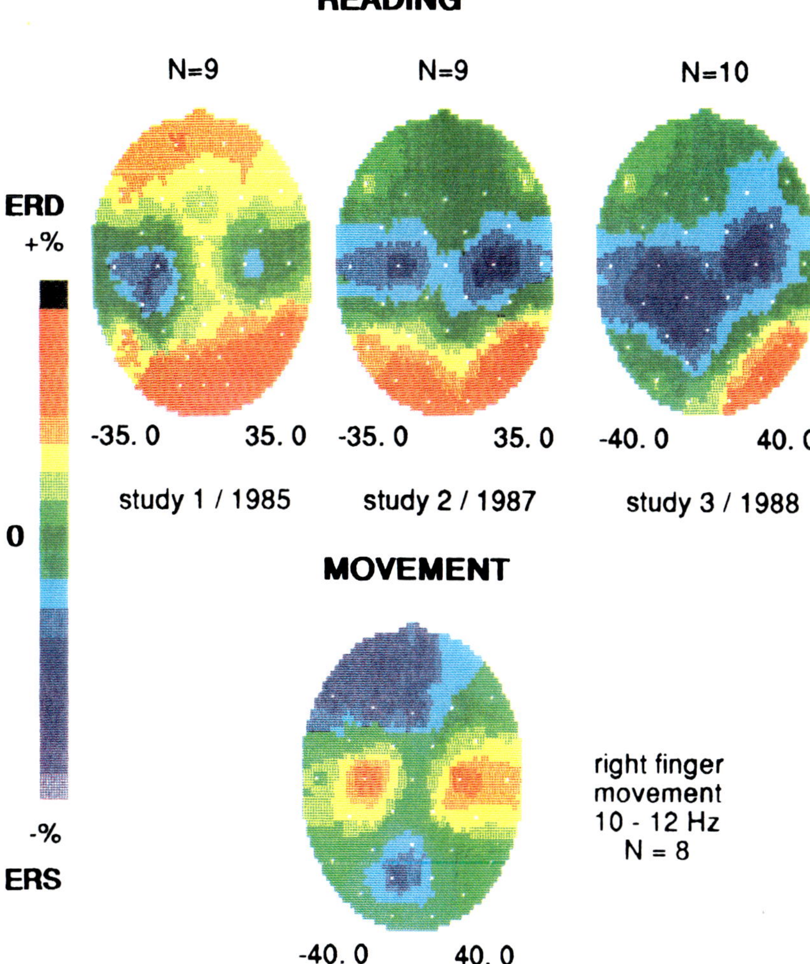

Figure 3. Grand average ERD maps calculated from three reading studies and one voluntary movement experiment. The number of subjects used in each study (N) and the range of power change are indicated for each map. "Red" indicates areas with power decrease or ERD and "blue" areas with power increase or ERS.

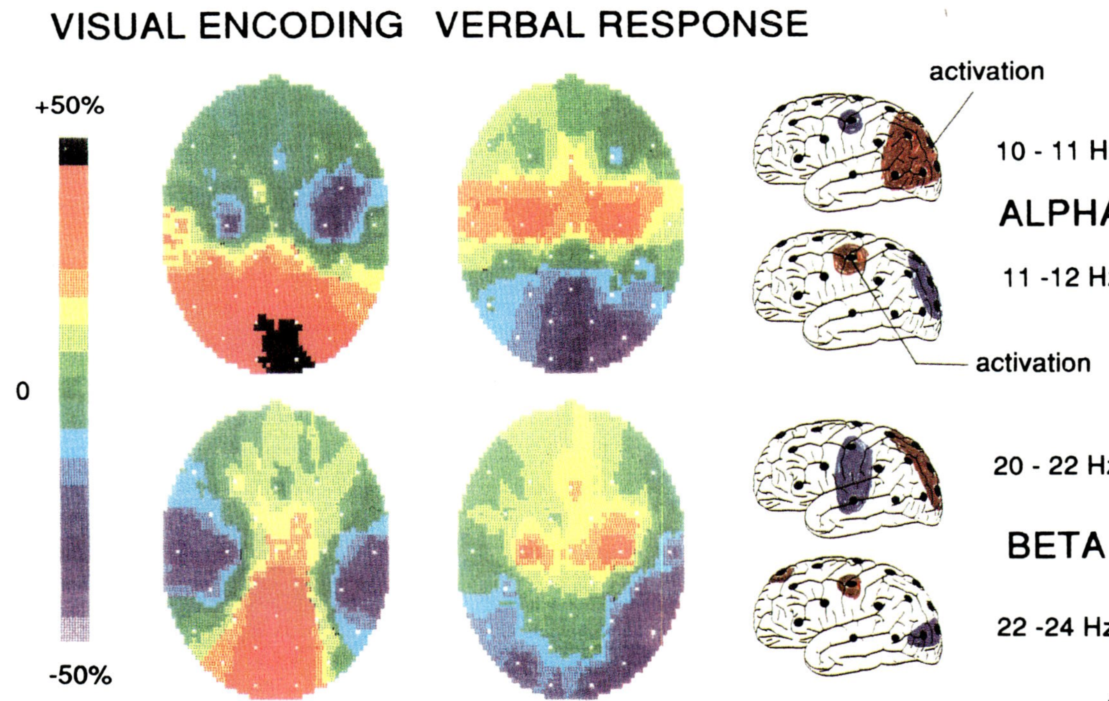

Figure 4. ERD maps calculated from data in the alpha and beta bands as indicated; subject S48. Each map represents a time interval of 125 ms. The maps on the left side were calculated during visual encoding and the maps on the right side during the verbal response. "Red" indicates areas with power decrease or ERD and "blue" areas with power increase or ERS. The position of the electrodes, including the areas with ERD and ERS, are marked in the "lateral brain" views on the right side.

Table 1. Changes in 10–12 Hz power within two time intervals during reading of words for six different electrode positions.[a]

	Left hemisphere				Right hemisphere	
	C_3	TPO_1	O_1	C_4	TPO_2	O_2
X	+29.66	+0.10	+1.02	+42.06	−26.94	−9.89
SE	8.72	12.98	12.26	12.05	10.75	11.98
$p <$	.01	n.s.	n.s.	.01	.05	.05
X	+29.34	−2.61	−0.87	+41.46	−30.88	−13.90
SE	9.41	13.73	13.39	12.24	10.02	11.18
$p <$	.01	n.s.	n.s.	.01	.01	.05

In %, referred to the references interval in which power is assumed to be 100%.
[a] The upper part of the table represents data from the time interval 375–500 ms after reading onset; the lower part represents data from 500–625 ms. Data from studies II and III (19 subjects). The significance of power changes (Wilcoxon text) is indicated.

attenuation of central localized mu rhythms found during voluntary finger movements (see example in Fig. 3 and Pfurtscheller and Berghold, 1989). Since the localization and form of the alpha power enhancement pattern during reading and the alpha power attenuation pattern during movement are quite similar, it can be speculated that the mu rhythm is desynchronized or blocked during planning or execution of motor acts and becomes synchronized during visual processing and immobility.

Analysis of Narrow Frequency Bands

To obtain a better understanding of the phenomena of ERD and ERS, 1-Hz and 2-Hz bands in the alpha and beta range were analyzed in some of the subjects of study III. EEG data from the reading and classification experiments were transformed according to a local average reference to get a more localized ERD pattern during motor activity (Pfurtscheller et al., 1988). The ERD maps from one subject are displayed in Figure 4, representing the reactivity in four frequency bands during reading (left side of Fig. 4) and 700 ms later, during the verbal response (right side of Fig. 4). It is of interest to note that the EEG reactivity during visual encoding was largest in the 10–11-Hz band, whereas the reactivity during the verbal response was maximal in the 11–12-Hz band.

Analysis of 2-Hz bands in the beta range revealed similar ERD maps (Fig. 4, lower part) as found in the alpha band, but nevertheless the areas of desynchronization and synchronization, respectively, were not exactly the same for both bands. In general, alpha desynchronization is accompanied by beta desynchronization, and alpha synchronization by beta synchronization, when the appropriate narrow frequency bands are analyzed.

The similarities and differences between alpha and beta reactivity pattern become more evident when the time courses are displayed (Fig. 5, same EEG

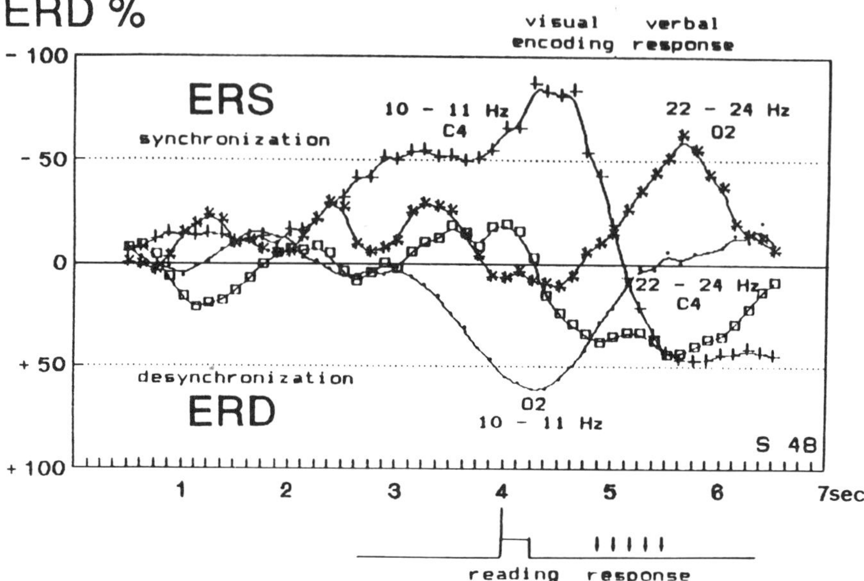

Figure 5. ERD time courses for electrodes C_4 and O_2 displaying changes in alpha and beta power; subject S48. The frequency bands analyzed are marked. Note the contrary behavior of alpha and beta power over central and occipital areas.

data as used in Fig. 4). Figure 5 indicates that ERD and ERS in the 10–11-Hz band start 1 to 2 s before reading and reach their maxima during reading. In contrast to this, the ERD and ERS in the 22–24-Hz band do not start before reading and are most prominent during the verbal response.

The topographical patterns and time courses displayed in Figures 4 and 5 give evidence that neural structures responsible for alpha and beta wave generation do not have the same neural mass and are not activated at the exact same time, but can nevertheless demonstrate similar spatial properties.

Discussion and Final Conclusions

Based on the data reported from three studies with 28 subjects, we can conclude that brain areas involved in the processing of sensory information, planning, or execution of movement or speech display desynchronized or blocked alpha band and/or beta rhythms. Desynchronization is therefore a sign of excited neural mass or activated cortical areas. Cortical areas not activated or not directly involved in performing a task, such as the motor cortex during reading or the visual cortex during movement, can display synchronized or enhanced alpha band and/or beta rhythms. Thus, synchronization of alpha and/or beta waves can be characteristic for inhibited neural mass or a cortical area at rest or in an "idling" state; Morrell (1966) speculated that stimulus-provoked alpha rhythms may be a sign of a central inhibitory process.

Somatosensory rhythms have been identified in the somatic area of normal cats and monkeys. They were synchronized during motionless visual attention and desynchronized by the slightest body movement (Rougeul et al., 1974, 1979); these rhythms were observed in monkeys on restricted foci over the hand area and over the parietal cortex. It is of interest that visual stimulation in an immobile animal can elicit a somatoparietal rhythm. Characteristic for these experiments is the strict localization of the synchronized rhythms to the cortical fields involved in the processing of somatic information or for motor programming.

The synchronization of central and/or parietal localized beta rhythms in animal experiments during immobilization is probably caused by a similar neuronal generator mechanism to that responsible for the synchronization of the mu rhythm in man during visual stimulation. All these data indicate that cortical areas not directly involved in performing a task can display synchronized activity. When such areas are activated, the intrinsic rhythms desynchronize. Another example of synchronized activity are the high-voltage (8–10 Hz) spindles in rats. They displayed the highest amplitude over the sensorimotor area while the rat was motionless, and were desynchronized during cortical activation (Buszaki et al., 1988).

In contrast to the desynchronization of alpha or beta frequency components as signs of excited neural mass, there can also be an induced 40-Hz oscillation after visual stimulation in the cat's visual areas (Eckhorn et al., 1988; Gray and Singer, 1989). These 40-Hz oscillations are found in the orientation-specific cortical columns as first described by Hubel and Wiesel (1962). For us, it does not appear to be an arbitrary coincidence that the 40-Hz synchronization (actual frequency in cats from 35–85 Hz) starts about 140 ms after simulus onset (Eckhorn et al., 1989), exactly within the time period when the alpha rhythm starts to desynchronize. It can be hypothesized that alpha desynchronization is a prerequisite for 40-Hz synchronization. The 40-Hz oscillations seem to be directly related to encoding and feature linking of visual stimuli (Eckhorn et al., 1988; Gray et al., 1989). The desynchronization of occipital alpha waves during the reading task reaches its maximum about 400 ms after stimulation onset and then gradually decreases. This time of about 400 ms is needed to complete encoding processes such as encoding of lines and their orientation, letters, words, and, finally, semantic encoding (Klimesch, 1988). For a conscious perception of a word that has been read, the occipital alpha desynchronization seems to be necessary. Therefore, it is not surprising that no alpha desynchronization is found in comatose patients after visual stimulation (Pfurtscheller et al., 1983).

In multichannel EEG data, synchronized and desynchronized alpha band activity can be found simultaneously for short time periods at different electrode locations. This fact can help to explain contradictory results on alpha enhancement and alpha attenuation based on a limited number of EEG channels (Galin et al., 1978; Ornstein et al., 1980). Special caution is necessary in interpreting centro-occipital or parieto-occipital EEG recordings because central and occipital areas can behave quite differently, in terms of the generation of alpha band activity, at the same moment of time.

The stimulus-evoked desynchronization of alpha and beta frequency components can be either localized to one scalp electrode or more widespread, appearing on several different recording sites. The bioelectrical activity measured with one scalp electrode represents the spatial average of the electrical potentials generated in underlying cortical tissue in the size of at least several square centimeters (Cooper et al., 1965). Amplitude changes in the form of an attenuation or enhancement of alpha waves mean that neural mass of at least some cm^2 changes its coherent activity. For the measurement of a stimulus-related increase or decrease of alpha or beta waves in scalp EEG, the synchronization or desynchronization of thousands of cortical modules is a necessary prerequisite.

From the different bioelectrical reactions after visual stimulation—event-related alpha desynchronization and stimulus-induced 40-Hz oscillations in the visual cortex—it can be concluded that desynchronization is not exclusively a sign of cortical activation. Forty-Hz oscillation strongly depends on the cortical organization of the columns after ocular stimulation and may provide a general mechanism for feature-linking via synchronous activity between different cortical columns. Desynchronization of upper alpha frequency components may be a prerequisite for 40-Hz oscillations and may reflect further processing of visual information including memory access and conscious visual experience. In contrast to upper alpha band desynchronization, lower alpha band desynchronization is widespread, longer lasting (up to some seconds), and can typically be found even before visual stimulation; it probably reflects processes of expectation and attention.

Different frequency components in the EEG from about 7 to 80 Hz can display stimulus-induced patterns of synchronization or desynchronization of different duration, topographical display, and area size. It seems that with increasing frequency, the reactive cortical area becomes more circumscribed and localized, the duration of EEG reactivity becomes shorter, and the size of facilitated neural mass decreases.

Acknowledgment. The authors would like to thank Dr. Schimke and Mr. Mohl for their help in data acquisition and processing and Mag. Clara Kirschner for preparing the manuscript. Supported by the "Fonds zur Förderung der wissenschaftlichen Forschung" in Austria, projects S49 MED -02 and -04.

References

Andersen P, Andersson SA (1968): Thalamic origin of cortical rhythmic activity. In: *The Neuronal Generation of the EEG. Handbook of Electroencephalography and Clinical Neurophysiology*, Creutzfeldt O, ed. Amsterdam: Elsevier, 2c:90–118

Aranibar A, Pfurtscheller G (1978): On and off effects in the background EEG during one-second photic stimulation. *Electroencephalogr Clin Neurophysiol* 44:307–316

Berger H (1930): Über das Elektrenkephalogramm des Menschen II. *J Psychol Neurol* 40:160–179

Buchsbaum MS, Rigal F, Coppola R, Cappelleti J, King AC, Johnson J (1982): A new system for gray-level surface distribution maps of electrical activity. *Electroencephalogr Clin Neurophysiol* 53:237–242

Buzsaki G, Bickford RG, Ponomareff G, Thal LJ, Mandel R, Gage FH (1988): Nucleus basalis and thalamic control of neocortical activity in the freely moving rat. *J Neurosci* 8(11):4007–4026

Chatrian GE, Petersen MC, Lazarte JA (1959): The blocking of the rolandic wicket rhythm and some central changes related to movement. *Electroencephalogr Clin Neurophysiol* 11:497–510

Cooper R, Winter AL, Crow HJ, Walter WG (1965): Comparison of subcortical, cortical and scalp activity using chronically indwelling electrodes in man. *Electroencephalogr Clin Neurophysiol* 18:217–228

Creutzfeldt O, Grünewald G, Simonova O, and Schmitz H (1969): Changes of the basic rhythms of the EEG during the performance of mental and visuomotor tasks. In: *Attention in Neurophysiology*, Evans CR, Mulholland TB, eds. London: Butterworth, pp 148–168

Eckhorn R, Bauer R, Jordan W, Brosch M, Kruse W, Munk M, Reitboeck HJ (1988): Coherent Oscillations: A Mechanism of feature linking in the visual cortex? *Biol Cybern* 60:121–130

Eckhorn R, Reitboeck HJ, Arndt M, Dicke P (1989): A neural network for feature linking via synchronous activity: results from cat visual cortex and from simulations. In: *Models of Brain Function*, Cotterill RMJ, ed. Cambridge: University Press, 255–272

Galin D, Johnstone J, Herron J (1978): Effects of task difficulty on EEG measures of cerebral engagement. *Neuropsychologia* 16:461–472

Gastaut H, Terzian H, Gastaut Y (1952): Etude d'une activité électroencéphalographique méconnue: le rythme rolandique en arceau. *Marseille Méd* 89:296–310

Gray CM, König P, Engel AK, and Singer W (1989): Oscillatory responses in cat visual cortex exhibit inter-columnar synchronization which reflects global stimulus properties. Nature 338:334–335

Gray CM, Singer W (1989): Stimulus-specific neuronal oscillations in orientation columns of cat visual cortex. *Proc Natl Acad Sci USA* 86:1698–1702

Hubel DH, Wiesel TN (1962): Receptive fields, binocular interaction, and functional architecture in the cat's visual cortex. *J Physiol* 160:106–154

Jasper HH, Andrews HL (1938): Electroencephalography III. Normal differentiations of occipital and precentral regions in man. *Arch Neurol Psychiatr* 39:96–115

Jasper HH, Penfield W (1949): Electrocorticograms in man: effect of the voluntary movement upon the electrical activity of the precentral gyrus. *Arch Psychiatr Z Neurol* 183:163–174

Klimesch W (1988): *Struktur und Aktivierung des Gedächtnisses: Das Vernetzungsmodell: Grundlagen und Elemente einer übergreifenden Theorie.* Toronto–Bern: Huber

Klimesch W, Pfurtscheller G, Mohl W (1988): ERD mapping and long-term memory: the temporal and topographical pattern of cortical activation. In: *Functional Brain Imaging*, Pfurtscheller, G, Lopes da Silva FH, eds. Toronto: Huber, pp 131–141

Klimesch W, Pfurtscheller G, Mohl W, Schimke H (1990a): Event-related desynchronization, ERD mapping and hemispheric differences for words and numbers. *Int J Psychophysiol* 8:297–308

Klimesch W, Pfurtscheller G, Schimke H, and Mohl W (1990b): Pre- and poststimulus processes in semantic classification as measured by event-related desynchronization. *J Psychophsiol* in press

Kreitman N, Shaw JC (1965): Experimental enhancement of alpha activity. *Electroencephalogr Clin Neurophysiol* 18:147–155

Lopes da Silva FH, van Lierop THMT, Schrijver CF, Storm van Leeuwen W (1973a): Organization of thalamic and cortical alpha rhythms: spectra and coherences. *Electroencephalogr Clin Neurophysiol* 35:627–639

Lopes da Silva FH, van Lierop THMT, Schrijver CF, Storm van Leeuwen W (1973b): Essential differences between alpha rhythms and barbiturate spindles: spectra and thalamo-cortical coherences. *Electroencephalogr Clin Neurophysiol* 35:641–645

Morrell LK (1966): Some characteristics of stimulus provoked alpha activity. *Electroencephalogr Clin Neurophysiol* 21:552–561

Moruzzi G, Magoun HW (1949): Brainstem reticular formation and activation of the EEG. *Electroencephalogr Clin Neurophysiol* 1:455–473

Ornstein R, Johnstone J, Herron J, Swencionis C (1980): Differential right hemisphere engagement in visuospatial tasks. *Neuropsychologia* 18:49–64

Pfurtscheller G, Aranibar A (1977): Event-related cortical desynchronization detected by power measurements of scalp EEG. *Electroencepalogr Clin Neurophysiol* 42:817–826

Pfurtscheller G, Aranibar A (1979): Evaluation of event-related desynchronization (ERD) preceding and following voluntary self-paced movement. *Electroencephalogr Clin Neurophysiol* 46:138–146

Pfurtscheller G (1981): Central beta rhythm during sensory motor activities in man. *Electroencephalogr Clin Neurophysiol* 51:253–264

Pfurtscheller G, Schwarz G, Pfurtscheller B, List W (1983): Quantification of spindles in comatose patients. *Electroencephalogr Clin Neurophysiol* 56:114–116

Pfurtscheller G, Steffan J, Maresch H (1988): ERD mapping and functional topography: temporal and spatial aspects. In: *Functional Brain Imaging*, Pfurtscheller G, Lopes da Silva FH, eds. Toronto: Huber, pp. 117–130

Pfurtscheller G, Berghold A (1989): Patterns of cortical activation during planning of voluntary movement. *Electroencephalogr Clin Neurophysiol* 72:250–258

Pfurtscheller G, and Klimesch W (1989): Cortical activation pattern during reading and semantic classifications studied with dynamic ERD mapping. In: *Topographic Brain Mapping of EEG and Evoked Potentials*, Maurer K, ed. Berlin: Springer, pp 303–313

Rougeul A, Corvisier J, Letalle A (1974): Rythmes electrocorticaux caracteristiques de l'installation du sommeil naturel chez le chat. Leurs rapports avec le comportement moteur. *Electroencephalogr Clin Neurophysiol* 37:41–57

Rougeul A, Bouyer JJ, Dedet L, Debray O (1979): Fast somato-parietal rhythms during combined focal attention and immobility in baboon and squirrel monkey. *Electroencephalogr Clin Neurophysiol* 46:310–319

Sergeant J, Geuze R, van Winsum W (1987): Event-related desynchronization and P300. *Psychophysiology* 24(3):272–277

Steriade M, Llinas RR (1988): The functional states of the thalamus and the associated neuronal interplay. *Physiol Rev* 68(3):649–742

Magnetoencephalographic Evidence for Induced Rhythms

KNUD SAERMARK, KELD B. MIKKELSEN, and EROL BAŞAR

Induced rhythmic oscillations of neuronal activity in the brain is a fascinating subject that holds promise of being of importance in understanding pattern formation in the central neurons system (CNS). Since the pioneering work by Adrian and Matthews (1928) there have been a number of publications in this field (see chapter by Bullock, this volume). Such induced (i.e., stimulus- or event- induced) as opposed to driven rhythmic oscillations have been recently shown by means of electrode experiments in animals (Eckhorn et al., 1988; Freeman and van Dijk, 1987; Gray and Singer, 1987; Gray et al., 1989; see Gray et al. and Eckhorn et al., this volume) and the experimental recordings include single unit spike trains, local field potentials (LFP), and multiple unit activities. Of interest in this connection is the discovery by Llinas and co-workers (Llinas, 1989; Steriade and Llinas, 1988) of "autorhythmic" neurons capable of acting as oscillators with multiple eigenfrequencies (e.g., 6 and 10 Hz) or as resonators that may be excited in a resonant way. Also in this case the experimental results are based on electrode experiments essentially of single unit character.

The above-mentioned results indicate a connection between EEG recordings and single unit recordings. It is worth noting that the earlier work of Başar (for a review see Başar, 1980) based on intracranial as well as scalp electrode measurements, as a working hypothesis made use of the concept of a resonant excitation of EEG sources. In particular, it was assumed that evoked potentials could be regarded as a resonant excitation of EEG sources and a frequency-dependent enhancement factor was defined in terms of an rms value for a prestimulus interval (spontaneous activity) and a peak–peak value for a relevant poststimulus interval (evoked activity). It was also emphasized that the dynamic aspects of the extremely complicated brain structure necessitate a consideration not only of the (simple) average of the recorded epochs, but also of the individual single epochs. Thus, a selective averaging is called for.

In this chapter we present magnetoencephalographic evidence, however meager it may appear, for induced rhythmic activity in the brain. As biomagnetic measurements are less well known than conventional EEG measurements, a few introductory comments may be in order. Biomagnetic measurements are noninvasive and contactless measurements of a component of the magnetic field generated by sources in the subject under examination [for reviews see, e.g., Hari and Ilmoniemi (1986); Hoke (1988)].

The measurements are performed by means of a single- or multichannel SQUID system and precautions are taken (ideally a magnetically shielded room) to reduce ambient magnetic noise as much as possible. In magnetoencephalographic recordings (MEG) the instrument is positioned as close as possible to the skull, without touching (magnetic sensor to skull distance 1–1.5 cm), and the magnetic field component perpendicular to the skull is measured. It is now important to note that the sources for the magnetic field measured as specified above are intracellular currents in the neurons. This statement is exact for certain geometrical headshapes and for certain homogeneity requirements; in practice, however, it appears to be an excellent approximation. Thus, the measured magnetic field is in a dominant way determined by intracellular currents, whereas the volume currents (extracellular currents flowing in all directions) responsible for the conventionally measured EEG have no or negligible influence. As a source model one often uses a stationary, equivalent current dipole (ECD) and the measured field is then determined by the tangential component of the current dipole moment.

Comparing the magnetic measurements with the intracranial electrode measurements one notes obvious source differences. Although the sources underlying the various recordings (single and multiple unit spike trains, LFPs, magnetic) are, in a not too transparent way, related to each other, one must expect results that supplement each other rather than reproduce each other.

Spontaneous Oscillations

As the relation between spontaneous oscillations and induced rhythms is at the center of focus, we begin with a review of our results concerning the distribution of the spontaneous magnetic activity across the cortical surface. There is of course some intersubject variability and the results presented here will mainly refer to subjects having a rather pronounced alpha activity. In general the parameters of the measurement were: Time-epoch $T = 120$ s and sampling frequency $fs = 200$ Hz. As the available SQUID system allows for only seven simultaneously measured magnetic channels, one has to move the cryostat sequentially from one measuring position to the next in order to cover all of the skull area; this is of course a drawback, which can only partly be remedied by use of a (very expensive) 37-channel SQUID system recently made commercially available. The total number of measuring positions, and thus the total number of magnetic channels, varied from subject to subject.

To illustrate the spatial variation of the spontaneous activity we show in Figure 1 a contour plot of the rms value for the magnetic recordings bandpass filtered in the band 2–25 Hz. A total of 266 channels were used and the contour plot is shown in a stereographic projection onto the tangent plane at the vertex of the subject. The scales are in cm; thus the vertex is at the center (0, 0) while negative (positive) values on the vertical axis signify left (right)

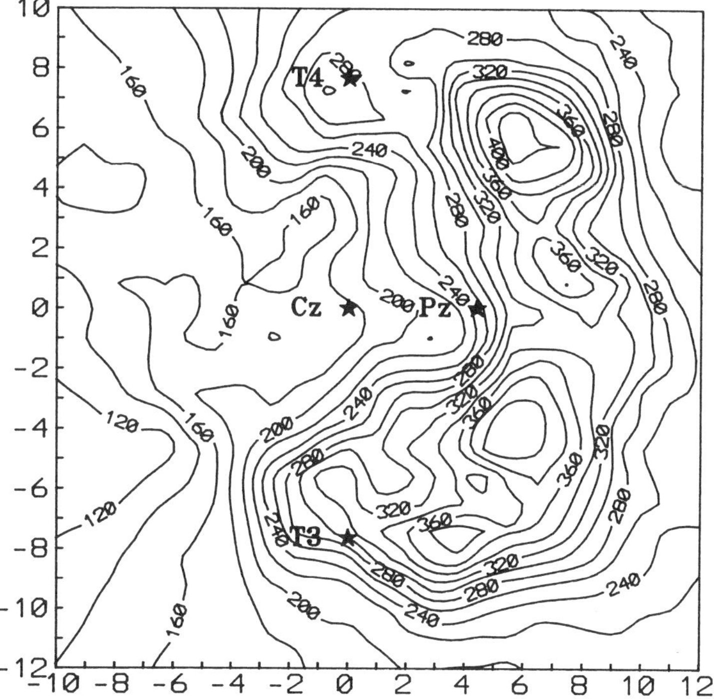

Figure 1. Contour plot for rms values (arbitrary units; 2–25 Hz) of spontaneous oscillations for a normal-subject. Stereographic projection; projection plane: tangent-plane to vertex. Scales: cm. Positive/negative ordinates: right/left hemisphere; negative/positive abscissae: anterior/posterior. A few 10/20 positions are shown as stars. There are 266 measuring channels uniformly distributed within the frame.

hemisphere and negative (positive) values on the horizontal axis signify anterior (posterior) regions. This convention is used throughout this chapter.

From Figure 1 one notes that the distribution of the rms values is almost symmetric across the two hemispheres, possibly with a slight left hemisphere dominance. Clearly, there are several local maxima; in particular, we draw attention to the local maximum observed at the position (0, −6) because the existence of this maximum will be of interest in the next section. An rms value, however, is determined by the total area below the spectral density curve and is thus not able to display the frequency content of a polychromatic recording. In Figures 2 and 3 we therefore show contour plots based on the amplitudes of the spectral density curve as observed at the fixed frequencies 10 and 20 Hz, respectively, from same subject and epochs. From Figure 2 one notes that the 10-Hz alpha activity is confined to the posterior regions of the two hemispheres, is rather symmetric with respect to the two hemispheres, and that the local maximum at (0, −6) still exists. In the 20-Hz regime displayed in Figure 3, on the other hand, one finds clearly developed and symmetrically located

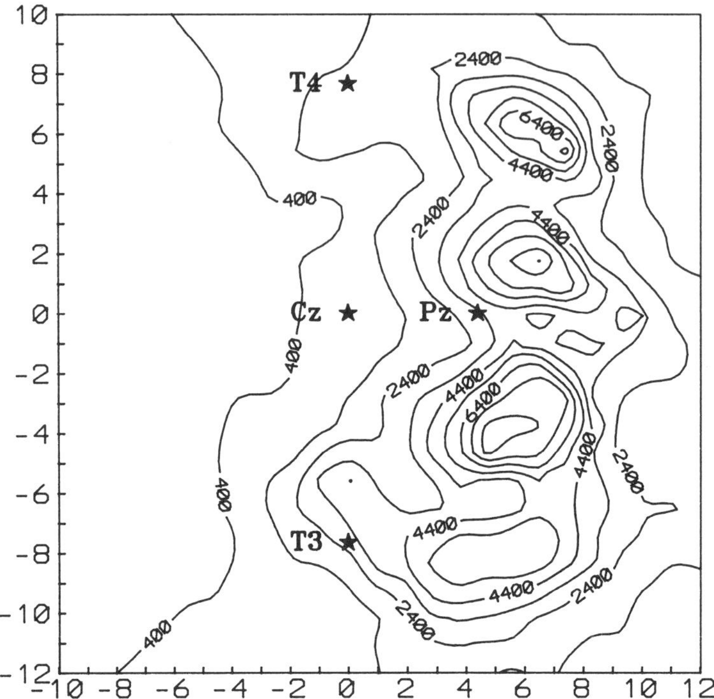

Figure 2. Contour plot for the amplitude of the spectral density as observed at 10 Hz, from the same subject and recordings as Fig. 6.1

maxima in the midtemporal regions and only weaker activity in frontal and occipital regions. The reason for focusing the attention on these two frequency values will become clear from the next section.

It is unfortunately not possible from contour plots of the type shown in Figures 1 through 3 to deduce secure information on the sources of the MEG recordings. For this purpose one would need isofield contour plots and, as the spontaneous activity is a rather global activity, that implies the use of a true multichannel SQUID system instead of the seven-channel system at our disposal. However, a comparison of Figure 2 with Figure 4 (bottom right)—to be discussed in the next section—may indicate that the sources for the alpha oscillations can be modeled as a collection of ECDs. For the present purpose, however, the noteworthy feature is the existence of the local maximum at the position around the point (0, −6) in Figures 1 and 2. As mentioned earlier, there is of course some intersubject variability; however, the features presented in Figures 1 and 2 appear to be typical for the subjects examined hitherto, at least for subjects with a pronounced alpha activity. The contour plot of Figure 3 (i.e., the distribution of the amplitude of the spectral density at the frequency 20 Hz) cannot, on the other hand, be interpreted in terms of an

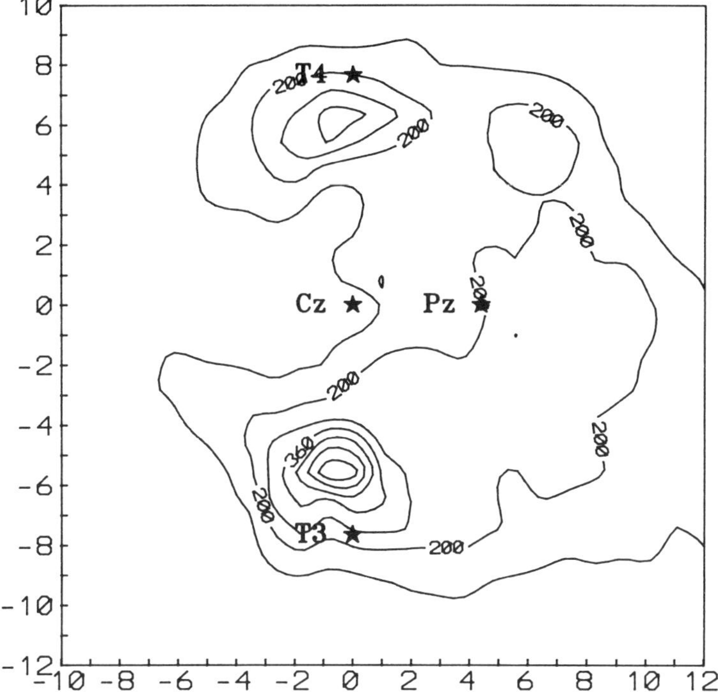

Figure 3. Contour plot for the amplitude of the spectral density as observed at 20 Hz, from the same subject and recordings as Figure 6.1

equivalent current dipole. Here a more complicated source structure is needed, possibly in the form of a closed current loop giving rise to a magnetic moment oriented more or less perpendicular to the skull.

Evoked Fields and Induced Rhythms

We now turn to induced rhythms as observed in connection with evoked magnetic fields. We here confine ourselves to results obtained by the use of auditory stimuli applied monaurally. Several different types of stimuli (tone burst, verbal stimuli, clicks, frequency-glide stimuli, etc.) have been used but the results presented here are based on tone-burst experiments. As a hallmark for the existence of induced rhythms, the observed oscillations should be not driven; they are preferably of a duration longer than the stimulus period and time-locked to the onset of the stimulus. We present results based on (simple) averages of the recorded epochs as well as on single epochs.

There is a general consensus that the source for the auditory evoked N100 magnetic field can be well represented by an ECD located in or close to the

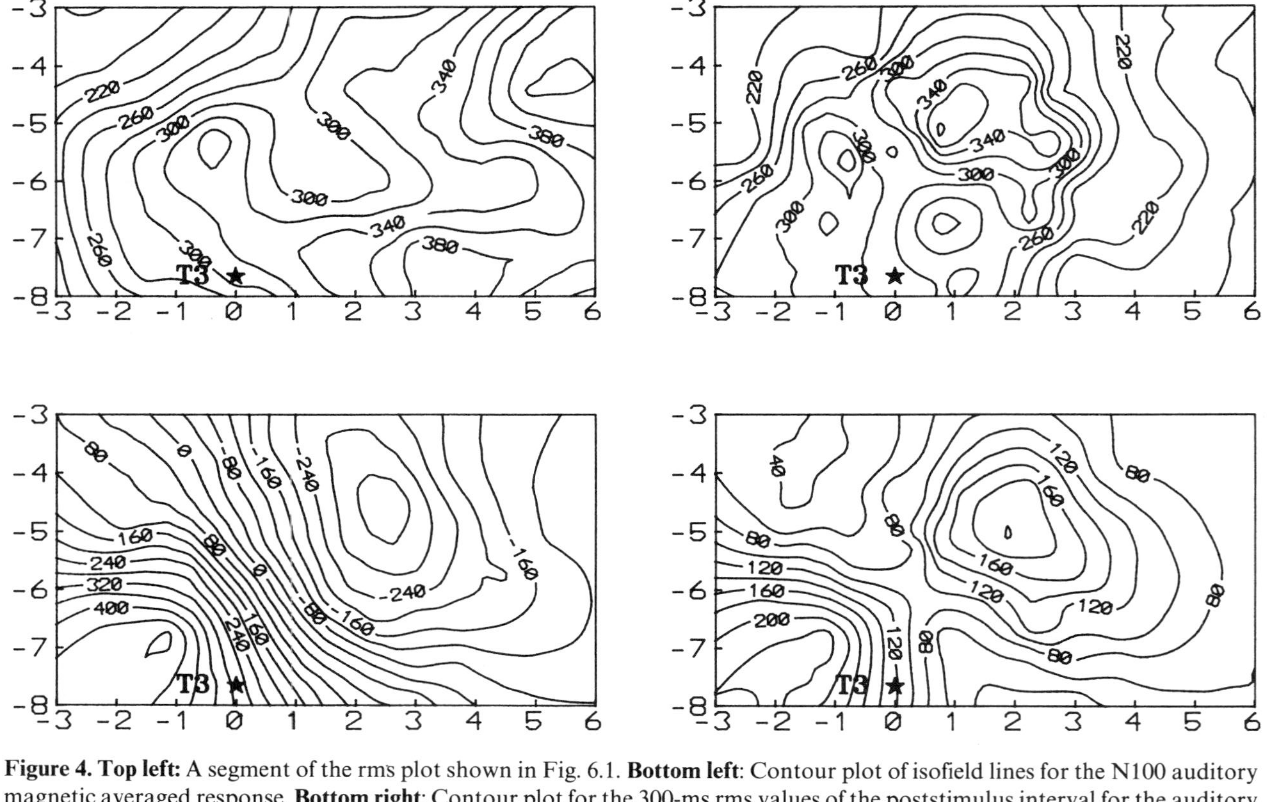

Figure 4. Top left: A segment of the rms plot shown in Fig. 6.1. **Bottom left**: Contour plot of isofield lines for the N100 auditory magnetic averaged response. **Bottom right**: Contour plot for the 300-ms rms values of the poststimulus interval for the auditory magnetic response. **Top right**: Contour plot for the 2–25 Hz rms values of the 300-ms pre-stimulus interval for the auditory magnetic evoked response measurement. All plots are for the same subject.

primary auditory cortex. To illustrate this we show in Figure 4 (bottom left) an isofield contour plot for the N100 signal (stimulus: 1 kHz tone burst of duration 500 ms, 100 epochs, and random interstimulus interval). This experimental plot is extremely well fitted by means of an ECD (correlation coefficient with dipole fit 0.985). This does not imply, however, that deviations from a model consisting of a single equivalent dipole cannot exist. To facilitate comparison especially with Figure 2 we further show in Figure 4 (bottom right) a contour plot for the rms values of the poststimulus (300 ms) period of the same data. Clearly, the topological structure shown there, where as mentioned the underlying signal source is known to be well approximated by an ECD, is reminiscent of the topological structure of at least the right hemisphere occipital part of Figure 2, whereas there may be some differences as regards the left hemisphere part of Figure 2. This similarity possibly allows for the conclusion that the source structure of the spontaneous alpha oscillations displayed in Figure 2 can be approximated by a collection of a small number of (localized) ECDs. For comparison we also show in Figure 4 (top left) a smaller segment of Figure 2, and Figure 4 (top right) a contour plot of the rms value for the prestimulus (300 ms) interval of the evoked response experiment.

A comparison of Figure 4 with Figures 1 and 2 now brings out the interesting observation that the local maximum observed at the position (0, -6) in Figures 1 and 2 nearly coincides with the location of the ECD, which is halfway between the two extremes in Figure 4 (bottom left), for the auditory evoked magnetic field. This is also, and more clearly, seen from a comparison of Figure 4 (top left) and Figure 4 (bottom left). The ECD position is maybe shifted slightly in the anterior direction; however, within the present experimental accuracy this cannot be claimed. This coincidence is seen, not only for this subject, but at least for all subjects showing pronounced alpha activity. The significance of the coincidence is not obvious and remains to be clarified. It does not mean that the auditory evoked ECD source position coincides with the unknown position of the alpha source, but it could indicate that there is a relatively close connection between the two types of sources. To substantiate this statement we now consider some results that we believe show the existence of induced rhythmic oscillations at alpha frequencies in connection with auditory evoked magnetic fields (N100/P200).

We first show, in Figure 5, the magnetic N100/P200 complex as observed by means of a first-order single-channel SQUID system. The curves shown are grand averages of the results of five measuring sessions performed within half a year on one subject. The measurements are here taken at 10 positions along a track passing through T4 and being parallel to the T4-Nasion line (Stimulus: 1 kHz tone burst, duration 500 ms, intensity 60 dB above psychoacoustic threshold, random inter stimulus interval, 60 epochs per measuring point). The data have been low pass filtered in the band DC to 25 Hz. From Figure 5 one notes two facts. First, the latency of the N100 signal shows a noticeable spatial variation especially occurring close to the point of polarity reversal, (i.e., above the ECD position). This latency variation has been

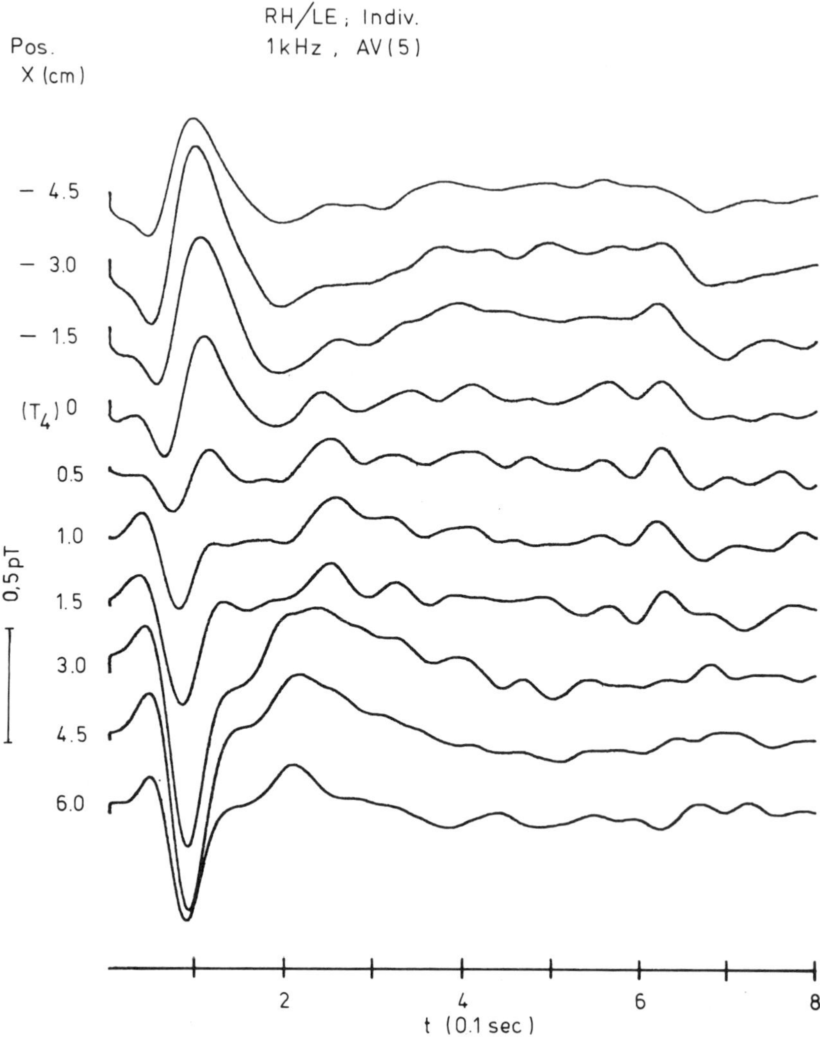

Figure 5. Auditory magnetic response observed along a track through T_4 and nasion. Grand average of five measuring sessions performed within 6 months on one subject. Single channel instrument. Posterior/anterior: negative/positive.

noted earlier (Elberling et al., 1982) and briefly discussed (Saermark, 1983, 1988) and will be dealt with eleswhere. Secondly, one notes a set of weak oscillations, of fast fourier transform (FFT) frequency 13.5 Hz, which are time-locked to the stimulus onset and extend well outside the stimulus duration of 500 ms. The oscillations further appear to be phase-locked to the stimulus in the sense that the oscillation maxima/minima at the different spatial positions occur at the same time positions. Finally, the amplitude of the oscillations is largest close to the point of polarity reversal of the N100 signal ($x = 0.5$ cm). The oscillatory behavior may be made more visible by pairwise additions of the traces in Figure 5 (i.e., -4.5 and 6; -3 and 4.5; etc.); if the measuring positions were strictly symmetric with respect to the dipole position the N100 complex would be eliminated and only the oscillatory behavior remain. Proceeding in this way one finds that the above statements concerning time- and phase-locking to the stimulus are substantiated.

The recordings shown in Figure 5 refer to right hemisphere measurements and are for a subject different from the one of Figures 1 through 4. We return now to left hemisphere measurements (contralateral stimulation) and consider results from a third subject obtained by means of a seven-channel SQUID system. In Figure 6 the two columns marked 0 and 1 refer to two measuring positions, one (pos. 0) with the center coil M1 positioned close to the anterior extreme of the dipolar isofield plot, the other (pos. 1) with the center coil M1 close to the position of the dipole itself (cf. Fig. 4). Each recording in these columns is a simple average of 100 epochs and are "raw" data (bandpass filtered in the band 1–30 Hz) showing a pre- and poststimulus region separated by the dotted line. In column 0, the N100 complex is well developed, but varies in amplitude due to the different spatial positions of the seven measuring coils, whereas there is almost no sign of a regular oscillatory background. In column 1, on the other hand, the N100 complex is not visible, but now there is a clear indication of an oscillatory background. For the same two measuring positions columns 2 and 3, corresponding, respectively, to columns 0 and 1, show the data bandpass filtered in the alpha band 8 to 13 Hz. Column 3 gives rise to the same observation as Figure 5: when the measuring position is close to the ECD position there occurs an excitation of an oscillatory character time-locked to the stimulus onset and with a frequency in the alpha range. A closer inspection further reveals at least a tendency also to a phase-locking in the sense described earlier. For the measuring position of column 2 (anterior extreme in the dipolar isofield plot) this excitation is strongly reduced, in fact, almost nonexisting.

Above, the phrase "with a frequency in the alpha range" was used. The precise value of the frequency is subject-dependent. For comparison with spontaneous oscillations we show in Figure 7 spectral density curves for the poststimulus interval for 42 channels [covering the dipolar region of Figure 4 (bottom left)] and for the subject of Figures 1 through 4 (stimulus, 1 kHz toneburst of 500 ms duration, 100 epochs, 4 s interstimulus interval). The spectral density was evaluated by means of a maximum entropy method, and the curves shown are average values for the 100 epochs. Evidently, there is a "resonant" frequency close to 10 Hz (dotted line) with a spatially varying amplitude. Further, one also observes a peak around 20 to 21 Hz, but this time only at some of the positions, and there may be indications of a small "bump" around 14 to 15 Hz. These observations are in good agreement with the contour plots in Figures 1 through 3.

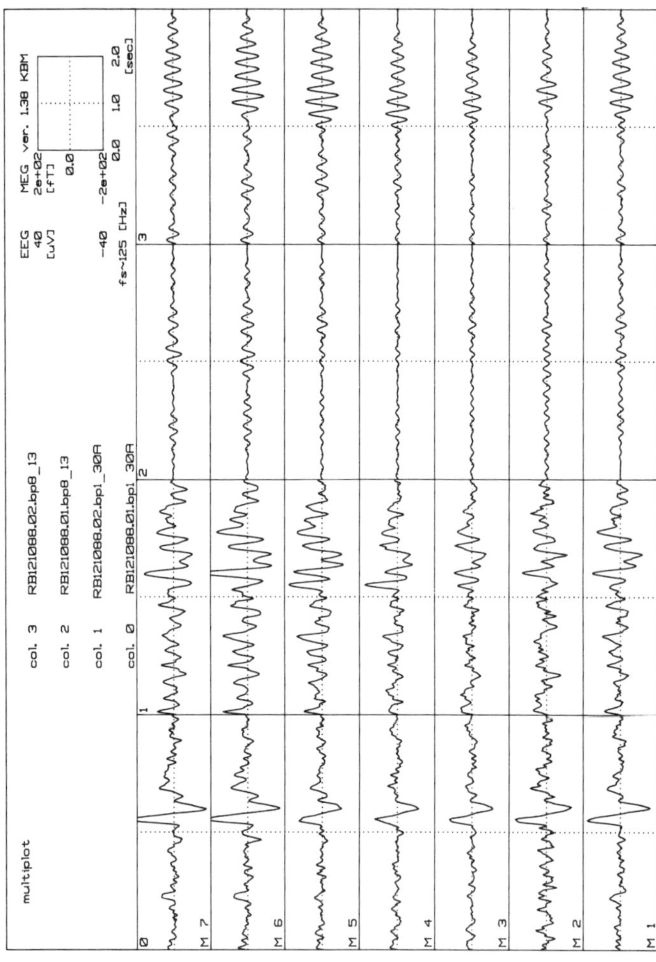

Figure 6. Magnetic recordings of evoked averaged response observed at two cryostat positions. Dotted line: stimulation time; pre- and poststimulus intervals: 500 ms. Column 0: Cryostat position at the extreme value of N100; 1–30 Hz bandpass filtered data. Column 1: Cryostat position right above the equivalent current dipole (polarity reversal of N100); 1–30 Hz bandpass filtered data. Column 2: As in column 0, but for 8–13 Hz bandpass filtered data. Column 3: As in column 1, but for 8–13 Hz bandpass filtered data.

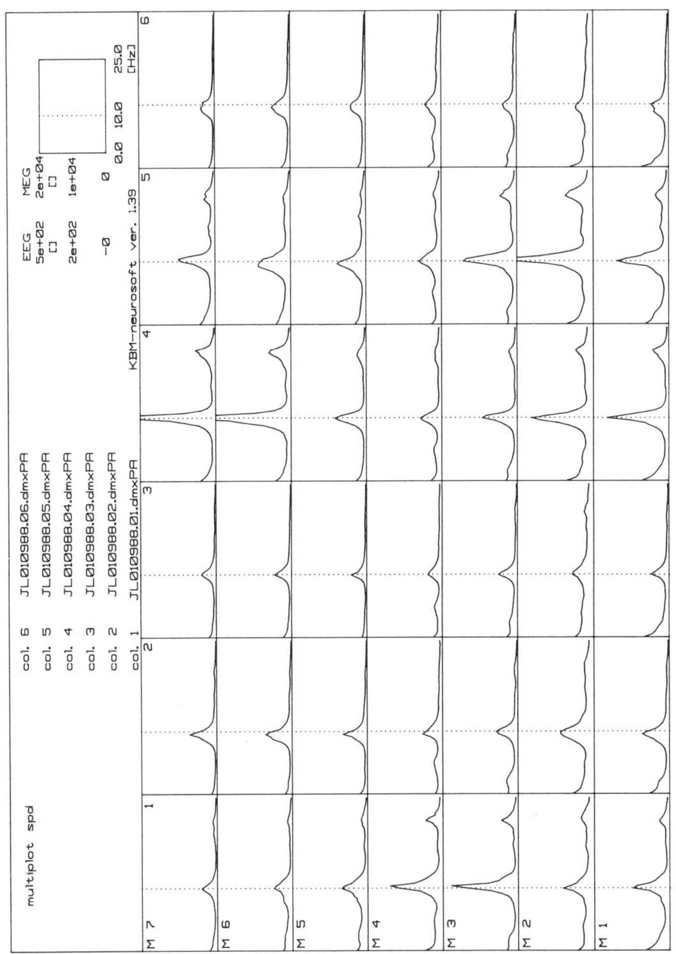

Figure 7. Spectral density (maximum entropy method) for each of 42 channel positions used in the magnetic evoked response experiment resulting in the contour plot shown in Fig. 4.

We briefly summarize the above results as follows. In experiments on auditory evoked magnetic fields (tone burst stimuli) there appears to be a simultaneous excitation 1) of an evoked response rather well modeled by an ECD located at or close to the primary auditory cortex and the dipole position for the N100 and P200 signals appear to (nearly) coincide, and 2) of an oscillatory response with a dominant frequency in the "alpha range" the source of which does not coincide with the ECD, but may or may not be related to the source for the spontaneous (alpha) activity in particular the generators of the local maximum of Figures 1 and 2. Whether or not the two sources are causally connected cannot be determined on the basis of existing evidence. In Başar's original work (see, e.g., Başar, 1980) on evoked potentials he hypothesized that the evoked response could be conceived of as an excitation of the generators of the spontaneous activity and he introduced a frequency window–dependent enhancement factor to describe this relation. On the basis of the biomagnetic experiments it has, however, not been possible in a consistent way to determine such enhancement factors. This does not, of course, exclude the possibility of a causal connection between the two types of signals, but on the face value of the existing evidence we are inclined to consider them as simultaneously excited but independent phenomena.

In the foregoing we have based the consideration mainly on contour plots. In the following we illustrate how the same conclusions follow from the time-domain recordings.

Induced Theta and Alpha Rhythmicities

Başar et al. (this volume) discuss the possibility of recording induced brain rhythmicities in the alpha, theta, delta, and 40-Hz ranges in adequately designed experiments, and show that a number of evoked potential single sweeps contain rhythmicities in the theta and alpha frequency range. Since the spatial resolution of experiments on magnetic evoked fields is significantly higher than that of scalp recording on evoked electrical potentials, there should be a possibility of observing induced rhythmicities in at least the alpha and/or theta frequency also in time recordings of auditory evoked magnetic fields. In order to examine this, we performed a series of experiments on 15 subjects. However, in the following we shall describe the results of only one experiment considered to be representative for most of the subjects under study. According to the nature of the present volume we do not give a detailed account and statistical evaluation of the experimental results. We remark, however, that in a recent communication [see Mikkelsen et al. (1989)], we noted a type of alpha enhancement observed at a temporal location and, at the same time, within a spatial distance of only 2 cm, a type of "alpha blocking." Using the experimental procedure described earlier we recorded for each subject the magnetic evoked fields at a number of cryostat positions. The stimulus was a 1-kHz tone burst at 60 dB HL intensity. For each channel position the FFT amplitude frequency characteristic for the averaged auditory evoked fields was computed (for details of the method see Başar et al., 1979 and Başar et al., this volume). Depending on the recording position the amplitude frequency characteristic showed a distinct maximum at 5 to 7 Hz or a sharp peak at 9 to 10 Hz in temporal locations, and sometimes a compound 5- to 15- Hz to structure.

The advantage of using magnetic recordings (instead of electrical recordings) in the computation of amplitude frequency characteristics is clearly seen from Figure 8. The very pronounced change in the frequency distributions—as a consequence of a spatial displacement of only a few cm—cannot be seen on the basis of electrical recordings from the scalp. How does the evoked response appear in the time domain for two such different frequency characteristics? Figure 9A shows the transient evoked response for the measurement giving rise to the distinct theta maximum in Figure 8A, and Figure 9B illustrates the evoked response (for the same subject) for the measurement giving rise to the high, dominant peak in the alpha-frequency range in Figure 8B. Figure 9 also shows the recorded data band pass filtered in the frequency range of 4 to 10 Hz and in the frequency range of 8 to 13 Hz, respectively. A comparison of the two pair of curves in Figure 9 clearly reveals a rhythmicity in the 10-Hz frequency range corresponding to the sharp alpha peak in the frequency distribution of Figure 8B and a damped theta rhythmicity corresponding to the theta peak in the frequency distribution of Figure 8A. It should also be emphasized that the averaged magnetic response in these cases show almost congruent time courses without any filtering. We add, that an analysis of single sweep responses—as opposed to the averaged response shown in Figures 8 and 9—reveals a large number of sweeps having the same type of oscillatory wave forms in the alpha or theta frequency range. This will be discussed elsewhere.

Discussion

The subject of induced rhythms is both extremely fascinating and important, but it is at the same time a very difficult experimental problem. Whereas the conclusion drawn from the electrode experiments mentioned in the introduction are very convincing, we wish to emphasize that the magnetoencephalographic data on induced rhythms presented here must be regarded only as evidence. We believe, however, that the data do show a (resonant) excitation of rhythmic oscillations time-locked to the stimulus. We have here focused on auditory stimuli of the tone burst type and on (mostly) frequencies in the "alpha range" and we tried to show that the generators of the induced rhythmic activity are closely related to the generators of the spontaneous alpha activity. Our data do indicate excitation also in other frequency bands such as 20 to 22 Hz (cf. the peak in the spectral density curves of Fig. 7), and in an inconclusive way also at the famous 40-Hz region. Our use of auditory stimuli

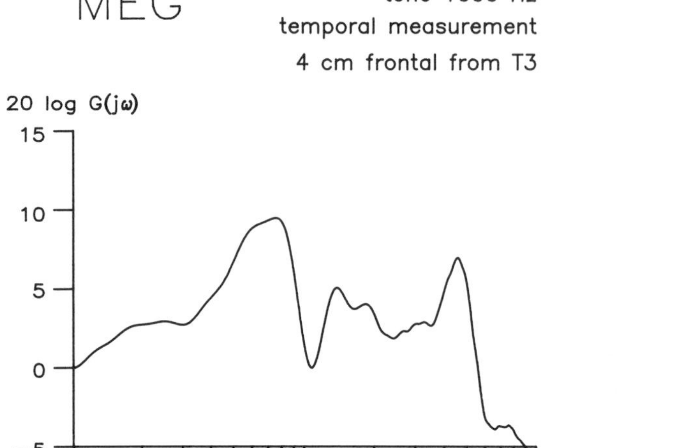

(A)

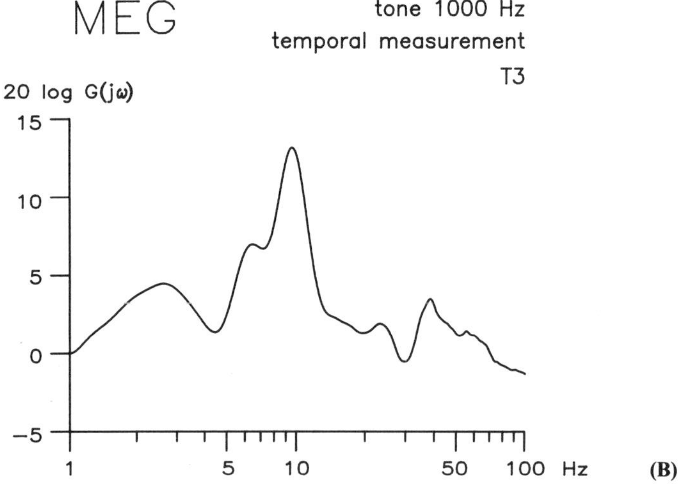

(B)

Figure 8. A: Amplitude frequency characteristic computed by means of FFT from transient evoked magnetic field for a normal subject. Stimulation: 1-kHz tone burst, 60 dB HL. Location: 4 cm frontal from T_3. **B**: As in A, but for the temporal lobe location: T_3.

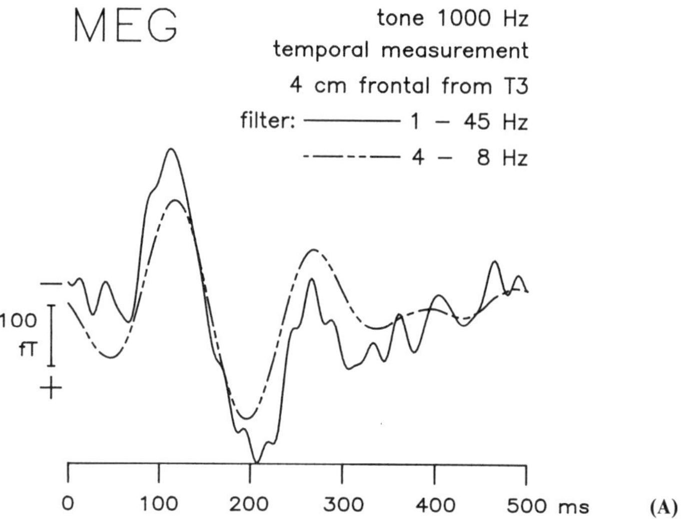

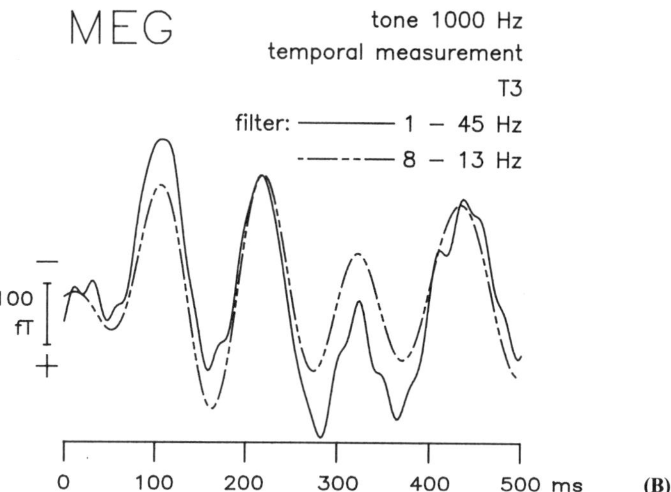

Figure 9. A: Transient evoked magnetic field measured at a position 4 cm frontal from T_3. **B:** Transient evoked magnetic field measured at the temporal position T_3. Same subject as in A. *Dashed curves*: data bandpass filtered in the band 1–45 Hz. *Solid curves*: data bandpass filtered in the bands 4–8 Hz, respectively 8–13 Hz.

in contrast to the visual stimuli used in the electrode experiments is hardly a difference of great significance as the existence of induced rhythmic activity might be assumed to be a general "brain property" (incidentally, we have—unsystematically—performed some visual experiments and further work is in progress).

In the electrode experiments one observes (see, e.g., the summary in Eckhorn et al., 1989 and Eckhorn et al., this volume) synchronization of induced (not time-locked) oscillations even between assemblies of different cortical areas (A17, A18) at positions where common single-cell tuning properties are present. In this connection we remark that the phase-locking (i.e., synchronization) observed in Figures 5 and 6 cannot be interpreted in this way even if the mutual separation between the magnetic channels is 2 cm; the phase-locking means, rather, that the rhythmic signals picked up by the various magnetic channels are due to a single source complex.

Despite the differences mentioned above, we believe that the magnetoencephalographic evidence presented here indicates that the observed time-locked stimulus-induced rhythmic activity is basically of "the same type" as the one observed by the electrode experiments. If this is correct, and if we are correct in our claim that the rhythmic activity observed in the alpha region is due to a resonant excitation of the sources of spontaneous alpha waves (more generally spontaneous oscillations in general) by sensory stimulation, then an interesting possibility for studying basic CNS functioning exists.

Acknowledgment. We gratefully acknowledge valuable discussions and assistance from C.K. Bak and J. Lebech.

References

Adrian ED, Matthews R (1928): The action of light on the eye. Part III The interaction of retinal neurons. *J Physiol* 65:273–298

Başar E (1980): *EEG–Brain Dynamics. Relation Between EEG and Brain Evoked Potentials.* Amsterdam: Elsevier/North-Holland

Eckhorn R, Bauer R, Jordan W, Brosch M, Kruse W, Munck M, Reitboek HJ (1988): Are form- and motion-aspects linked in visual cortex by stimulus-evoked resonances. Multiple electrode and cross-correlation analysis in cat visual cortex. EBBS-Workshop on Visual Processing of Form and Motion, Tubingen, Confer Vol, p 7

Eckhorn R, Reitboek HJ, Arndt M, Dicke P (1989): A neural network for feature linking via asynchronous activity: results from cat visual cortex and from simulations. In: *Models of Brain Function* Cotterill RMJ, ed. Cambridge: Cambridge University Press pp 255–272

Elberling C, Bak C, Kofoed B, Lebech J, Saermark K (1982): Auditory magnetic fields. Source location and 'Tonotopical Organization' in the right hemisphere of the human brain. *Scand Audiol* 11:61–65

Freeman WJ, van Dijk BW (1987): Spatial patterns of visual cortical fast EEG during conditioned reflex in a rhesus monkey. *Brain Res* 422:267–276

Gray CM, Singer W (1987): Stimulus-dependent neuronal oscillations in the cat visual cortex area 17. 2nd IBRO-Congrs. Neurosci Suppl, 1301P

Gray CM, Konig P, Engel AK, Singer W (1989): Oscillatory responses in cat visual cortex exhibit inter-columnar synchronization which reflects global stimulus properties. *Nature* 338:334–337

Hari R, Ilmoniemi RJ (1986): Cerebral magnetic fields. *CRC Crit Rev Biomed Eng* 14:93–126

Hoke M (1988): Squid-based measuring technique—a challenge for the functional diagnostics in medicine. In: *The Art of Measurement. Metrology in Fundamental and Applied Physics*, Kramer B, ed. Weinhelm: VCH Verlagsgesellschaft pp 287–335

Llinas RR (1989): The intrinsic electrophysiological properties of mammalian neurons: insights into central nervous system function. *Science* 242:1654–1664

Mikkelsen KB, Saermark K, Lebech J, Bak CK, Başar E (1989): Selective averaging in auditory magnetic field experiments. In: *Advances in Biomagnetism* Williamson SJ, Hoke M, Stroink G, Kotani M, eds. New York: Plenum Press, pp 93–96

Saermark K (1983): Some tentative model considerations based on experimental neuromagnetic data. *Il Nuovo Cimento* 2D:438–459

Saermark K, Lebech J, Bak CK (1988): Magnetic fields from the human auditory cortex. In: *Springer Series in Brain dynamics 1* Başar E, ed. Berlin–Heidelberg: Springer–Verlag pp 299–304

Steriade M, Llinas RR (1988): The functional states of the thalamus and the associated neuronal interplay. *Physiol Rev* 68:649–742

Rostrocaudal Scan in Human Brain: A Global Characteristic of the 40-Hz Response During Sensory Input

RODOLFO R. LLINÁS and URS RIBARY

Cortical oscillatory activity in the 40-Hz range has been observed in man during cognitive tasks and following sensory stimulation, as analyzed by electroencephalographic (EEG) and magnetoencephalographic (MEG) means (Galambos et al., 1981; Maekelae and Hari, 1987; Sheer, 1989; Weinberg et al., 1988). Such oscillatory activity is not unique to man but has been seen in many mammalian forms during attentive states (Bouyer et al, 1987) and during physiological stimulation of the olfactory (Bressler and Freeman, 1980) or the visual systems (Eckhorn et al., 1988; Gray and Singer, 1989). However, these 40-Hz activity recording were restricted to localized brain areas and on occasion to small cell groups, to include a few cortical columns. Even in those studies where EEG and MEG recordings were attained, data analysis was restricted to a single time slice at the maximum positive or negative peak of an averaged evoked response. Nevertheless, these studies indicate that 40-Hz coherent neuronal activity large enough to be detected from the scalp is generated during cognitive tasks (cf. Sheer, 1989).

We felt, however, that the 40-Hz oscillatory activity observed in various brain regions could reflect more general processes that could be (at least in part), responsible for the conjunctive nature of the cognitive properties of brain functions. We thus hypothesized that the 40-Hz oscillatory activity could reflect certain patterns and share characteristics that are common to much cortical function (Ribary et al, 1988). It was further proposed that the 40-Hz activity reflected the resonant properties of the thalamocortical system, which is itself endowed with intrinsic 40-Hz oscillatory activity (Ribary et al, 1989; Llinas, 1990; Ribary and Llinas, 1990; Llinás et al, 1991; Ribary et al., 1991).

Recently we have utilized a multichannel magnetic recording to investigate the global organization of the human 40-Hz response over an entire cerebral hemisphere. This approach offers a unique noninvasive methodology capable of localizing and monitoring human brain function in real time (Ribary et al., 1989; Suk et al. 1991; Yamamoto et al., 1988).

Global Organization of 40-Hz Oscillatory Activity in Humans

In these experiments the 14-channel MEG system (BTi) was used to record and analyze the spatial and temporal organization of 40-Hz activity over a cerebral hemisphere during auditory processing in healthy adult subjects. The neuromagnetic measuring system consists of a magnetically shielded room, two cryogenic dewars with seven magnetic sensors each, and a probe-position indicator. The latter determines the position and orientation of the sensors with respect to digitized points over the head (Yamamoto et al., 1988). The recordings were obtained from the right cerebral hemisphere. The two dewars (14 sensors) were used simultaneously to obtain the first 28 sets of responses, while the last seven were obtained using one dewar in the center of the recorded area to complete the 35 recording sites.

The stimuli comprised frequency-modulated tones of 300 ms duration starting at any frequency between 50 and 350 Hz. This modulation swept upward or downward within this range. This procedure was implemented in order to enable us to identify features of the 40-Hz response that were independent of the characteristics of any specific stimulus. The stimulus was binaurally presented at random time intervals and at various intensities ranging from threshold to around 40 dB above threshold. The gated sinusoidal waves could be triggered such that each stimulus would begin with a wave form starting from zero (congruent) or randomly such that the stimulus could begin with a rapid transient (not congruent). No differences in response were detected between these two forms of stimulation.

As stated above, three runs were required for each subject in order to record all 35 positions. During each run 800 epochs were collected from each recording site and averaged. MEG data were recorded using a bandpass filter from 1 to 100 Hz. The epochs were examined offline after bandpassing through a 35- to 45-Hz filter and compared with data, bandpassing through a 25- to 35-Hz and through a 45- to 55-Hz filter. The onset of the stimulus was used to trigger the averaging paradigm.

Fast Fourier transformation (FFT) of averaged MEG data recorded between 1 and 100 Hz showed an increased activity in the higher frequency range between 30 and 50 Hz during auditory processing, with a peak around 40 Hz. In addition, filtered data (35–45 Hz) indicated that synchronized 40-Hz activity was recorded over the entire hemisphere during auditory processing. The largest signal was seen over the lateral occipital, temporal, and frontal areas. Whereas the 40-Hz background wanders in and out of phase among the channels of the probe, it was clearly phase-locked in synchrony among the channels for periods of over 100 to 200 ms after onset of stimulus. Such phase-locking was observable within the area of a single probe (≈ 25 cm^2) (Fig. 1). Similar findings, showing temporal and spatial coherence, were obtained for each of the five probe positions. The phase-locking relative to the stimulus time zero was found to be independent of the absolute amplitude of the response at any site. Significantly, large phase differences in the 40-Hz activity were consistently found between the five probe locations (Fig. 2). There was a small but clear phase shift among the seven channels of each probe that could be followed as a continuous event over the distance along the entire hemisphere (Fig. 2). These phase shifts were consistent around 40 Hz

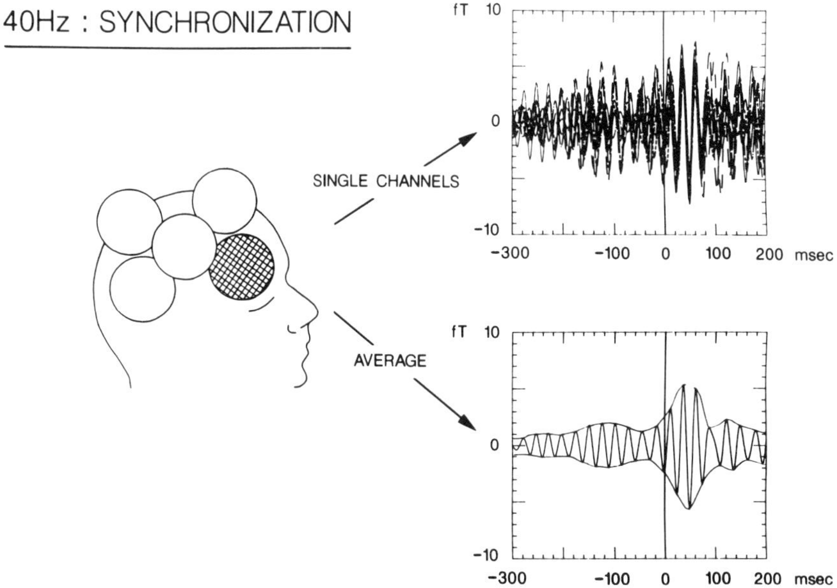

Figure 1. Synchronization of human magnetic 40-Hz oscillatory activity during auditory processing (independent of any stimulus presentation rate), within seven single channels of one probe, placed over lower frontal areas. The graph on the top right indicates a superimposition of 40-Hz activities, time-locked to the stimulus start, recorded from the seven channels. On lower right, the graph indicates an average of all seven channel responses, demonstrating the phase-lock over a larger area (around 25 cm^2).

(35–45 Hz) and disappeared in lower (25–35 Hz) or higher frequency bands (45–55 Hz). This continuous phase shift of the oscillatory activity, within a prime frequency band around 40 Hz, occurred from the frontal to the occipital pole of the hemisphere and corresponded to a shift of the 40-Hz cycle of about 4 to 6 ms from front to back. This phase shift was solely responsible for this dynamic sweep pattern in 40-Hz magnetic activity. At each moment in time, a field pattern consisting of a positive and a negative peak was observed and found to "rotate" continuously over the hemisphere, including the frontal, temporal, parietal, and occipital cortices. We define this rostrocaudal sweep as the phase shift of the positive components of this bipolar field. This shift thus defined is seen to commence, after an initial magnetic silence, over the superior frontal cortex (position 1, Fig. 2), and to traverse over parietal, parieto-occipital (position 2), to occipito-temporal areas (position 3). This rostrocaudal shift is accompanied by a concurrent shift of the negative components in the opposite direction (with a phase difference of about 180°) over the temporal pole (position 4) to inferior or orbitofrontal areas (position 5).

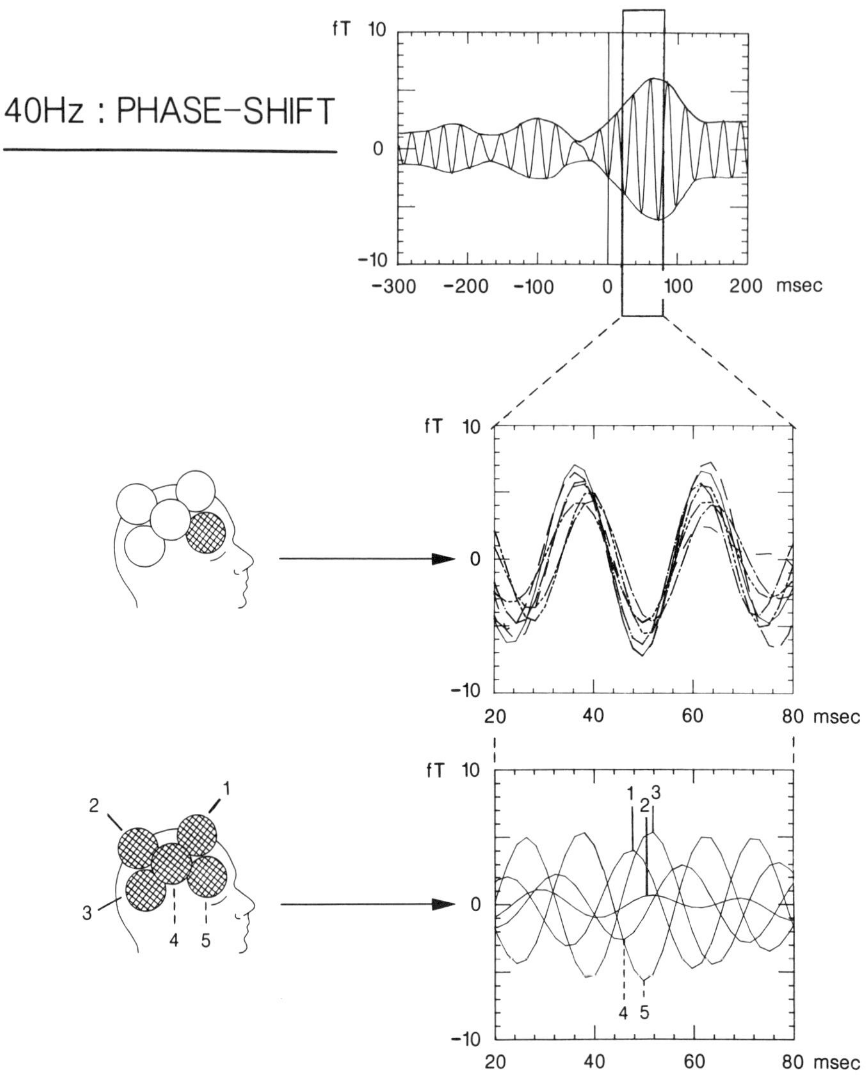

Figure 2. Phase shift of human magnetic 40-Hz oscillatory activity during auditory processing. The time period between 20 and 80 ms after the start of presentation of the auditory stimuli is shown enlarged in the middle and lower panels. The middle panel shows the superimposition of seven channels (sensors) from one probe (inferior frontal, hatched in sketch at left; simultaneous records) and demonstrates small differences in phase within this region. The lowest panel shows the superimposition of average responses from all sensors in each of the five probe positions (hatched and numbered at left; nonsimultaneous records) and demonstrates large, consistent phase shifts from region to region, indicating a continuous rostrocaudal phase shift over the hemisphere.

Discussion

Our recent MEG data indicate that 40-Hz oscillatory activity is synchronized over large cortical areas during auditory processing in man. In addition, these data point to a global organization of the 40-Hz activity over the hemisphere indicating that certain aspects of the auditory processing by the brain may be independent of the properties of the stimuli per se. The finding suggests that, in addition to the processing of the specific properties of the stimuli via auditory pathways, the brain may use a parallel, more global mechanism that allows the stimulus to be placed in temporal context with respect to the intrinsic functional state of the brain at the time the stimulus was presented.

Indeed as expected from the above statement, the 40-Hz activity recorded during auditory processing shows a highly organized spatial and temporal pattern of neuronal oscillation and resonance. The spatiotemporal magnetic field pattern, consisting of a positive–negative field, suggested the presence of a coherent rostrocaudal sweep of activity repeating every 12.5 ms due to a continuous phase shift over the hemisphere (Fig. 2). In addition to the above, preliminary data from studies underway indicate that similar 40-Hz phase shifts and dynamic pattern can be detected in nonaveraged, single epochs during auditory processing, using a 37-channel MEG system (BTi) with a lower noise level and improved sensor equipment. Further support for the sweep hypothesis is provided by the fact that this sweep of a positive–negative magnetic field was absent below or above 40 Hz, as analyzed by using a lower (25–35 Hz) or higher frequency band filter (45–55 Hz). Finally, preliminary data obtained with a 37-channel MEG system (BTi), before auditory stimulation, indicate the presence of brain scanning even during the nonactivated period.

These findings strongly suggest that the 40-Hz activities reflect an internal oscillator, which undergoes a reset at the start of the auditory stimulus and results in a time-locked spatiotemporal coherence from one epoch to the other with respect to the start of stimulation. It is interesting to note that a high variance was found around 40 Hz during auditory processing. This increase was followed by a decrease and a subsequent increase in variance, indicating coherent and "decoupled" oscillatory 40-Hz activity as a function over time and space.

In short, then, these findings indicate the presence of a scanning-like process most probably of intrinsic origin that covers much of the brain surface with a focus on the activated sensory area. Such scanning, we propose, occurs through thalamocortical-resonant synaptic interactions (Llinás, 1990). The thalamus we propose may activate the cortex in a coherent manner such that a wave of electrical activity "sweeps" the cortical mass from its frontal to occipital poles. Such sweep must be accompanied by a radial activity in the corticothalamic axis as it progresses over the cortex in the rostrocaudal direction (Fig. 3).

Although the morphological basis for such sweep has not been identified, several possibilities may be mentioned. One site of origin may be the reticular

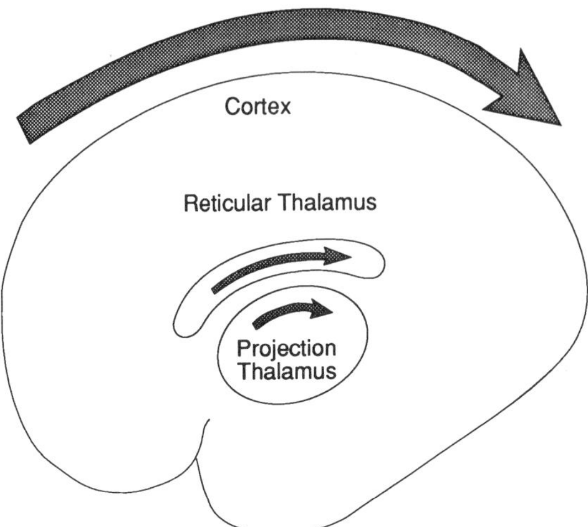

Figure 3. Schematic diagram of the macroscopical organization of the coherent 40-Hz response in the human. The results presented suggest that a coherent rostro-caudal sweep in the phase-shift of the 40-Hz coherent activity occurs every 12.5 ms over the cerebral hemisphere, as indicated by the large arrow over the cortex. We propose that such brain scan is produced by reciprocal neuronal interactions, probably at the reticular nucleus, which produces an organized continuous wave of activity in that nucleus (*arrow*). This sequential activation of the reticular nucleus serves to generate a similar response in the projection thalamus (*arrow*) and via the thalamocortical pathway a similar activity in the cortex. For more details see text.

nucleus of the thalamus, which sends inhibitory projections to the dorsal thalamus as well as recurrent collaterals back to itself (Steriade et al, 1990). Such a negative feedback circuit could, in principle, allow the organized conduction of an inhibitory wave along the rostrocaudal length of the reticular nucleus. The extensive connectivity of this nucleus onto the dorsal thalamus would allow a similar wave of coherent activity to be conducted by the thalamocortical projection system, thereby implementing the scanning process. In addition, the intralaminar nucleus of the thalamus and the pulvinar also projects over sufficiently extensive regions of the cortex (Steriade et al., 1990) to be possible candidates for such scanning or function.

It must be emphasized at this point, however, that the above speculations notwithstanding, the mechanism for this coherent 40-Hz activation of the cortex may ultimately involve feedback resonance between many areas in the cortex and their thalamic counterparts. The fact that our studies indicate a very consistent and stereotyped rostrocaudal organization of brain activity that is observable in individuals of different ages is indicative of the robustness of this phenomenon (Ribary et al, 1989). Moreover, for a given individual the pattern of the phase shift is superimposable from one scan to the next, indicating that a set of well defined constraints must be present in its generation.

At this time all that may be proposed is that the 40-Hz response described here and in previous papers (Ribary et al, 1989) represents a spatially and temporally organized coherent cortical activity. This "brain scan" seems to be reinforced by activities in the corticothalamic pathways, with a focus on the activated sensory area. Ultimately this coherent 40-Hz activity may serve as the basis for the conjunctive property that characterizes the unity of cognitive experience.

Summary

Studies on the auditory system in humans, using the MEG technique, indicate synchronized 40-Hz oscillatory activities, which are highly organized in space and time. We hypothesize that this coherent sweep of 40-Hz response could reflect a scanning of the brain with a focus on the activated sensory area, in order to generate a single percept from multiple sensory components.

Acknowledgments. The authors acknowledge the continued support of Biomagnetic Technologies Inc. (BTi)

References

Bouyer JJ, Montaron MF, Vahnee JM, Albert MP, Rougeul A. (1987): Anatomical localization of cortical beta rhythms in cat. *Neuroscience* 22:863–869

Bressler SL, Freeman, WJ (1980): Frequency analysis of olfactory system EEG in cat, rabbit and rat. *Electroencephalogr Clin Neurophysiol* 50:19–24

Eckhorn R, Bauer R, Jordan W, Brosch M, Kruse W, Munk M, Reitboeck HJ (1988): Coherent oscillations: A mechanism of feature linking in the visual cortex? *Biol Cybern* 60:121–130

Galambos R, Makeig S, Talmachoff PJ (1981): A 40Hz auditory potential recorded from the human scalp. *Proc Natl Acad Sci* 78:2643–2647

Gray CM, Singer W (1989): Stimulus-specific neuronal oscillations in orientation columns of cat visual cortex. *Proc Natl Acad Sci*, 86:1698–1702

Llinas R (1990): Intrinsic electrical properties of mammalian neurons and cns function. *Fidia Research Foundation Neuroscience Award Lectures* 4:173–192

Llinas R, Grace AA, Yarom Y (1991): In vitro neurons in mammalian cortical layer 4 exhibit intrinsic activity in the 10- to 50-Hz frequency range. *Proc Natl Acad Sci USA* 88:897–901

Maekelae JP, Hari R (1987): Evidence for cortical origin of the 40Hz auditory evoked response in man. *Electroencephalogr Clin Neurophysiol* 66:539–546

Ribary U, Ioannides AA, Singh KD, Hasson R and Llinas R. Magnetic field tomography (MFT) of coherent thalamo-cortical 40-Hz oscillation in humans. *Proc Natl Acad Sci* 88:11037–11041, 1991.

Ribary U, Llinas R (1990): The spatial and temporal organization of the 40Hz response in human as analyzed by magnetic recording (MEG). *Eur J Neurosci* 3(Suppl.): 51 (1229)

Ribary U, Llinas R, Kluger A, Suk J, Ferris SH (1989): Neuropathological dynamics of magnetic, auditory, steady-state responses in Alzheimer's disease. In: *Advances in Biomagnetism*, Williamson S, Hoke M, Stroink G, Kotani M, eds. New York: Plenum Press, pp 311–314

Ribary U, Weinberg H, Cheyne D, Johnson B, Holliday S, Ancill RJ (1988): EEG and MEG (magnetoencephalography) mapping for indexing pathological changes in human brain. *Eur J Neurosci* 1(Suppl.): 44.17

Sheer DE, (1989): Sensory and cognitive 40Hz event related potentials: Behavioral correlates, brain function and clinical application. In: *Brain Dynamics*, Başar E, Bullock TH, eds. Berlin: Springer–Verlag, pp 339–374

Steriade M, Jones EG, Llinas R (1990): *Thalamic Oscillations and Signalling*. Neuroscience Research Foundation Inc. New York: John Wiley & Sons

Suk J, Ribary U, Cappell J, Yamamoto T, Llinas R (1991): Anatomical localization revealed by MEG recordings of the human somatosensory system. *Electroencephalogr Clin Neurophysiol* 78: 185–196, 1991

Weinberg H, Cheyne D, Brickett P, Gordon R, Harrop R (1988): An interaction of cortical sources associated with simultaneous auditory and somesthetic stimulation. In: *Functional Brain Imaging*, Pfurtscheller G, Lopes da Silva FH, eds. Toronto: Hans Huber Publishers, pp 83–88

Yamamoto T, Williamson S, Kaufman L, Nicholson C, Llinas R (1988): Magnetic localization of neuronal activity in the human brain. *Proc Natl Acad Sci* 85: 8732–8736

Evoked Potentials: Ensembles of Brain Induced Rhythmicities in the Alpha, Theta and Gamma Ranges

EROL BAŞAR, CANAN BAŞAR-EROGLU, RALPH PARNEFJORD, ELKE RAHN and MARTIN SCHÜRMANN

Summary

This chapter is based on our working hypothesis interpreting the evoked potential (EP) as a stimulus-induced synchronization and enhancement of the spontaneous EEG activity (Başar 1980). According to this hypothesis, the superposition of evoked rhythmicities in several frequency channels can give rise to the compound EP (an example is given in the appendix to this chapter).

Possible functional correlates of evoked rhythmicities in distinct frequency ranges may emerge from a variety of experimental results:

(1) When external sensory stimuli of different modalities are applied to cats, the following observation was made in recordings from primary sensory cortical areas: damped alpha rhythmicities upon adequate stimuli were enhanced whereas alpha rhythmicities upon inadequate stimuli were less marked.

(2) When auditory stimuli with an intensity near the hearing threshold were applied to human subjects, rhythmicities of slow frequency were observed. These slow frequency rhythmicities may reflect the process of decision making for the detection of a tone.

(3) During an "omitted stimulus" paradigm, 40 Hz responses with a latency in the 300 ms range were recorded in cat hippocampus. The 40 Hz responses were associated with P300 responses.

(4) When human subjects had to perform a time prediction task, alpha waves prior to the cognitive target showed higher amplitudes and phase coupling in anticipation of the target.

In summary, high cooperation or synergy in neural tissues—as may be attained in special paradigms—is possibly a prerequisite for the recording of "homogeneous" rhythmicities restricted to distinct frequency channels.

Supported by grants BA 831/5-1 and BA 943/1-1 of the Deutsche Forschungsgemeinschaft (DFG).

Abbreviations: EEG, electroencephalogram; EP, evoked potential; ERP, event-related potential; AFC, amplitude frequency characteristics.

Working Hypothesis on the Relationship Between Evoked Potentials and the Electroencephalogram

For about 15 years our research group has published several reports about a working hypothesis on the brain's electroencephalogram (EEG) and evoked potentials (EPs). This hypothesis has several issues that are interrelated. In our view, the conventional averaged EP, which is widely used and very popular, was considered only as a rough estimate of brain's EEG response, and it was claimed that the averaged EP does not take into account dynamic changes in the brain's intrinsic activity. On the contrary, both single EPs and EP-like EEG segments probably resulting from hidden sensory or cognitive stimulation were considered as the brain's quasi-invariant resonant modes containing important brain frequency codes related to central nervous system function (Başar, 1980, 1983; Başar and Stampfer, 1985; Stampfer and Başar, 1985).

The hypothesis explained in several books and papers can be summarized as follows:

1. The EEG consists of the activity of an ensemble of generators producing rhythmic activity in several frequency ranges. These oscillators are active usually in a random way; however, by application of sensory stimulation these generators are coupled and act together in a coherent way. This synchronization and enhancement of EEG activity gives rise to an "evoked" or "induced rhythmicity" (Başar, 1980: "alpha response," "theta response," "40 Hz (gamma) response," etc.). As an analogy to this event, Figures 1A and 1B show the reordering of elementary magnets in a magnetic field and the schematic analogy with phase ordering of neural populations. This analogy was used to explain the already known entropy transitions in physical systems and to extrapolate the same entropy transition process to the level of neural tissue. Evoked potentials representing ensembles of neural population responses were considered as a result of transition from a disordered to an ordered state, as illustrated in Figure 1B. (For details of this analogy also in the view of synergetics, see Başar 1980, 1983; Başar et al., 1991.)

2. These rhythmicities may also occur without defined physical stimulation but may be triggered by hidden sources, for example as a result of cognitive loading (Başar et al., 1989). In other words, according to our general hypothesis, coherent EEG states were considered as internally induced rhythmicities, similar to EPs but without known causal events.

3. The superposition of induced or evoked oscillations in various EEG frequency channels (4 Hz, 10 Hz, 20 Hz, 40 Hz, etc.) gives rise to the compound EP. These frequency channels are related to the main peaks in the amplitude frequency characteristics (AFC) computed from the compound EP (the method for the computation of the AFCs is explained in details below). To analyze EPs we have used response adaptive digital filters—without creating phase shift—with limits chosen adequately according to the main

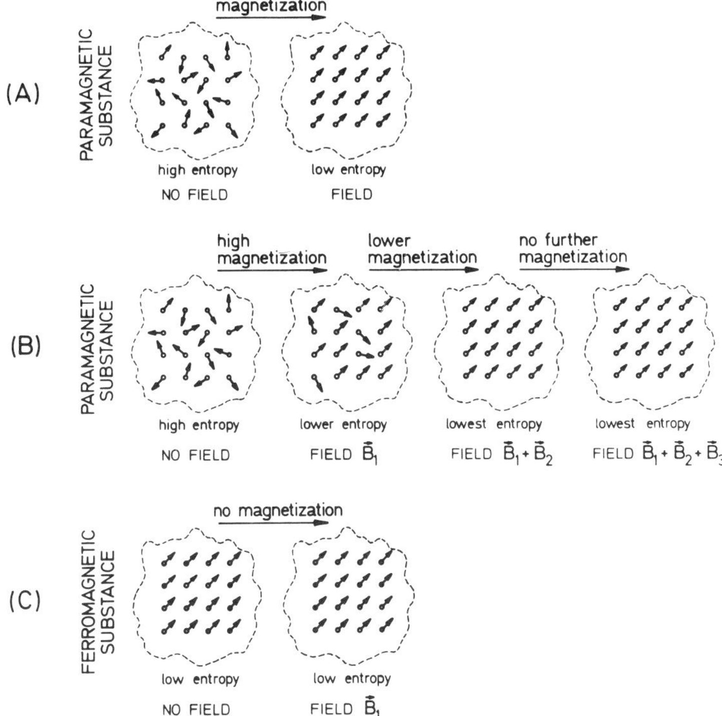

Figure 1. A: Evoked magnetization of paramagnetic and ferromagnetic substances on excitation by externally applied magnetic fields. Vector represents moments of elementary magnets in magnetic substance.

A: Let us suppose that we have a box full of atoms or molecules with permanent magnetic moments, i.e., a gas, a liquid, or a crystal. When there is no magnetic field B, the molecules are kicked around by thermal motions. When there is a magnetic field, however, it lines up the little magnets. The magnetization ($\vec{M}$) of a material is the net magnetic moment per unit volume, i.e., the vector sum of all the atomic magnetic moments in a unit volume. The induced (evoked) magnetization ($\vec{M}$) is proportional to the magnetic field $\vec{B}$. This is the phenomenon of paramagnetism. The ratio of the magnetization to the electric field is the magnetic susceptibility. At a fixed temperature, the entropy of a system of magnetic moments is lowered by the magnetic field.

B: If we apply to a system of magnetic moments exposed to a preliminary field $\vec{B}_1$ a second field $\vec{B}_2$, the magnetization caused by $\vec{B}_2$ will be lower than that caused by $\vec{B}_1$.

C: Similarly, the magnetization caused by the same field $\vec{B}_1$ to a ferromagnetic substance (i.e., to a system with larger spontaneous magnetization) will be lower.

In other words, in a system of magnetic moments with high entropy, the magnetization of the system will be larger than that in a system of magnetic moments with lower entropy.

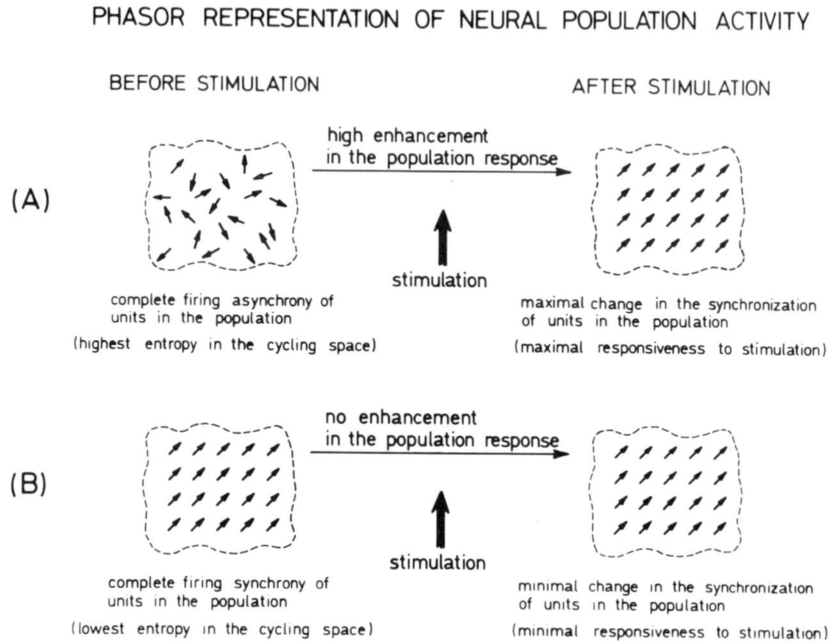

Figure 1. B: A phasor representation of neural population activity. The phasor represents the state of individual neural elements in the physicochemical cycling space, in analogy with the moment vectors of the elementary magnets in a magnetic field.

AFC peaks. By using such filters we can visualize an enhancement following the stimulation and a damped sinusoidal waveform that we have called "evoked theta/evoked alpha" or "evoked 40 Hz" depending on the frequency of these damped oscillations. To give a more detailed example of our analysis procedure, the appendix deals with thc supcrposition of oscillatory response potentials in the frequency ranges mentioned above (4 Hz, 10 Hz, 20 Hz, and 40 Hz) in the case of a cat hippocampal EP.

The description of resonance phenomena in neural tissues in various frequency ranges has gained emphasis. New reports concerning the cellular level (Llinás, 1988; Gray and Singer, 1987, 1989; Gray et al., 1989; Eckhorn et al., 1988; Dinse et al., 1991) agree in proposing the important role of resonance phenomena in brain signaling.

In the past 10 years during which this hypothesis has been discussed, some of the criticism was centered on the following issue: The interpretation of EPs as a superposition of evoked rhythmicities of various frequencies might be a hypothetical one—how can one demonstrate that these rhythmicities predicted by using digital filters are correlated with real rhythmicities?

In this chapter we summarize some of our strategies that are already published or will soon be published. We shall not only consider the objection mentioned above, but also try to find possible functional correlates of induced rhythmicities.

Examples of Induced Rhythmicities

After introducing our methods, we will present examples of induced rhythmicities to be observed in EPs, event-related potentials ERPs, and related fields. These examples will be classified by the events giving rise to the respective potentials: rhythmicities due to external events will be dealt with as well as rhythmicities due to internal or cognitive events.

Outline of our methodology to study resonances and induced rhythmicities in neural tissues

Resonance is the response that may be expected of underdamped systems when a periodic signal of a characteristic frequency is applied to the system. The response is characterized by a "surprisingly" large output amplitude for relatively small input amplitudes; that is, the gain is large.

Resonance phenomena or responses to forced oscillations can be analyzed in the direct empirical way as follows: A sinusoidal signal of a frequency f is applied to the system. After a certain period sufficient for the damping of the transient, only forced oscillations will remain, having the frequency of the signal. Then the amplitude of the applied signal (input), the amplitude of the forced oscillations (output), and the phase difference between input and output will be measured. Gradually increasing the frequency from $f = 0$ to $f = f_0$, the output amplitude relative to the input amplitude and the phase differences will be measured as a function of frequency (amplitude characteristics and phase characteristics, respectively; Solodovnikov, 1960).

Although this approach reveals the natural frequencies of a system, only a few workers have investigated the behavior of the EEG response using sinusoidally modulated light and sound signals (for details on pioneering experiments, see van der Tweel, 1961). Difficulties result from the requirement for evoked responses to sinus signals of over at least three decades of stimulation frequencies, evoked responses in each stimulation frequency being averaged using at least 200 stimuli. Another difficulty comes from the frequent changes in brain activity stages: they may change within a few minutes and have a limited duration, which is not sufficient for the application of sinusoidal stimuli of different frequencies. There is, however, another way of obtaining the frequency characteristics of a system, called "transient response frequency characteristics method": according to general systems theory, all information concerning the frequency characteristics of a linear system is contained in the transient response of the system and vice versa. In other words, knowledge of the transient response of the system allows one to predict how this system would react to different stimulation frequencies, if the stimulating signal were sinusoidally modulated. If the step response $c(t)$ of the system, in our case, the sensory evoked potential, is known, the frequency characteristics, $G(j\omega)$ of this system can be obtained with a Laplace transform, that is, a one-sided Fourier transform:

$$G(j\omega) = \int_0^\infty \frac{d\{c(t)\}}{dt} \exp(-j\omega t)dt$$

($\omega = 2\pi f$, where f is the frequency of the input signal).

The frequency characteristics $G(j\omega)$, including the information of amplitude changes of forced oscillations and the phase angle, is also called the frequency response function. It is a special case of the transfer function and is, in practice, identical with the transfer function (Bendat and Piersol, 1968). The amplitude frequency characteristics $G(j\omega)$ and the phase angle $\phi(\omega)$ can be obtained by numerical evaluation (using a fast Fourier transform) with the help of a digital computer.

Although this transform is valid only for linear systems, it can be applied to nonlinear systems as a first approach (Başar, 1980): the errors due to system nonlinearities are smaller than errors resulting from the length of measurements in sinusoidal stimulation experiments given the rapid transitions of the brain's activity from one stage to another.

Finally, a limitation of this approach has to be mentioned: by application of sensory stimuli, the brain is not directly excited with the proper input signal—there are physiological transducers (cochlea, retina, skin) between the input signal and the measured electrical output. Therefore, a direct comparison of the input and output signal is impossible; instead, the relative output amplitudes, or the magnitude of the maxima in the amplitude characteristics, are to be compared.

The experiments summarized in this chapter included both scalp recordings from human subjects and intracranial recordings from chronically implanted electrodes in freely moving cats.

The methodology to evaluate EPs, AFCs, and digitally filtered data was described previously (e.g., Başar, 1980). The essential steps are as follows:

Recording of EEG–EP epochs: With every stimulus presented, a segment of EEG activity preceding and the EP following the stimulus were digitized and stored on computer disc memory. This operation was repeated about 100 times.

Selective averaging of EPs: The stored raw single EEG–EP epochs were selected with specified criteria after the recording session; EEG segments showing movement artifacts, sleep spindles, or slow waves were eliminated.

Amplitude frequency characteristics: These were computed according to the formula given above.

Digital filtering: EP frequency components were computed using digital filters without phase shift (Başar and Ungan, 1973). The limits of the used passband filters are not arbitrarily chosen. Filters are applied only for selec-

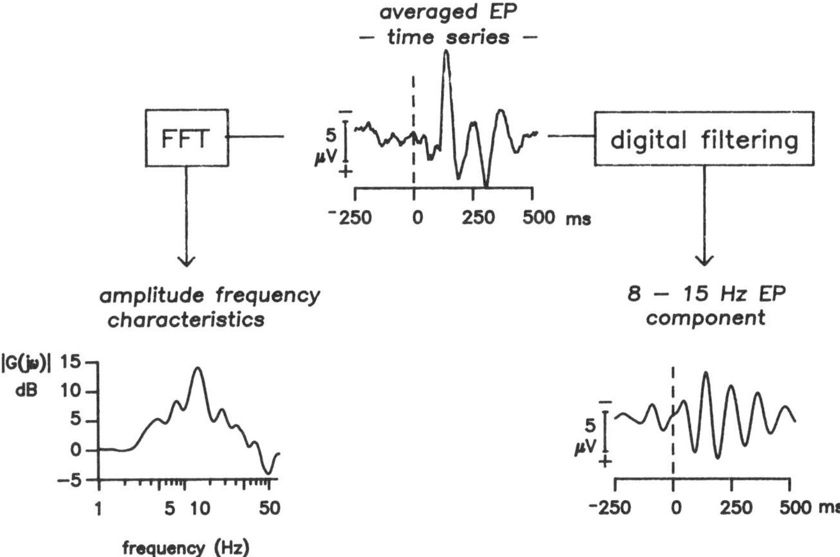

Figure 2. Methods of frequency domain analysis of EPs: selective averaging gives the transient averaged EP (*top*). From the EP the amplitude frequency characteristics (*bottom left*) and the filtered averaged EP (*bottom right*) are computed. Note that the filter limits have to be chosen adequately according to the amplitude frequency characteristics. FFT, fast Fourier transform.

tivity channels, or tuning frequencies indicated by clear peakings in the amplitude frequency characteristics.

For a detailed example for the decision of the choice of the filters, which are adapted to AFC, see the Appendix.

The essential mathematical procedures applied are schematically illustrated in Figure 2.

Examples of rhythmicities induced by external events

As outlined in the introduction, the potential changes effected by external events, in this case, auditory or visual stimulation of a human subject or experimental animal, can be interpreted as induced rhythmicities.

Light-induced rhythmicities in the visual cortex of the cat brain. Our first examples of induced rhythmicities refer to intracranial recordings from the cat cortex (Fig. 3: mean value AFCs from 12 experiments with six cats; two experiments were performed with each of the cats). Analysis of the visual EP recorded from the cat visual cortex (area 17) depicted AFCs with a maximum or with a dominant peak at 12 Hz (Fig. 3B; for AFCs of auditory EPs, Fig. 3A; see Başar et al., 1991). Similar findings are contained also in the visual evoked

AMPLITUDE FREQUENCY CHARACTERISTICS
Grand Average N = 12

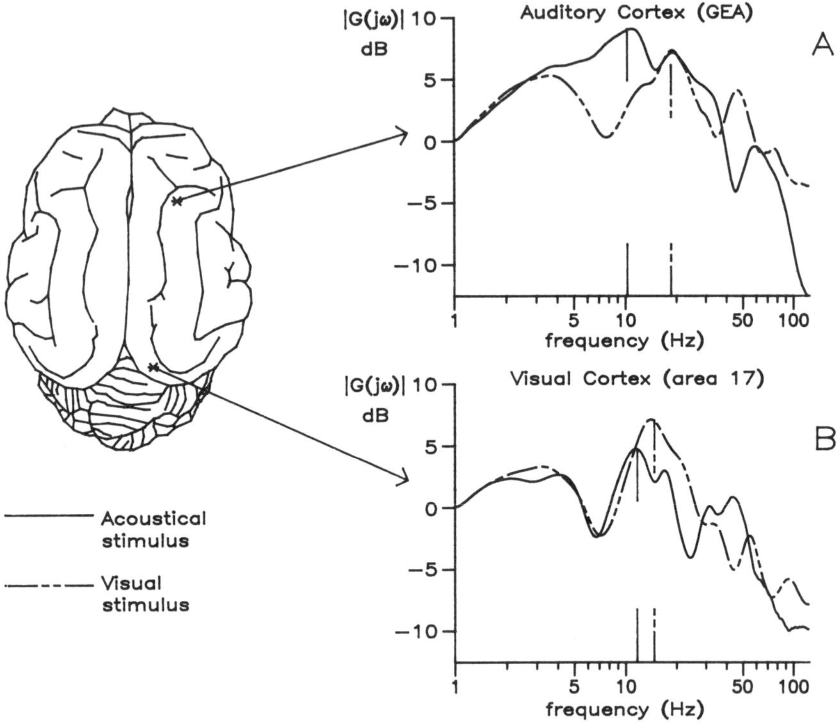

Figure 3. Amplitude frequency characteristics computed from cat auditory and visual EPs (grand averages of $N = 12$ experiments with six cats). Along the abscissa: frequency in logarithmic scale; along the ordinate: amplitude in relative units (decibels, dB). EPs were recorded from (**A**) the auditory cortex and (**B**) the visual cortex of the cat brain.

response from the human recorded in the occipital area (Başar 1980; Başar et al., 1991; Schürmann and Başar, in preparation).

In our previous work we have defined resonance phenomena of the brain as an enhancement and synchronization of EEG in the conventional EEG frequency bands on sensory or cognitive stimulation. Therefore, we now show a single sweep analysis of EEG and EPs filtered in the frequency range between 8 and 14 Hz. Figure 4A illustrates single EEG–EP epochs (prestimulus EEG segment and visual/auditory EP) recorded in the cat visual cortex. Single visual EPs (right column) showed great enhancements of 10-Hz activity, their waveforms being rather similar to one another.

Despite recent results concerning induced rhythmicities in cellular record-

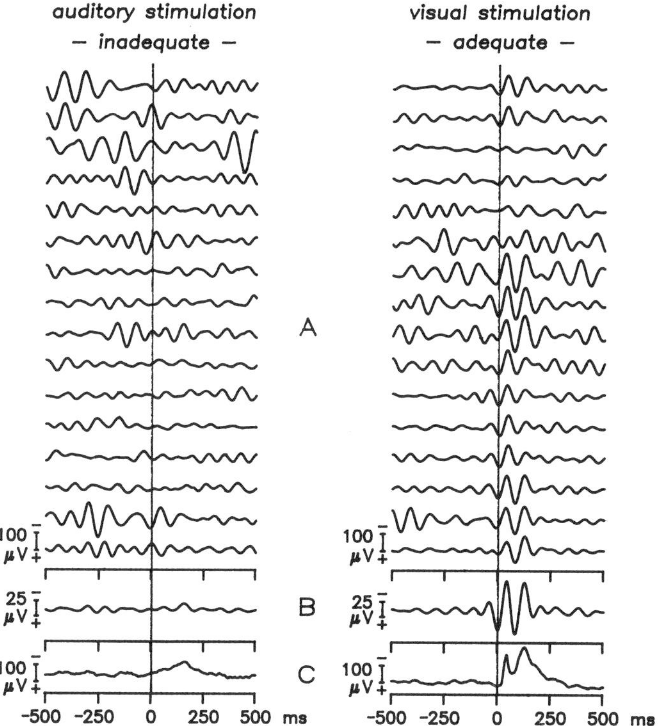

Figure 4. A: EEG–EP epochs filtered in the 8–14 Hz range (**A**); averaged EP filtered in the 8–4 Hz range (**B**); unfiltered averaged EP (**C**). Cat intracranial recordings from the visual cortex. **Left column**: auditory stimulation **Right column**: visual stimulation (see text for details).

ings (see earlier), one might ask whether the filtering procedure gives rise to this type of enhancement. There are two arguments against this criticism. First, even the averaged visual EP without filtering (at the bottom of the illustration) suggests by the two waves a possible portion of a 10-Hz oscillatory waveform. Second, at the left side of the illustration there are single sweeps of auditory EPs filtered in the same frequency range between 8 and 14 Hz, also recorded in the visual cortex. We refer to such measurements as "cross-modality" experiments (cf. Hartline, 1987). Auditory stimulation does not elicit any significant 10-Hz enhancement in the visual cortex. As we have discussed elsewhere (Başar et al., 1991) and will be the discussion of several papers, the inadequate stimulation in cross-modality experiments does evoke mostly a theta resonance or rhythmic theta activities in the cortex. We also have shown in our earlier publications (Başar, 1988) that in a number of human single

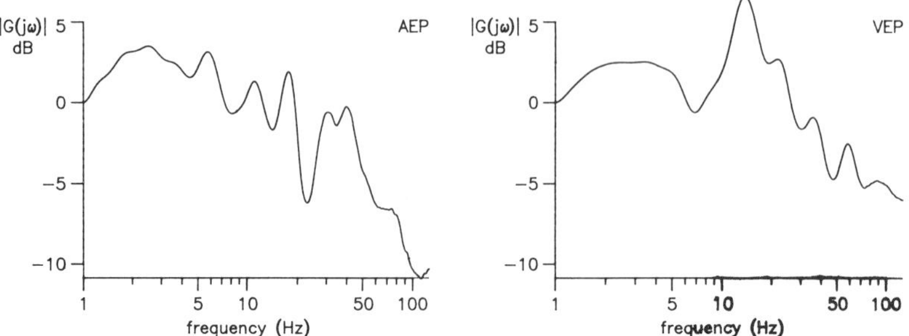

Figure 4. B: Amplitude frequency characteristics computed from the averaged EPs shown in Fig. 4A. **Left**: AFC computed from the auditory EP. **Right**: AFC computed from the visual EP.

sweep EPs, recorded from occipital scalp positions, damped oscillatory waveforms of about 10 Hz similar to those shown in the right column of Figure 4A can be recorded.

We only briefly mention cross-modality recordings from the auditory cortex (gyrus ectosylvianus anterior) of the cat brain. In such experiments we observed a complementary effect: large alpha enhancements—damped oscillatory wave forms in the 9- to 10-Hz frequency range—were present in auditory EP recordings. In visual EP recordings from the auditory cortex such alpha enhancements were not observed.

We learned from these experiments that such damped alpha activity is not present in all parts of the brain or elicited by all types of stimuli: it is only by the combination of EP analysis including Fourier transform and digital filtering, of adequate stimuli, and of appropriate electrode positions that such activities can be recorded.

Figure 4B illustrates the AFCs computed from the two EPs shown at the bottom of Figure 4A; that is, EPs recorded from the visual cortex of the same cat but obtained with different sensory modalities. The AFC computed from the visual EP (right) has a prominent maximum at around 12 Hz (approx. 7 dB). The response to auditory stimulation (left) is, on the contrary, highly attenuated in the 10-Hz frequency range. Both responses are, however, similar in the 1- to 5-Hz frequency range. This comparison, together with the results of Figure 4A, underlines the following properties of neural tissues under study: In the 10-Hz frequency range (filter limits: 8–14 Hz) the recorded large enhancements of single visual EPs in the visual cortex are also reflected in the AFC in the shape of a dominant 12-Hz peak. In the language of systems theory, significant (sharp) peaks in the amplitude characteristics of the transfer function characterize resonant behavior of the studied system. One may also express this behavior as tuning of the "device," or one might express the resonant frequency channels as the "natural frequencies" of the system. In our case we may say that neural tissues in the occipital cortex are tuned to respond with 12 Hz and 1 to 5 Hz to adequate (visual) stimuli and with 1 to 5 Hz to inadequate (auditory) stimuli. The response magnitudes to both visual and auditory stimulation are similar in the low 1- to 5-Hz frequency range. It is important to note that the 10- to 12-Hz response peak has almost disappeared in the case of inadequate (auditory) stimuli, which, in turn, did not evoke alpha enhancements in single EEG–EP epochs of Figure 4A. This phenomenon is more marked in experiments with a single cat in comparison to mean value curves of Figure 3B. In this chapter we do not describe the cortical gamma response (40-Hz range) to sensory stimuli.

Low frequency rhythmicities induced by tones at the hearing threshold. We have performed experiments at the human hearing threshold with the following paradigm: subjects had to pay attention to acoustical stimuli (2000-Hz tone burst). The threshold was defined in a preexperimental trial as the sound pressure level where about half of the tones presented were indicated as heard. For the description of similar experiments see Picton et al. (1976), with the exception that in our paradigm no background noise was needed, thus avoiding the difficulty of ascertaining the difference between selective attention, background noise, and target tones and actual threshold perception. Some yet unpublished results are presented below (Parnefjord and Başar, in preparation).

In Figure 5 a typical AFC of one of the subjects is given. In comparison to the AFC computed from responses to 80 dB tones (dashed curve), the prominent maximum at 10 Hz disappears. However, a dominant peak between 1

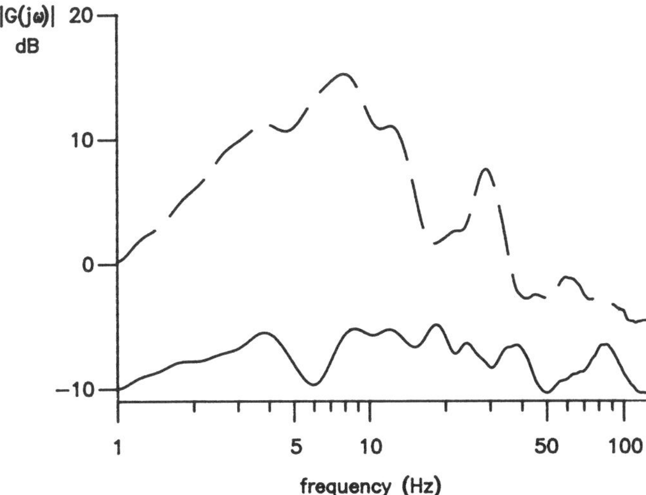

Figure 5. Amplitude frequency characteristics computed from averaged responses to 2000 Hz, 80 dB tones (*dashed curve*) and from responses to tones at the subject's auditory threshold (*continuous curve*), respectively.

and 4 Hz remains in the case of stimulation at the auditory threshold (continuous curve). This AFC of the single subject can be considered as representative for all subjects, since in the detection task the 1- to 4-Hz peak was present in the amplitude frequency characteristics of 8 subjects out of 10.

Another subject showed a behavior often encountered in experiments depending on the degree of cooperation of subjects. Being a staff member and having great ambition to produce good results, she carefully paid attention in order to detect all the tones at her hearing threshold. Figure 6C shows the averaged EP (wide-band filtered) at the threshold level for the tones that were heard. The averaged response shows a high amplitude oscillation in the range of 20 μv peak-to-peak. The filtered averaged curve (1–3-Hz filter, Fig. 6B)

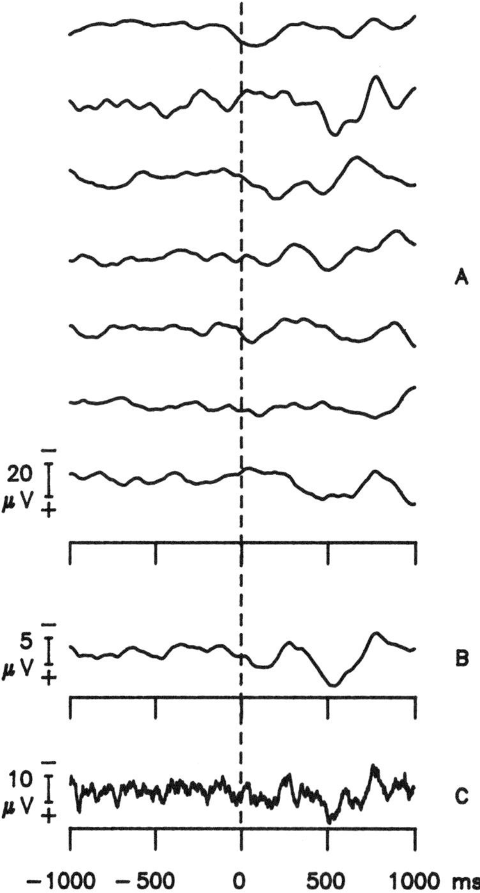

Figure 6. Responses to tones at the auditory threshold that were indicated as heard: (**A**) filtered single EEG–EP epochs (1–3 Hz); (**B**) filtered averaged EP (1–3 Hz); (**C**) wide-band filtered averaged EP.

resembles a slow wave oscillation that we call an "induced rhythmicity at the auditory threshold." Figure 6A also shows sweeps showing this behavior. In other words, the entire time course of the EP was dominated by this slow wave oscillation with an almost homogeneous frequency content. Five of the 10 subjects under analysis showed a similar behavior; however, the time-locking of the 1- to 3-Hz oscillation was different in all the subjects.

What is the implication of such experiments? In particular circumstances, when the human subjects try to perform a signal detection task, they produce slow induced rhythmicities which occur even at very low stimulation intensity. This means that the electrical signal emitted from the brain is an induced rhythmicity—visible without filtering—based on signal detection and perception at the hearing threshold. Certainly this signal detection also comprises "decision making" by the subject.

Examples of rhythmicities induced by internal events

Rhythmicities cannot be induced only by external events, as in the examples given above. Event-related potentials like those elicited by the omission of stimuli can be interpreted as internal (or cognitive) induced rhythmicities. A further example of such rhythmicities is an experiment in which the prestimulus EEG becomes phase-locked to an expected target.

P300–40-Hz compound responses induced by omitted stimuli. We have recently published several results concerning event-related responses (especially N200–P300 components) in hippocampus of freely behaving cats (Başar-Eroglu and Başar, 1987, 1991; Başar-Eroglu, 1990; Başar-Eroglu et al., 1991a, 1991b). The paradigm used was the following: The cats heard tones of 2000 Hz and 80 dB with regular intervals over a long period of time. In the second stage of the experiment every fifth of these tones was omitted.

In the course of such experiments, we observed induced 40-Hz rhythmicities in the cat hippocampus. Figure 7A shows about 10 single EEG epochs—responses to omitted stimuli—recorded during an experimental session and digitally filtered with a passband of 30 to 50 Hz. The average of 50 sweeps (filtered 30–50 Hz) from the same experimental session is also shown in Figure 7A. At the lowermost row is the wide band filtered event-related potential, which shows marked peaks: a negative one around 200 ms and a positive one around 300 ms. The analogy between this waveform and Sutton's event-related potential "P300" (Sutton et al., 1965) has been pointed out previously (Başar-Eroglu and Başar, 1987; Başar-Eroglu, 1990). Without filtering it is not possible to recognize the 40-Hz component, which is probably masked by the low frequency activity and which we call "40-Hz response with P300 latency." However, the filtered single epochs and the averaged curve show a 40-Hz burst around 270 to 300 ms following the omitted (target) stimulation. The observation of single sweeps shows that in a large number of single sweeps, in fact, a 40-Hz wave packet can be seen. The maximal peak-to-peak

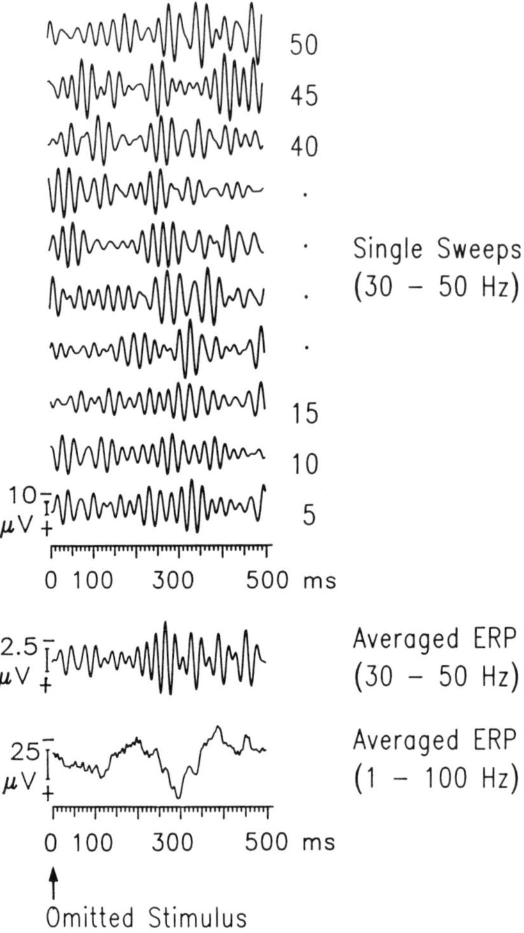

Figure 7. A: Single event-related potentials recorded during a "P300" session, filtered averaged ERP, and wide-band filtered averaged ERP; cat hippocampal electrodes.

amplitudes of 40-Hz wave packets usually do not exceed 50 μV; as a rule they were in the range of 20 μV. The time-locking is weak.

For all the cats we have grouped single ERP epochs into two groups in order to reduce the probability that the results might be contaminated by some accidental peaks. Figure 7B shows a superposition of the mean value of two groups of ERP epochs that were registered in the first half and in the second half of the experiments, respectively. It is a good congruency of curves between 250 and 300 ms following the target (omitted tones). In 80% of the cases the 40-Hz oscillations (peak-to-peak amplitudes) have larger values in the second half of the experiments. This behavior is reflected in slight differences of the two mean value curves.

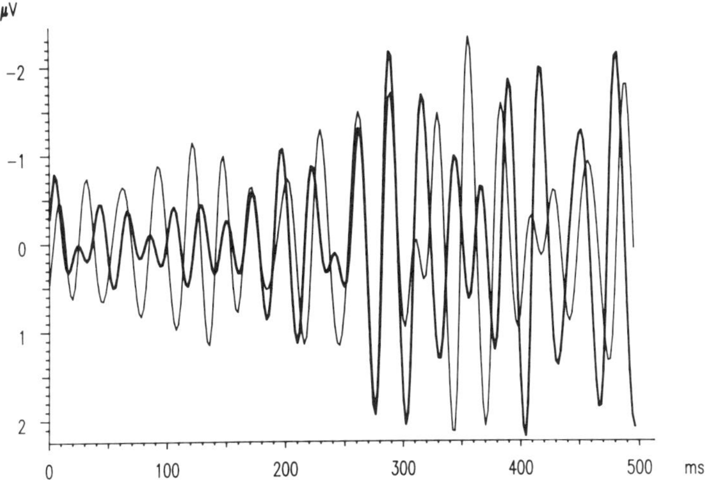

Figure 7. B: Averaged event-related potentials recorded during a "P300" session; filter limits: 30–50 Hz. *Thin line*: subset A (epochs from the beginning of the experiment); *heavy line*: subset B (epochs from the end of the experiment).

Figure 8 illustrates results of experiments from eight cats (filtered curves: 30–50 Hz). This illustration shows that in all the cats in the CA3 region of the hippocampus a significant 40-Hz packet at around 300 ms was recorded. The position of the 40-Hz packet had some fluctuations with respect to the time axis.

Differences between recordings of the 40-Hz responses (with P300 latency) from different layers of the hippocampus were dealt with in a previous report (Başar-Eroglu and Başar, 1991). Figure 9 presents such recordings and facilitates the comparison of wide-band filtered curves with curves filtered in the 30- to 50-Hz range.

Internally induced 10-Hz event-related rhythms. As outlined above, an external stimulus (e.g., a light flash eliciting 10-Hz enhancement) can induce the transition from a disordered to an ordered state of the brain (see analogy in Figure 1B). We also can evoke a 40-Hz response with sharp onset light or acoustical stimulation and so on. At this point an important question is: Can we find a way to put the brain in such coherent states of EEG activity without external sensory stimulation? Can we find a sensory-cognitive task to produce coherent internal EPs, or better, internal event-related potentials?

Since the first measurement of the event-related potential "P300" by Sutton et al. (1965), several paradigms have been used in order to correlate cognitive tasks and behavior with slow waves of the brain. However, there are only few reports that analyze prestimulus EEG activity during these tasks. Our earlier research, which demonstrated the correlation between EEG and EPs, led us to start experiments that also indicated a strong relation between prestimulus

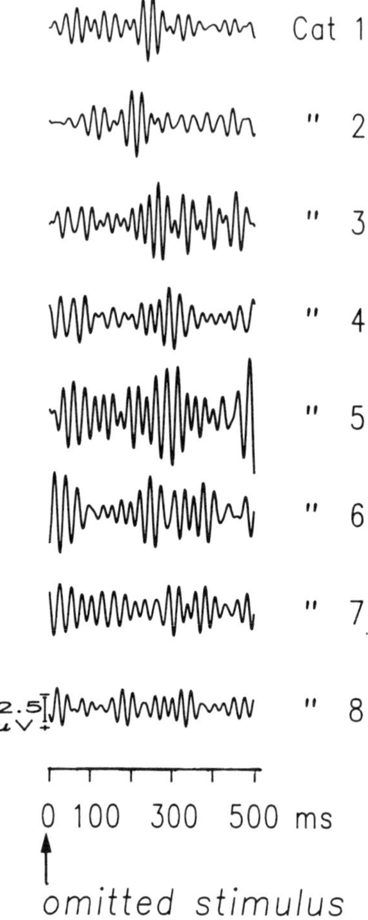

Figure 8. Filtered averaged event-related potentials (30–50 Hz) from the CA3 region of the hippocampus. Recordings from eight cats.

EEG and P300 (Başar et al., 1984; Başar and Stampfer, 1985; Stampfer and Başar, 1985). We observed that during the application of various event-related paradigms the prestimulus EEG tends to attain a phase-ordered pattern before expected stimulation.

Our preliminary experiments have now been extended to measure the event-related EEG before a cognitive task with a new paradigm. Our results demonstrated the existence of regular, phase-ordered prestimulus EEG rhythms, which tend to show a repeatable pattern formation preceding successful cognitive tasks.

Experiments were carried out with 16 volunteer healthy subjects, mostly students aged 19 to 21 years. The EEG has been recorded in vertex, parietal,

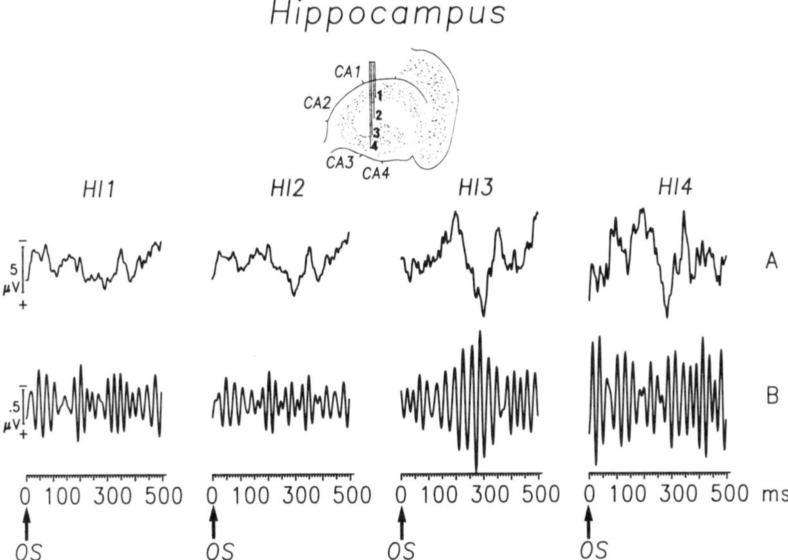

Figure 9. Multielectrode positions 1–4 for measurements in hippocampal layers CA1–CA4. **Middle**: wide-band filtered averaged event-related potentials ($N = 8$ cats). **Bottom**: averaged event-related potentials ($N = 8$ cats), filtered in the 30–50 Hz range. OS, omitted stimulus.

and occipital locations against an earlobe reference (C_z, P_3, P_4, O_1, and O_2 in the 10–20 system). The subjects sat in a soundproof and echo-free room dimly illuminated. As auditory stimuli 2000 Hz 80 dB tones of 800 ms duration were applied with regular intervals of 2600 ms. Every third or fourth tone was omitted. The subjects were asked to predict and to mark mentally the time of occurrence of the omitted signals.

When subjects had learned and successfully followed the regular sequence of the tones including the cognitive target, they were usually able to increase their attention. Then, rhythmic prestimulus EEG patterns could be observed. Most of the subjects reported that at the beginning of an experimental session with repetitive signals they had difficulties in predicting the time of occurrence of the stimulus omission. Usually, in the second half of the experiment they were able to predict the time of occurrence of the stimulus omission. Accordingly, we selectively averaged approximately 10 prestimulus EEG epochs from the beginning of the experiment ("first 10") and 10 such epochs from the end of the experiment ("last 10"). Figure 10 illustrates comparatively the averages of the first and the last 10 prestimulus EEG epochs (digitally filtered: 1–25 Hz) that were recorded at the vertex of a subject who reported that at the beginning of the experiment he felt unsure and diffuse. Toward the end of the experimental session he became more concentrated, and thus performed his task much better. The average of the last 10 sweeps depicted a regular

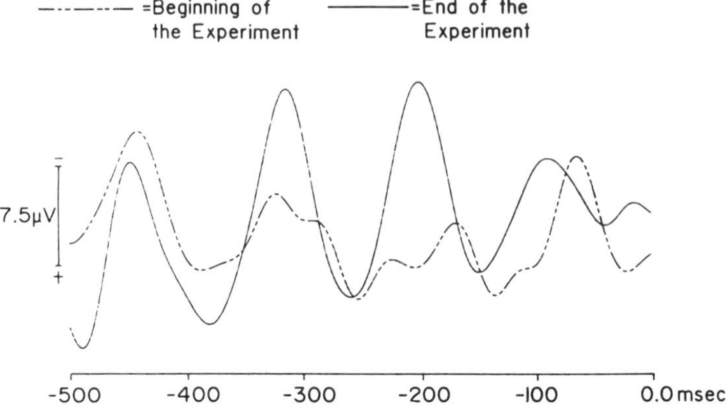

Figure 10. Averages of the first and last 10 prestimulus EEG segments in a "repeatable pattern formation" experiment (see text). Vertex recording, filtered in the 1–25 Hz range.

rhythmic behavior with large amplitudes. The first 10 sweeps tend also to the same rhythmicity, but the average is less regular and has low amplitudes.

In addition, the superposition of single sweeps demonstrates the formation of repeatable patterns: Figure 11 shows approximately 10 prestimulus EEG epochs at the end (A) and at the beginning (B) of an experiment. At the end of the experiment repeatable patterns were observed, whereas at the beginning no coherent state was attained. The superposition of the last nine sweeps for another subject is illustrated in Figure 12 (single sweeps recorded from vertex and parietal leads; digitally filtered: 7–13 Hz).

These experiments and our earlier results Başar, 1988) have shown that during cognitive tasks it is possible to measure almost reproducible EEG patterns in subjects expecting defined repetitive sensory stimuli. While paying attention to an omitted stimulus, the subjects probably anticipated with 10-Hz waves time-locked to the stimulus, showing almost reproducible patterns. We use the expression "quasideterministic EEG" for the recurrently emitted, almost reproducible EEG patterns. Our interpretation is as follows: The occurrence of such EEG patterns—and possibly similar patterns in other frequency ranges—may be linked to a short-term memory process that is tentatively denoted as "dynamic memory" (Başar, 1988).

In this chapter we included only a few examples of repeatable EEG alpha patterns time-locked to a stimulus. Such dynamic patterns were also described using light targets and occipital recordings. Such dynamic alpha templates do not exist when the probability of occurrence of the target is low; in other words, when the sequence of the target stimuli is less regular, the single target stimulus thus being less predictable, as was shown by Başar et al. (1989) using correlation analysis and several paradigms.

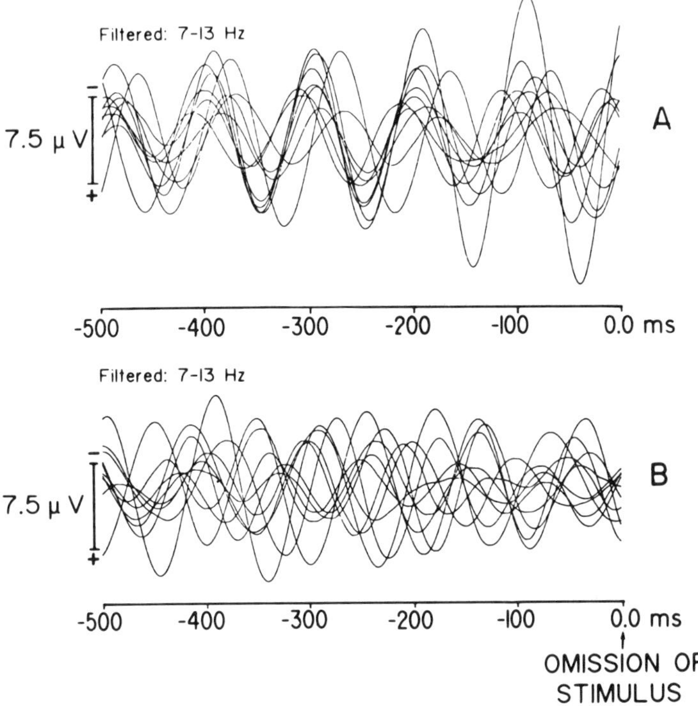

Figure 11. A: Approximately 10 prestimulus EEG sweeps at the end of a "repeatable pattern formation" experiment. **B:** Approximately 10 prestimulus EEG sweeps at the beginning of the experiment. Vertex recording, all sweeps filtered in the 7–13 Hz range.

Discussion

In this chapter we have given examples of internal induced rhythms or external sensory-induced rhythmicities obtained with various paradigms and under different experimental conditions.

Emitted versus sensory-induced rhythmicities: are they distinct entities?

Experiments including certain types of cognitive targets like those outlined in the previous sections make it possible to show brain responsiveness (or resonances) to various stimuli in one of the known EEG frequency channels (i.e., in frequency channels in which the brain is able to show spontaneous rhythmic activity). The hippocampus of the cat brain gave rise to emitted 40-Hz activity with a latency of around 300 ms following omitted stimuli. In human experiments a sound or light cognitive target induced alpha rhythmicities before target. The occipital cortex responds to light stimulation with 12-Hz

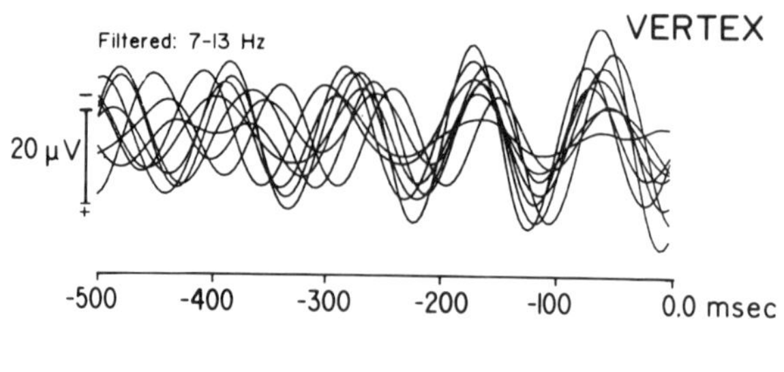

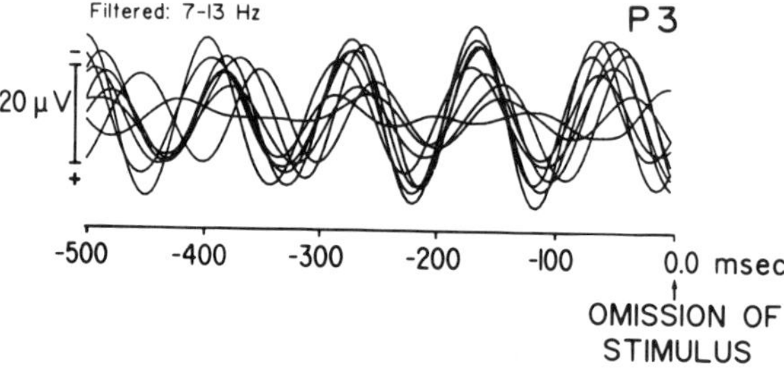

Figure 12. The last nine sweeps of a "repeatable pattern formation" experiment. Vertex (Cz) and parietal (P3) recordings filtered in the 7–13-Hz range.

oscillatory wave forms, whereas the auditory cortex does not. At the hearing threshold human subjects do elicit very slow rhythmicities around 2 Hz. We interpreted the 2-Hz induced rhythmicities tentatively as induced rhythms during signal detection or decision making.

Başar (1980) stated that event-related potentials of the brain and the sensory EPs consist of a superposition of various enhanced and time-locked EEG responses. The EP contains fragments of time-locked and enhanced EEG activities in all possible EEG frequency bands. In this chapter we have selected paradigms and special experiments, reduced the ensemble of external and cognitive conditions, and decreased the sensory cognitive tasks to special situations in which the brain should be involved with one of the tasks in which one dominant rhythmicity could be detected. This combination may be regarded as a new step undertaken in this field.

Furthermore, in our strategy to interpret brain rhythmicities (induced or spontaneous) we want to state that it is not yet possible to correlate rhythmicities in various frequencies with a unique function of the central nervous system (see also Epilogue of this volume). As to our experiments, there are also topological differences: significant 12-Hz rhythmicities in the cat visual cortex can be induced only by visual stimulation, whereas in the auditory cortex ample 10-Hz rhythmicities (or resonances) can be elicited only by auditory stimulation (Başar et al., 1991). Forty-Hz rhythmic responses were elicited by auditory or visual stimulation in various parts of the brain (Başar, 1980, 1987), but in some given experiments and in a given brain structure (hippocampus) the 40-Hz activity is recorded together with the so-called P300 wave. The induced alpha rhythmicities are not only evoked by light stimulation but also induced during experiments where subjects perform a mental effort in order to mark mentally a light target or an acoustical target.

Rhythmicities as building blocks

According to our hypothesis, spontaneous EEG rhythmicities, probably due to hidden sources, or induced rhythmicities appear during various types of behavioral and sensory conditions. Occurrence of several types of cognitive, sensory, or motor behavior may induce all these rhythmicities together. Accordingly, we consider various rhythmic activities in several parts of the brain as "building blocks" that accompany physiological and psychological events. [The expression "building block" was used in a recent study by Lehmann (1989) to correlate "EEG microstates" with states of perception, cognition, and emotion.] Only their combination should be considered as a representation of complex behavior. Further, only in special cases of simple behavior in which the brain has a state of high cooperation or synergy is it possible to isolate rhythms with a unique frequency (see earlier).

As mentioned above, there is a remarkable relationship between presented results and recent findings at the cellular level: stimulus-specific oscillations in the 40-Hz range were reported by Gray and Singer (1987; Gray et al., 1989) as well as by Eckhorn et al. (1988). Gray et al. (1990) recently published experiments comparing stimulus-dependent neuronal oscillations in cat visual cortex. The new data of these authors indicate that moving stimuli were much more effective in evoking oscillatory responses than were stationary stimuli. In no instance, using either stationary or moving stimuli, was the phase of the oscillatory response phase-locked to the stimulus. Gray et al. (1990) claim a functional hetereogenity among cells within striate cortex based on their temporal firing patterns and show evidence that the temporal pattern of cellular oscillatory activity is influenced by changes in stimulus properties.

Analyzing the responses to simple flashed stimuli, Dinse et al. (1991) found that the vast majority of neurons in the visual cortex of the cat exhibit complex temporally modulated responses that can be characterized as damped aperiodic oscillations in the range of 8 to 12 Hz. Intracellular recordings of 6 and 10 Hz rhythms, respectively, in thalamic cells remain to be mentioned as well (Llinás, 1988).

Conclusion

Several paradigms or strategies, summarized in this report and its appendix, were applied in order to reach a unique goal: to point out that the EEG serves as a functionally relevant signal (or operator) in various frequency channels that can be brought to resonant behavior depending on functional brain states. Such properties of the EEG were observed in field potential measurements from both the human scalp and from cat intracranial electrode sites. We emphasize that the EEG operators are functionally significant if 1- to 4-Hz, 4- to 7-Hz, 8- to 13-Hz, or 40-Hz activities can be brought to a resonant state with a high degree of synchrony. The time-locking of an internally induced EEG fragment may depend on the specific behavior (e.g., induced alpha templates before a cognitive target, 40-Hz induced rhythmicities with 300-ms latency in hippocampus during cognitive tasks). Rhythmicities of 12 Hz can also be induced with light flashes in the visual cortex of the cat or in occipital recordings of human subjects. The same stimulation elicits completely different alpha resonances in the auditory cortex. These results show topographic aspects of EEG operators.

In recent years the analysis of induced rhythmicities of the brain gained tremendous importance in the search for brain functions following with the discoveries of approximately 40-Hz, 10-Hz, and 5-Hz oscillatory responses at the single cell level (e.g., Gray and Singer, 1987; Gray et al., 1989, 1990; Eckhorn et al., 1988; Llinás, 1988; for a summary and discussion, see Bullock, this volume and Başar, Epilogue to this volume). We assume that the analysis of EPs performed within the scope of resonance phenomena and/or induced rhythmicities can be developed into a most important tool to understand and to interrelate sensory and cognitive functions of the brain. Once the physiological significance of 10-Hz and 40-Hz resonance phenomena is established, the type of component analysis here presented provides an excellent possibility to describe functional states of the intact brain during consciousness. We assume that by using such methods the analysis of EEG, sensory EPs, and event-related potentials will experience a renaissance in the search of brain function.

The approach with the tools of chaotic dynamics gave mathematical evidence that EEG is not necessarily a noisy state, but a "hot signal" related to tasks. For a review of chaotic dynamics of EEG we refer to the Epilogue of this volume and to references (e.g., Babloyantz et al., 1985; Başar, 1990; Bullock, 1990).

Acknowledgments. We are grateful to F. Greitschus for expert software development, to B. Stier for excellent technical assistance, and to J. Djordjevic for careful secretarial work.

References

Babloyantz A, Nicolis C, Salazar M (1985): Evidence of chaotic dynamics during the sleep cycle. *Phys Lett [A]* 111:152–156

Başar E (1980): *EEG Brain Dynamics. Relation between EEG and brain evoked potentials.* Amsterdam: Elsevier

Başar E (1983): Toward a physical approach to integrative physiology. I. Brain dynamics and physical causality. *Am J Physiol* 254:R510–R533

Başar E (1988): EEG-dynamics and evoked potentials in sensory and cognitive processing by the brain. In: *Dynamics of Sensory and Cognitive Processing by the Brain*, Başar E, ed. Berlin–Heidelberg–New York: Springer–Verlag pp. 30–55

Başar E, Başar-Eroglu C, Rahn E, Schürmann M (1991): Sensory and cognitive components of brain resonance responses: an analysis of responsiveness in human and cat brain upon visual and auditory stimulation. *Acta Otolaryngol [Stockholm]* (in press) pp. 43–77

Başar E, Başar-Eroglu C, Röschke J, Schütt A (1989): The EEG is a quasi-deterministic signal anticipating sensory-cognitive tasks. In: *Brain Dynamics*, Başar E, Bullock TH, eds. Berlin–Heidelberg–New York: Springer–Verlag

Başar E, Başar-Eroglu C, Rosen B, Schütt A (1984): A new approach to endogenous event-related potentials in man: relation between EEG and P300-wave. *Int J Neurosci* 24:1–21

Başar E, Stampfer HG (1985): Important associations among EEG-dynamics, event-related potentials, short-term memory and learning. *Int J Neurosci* 26:161–180

Başar E, Ungan P (1973): A component analysis and principles derived for the understanding of evoked potentials of the brain: a study in the hippocampus. *Kybernetik* 12:133–140

Başar-Eroglu C (1991): *Eine vergleichende Studie corticaler und subcorticaler ereigniskorrelierter Potentiale des Katzengehirns.* Habilitationsschrift, Medizinische Universität zu Lübeck

Başar-Eroglu C, Başar E (1987): Endogenous components of event related potentials in hippocampus: an analysis with freely moving cats. In: *Current Trends in Event-Related Potential Research*, Johnson R Jr, Rohrbaugh JW, Parasuraman R, eds. Amsterdam: Elsevier pp. 440–449

Başar-Eroglu C, Başar E (1991): A compound P300—40 Hz response of the cat hippocampus. *Int J Neurosci* 60:227–237

Başar-Eroglu C, Başar E, Schmielau F (1991b): P300 in freely moving cats with intracranial electrodes. *Int J Neurosci* 60:215–216

Başar-Eroglu C, Schmielau F, Schramm U, Schult J (1991a): P300 response of hippocampus with multielectrodes in cats. *Int J Neurosci* 60:239–248

Bendat JS, Piersol AG (1968): *Measurement and Analysis of Random Data.* New York: John Wiley

Bullock TH (1990): An agenda for research on chaotic dynamics. In: *Chaos in Brain Function*, Başar E, ed. Berlin–Heidelberg–New York: Springer pp 31–41

Dinse HRO, Krüger K, Best J (1991): Temporal structure of cortical information processing: cortical architecture, oscillations, and non-separability of spatio-temporal receptive field organization. In: *Neural Cooperativity—Models and Experiments*, Krüger J, ed. (in press)

Eckhorn R, Bauer R, Jordan W, Brosch M, Kruse W, Munk M, Reitboeck HJ (1988): Coherent oscillations: a mechanism of feature linking in the visual cortex? *Biol Cybern* 60:121–130

Gray CM, Singer W (1987): Stimulus-specific neuronal oscillations in the cat visual cortex: a cortical function unit. *Soc Neurosci Abst* 404:3

Gray CM, König P, Engel AK, Singer W (1989): Oscillatory responses in cat visual cortex exhibit inter-columnar synchronization which reflect global stimulus properties. *Nature* 338:334–337

Gray CM, Engel AK, König, Singer W (1990): Stimulus-dependent neuronal oscillations in cat visual cortex: receptive field properties and feature dependence. *Eur J Neurosci* 2:607–619

Hartline PM (1987): Multisensory convergence. In: *Encyclopedia of Neuroscience*, Adelman G, ed. Boston–Basel–Stuttgart: Birkhäuser

Lehmann D (1989): Microstates of the brain in EEG and ERP mapping studies. In: *Brain Dynamics*. Başar E, Bullock TH, eds. Berlin–Heidelberg–New York: Springer–Verlag

Llinás RR (1988): The intrinsic electrophysiological properties of mammalian neurons: insights into central nervous system function. *Science* 242:1654–1664

Picton TW, Hillyard SA, Galambos R (1976): Habituation and attention in the auditory system. In: *Auditory System: Clinical and Special Topics*, Keidel WD, Neff WD, eds. Berlin–Heidelberg–New York: Springer (*Handbook of Sensory Physiology*, vol. V/3)

Solodovnikov VV (1960): *Introduction to the Statistical Dynamics of Automatic Control Systems*. New York: Dover

Stampfer HG, Başar E (1985): Does frequency analysis lead to a better understanding of human event-related potentials? *Int J Neurosci* 26:181–196

Sutton S, Braren M, John ER, Zubin J (1965): Evoked potential correlates of stimulus uncertainty. *Science* 150:1187–1188

van der Tweel LH (1961): Some problems in vision regarded with respect to linearity and frequency response. *Ann N Y Acad Sci* 89:829–856

Appendix

Contribution of different evoked potential components to the original averaged EP

Usually the average evoked response is described in terms of several arbitrarily defined components such as peak (wave) latencies, wave magnitudes, and so forth. These arbitrarily defined components generally depend on the location of the recording electrode, behavioral state or sleep stage of the subject under study, and on the nature of the stimulating signal. Therefore, the interpretation of these arbitrarily defined components is difficult and generally does not allow comparisons between EPs of different brain structures or between EPs obtained under different experimental conditions.

The following analysis brings a new point of view to the understanding of time courses of evoked potentials. Figure A1(A) shows a typical hippocampal evoked potential, and Figure A1(B) shows the AFC obtained using the transient evoked response of Figure A1(A). The frequency limits of the filters are chosen in such a way that they fit with minima of amplitudes in the amplitude frequency characteristics (adaptive filtering).

The filtered averaged EPs obtained by applying pass-band and stop-band filters covering the same frequency ranges are shown together in Figure A2. One can easily follow the influence of various frequency components on a single wave and also see how different waves are affected by the same oscillatory response component in this figure. For a detailed description, the entire averaged EP is divided into time sections T_1, T_2, T_3, and T_4.

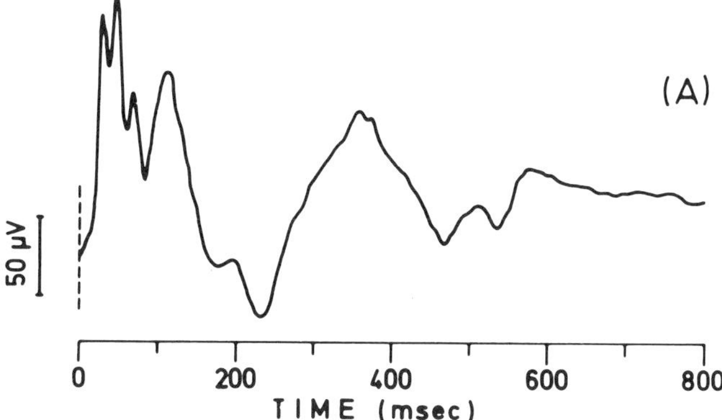

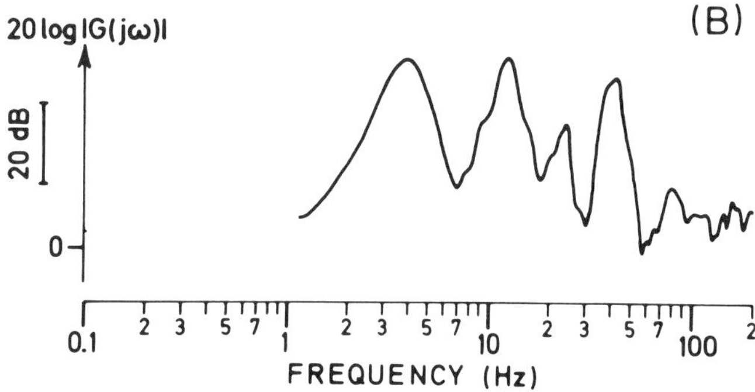

Figure A1. A: Selectively averaged EP recorded from the right dorsal hippocampus of the cat by auditory stimulation in the form of a step function (tone burst of 2000 Hz and 3 s duration). Upward deflections indicate negativity of the hippocampus electrode. Thirty-two responses averaged by means of an averaging computer. **B:** Amplitude frequency characteristic computed using the transient evoked response of A. Along the abscissa is the frequency in logarithmic scale, along the ordinate the relative amplitude in decibels.

Section T_1: This time section of the averaged EP is formed mainly by the components of 8 to 18 Hz and 30 to 55 Hz. Other components have minor contributions. It is seen by comparing the curves in C that the elimination of the 18- to 30-Hz component slightly modifies the relative amplitude positions of waves I and III. The effect of the frequencies higher than 55 Hz is almost negligible (compare the curves in E). The effect of the 0- to 8-Hz component is merely an upward shift of the entire curve in this section (compare the curves in A). But, the removal of the 8- to 18-Hz component causes essential alterations: Wave V, which is originally the smallest negative wave in this section, becomes the largest negative wave of the entire averaged EP (compare the

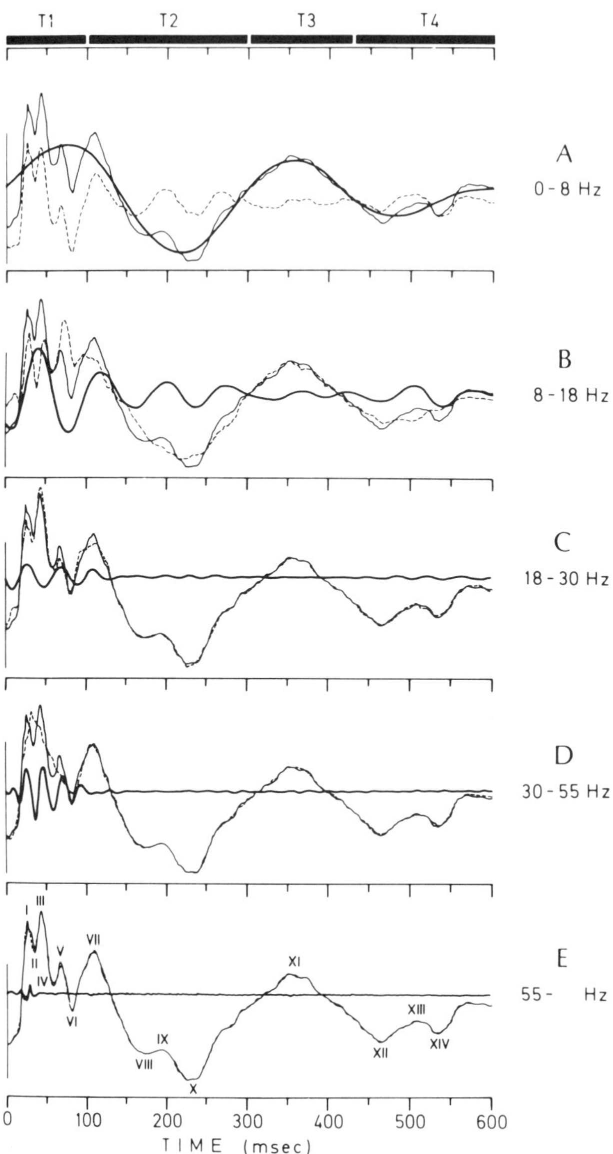

Figure A2. Filtering of the hippocampal selectively averaged EP shown in Fig. A1.A with different stop-band and passband filters. Negativity upward. Heavy solid curves are filtered averaged EPs obtained with application of pass-band filters. Dashed curves are filtered averaged EPs obtained with application of stop-band filters. The band limits (shown in the right side of averaged EPs) are chosen according to minimal values of the hippocampal amplitude characteristics shown in Fig. A1.B. The original selectively averaged EP is shown in thin solid curves for comparison with all the filtered averaged EPs. Time sections $T_1 \ldots T_4$ are shown at the top of the illustration. Roman numerals in the bottom panel indicate the successive peaks and valleys.

curves in B). This is because wave V is pulled down by this component while the same component enhances the negativity of waves I and III. On the other hand, all the positive and negative waves from I to VI appear to be the result of one single component of 30 to 55 Hz, since all these waves disappear when this component is filtered out by a stop-band filter (compare the curves in D).

Section T_2: Wave VII is a compound wave resulting from the components of 8 to 18 Hz and 18 to 30 Hz. This wave is affected when any of these components is filtered out. The contribution from the 8 to 18-Hz frequency band, however, is more significant than the others (compare the curves in B and C). As a matter of fact, all the waves from VII to X are due to the component of 8 to 18 Hz, since all of them are extinguished by removing this component from the averaged EP (see the dashed curve in A). Wave IX, which is far more positive than wave VII due to the theta component in the recorded averaged EP, reaches the same level of negativity as wave VII upon elimination of this component (compare the curves in A). Elimination of the 0- to 8-Hz component, furthermore, discloses a negative wave at about 270 ms (see the dashed curve in A). This negative wave, which is contributed by the alpha response of 8 to 18 Hz (see the heavy curve in B), cannot be recognized in the compound averaged EP because this wave can only cause a small change in the slope of the theta component.

Section T_3: The course of the averaged EP in this time section is determined only by the theta component. Because the filtered averaged EP obtained by filtering out this component is almost a straight line in this section (see the dashed curve in A). One can reach the same conclusion, however, by seeing that the only component that has a significant deviation from the baseline is the one in A, giving rise to wave XI.

Section T_4: This is another time section where the theta (4 Hz) and alpha (8–18 Hz) response components determine the course of the recorded averaged EP together, like in time section T_2. The waves XII, XIII, and XIV of the alpha component are superimposed on the positive valley of the theta component. When one of these two components is eliminated by stop-band filtering, the other one remains as the only component (compare the curves in A and B). The other components of the averaged EP do not show any deviation from the baseline in this time section.

The example shown here points out exactly how the grossly recorded evoked potentials are influenced and formed by different frequency components. Moreover, the fact that it is difficult to obtain evoked potentials having always the exact same shape can be understood clearly by consideration of the above. Since the equilibrium of contribution from different components changes perpetually, stability of AEPs cannot be expected.

Neural correlates of the 4-Hz, 8- to 18-Hz, and 30- to 55-Hz components were covered in detail in previous publications (Başar, 1980).

Predictions on Neocortical Dynamics Derived from Studies in Paleocortex

WALTER J. FREEMAN

Studies for more than six decades of oscillations in the ranges of theta (3–7 Hz), alpha (8–12 Hz), and beta (13–25 Hz) activity have created an immense data base but have given little understanding of their neurogenesis. In contrast, the neurodynamics of gamma activity (25–90 Hz) is better understood, but measurements in neocortex have been relatively few. This has been due partly to its contamination by nonneural potentials, especially by electrode noise and by electromyographic (EMG) potentials from the scalp muscles during noninvasive recordings from humans, and partly to its characteristics of broad spectrum, aperiodicity, and low amplitude.

A seeming exception is the "40-Hz" activity that has been reported in more than 1000 publications in the past three decades in human scalp recordings of endogenous (Sheer, 1976) and evoked (Galambos et al., 1981) oscillations and in paleocortical recordings from humans (Lesse, 1957) and animals (Freeman, 1975). Although bursts at or near 40 Hz are not uncommon in brain recordings, they are more likely to occur elsewhere in the broad gamma range and to show substantial frequency modulation within and between bursts. Studies of the spatial patterns of gamma activity in the olfactory system have shown that perceptual information is present in the amplitude modulation of widespread aperiodic waveforms (Bressler, 1987; Freeman, 1987a; Skarda and Freeman, 1987). Recent developments in the analysis of neocortical oscillations have shown that behavioral information is also manifested in the spatial patterns of activity in the somatosensory (Freeman and Maurer, 1989) and visual (Freeman and van Dijk, 1987) cortices. It has also been demonstrated for single neurons in visual cortex that nerve impulses, which are evoked by patterned stimulation of the retina, are phase-locked to narrow-band oscillations in local field potentials (LFPs, also known as electroencephalograms, EEGs, dendritic currents, or brain waves) (Eckhorn et al., 1988; Gray et al., 1989). These findings provide strong evidence that induced oscillations in the gamma range give direct access to neural mechanisms of cortical information processing. Therefore, they merit intensive study, analysis, and modeling.

The intrinsic biophysical properties, behavioral correlates, and nonlinear dynamics of gamma activity are comparatively well understood for the oscillations of paleocortex (Freeman, 1975, 1987a, 1987b, 1990a, 1990b). A review of these studies may help to clarify the problems that are arising in neocortical studies and to suggest methods and data that will be needed to solve them. Unquestionably the mammalian neocortex is more complex in all aspects, which is reason to take advantage of existing knowledge. This chapter sets forth nine predictions regarding experimental findings to come from neocortical studies. It is hoped that they may assist development of dynamic models of the functions of neocortex in perceptual and goal-directed behavior.

Classes of Stable State Manifested by Basal Cortical Activity

The basic cytoarchitecture of the neocortex (Ramon y Cajal, 1909–1911; Sholl, 1956) gives strong reason to suppose that populations of cortical neurons support macroscopic patterns of neural activity that cover large areas of cortex (Freeman, 1975, 1987a). Each of the immense numbers of neurons is synaptically connected to many thousands of other neurons by afferent and efferent endings. There are no small numbers of privileged pathways, nor are there more than a small handful of the crisp histological boundaries found in paleocortex within or between the numerous cytoarchitectonically and neurochemically defined neocortical areas. The linear integrative and cable delay properties of the dendrites of cortical neurons provide for smoothing of the thousands of action potentials arriving each second. The spatial divergence of output along with axonal delays provide for the coupling of neurons into populations over wide areas. Saturation nonlinearities from thresholds and refractory periods at the trigger zones of all of the neurons provide global stability by setting bounds to the amplitudes of activity in all parts.

For these reasons, neocortical populations are predicted to comprise distributed nonlinear operators that can be described by coupled ordinary nonlinear differential equations. As such, they have three classes of stable states, each of which is characterized by a type of attractor. The simplest is an equilibrium state with a point attractor, which is manifested by steady and nonfluctuating output. This state occurs in cortex under very deep anesthesia (Freeman, 1975) and following surgical isolation for *in vivo* (Burns, 1958) and *in vitro* cortical preparations. The second class is a repetitive state with a limit cycle attractor, which may be manifested by periodic oscillation of cortical neurons. The third and more general class is a stable chaotic state with a strange attractor, which is manifested by aperiodic, broad spectrum activity, often with recurring near-periodic bursts (Thompson and Stewart, 1986). Activity in this state may superficially have the appearance of noise, even though it is deterministic, not stochastic, and is limited to a restricted region of the state space, thereby delineating an attractor. A still more general class of states includes those that are chaotic but unstable, in the sense that the activity is continually evolving and does not serve to delineate a stable attractor.

The greater part of neocortical activity appears to be aperiodic and unpredictable. Even the relatively narrow-band theta and alpha activities on close inspection are seen to be erratic and not sinusoidal, possibly chaotic (Skarda and Freeman, 1987). Judgment from recordings as to class is difficult. The population activity of neocortex is observed in two forms: multiple unit activity (MUA) from well placed microelectrodes and extracellularly summed dendritic potentials in the form of LFPs. Aperiodic activity alone, regardless of whether it is MUA or LFP, is not a clear indicator of chaos because switching transients, exogenous perturbations, and penetrating electric currents that are of noncortical origin in the cortex may cloud an underlying point or limit cycle attractor. Every recording from a biological system contains uncontrolled fluctuation, some of it due to the electrodes and the amplifiers, and some of it due to the mixing of currents in the extracellular medium from multiple neural populations. (Interpreting LFPs is like trying to listen to one person at a time in a room full of people talking, while heavy traffic moves by the windows.) The brain is also subject to repeated bombardment by sensory stimuli, and it is subject to sudden changes in its state called bifurcations, the causes for which may be endogenous or exogenous. Any designated segment of recording may represent the transitory oscillation of cortical populations as they asymptotically approach a point or limit cycle attractor, or it may represent the steady state summed output of one or more chaotic generators, all the while mixed with and perturbed by uncontrolled inputs of unknown origins. Conventional methods used to distinguish and measure these cases, such as phase portraits, Poincare plots, and the calculation of correlation dimensions, Lyapunov exponents, and related quantities (Thompson and Stewart, 1986) are not appropriate for nonautonomous systems (Grassberger and Procaccia, 1983). (An open system is autonomous when it is left to feed and excrete at its own pace without external stimulation, guidance, or control.) Areas of neocortex in waking and behaving experimental subjects cannot be autonomous, but they may become nearly so when the subjects are awake but inactive and not processing information.

Two instances of near-autonomy have been found in the olfactory system. One is a partial complex seizure that resembles petit mal in humans. The other is a state of relaxed and nonmotivated waking, in which for periods of seconds to minutes experimental animals are seen to have low amplitude aperiodic LFP activity. The spectrum shows a linear decrease in log power with increasing log frequency, that is, "1/f", except for a low frequency fluctuation that may be imposed by respiration. The activity of this state has been simulated with the solutions to a network of nonlinear ordinary differential equations that is modeled on the anatomy and physiology of the olfactory system (Freeman, 1987b). Calculation of the correlation dimensions (Grassberger and Procaccia, 1983) of the real and simulated LFPs agree with each other in giving low values (Freeman, 1987a, 1988). These findings suggest that in this state, after the activity that relates to respiratory perturbation and to high frequency electrode noise has been removed by bandpass filtering, the remaining gamma activity manifests a low dimensional chaotic attractor for the entire central olfactory system.

I predict that a similar state will be identified in various parts of the neocortex in waking but nonmotivated subjects, provided that the theta and alpha activities are dealt with so as not to obscure the intrinsic cortical dynamics. I further predict that when it has been identified this state may provide a beachhead for using deterministic chaotic dynamics to investigate its properties in more complex behavioral conditions, including the dimensions and the geometrical properties of its attractors (Freeman, 1987a, 1987b, 1988).

Oscillations in the Probabilities of Neuronal Firing

An important question to address is whether oscillations, either periodic or chaotic, are to be found in pulse trains from single neurons and from multiple neurons in local neighborhoods. Several experimental techniques are available to search for oscillations, including the use of autocorrelation, cross-correlation between pairs of pulse trains (individual or MUA), pairs of LFP traces, or combinations of these such as spike-triggered averaging of LFPs. The most sensitive method is to calculate the probability of unit firing conditional on the LFP. When this function is normalized to the mean firing rate, it is called the normalized conditional pulse probability density, or NCPD (Freeman, 1975, 1979). The NCPD as a function of time is called the pulse probability wave, and the dependency of the NCPD on LFP amplitude is called the experimental sigmoid curve (Freeman, 1975; Eeckman, 1988).

Several experimental problems attend the derivation of unit cross-correlation functions and NCPD tables. Chief among them are the difficulties of determining the cells of origin of the several electrical signs and their degrees of mixing of populations of different kinds. A pulse train that has been verified to come from a single neuron by the refractory periods in its interval histogram does not pose this problem, but a recording of MUA may or may not come from populations that are all excitatory or all inhibitory. Similarly, recordings of LFPs may be derived from one population or from a mixture of dendritic currents of multiple overlapping or interacting populations. Here it is necessary to know the cytoarchitectures of the component populations, the connectivities of their feedback loops, and the geometries of their extracellular fields. These properties are well known for several areas of paleocortex but less so for any area of neocortex. The identification of the cells of origin, that is, the sites of electromotive forces of the dendritic currents that reveal oscillations in the gamma range, requires use of current source density and other volume conductor techniques (Freeman, 1975; Mitzdorf, 1987; van Rotterdam, 1987). It must be done for further development of neocortical neurodynamics.

Also, single and multiple neurons in a given population can simultaneously participate in more than one interactive neural system. One form of evidence is the presence of activity in different frequency ranges relating to differing aspects of behavior. For example, in studies of paleocortex it has been necessary to remove low frequency LFP activity relating to the respiratory system in order to study the NCPD in the gamma range that is intrinsic to odor classification by the central olfactory system. Hence, it is desirable to compute power spectra of the LFP trace before calculating the NCPD and to bandpass filter the trace around selected ranges.

I predict that when high amplitude, low frequency activity, particularly the theta and alpha waves, has been segregated from activity in the beta and gamma ranges of neocortical LFPs, and the band-limited traces are decomposed into the outputs of defined populations, a large majority of neocortical neurons will be found to yield well defined pulse probability waves and experimental sigmoid curves.

Phase Lags of 90° in Neural Negative Feedback Loops

A basic question to be answered early in studies of induced oscillations is whether they arise by coupling of neurons that oscillate as individuals or by synaptic interactions among neurons that do not oscillate as individuals. Substantial experimental evidence has been accumulated showing that individual neurons can and do generate periodic axonal and dendritic activity, and this conclusion is supported by numerous models derived from the Hodgkin–Huxley system (e.g., Llinas, 1988). However, several observations from paleocortex indicate that in normal physiological states the oscillations of individual neurons cannot account for gamma activity. One finding is that the typical firing rates of almost all cortical neurons are substantially less than the frequencies of oscillation in the gamma range. Another finding is that the interval histograms of single neural pulse trains commonly conform to the Poisson distribution and do not show peaks near intervals of 25 ms that would correspond to spectral peaks near 40 Hz. Yet another finding is that the time series of unaveraged recordings of LFPs show marked variations in frequency over the short term, which is not easily compatible with concepts of resonance and entrainment of individual neuronal oscillators. Moreover, it is well established that isolated slabs of neocortex (Burns, 1958) and paleocortex (Becker and Freeman, 1968) with intact blood supply but without extrinsic neural connections tend to remain silent and nonoscillatory, despite the integrity of their chemical milieux.

The most compelling evidence for interneuronal feedback as the basis for cortical oscillations is the existence of quarter-cycle phase lags between neurons situated close to each other in local areas of cortex. The analysis and modeling of cortical systems of coupled excitatory and inhibitory neurons show that the outputs of the two kinds of neurons should have a characteristic pattern, in which they both oscillate at the same instantaneous frequency, but with the inhibitory output lagging the excitatory output by approximately a quarter cycle (Freeman, 1975; Eeckman and Freeman, 1990). The quarter-cycle delay arises because each cycle of the oscillation has four steps: 1) excitation of the excitatory neurons, 2) excitation of the inhibitory neurons (one-fourth cycle later), 3) inhibition of the excitatory neurons, and 4) disexcitation of the inhibitory neurons, which leads to disinhibition (reexcitation) of the excitatory neurons and the start of the next cycle. Therefore, each maximum of activity by excitatory cells is preceded by a minimum of inhibitory cell activity one quarter cycle beforehand, and it is followed by a maximum of inhibitory cell activity one quarter cycle afterward. This analysis can also account for the common frequency of "40 Hz" in parts of the cortex for which the mean passive membrane time constant is 4.5 ms and the dendritic cable delay averages 1.3 ms, because 4 steps times 5.8 ms gives 23 ms, which corresponds approximately to the wavelength of 40 Hz.

An important consideration here is my basic premise that the macroscopic interactions that lead to spatially distributed oscillations are carried on by axonal transmission and synaptic integration and not by chemomodulatory diffusions, electric fields, or ephaptic influences that might take place in dendritic bundles, nests, discoids, barrels, and glomeruli. Only axons have the speed and range of transmission that can account for large scale neural cooperativity, and if synapses on dendrites are not the main basis for neural integration, it is difficult to see why the brain puts more than 90% of its energy into operating them. If oscillations are cooperative, then the lags introduced by dendritic integration must be expected and accounted for in the form of a phase lag for each oscillatory network.

This phase relationship has been found in every cortical system in which it has been sought, which includes all parts of the central olfactory system (Freeman, 1975), the entorhinal cortex (Eeckman and Freeman, 1990), and the hippocampus (Horowitz, 1972). The inhibitory interneurons are generally smaller and may be less numerous, and it is therefore more difficult to detect and measure their pulse trains. These difficulties may account for the fact that reports on them in other areas of neocortex have not yet been forthcoming. It may, moreover, be problematic to predict which populations the two signals should be assigned to.

This point can be illustrated by comparing the properties of the olfactory bulb with those of the various parts of the olfactory cortex. The dominant LFPs of the bulb predominantly manifest the dendritic currents of the inhibitory interneurons, and the bulbar action potentials come mainly from excitatory cells. The waves of the LFPs therefore lag behind the oscillations in cell firing probability, as predicted from negative feedback analyses. In contrast, in the olfactory cortex the dominant LFPs are generated by the excitatory neurons. Two classes of unit activity are found. For some cells (excitatory) the firing probability oscillates in phase with the LFPs, and for others (inhibitory) there is a 90° phase lag on average. Yet another phase relation emerges in the hippocampus, where the peaks in unit firing lead peaks in the oscillation in LFPs (Horowitz, 1972). This phase relation poses an unresolved problem. Either the units come from pyramidal cells (excitatory), the LFPs come from inhibitory interneurons, and the oscillations are endogenous (as in the bulb), or the units come from entorhinal afferent axons, the LFPs from pyramidal cells, and the oscillations are exogenous (as in the pyriform cortex).

A similar problem arises in the visual cortex, where a class of units has yet to be defined in terms of lead or lag with respect to the dominant population of units that appears to fire in phase with the LFPs. It seems likely that the main generators of neocortical LFPs that are recorded monopolarly with electrodes placed on the pial or dural surface are the pyramidal cells in layers III and V (Mitzdorf, 1987). These cells appear to be excitatory and to receive sensory afferent axons. They should therefore constitute the feedforward limb. By volume conductor theory their pulse probability waves should be in phase with the LFP oscillation (Freeman, 1975). Recent observations on the visual cortex Eckhorn et al., 1988; Gray et al., 1989) bear this out for that area of neocortex. The peaks of firing of Golgi type II neurons by this interpretation should lag the peaks of the LFPs. But if the peaks of firing are found to lead the peaks of the LFPs, then either the LFPs are generated by the inhibitory interneurons, or the neurons with phase lead are afferent axons, and the cortical oscillations are likely to be exogenous. Caution is advised in any case, because there are other factors that contribute to determining the frequencies and phases of cortical oscillations and the amplitudes of basal and induced activities (Freeman, 1990b), such as the existence of mutually excitatory and mutually inhibitory feedback loops in cortex in addition to negative feedback loops (Freeman, 1975). Nevertheless, I predict that pulse probability waves will also be found for inhibitory interneurons in all areas of neocortex, and that these waves will be found to lag the local LFP oscillations by approximately a quarter cycle in visual cortex and all other areas of neocortex.

Open Loop Time Constants of Neocortical Populations

An important premise for the prediction of the quarter cycle phase lag is that the open loop time constants of the excitatory and inhibitory neurons should be approximately or precisely equal. This premise has been experimentally tested and verified for selected parts of the paleocortex (Freeman, 1975), but not yet for any part of the neocortex. This lack of information about the open loop time constants is an unfortunate shortcoming in cortical neurodynamics. An elementary dictum in the study of feedback control systems is the requirement that the loops must be opened, and the delays in each limb of the system must be evaluated precisely, in order to be able to evaluate the closed loop gains from the closed loop time constants, which are taken from the frequencies of oscillation.

The technique for obtaining open loop responses is clearly defined (Freeman, 1964, 1972, 1975). A level of anesthesia is induced by any general or local anesthetic sufficient to suppress the background activity of an area of cortex without killing the cells, and the compound dendritic response to afferent axonal electrical stimulation is recorded extracellularly. This has the form of a summed extracellular excitatory postsynaptic potential (EPSP) from a population of neurons. It has a rapid rise time determined by synaptic and dendritic cable delays and a slower decay time determined by the passive electrical properties of the neuronal membrane. The time constants in the olfactory system have been shown not to vary during the induction of or recovery from deep anesthesia.

There is no strong reason to doubt that these molecular and biophysical properties of passive membrane are essentially the same for cortical excitatory and inhibitory neurons, so that I predict that the phase lag between their outputs should be approximately a quarter cycle. The fact that activity is commonly near "40 Hz" suggests that the open loop neocortical responses will have rise and decay times similar to those for the open loop responses of paleocortical populations (respectively, approximately 1.3 ms and 4.5 ms). Because these parameters are so important for the interpretation of cortical data and the modeling of cortical dynamics, the experimental evaluation of the open loop time constants of neocortical populations should have high priority in the study of cortical neurodynamics.

The Asymmetric Sigmoid Curve: The Nonlinearity of Populations

Precise formulation of the nonlinear gain function that is commonly called the "sigmoid curve" or "squash function" is essential for analysis and simulation of cortical neurodynamics. This function represents the static nonlinearity that governs the transformation in neural populations of the dendritic current amplitudes to pulse frequencies at trigger zones (Freeman, 1975). It is a crucial determinant of the stability properties of cortical populations, because it enables rapid and repetitive state changes in relation to behavior (Freeman, 1968; Grossberg, 1973), and it defines the domain in which these state changes take place, owing to long-term limitations on neural activity by thresholds (zero firing rates) and the hyperpolarizing afterpotentials that determine maximal firing rates.

This nonlinear gain function is based on experimentally derived NCPD tables. An equation has been derived to fit the NCPD as a function of LFP amplitude. It has a single parameter that simultaneously determines the mean and maximal firing rates and their maximal rates of change with increasing dendritic current (Freeman, 1979). Three premises are used in the derivation of the equation: 1) There is a factor in the membranes of neurons that increases exponentially the tendency to give action potentials with depolarization in the subthreshold range, the m factor in the Hodgkin–Huxley equations, 2) The firing rate tends asymptotically to a maximum that depends on the m factor, 3) Negative firing rates do not occur. The curve constituting the solution to the equation has been found to fit the experimental sigmoid curves of both excitatory and inhibitory neurons in all parts of the olfactory system and in the entorhinal cortex (Eeckman and Freeman, 1991).

In view of its simple determinants I predict that the asymmetric sigmoid curve will be found to hold for both excitatory and inhibitory neuron populations throughout the neocortex. Further, I predict that, as in the olfactory system, the single parameter in the equation that defines the mean, slope, and maximum of the curve will be found to increase with increasing behavioral arousal and motivation. A critical property of this curve is the location of the maximal slope (gain) on the excitatory side of the resting point. It is this asymmetry that enables areas of cortex to be destabilized by sustained afferent input. Also, the asymmetry allows modelers to use the input as a bifurcation parameter, as discussed below.

Bifurcation and the Segmentation of Neocortical Recordings

Among the more obvious properties of the activity of the olfactory system is the slow wave of the LFP with each inhalation and the accompanying surge of MUA, which induces a burst of oscillation. It is obvious that the olfactory system is under limbic control, with regard to the timing and pattern of inhalation (Freeman, 1990c). Careful examination of the spatial patterns of phase modulation of the dominant frequency components of the bursts in the olfactory bulb has shown that each burst has a unique phase pattern (Freeman and Baird, 1987). This phase property could occur only if each burst is formed by a bifurcation in the olfactory dynamical system during inhalation.

From our nonlinear models of olfactory dynamics, I conclude that the sigmoid nonlinearity endows the system with sensitivity to input. Thus, given the excitation provided by the surge of receptor action potentials with each inhalation, intrabulbar activity and interactions are both regeneratively increased beyond a point where a threshold is crossed. The system then jumps globally from one attractor to another one, and then to another attractor with exhalation; thereby in a waking and motivated subject the olfactory system undergoes bifurcation repeatedly with respiration. Therefore it is feasible to divide recordings of olfactory system activity into segments containing oscillatory "bursts" and interbursts. At respiratory rates in rabbits of 3 to 7/s each segment lasts on average 75 to 160 ms, during which the system can be regarded as stationary in respect to behavioral processing of odorant information within that burst (Freeman and Viana Di Prisco, 1986; Freeman and Grajski, 1987), in the sense that the system lies within the basin of an unchanging attractor. The bifurcation and the burst are seen whether or not an odorant stimulus is delivered to the nostrils, because the air always contains background odorants that serve for the identification of the status quo and for detection (but not identification) of novel odorants (Skarda and Freeman, 1987).

Similar time markers are not so apparent in neocortical recordings. The possibility that theta and alpha waves might manifest gating operations in neocortex has been suggested repeatedly over the past four decades, but there is still no vindicating experimental evidence on hand. Yet from our analysis of the spatial patterns of recordings from the visual cortex of the monkey (Freeman and van Dijk, 1987) and the human somatosensory cortex (Freeman and

Maurer, 1989), I am confident that similar spatial patterns will be found in most if not all areas of neocortex. That is, the neocortical LFPs will be found to manifest stationary states in respect to perceived inputs and goal-directed outputs of the brain, having durations between 75 and 300 ms. Candidates for segmentation markers include (but are not limited to) microsaccades in the visual system, finger tremor in the somatosensory system, and the abrupt shift in the spatial orientation of the global dipole in the human scalp EEG (Lehmann et al., 1987), which remains fixed for approximately 200 ms on average and then jumps randomly to a new orientation. I predict that within these time segments stationary space–time patterns of cortical activity will be revealed by multichannel recordings from waking subjects.

Spatial Patterns, Phase Coherence and Learning

Experimental data from the olfactory system (Bressler, 1984; Freeman and Skarda, 1985; Gray et al., 1986; Gray and Skinner, 1988b) have shown that odorant information is present in the spatial patterns of amplitude modulation of bursts that are induced by inhalation. These spatial patterns recur only with odorant conditioned stimuli (CSs), which the subject has been conditioned to discriminate by receiving reinforcement for a CS+ and not for an intermittently delivered CS−. The emergence of these spatial patterns is enabled by synaptic modifications, which our evidence shows have taken place between the mutually excitatory neurons in the olfactory bulb and cortex. These neurons that are selectively activated by odorant CS+'s are responsible for the sensitization of the system to learned stimuli, because they enormously facilitate regenerative feedback, destabilization, and bifurcation through the asymmetric sigmoid curve (Freeman, 1987b).

Our evidence from the visual cortex of a rhesus monkey indicates that basically the same mode of signal expression exists there as in olfaction (Freeman and van Dijk, 1987). I predict that this mode for the expression of cortical information will be found to hold for all parts of the neocortex, including primary sensory and motor areas and higher associational areas as well. That is, a common chaotic carrier wave in the broad gamma range will be found to comprise a substantial fraction of the variance of the LFPs recorded over areas of cortex up to 10 × 10 cm or more, and behavioral information will be found in the spatial patterns of amplitude modulation of the carrier. The spatial patterns will be subject to change with learning, when new discriminable stimuli are introduced, or when the contingencies of the reinforcement are modified. In each case when the learning situation is modified selectively, all of the extant and identified spatial patterns in that area are predicted to change concomitantly.

Further, in the design of behavioral experiments it is important to realize that these spatial patterns of the gamma carrier are not sensory—they are perceptual. That is, the behavioral correlate of each identifiable activity pattern is not some feature or collection of features of a stimulus; it is the significance of the stimulus as established by the history of reinforcement. This distinction has been shown in several ways in the olfactory system, most convincingly by training a thirsty rabbit to lick in response to a CS+ rewarded with water and not to lick in response to a CS− with no reward. When the reinforcement was switched to the previously unrewarded odorant and away from the old CS+, both bulbar activity patterns changed. So also did the pattern for the control state, which had no deliberate odorant stimuli. The control pattern serves the subjects as the basis for detecting the presence of novel stimuli by failing to be induced upon inhalation of unfamiliar odorants. It is a signal for the status quo, and its absence triggers an orienting reflex. On the basis of these data I predict that neocortical spatial patterns of gamma activity will be found to depend on learned associational properties of stimuli rather than on the stimuli per se.

The location of the modifiable synapses in the olfactory bulb and prepyriform cortex was identified experimentally. Animals were trained to perform an operant in response to electrical stimuli delivered to the lateral olfactory tract, while changes were measured in the waveforms of the bulbar and cortical potentials evoked by the stimuli. Modeling showed that the only class of synapse that could account for the changes in the evoked potentials with associational learning was the class of synapses between mutually excitatory neurons and not the class of synapses between the input pathway and the excitatory neurons (Freeman, 1968; Emery and Freeman, 1969). Subsequent reports by numerous investigators of neural networks (Amari, 1977; Anderson et al., 1977; Hopfield, 1982; Kohonen, 1984) have shown that reciprocal connections between excitatory elements in arrays are advantageous in associative memory systems. On these grounds I predict that the modifiable synapses in neocortex in associative learning will be found in the connections between selected classes of pyramidal cells that receive specific thalamic afferents. Further, I predict that the modification of these synapses will support the formation of nerve cell assemblies as described by Hebb (1949), and that the nerve cell assemblies will be found to mediate the selection by CSs of the appropriate basins of perceptual attractors.

Sources of Excitatory Bias for Neocortex

The hallmark of healthy brains in humans and in animals from every phylum is the basal or "spontaneous" activity that is found in all normal and most abnormal states. It is exceedingly robust. Yet many neurons that are isolated and left to themselves tend to fall into inactivity and depression. As already noted, this is obviously true of the neurons in isolated cortical slabs. It also holds for the neurons in the more central parts of the olfactory system when they are experimentally deafferented; that is, when the axons forming the lateral olfactory tract connecting the bulb to the anterior olfactory nucleus and prepyriform cortex are either surgically cut or temporarily inactivated by local anesthetics (Freeman, 1975) or by cryogenic blockade (Gray and Skinner, 1988a). The question arises, how does this "spontaneous" activity arise?

Simulations of the dynamics of the olfactory system have shown that the chaotic waveforms that replicate the basal "spontaneous" activity cannot be generated by parts that simulate isolated parts. The minimal configuration includes the olfactory bulb, anterior olfactory nucleus, and prepyriform cortex with long feedback paths interconnecting them (Freeman, 1987b). The same pattern of shutdown occurs in the model when the homologous disconnect is made between the bulb and the other two parts. These experimental and theoretical findings show that both the unit and LFP basal activities of all parts of the olfactory system are the manifestations of the global dynamics of the system. The converse is not the case; that is, LFPs are not the mere sums of local activities. The implication for neocortical studies is that normal cortical function must depend heavily on corticocortical and corticothalamic feedback pathways, and that perceptual functions such as those that take place during associative learning and memory should not be sought in isolated slabs.

The maintenance of "spontaneous" chaotic activity patterns in models of the olfactory system depends heavily on the use of subsidiary elements that simulate populations of neurons that are mutually excitatory. These elements provide a sustained excitatory input to the elements formed into negative feedback loops. This input constitutes a variable bias control. The intrinsic importance of the bias in the models suggests that an important component both in neocortex and in dynamic models of neocortex is a source of excitatory bias: that is, a sustained excitatory input to each local region of cortex. The implication from Burns' (1958) results with slabs is that a bias is required to maintain the basal activity. In the olfactory system the source of this bias has been identified as the externally situated interneurons in the olfactory bulb, the periglomerular cells. These neurons have been shown to form a mutually excitatory population that can stabilize itself without the need for inhibitory feedback. The periglomerular population provides continuing depolarizing bias to other excitatory neurons in the bulb, and they in turn maintain the background activity of the inhibitory interneurons in the bulb and of the neurons in other parts of the system to which the bulbar neurons project (Freeman, 1975; Martinez and Freeman, 1984; Rhoades and Freeman, 1990).

Modeling indicates that this interneuronal population is necessary not only for maintaining the chaotic basal activity in the olfactory system (Freeman, 1987b); it is also required for mediating varying states of arousal and motivation, and for enabling bifurcation to take place on the presentation of a stimulus and on the termination of the stimulus. An excitatory bias is essential not only to induce a burst of oscillation in the olfactory system but also to terminate the burst by withdrawal of the bias, so that a new odorant sample can be taken quickly. This aspect gives good reason to look for mutually excitatory populations as the source of low frequency bias potentials. It is unlikely that slow EPSPs can play this role because they cannot be so rapidly adjusted or turned off.

On these grounds a comparable source of depolarizing bias should be sought for other areas of paleocortex and of neocortex. It seems likely that the dentate fascia may play this role for the hippocampus. The source is not likely to be found within the cortex (as it is within the bulb) because if it were, then undercut areas would not tend to go silent. It is also unlikely to be found in specific thalamic projections, because the sensory relay neurons must transmit information with high spatial and temporal frequencies. Modeling indicates that biasing neurons should operate in low spatial and temporal frequency ranges. Among the more likely candidates for neocortical excitatory bias generators are the nonspecific thalamic reticular nuclei. These have long been implicated in the cortical arousal reaction (Jasper, 1960), which is deeply involved with induced rhythms of the brain. The fact that these nuclei have their own regulatory feedback mechanisms is suggested by the "recruiting response" (Dempsey and Morison, 1942); rhythmic electrical stimulation of thalamic reticular nuclei induces waxing and waning cortical evoked potentials. It is noteworthy that paleocortices do not show this pattern of response. Recruitment is a near-forgotten chapter in the history of neocortical studies that will surely be reopened. Excitatory and inhibitory biases in the olfactory bulb have been linked with centrifugal projections of cholinergic, dopaminergic, and norepinephrinergic projections, and possibly with neuropeptides. Any or all of these may play roles in neocortex that need to be clarified. What is essential is to recognize the nature of and need for biases.

Conclusion

Brain scientists have been seriously concerned with induced rhythms for well over a century, following the discovery of the central origin of the respiratory cycle and its modulation by Hering–Breuer reflexes (reviewed by Best and Taylor, 1950). Numerous hypotheses have been advanced to explain the basic fact that respiratory frequency and depth are controlled mainly by steady "bias" levels of pH and carbon dioxide in the brain, none of which is satisfactory. The bias control of rhythms is part of the larger problem of the nonlinear dynamics of distributed populations of neurons in cortex and brain stem alike, that generate and control locomotion, perception, emotion, and intellectual processes. Recent progress in theory and in computer technology has provided an abundance of models. The present difficulties lie mainly in experimental testing of proposed models in all of these areas of application. Success in any one will illuminate all of the others. The predictions offered in this chapter are intended to focus the attention of modelers on those properties of neocortex that may be decisive in constructing and testing workable models of the dynamics of perception.

Summary

Of the two main types of cerebral cortex the dynamics of the simpler three-layered paleocortex is better understood; however, the six-layered neocortex is more interesting, because it is the organ of intellect. In this report concepts from nonlinear dynamics that have been useful for understanding paleocortical rhythms are summarized, and nine predictions are made as to what will be found in forthcoming applications to the neocortex.

1. A stationary and nearly autonomous basal state is predicted for local areas of neocortex in waking, nonmotivated subjects. It is characterized by aperiodic, broad spectrum activity above 25 Hz.. This activity will be optimal for applications of the theory of chaos to neocortical dynamics.
2. Oscillations in the firing probabilities of neurons at the frequencies of local field potentials are predicted for a majority of cortical neurons.
3. Neocortical oscillations are predicted to arise by feedback between excitatory and inhibitory neurons and not by coupling of oscillatory neurons. This will be proven by phase relations, in which the inhibitory outputs will be shown to lag excitatory outputs by about a quarter cycle.
4. The open loop time constants of excitatory and inhibitory neocortical populations, which must be measured in order to model the cortex, are predicted to approximate each other and those of paleocortical populations, which are circa 4.5 ms (passive membrane) and 1.3 ms (lumped dendritic delay).
5. The asymmetric sigmoid curve that describes the relation between dendritic current and axonal firing probability and that constitutes the static nonlinearity of paleocortical populations is predicted to hold for both the excitatory and inhibitory neural populations in the neocortex.
6. Stationary states are predicted to exist in local areas of cortex having durations of 100 to 300 ms and spatial patterns like frames in a movie.
7. Perceptual information as distinct from sensory-evoked activity is predicted to exist primarily in the spatial patterns of amplitude modulation of carrier waves with frequencies above 25 Hz but secondarily in other spectral ranges such as alpha and theta owing to gating and biassing mechanisms.
8. Changes in these spatial patterns are predicted to occur in associative learning that are based on changes in the excitatory synapses of pyramidal cells onto other pyramidal cells, in accordance with a Hebb rule.
9. A variable excitatory bias is predicted to exist for each cortical area as an essential basis for its dynamic control. A likely source is from mutually excitatory neurons in "non-specific" thalamic reticular nuclei.

Acknowledgments. Supported by grant MH06686 from the National Institute of Mental Health. I am grateful to Cathleen Barczys for critical review of this manuscript.

References

Amari S (1977): Neural theory of association and concept formation. *Biol Cybern* 26:175–185

Anderson JA, Silverstein JW, Ritz SR, Jones RS (1977): Distinctive features, categorical perception, and probability learning: Some applications of a neural model. *Psychol Rev* 84:413–451

Becker CJ, Freeman WJ (1968): Prepyriform electrical activity after loss of peripheral or central input or both. *Physiol Behav* 3:597–599

Best CH, Taylor NB (1950): *The Physiological Basis of Medical Practice*, 5th ed. Baltimore MD: Williams and Wilkins, pp 407–410

Bressler SL (1984): Spatial organization of EEGs from olfactory bulb and cortex. *Electroencephalogr Clin Neurophysiol* 57:270–276.

Bressler SL (1987): Changes in electrical activity of rabbit olfactory bulb and cortex to conditioned odor stimulation. *J Neurophysiol* 102:740–747

Burns BD (1958): *The Mammalian Cerebral Cortex*. Baltimore MD: Williams and Wilkins

Dempsey EW, Morison RS (1942): The electrical activity of thalamocortical relay systems. *Am J Physiol* 138:283–289

Eckhorn R, Bauer B, Jordan W, Brosch M, Kruse W, Munk M, Reitboeck HJ (1988): Coherent oscillations: a mechanism of feature linking in visual cortex? *Biol Cybern* 60:121–130

Eeckman FH (1988): Statistical correlations between unit firings and cortical EEG. Ph.D. Thesis in Physiology, University of California at Berkeley

Eeckman FH, Freeman WJ (1990): Correlations between unit firing and EEG in the rat olfactory system. *Brain Res* 528:238–244

Eeckman FH, Freeman WJ (1991): Asymmetric sigmoid nonlinearity in the rat olfactory system. *Brain Res* in press

Emery JD, Freeman WJ (1969): Pattern analysis of cortical evoked potential parameters during attention changes. *Physiol Behav* 4:67–77

Freeman WJ (1964): A linear distributed feedback model for prepyriform cortex. *Exp Neurol* 10:525–547

Freeman WJ (1968): Analog simulation of prepyriform cortex in the cat. *Math BioSci* 2:181–190

Freeman WJ (1972): Measurement of open-loop responses to electrical stimulation in olfactory bulb of cat. *J Neurophysiol* 35:745–761

Freeman WJ (1975): *Mass Action in the Nervous System*. New York; Academic Press

Freeman WJ (1979): Nonlinear gain mediating cortical stimulus-response relations. *Biol Cybern* 33:237–247

Freeman WJ (1987a): Techniques used in the search for the physiological basis of the EEG. In: *Handbook of Electroencephalography and Clinical Neurophysiology*, Gevins AS, Remond A, eds. vol 3A, Part 2. Amsterdam: Elsevier

Freeman WJ (1987b): Simulation of chaotic EEG patterns with a dynamic model of the olfactory system. *Biol Cybern* 56:139–150

Freeman WJ (1988): Strange attractors that govern mammalian brain dynamics shown by trajectories of electroencephalographic (EEG) potential. *IEEE Trans Circ & Syst* 35:781–783

Freeman WJ (1990a): On the problem of anomalous dispersion in chaoto-chaotic phase transitions of neural masses, and its significance for the management of information in brains. In: *Synergetics of Cognition*, Haken H, Stadler M, eds. Berlin: Springer–Verlag, pp 126–143

Freeman WJ (1990b): Colligation of the distributions of amplitude-dependent characteristic frequencies among coupled cortical oscillators. In: *NEC Research Institute Symposium*, vol 1, Gear CW, ed. New York: Society of Industrial and Applied Mathematics Ch 5, pp 69–103

Freeman WJ (1990c): On the fallacy of assigning an origin to consciousness. In: *Machinery of the Mind*, John ER, ed. Cambridge MA: Birkhaeuser Boston Inc. Ch 2, pp 14–26

Freeman WJ, Baird B (1987): Relation of olfactory EEG to behavior: Spatial analysis. *Behav Neurosci* 101:393–408

Freeman WJ, Grajski KA (1987): Relation of olfactory EEG to behavior: Factor analysis. *Behav Neurosci* 101:766–777

Freeman WJ, Maurer K (1989): Advances in brain theory give new directions to the use of the technologies of brain mapping in behavioral studies. In: *Topographic Mapping of EEG and Evoked Potentials*, Maurer K, ed. Berlin: Springer–Verlag

Freeman WJ, Skarda CA (1985): Spatial EEG patterns, non-linear dynamics and perception: the neo-Sherringtonian view. *Brain Res Rev* 10:147–175

Freeman WJ, Van Dijk B (1987): Spatial patterns of visual cortical fast EEG during conditioned reflex in a rhesus monkey. *Brain Res* 422:267–276

Freeman WJ, Viana Di Prisco G (1986): Relation of olfactory EEG to behavior: time series analysis. *Behav Neurosci* 100:753–763

Galambos R, Makeig S, Talmachoff P (1981): A new auditory potential recorded from the human scalp. *Proc Natl Acad Sci USA* 78:2643–2647

Grassberger P, Procaccia I (1983): Measuring the strangeness of strange attractors. *Physica* 9D:189–205

Gray CM, Freeman WJ, Skinner JE (1986): Chemical dependencies of learning in the rabbit olfactory bulb: acquisition of the transient spatial-pattern change depends on norepinephrine. *Behav Neurosci* 100:585–596

Gray CM, Koenig P, Engel KA, Singer W (1989): Oscillatory responses in cat visual cortex exhibit intercolumnar synchronization which reflects global stimulus properties. *Nature* 338:334–337

Gray CM, Skinner JE (1988a): Centrifugal regulation of neuronal activity in the olfactory bulb of the waking rabbit as revealed by reversible cryogenic blockade. *Exper Brain Res* 69:378–386

Gray CM, Skinner JE (1988b): Field potential response changes in the rabbit olfactory bulb accompany behavioral habituation during repeated presentation of unreinforced odors. *Exper Brain Res* 73:189–197

Grossberg S (1973): Contour enhancement, short term memory, and constancies in reverberating neural networks. *Stud Appl Math* 52:213–257

Hebb DO (1949): *The Organization of Behavior: A Neuropsychological Theory*. New York: Wiley

Hopfield JJ (1982): Neuronal networks and physical systems with emergent collective computational abilities. *Proc Natl Acad Sci* 81:3058–3092

Horowitz JM (1972): Evoked activity of single units and neural populations in the hippocampus of the cat. *Electroencephalogr Clin Neurophysiol* 32:227–240

Jasper HH (1960): Unspecific thalamocortical relations. In: *Neurophysiology Section,*

Handbook of Physiology, vol. 2, Magoun HW ed. Baltimore MD: Williams and Wilkins, pp 1307–1321

Kohonen T (1984): *Self-Organization and Associative Memory*. Berlin: Springer-Verlag

Lehmann D, Ozaki H, Pal I (1987): EEG alpha map series: brain micro-states by space-oriented adaptive segmentation. *Electroencephalogr Clin Neurophysiol* 67: 271–288

Lesse H (1957): Amygdaloid activity during a conditioned response. *Proc. Fourth International Congress of Electroencephalography and Clinical Neurophysiology*, Brussels, pp 99–100

Llinas RR (1988): The intrinsic electrophysiological properties of mammalian neurons: insights into central nervous system function. *Science* 242:1654–1664

Martinez DM, Freeman WJ (1984): Periglomerular cell action on mitral cell in olfactory bulb shown by current source density analysis. *Brain Res* 308:223–233

Mitzdorf U (1987): Properties of the evoked potential generators: current source-density analysis of evoked potentials in cat cortex. *Int J Neurosci* 33:33–59

Ramon y Cajal S (1909–1911): *Histologie du Systeme Nerveux de l'Homme et des Vertebres*, vols. I, II. Paris: Maloine

Rhoades BK, Freeman WJ (1990): GABAergic modulation of EEG and evoked potentials in the rat olfactory bulb. Abstracts, American Chemosensory Society

Sheer D (1976): Focussed arousal and 40-Hz EEG. In *The Neuropsychology of Learning Disorders: Theoretical Approaches*, Knights RM, Baker DJ, eds. Baltimore, MD: University Park Press, pp 71–87

Sholl DA (1956): *The Organization of the Cerebral Cortex*. New York: Wiley

Thompson JMT, Stewart HB (1986): *Nonlinear Dynamics and Chaos*. New York: Wiley

Skarda CA, Freeman WJ (1987): How brains make chaos in order to make sense of the world. *Brain Behav Sci* 10:161–195

van Rotterdam A (1987): Electrical and magnetic fields of the brain computed by way of a discrete systems analytical approach: theory and validation. *Biol Cybern* 57: 301–311

A Comparison of Certain Gamma Band (40-HZ) Brain Rhythms in Cat and Man

ROBERT GALAMBOS

Human and Cat Rhythms Compared

I still recall my astonishment when I learned that if you open your eyes the electroencephalogram (EEG) alpha waves will disappear, and that if then you close them the alpha waves will reappear. The year was 1934, and I have been hoping ever since to learn what causes the 10-Hz rhythm in the first place, and then what brain process turns it off and on. The editors of this book have asked me to compare another human brain rhythm—in the region of 40 Hz this time—with a cat rhythm in the same frequency range that is discussed elsewhere in this volume by Gray and Singer and their colleagues, and by Eckhorn and his colleagues. I do as much as I can to oblige them in what follows, first describing some properties of the human 40-Hz phenomena, then comparing these with the microelectrode data from the cat. After concluding that the two differ in several ways, I branch out to consider the general problem of brain rhythms briefly, and to speculate on their possible physiological origins and functions.

The human steady-state response

Examples of human evoked potentials (EPs) elicited by flash, click, and tactile stimuli delivered at a rate of 32 per second appear in Figure 1. Known also as steady-state responses (SSRs), these EPs were recorded using standard EEG procedures from the scalp of an adult male. Each trace averages responses to nearly 6000 stimuli (3 min worth), and replications of each condition are superimposed. The vertical lines show when the stimuli were delivered. Stimulus intensity was adjusted in each case so as to yield a response amplitude of approximately 1 μV at the electrode located on top of the head (C_z). The three other channels recorded SSRs obtained near the cortical termination of the visual (O_z), tactile (C_3), and auditory (T_3) modalities. Several features of these SSRs are notable:

1. Human EPs to stimuli delivered at high stimulus rates are not unique to the visual modality.
2. In the three modalities they all resemble sinusoids and are similar in amplitude.

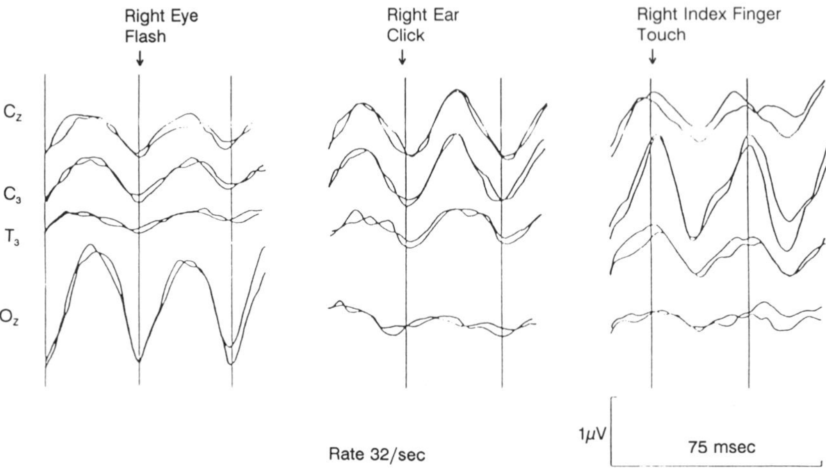

Figure 1. Steady-state responses (SSRs) to stimuli: one subject, three modalities, one experimental session. Computer-generated square waves activated either a Grass strobe unit to produce flashes, an earphone to produce clicks, or a vibrator touching the tip of a forefinger, at a rate of 32 Hz. The two vertical lines in each segment (only one bears an arrow) mark the moments of stimulus delivery. Conventional EEG electrodes, applied according to the 10-20 system and referenced to the neck were connected to amplifiers (gain 50,000, bandpass 0.3–300) and a Nicolet Med80 computer. The text supplies additional details.

3. The interval between moment of stimulus delivery and baseline crossing of the response is not identical for the three modalities; this phase difference is at least in part related to the differences in distance, and therefore in conduction time, between the sense organ stimulated and its response generator in the brain.
4. Visual and tactile amplitudes are largest at the scalp electrode that overlies the cortical region to which the modality projects. (Auditory EPs do not follow this rule because their presumed generator lies hidden in the sylvian sulcus.)
5. From the fact that the stimulus rate was 32, not 40 Hz, the reader can correctly infer that SSRs are not sharply tuned in any of the modalities; the optimal stimulus rate regularly lies near 40 Hz, but adjacent rates are always more or less effective. To recognize this fact, and in agreement with a solution Bressler recently advocated (Bressler, 1990), I replace "40 Hz" with "gamma band" throughout what follows, and define in the appended Glossary the related terminolgy to be used. The pioneers in EEG research invented the term gamma for spontaneous EEG frequencies in the 35- to 50-Hz region; any bandpass selected will be arbitrary, and mine is to be 25 to 110 Hz, which resembles that used by Eckhorn et al., (1988).

Some properties of the auditory SSRs

For a general discussion of SSRs like those of Figure 1 see Regan (1989), who was among the first to research the visual variety. However, much of the recent work by us and others has been on the auditory SSRs (e.g., Galambos et al., 1981; Brown and Shallop, 1982; Stapells et al., 1984; Linden et al., 1985; Kankkunen and Rosenhall, 1985; Rees et al., 1986; Jerger et al., 1986; Picton et al., 1987; Galambos and Makeig, 1988; Makeig and Galambos, 1989a, 1989b; Makeig, 1990). The following figures, which illustrate their most important properties, come mostly from unpublished experiments Scott Makeig and I have performed.

Figure 2 demonstrates the effect of sleep on auditory SSR amplitude. It is made up of pairs of wave shapes like those in Figure 1 linked one after another in real time. Shown expanded in the bottom row, each response pair is

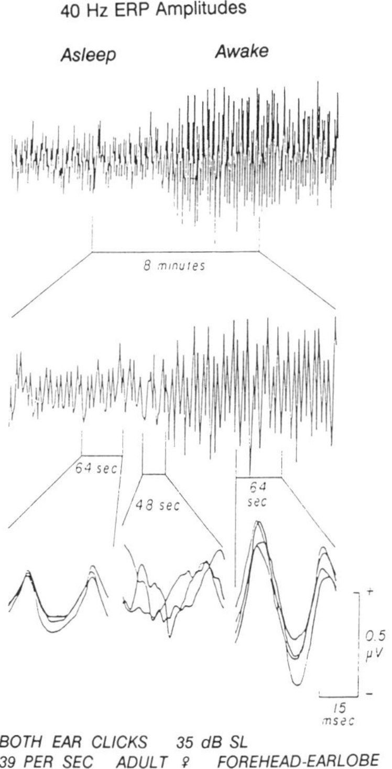

Figure 2. Auditory SSRs monitor the transition from sleep to wakefulness during a postprandial nap. Stimulus, recording, and averaging conventions as in Fig. 1. Faint clicks, delivered at a rate of 39 Hz through hearing aid earphones, activated the brain throughout. When sleeping, the subject generated between two and three times less energy at the stimulus rate than when awake.

the averaged response to monaural clicks delivered at 39 Hz for 16 s. The subject, a female adult instructed to stay awake while lying down with eyes closed in a quiet, dark room after lunch, dozed off and woke up repeatedly during an experiment lasting about half an hour. From top to bottom, Figure 2 shows with progressively greater time resolution the SSR changes taking place during one of the awakenings.

The auditory SSR amplitude is attenuated by 50% or more in sleep, and promptly restored upon wakening. It is also clear, from all-night experiments where sleep stage and SSR amplitude were evaluated at the same time, that the two are only weakly correlated; in one 8-h session both the largest and the smallest SSR amplitudes were obtained during rapid eye movement (REM) stages (unpublished data). We name the process responsible for the amplitude modulation of Figure 2 a *modulator* and have identified, in addition to the sleep-induced variety, the stimulus-induced and the spontaneous "minute rhythm" (i.e., 20–120 s) modulators (Galambos and Makeig, 1988). The physiological mechanism(s) responsible for these impressive variations in SSR amplitude are unknown.

SSR measurements and their applications

Fourier analysis is a convenient way to quantify periodic signals such as those in Figure 1. In our procedure, the Discrete Fourier Transform algorithm (DFT; Regan, 1989) calculates the sine wave that best matches the more or less noisy one recorded at the scalp. This DFT is a complex number that changes in characteristic ways when perturbations are introduced into the stimulus train producing the SSR; the resulting complex event-related potential (CERP) is currently under study as a possible method for measuring brain events correlated with cognitive behaviors (Makeig and Galambos, 1989; Rohrbaugh et al., 1990).

In another application, numbers representing the SSR amplitude (in μV) and phase (in degrees relative to the moment of stimulus delivery) are extracted from the DFT and plotted, as in Figure 3, as a function of the intensity level of the sounds presented to a listener. The plot reveals this general rule: louder sounds produce larger response amplitudes and shorter phase delays. The figure makes clear, furthermore, that both of these measures become untrustworthy at sound intensities close to the subject's threshold of hearing. This suggested to us that hearing threshold might be estimated objectively and simply by measuring the intensity-dependent changes in SSR amplitude and/or phase, and we have published experiments (Stapells et al., 1987, 1988) showing that for adults this is correct, give or take 5 to 10 dB.

Incidentally, the two lines labeled "noise" in Figure 3, one for each ear, show the averaged amplitude of eight spontaneous EEG frequencies, four above and four below the stimulus rate, spaced 1 Hz apart; this "noise" is a reasonably accurate estimate, we believe, of what the spontaneous EEG amplitude at the stimulus rate would have been in the absence of stimulation. If

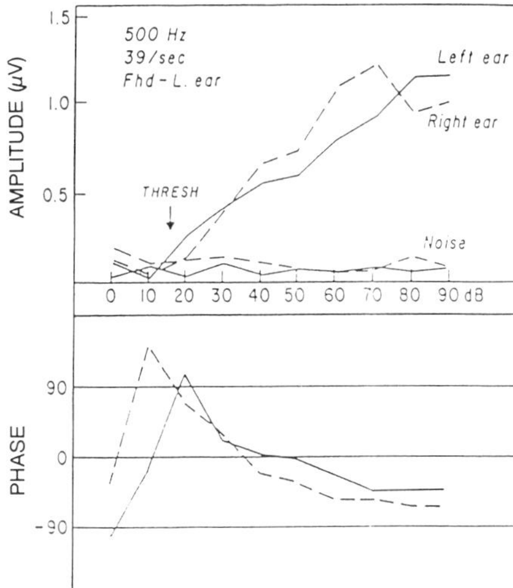

Figure 3. Estimation of hearing threshold using SSR amplitude and phase. Stimulus, recording, and averaging conventions resemble those in Figs. 1 and 2. Brief tone bursts (500 Hz) at 10 intensities were randomly delivered to one ear or the other in separate experiments. Fourier analysis of the resulting SSRs yielded the response amplitude and phase numbers plotted. Note the regular intensity-dependent changes in both measures at suprathreshold stimulus intensities, and their disappearance in the threshold region. The behavioral threshold (*arrow*) was the same for both ears. See text for more details.

this assumption is valid, all amplitude enhancements beyond this level must represent new 39-Hz energy produced by the stimulus, not merely phase-locking of the spontaneous energy already present at that frequency.

A short latency gamma band response follows both auditory and visual stimuli

A striking way in which human gamma band responses (GBRs) resemble the cat oscillatory responses is that both clicks and flashes evoke a train of five or more wavelets in the gamma band range. Figure 4 shows the auditory (A) and visual (B) GBRs recorded from a single subject; the top trace in each case is the wideband response, the middle trace the gamma band response filtered out of it, and the bottom trace what remains. The auditory and visual stimuli were both delivered at a rate of 1 per 10 s at the start of the trace. We recently reported briefly on click-evoked auditory GBRs like those in Figure 4A, which we then called the auditory 40-Hz band event-related potential (ERP) (Makeig and Galambos, 1989b). Figure 4B, the visual record, is the averaged response to about 60 red flashes delivered to my eyes. We have only just

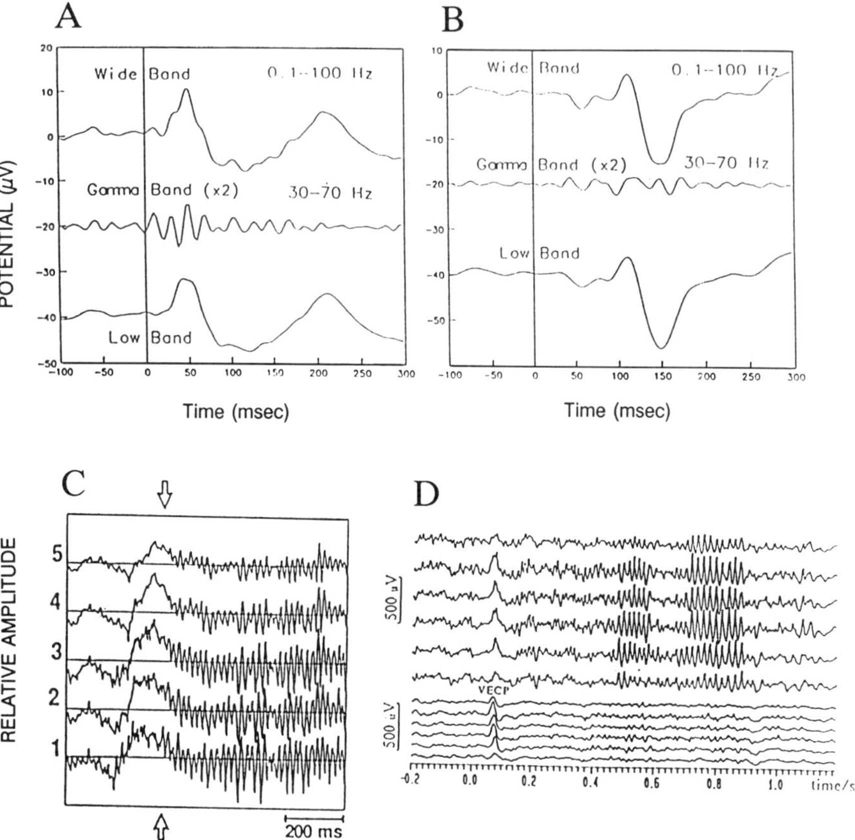

Figure 4. Gamma band responses (GBRs) from man and gamma band oscillations from the cat.
Click (**A**) and flash (**B**) responses from the human scalp; moving-stripe responses from cat cortex (**C, D**). **A, B**: **Upper trace** (wideband: 0.1–100 Hz bandpass) shows evoked potentials to stimuli applied at time zero; **Middle trace**: The GBR extracted from the upper trace by a gamma band filter (30–70 Hz bandpass) and displayed at twice the gain shown on the ordinate. **Bottom trace**: What remains of the Wideband response after removal of the GBR.
C, D: Responses to moving stripes obtained through microelectrodes from cat visual cortex. C is modified from Engle et al. (1990), D modified from Eckhorn et al. (1989); see text for details.

begun to study this visual phenomenon, which resembles one described by several others (see Cracco and Cracco, 1978 for a summary).

Evidently, each visual and auditory stimulus delivered to human subjects evokes a gamma band response, which is defined here as a train of short-latency (25 ms or less), small amplitude (about 1 μV maximum), wavelets in the 30- to 50-Hz range; this GBR lasts 120 ms or so and is precisely time-locked to each stimulus.

Figures 4C and D show that, contrary to what has just been said about human GBRs, the moment of stimulus onset does not time-lock the latency and phase of the cat oscillatory responses. Figure 4D, from a figure published by Eckhorn et al. (1990), shows these rhythms generated in cat cortex at the time black and white stripes were moved in front of the eyes. The six upper lines display events seen at six different microelectrode locations during a single stimulus presentation. In every channel a visual evoked cortical potential (VECP) appears about 100 ms after the stimulation begins, followed about 400 ms later by two successive oscillatory responses. The lower six lines show grand averages of 10 such records containing the oscillatory responses; the time-locked VECP is still visible in every channel, but the oscillations have been averaged toward zero. Figure 4C, from a figure published by Engel et al. (1990), shows similar oscillations elicited from cat cortex, this time at five microelectrode locations; the authors estimate them to begin at the open arrow, and as in Figure 4D, these are preceded by a large visual evoked cortical potential that onsets at an uncertain point perhaps 200 ms ahead of the open arrow.

Evidently each cat response has two parts: an early stimulus-locked slow-wave portion (e.g., the VECP) followed by a burst of waves that is remarkably tightly synchronized across the brain regions sampled. The fact that these waves are merely induced by, not time-locked to, the initiating stimuli means that the averaging process that is essential for revealing human GBRs eliminates the cat phenomenon.

Interim summary

Figure 4 illustrates two differences between the cat and human phenomena.

1. *Human GBRs are time-locked to the stimulus, but the cat rhythm is not.* Those who work with the cat rhythm agree that, as Figure 4C and D demonstrate, its onset latency, frequency, amplitude, and temporal phase are not time-locked to the moment of stimulation (summarized by Gray, this volume). As just noted, however, both the human GBR and the cat VECP do bear fixed relationships to the stimulus onset. Presumably the brain generators of stimulus-locked potentials differ from generators of the merely stimulus-induced potentials in important ways still to be defined.

2. *The human latency is shorter than the cat latency.* The human GBR is already well under way 50 ms after a flash or click has been delivered, whereas the cat rhythms begin several hundreds of milliseconds after stimulus onset (Fig. 4). The shortest cat latency I have seen showed oscillations delayed about 100 ms after stimulus onset, which in that instance was the abrupt illumination of a stationary bar optimally oriented for units isolated in area 18 (C.M. Gray, personal communication). If this is in fact the minimum cat latency recordable, it is at least double that of the human response, a discrepancy that would argue against assigning them a common physlologlcal origin.

This raises the question whether the cat cortex generates two gamma band oscillations, the second being analogous to the early, precisely time-locked human GBR. This human analogue, if there is one, would appear in the 200-ms poststimulus interval: I do not see it in the recordings of Figure 4, nor in the other records of the Gray and Singer and Eckhorn groups available to me. Perhaps a data analysis procedure like that used to extract human GBRs is required to settle the matter.

Two additional differences between human and cat rhythms can be cited.

3. *The anesthetic halothane affects the human and cat responses differently: The cat experiments being considered were performed under halothane anesthesia, a drug that abolishes the auditory GBR in man.* In human patients being prepared for an operation, Thornton et al. (1983) correlated the increasing halothane blood levels with the progressive deterioration and final disappearance of what is known as the middle latency auditory response (MLR). As we have reported (Makeig and Galambos, 1989b), this MLR is derived directly from the auditory GBR shown in Figure 4: as the interstimulus interval shortens with rise in stimulus rate, the GBR wavelet sequence begins to overlap on itself; at the 10-Hz rate this overlapping process produces the MLR, and at still higher rates it produces SSRs. Our preliminary studies suggest that a similar overlapping of the *visual* gamma band wavelets is responsible for visual SSRs like those in Figure 1. We do not know whether visual GBRs are like auditory GBRs in being depressed by halothane, but if they are, as seems likely, the cat and human generators would differ in this respect.

4. *The stimulus that generates the human GBR will not generate the cat rhythm.* Light flashes illuminating the entire retina produced the human GBR in Figure 4B. By contrast, one must present patterned visual stimuli in particular ways to produce the cat oscillatory response (Engel et al., 1990). No one to my knowledge has moved the oriented stripes that elicit the cat response in front of the human eye while recording from either scalp electrodes or from electrodes located on or in the visual cortex. The information such experiments might reveal, however, would not change what we already know, namely, the simple unpatterned flash that evokes human GBRs does not induce the cat oscillations.

Brain-Rhythm Generators: A Classification and Discussion

One must wonder, first of all, about the validity of the conclusion reached in the first section. For instance, different species are being compared, which is probably irrelevant, since cat and human brains almost certainly use similar mechanisms to process visual stimuli. However, the two brains processed different stimuli: red flashes into human eyes are not moving stripes across cat eyes, and one can be certain that no brain will process such dissimilar stimuli in exactly the same way. Then there is the difference in electrophysiological perspective: microelectrodes see details whereas scalp electrodes deliver some sort of "big picture." Finally, I have freely extrapolated hard data on auditory GBRs to the visual GBR about which relatively little is known, a procedure many will surely find objectionable. Without doubt, the editors asked me to examine two very different brief glimpses of the brain at work, and one of these is certainly distorted and incomplete.

In what follows I go beyond what I was asked to do to consider briefly the various problems the burgeoning field of brain rhythms presents for analysis.

The EEG gamma-band rhythms classified

The class of gamma band rhythms includes at least the following four types distinguished in the literature:

1. The *spontaneous* gamma waves, which at any given moment contribute a fraction of the total EEG energy a brain is generating.
2. The *induced* oscillations which, like those in Figure 4C and D, are initiated by but not tightly time-locked to a stimulus; gamma band activities induced by olfactory stimuli have received far more attention than any other variety (see Freeman, this volume).
3. The *evoked* gamma band response (GBR) which, as seen in Figure 4A and B, is both induced by and precisely time-locked to a stimulus. Başar (1980) and Başar-Eroglu and Başar (1991) have demonstrated that visual and auditory stimuli evoke these in many brain regions.
4. The *emitted* gamma band oscillations: these represent gamma band energy time-locked to a stimulus that has not been presented. The evidence for this improbable phenomenon was recently presented for man by Başar et al. (1989), for cat from hippocampal recordings by Eroglu-Başar and Başar (1991) (see Fig. 5D), and for nonmammalian vertebrates (the fish) by Bullock et al. (1990) (see Fig. 5C). Emitted oscillations in man are conceptually related to the "omitted P3" evoked potential, a slow-wave sequence that appears under scalp electrodes when human subjects detect the absence of an expected visual, auditory, or tactile stimulus. Explanations of these signs of stimulus anticipation usually postulate an internal timing system that predicts the occurrence of future events.

The EEG 10-Hz band rhythms classified

It is probably not coincidental that what is known about the EEG alpha rhythm fits rather neatly into the classification scheme just outlined.

1. Alpha is more than just a spontaneous rhythm; it is the prototype of spontaneous brain rhythms.
2. Alpha can be induced: Perhaps the reader will find credible the claim that induced alpha band rhythms are analogues of the gamma band rhythms induced by moving stripes and odors in the animal experiments. Consider closing the eyes in a lighted room: like turning off the lights, it reduces

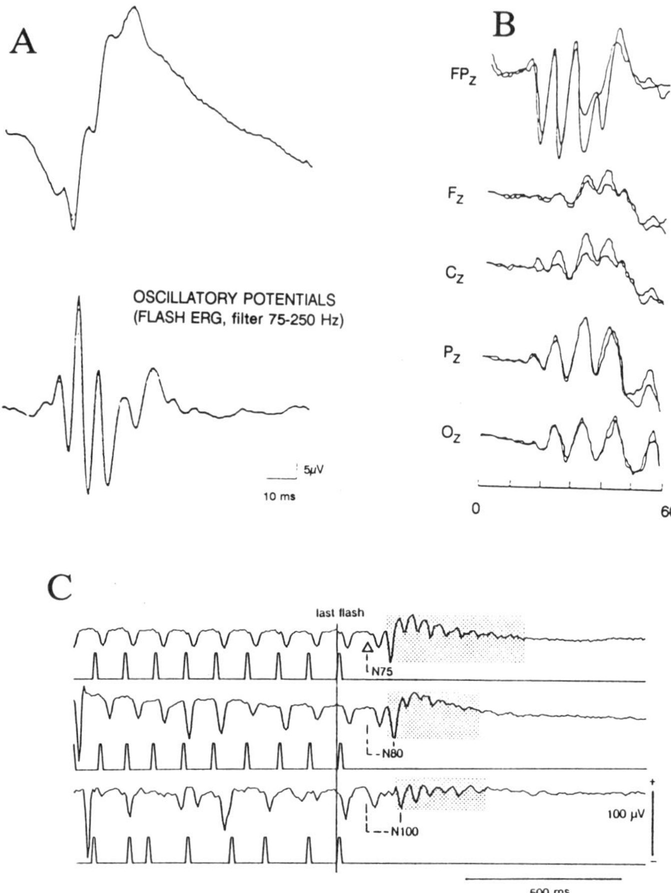

Figure 5. A sample of published gamma band rhythms.
A: The 100 Hz-band evoked retinal rhythm. The oscillatory potentials, below, were extracted from the human electroretinogram, above, by a high pass filter. Modified from Kergoat and Lovacik (1990).
B: The 100 Hz-band evoked rhythms from the human scalp. **Top to bottom**: Placement of the midline recording electrodes from the front (F_z) to the rear (O_z) of the head. Modified from Cracco and Cracco (1978).
C: The 15–30 Hz-band emitted potentials from the fish brain. **Top to bottom**: Three different experiments each showing (*upper line*) the response in the brain stem and (*lower line*) the moment flashes were delivered to the eye. The interstimulus interval is constant in the top experiment and jittered in the other two. The vertical line locates the last flash delivered and the shaded area covers the electrical activity emitted at approximately the time the next flash would have appeared. After Bullock et al. (1990). See text for further details.
D: Activity generated in the hippocampus of a freely moving cat at the moment single tone-bursts are *omitted from* a series being presented at the rate of one per 2.5 s.; the traces average 50 such stimulus omissions. The 30–50-Hz band response in the top trace has been extracted from the feline version of the human omitted-stimulus (P300) wave-complex in the bottom trace. Modified from Başar-Eroglu and Başar (1991).

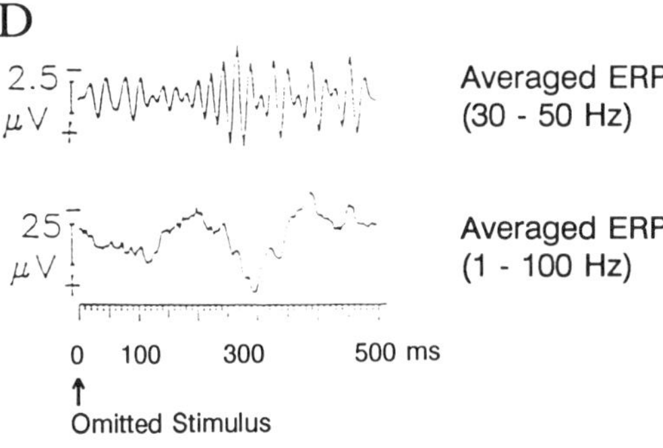

Figure 5 (*Continued*)

retinal illumination and initiates, or induces, an alpha band burst in the EEG. An example of alpha induced by (undefined) changes in internal state: the rhythm disappears the moment a subject follows the instruction "multiply 11 by 13," and it reappears as soon as the answer is delivered.

3. Alpha can certainly be evoked: Time-locking of alphalike rhythms to onset of light flashes was clearly described by M.A.B. Brazier more than 30 years ago in one of the earliest reports on human computer-averaged evoked responses (Brazier, 1960). The physiological basis of this phenomenon—a near–10-Hz periodic oscillation that continues for a second or so—remains unclear (see Mangun, this volume, for a summary). Brazier's discussion of her discovery has a familiar ring:

   > This finding of a rhythm phase-locked to the stimulus shows that the brain now has a rhythm that has been imposed on it through a sensory system. Has this imposed rhythm supplanted the "endogenous" one; or is it the same rhythm with a shift in phase to carry the message; or is the basic rhythm still there and this one added? In the latter case the brain would have its own rhythm against which to match this one for both frequency and phase. (p. 351)

   Substitute gamma band for the alpha band she had in mind, and her questions are the same ones several contributors to this volume ask.

4. Finally, alpha can be emitted: In the study where Başar et al. (1989) demonstrated anticipatory time-locking of gamma band energy, a well trained subject emitted time-locked bursts of alpha-band energy for up to a full second before the delivery of an expected target. By contrast to the modest evidence they advanced for anticipatory time-locking of waves in the gamma band, the alpha locking to the moment in the future when a target will be delivered is robust and highly significant statistically.

These comparisons prompt a possibly heuristic speculation: Because gamma band and alpha band rhythms behave similarly—that is, can be induced, time-locked, emitted, and so on—the physiological mechanisms through which they are generated and controlled, when revealed, will have much in common.

The plethora of stimulus-induced rhythms

In his introductory chapter to this volume Bullock pointed to human and animal rhythms other than those in the 10-Hz and 40-Hz bands. The three visual examples that follow, which range in frequency from the approximate 100-Hz, or high gamma band to the low gamma band (or mixed beta gamma) range, will illustrate still other rhythmic phenomena that await inclusion into —or exclusion from—schemes that relate rhythmic responses to perceptual and cognitive performance.

1. Figure 5A shows the five to seven near–100-Hz wavelets (called oscillatory potentials; OP) present in the electroretinogram (Cracco and Cracco, 1978; Bartel et al., 1990; Kergoat and Lovasik, 1990). A similar stimulus-locked high gamma band phenomenon has also been repeatedly documented in human scalp recordings [Fig. 5B; Cracco and Cracco (1978) and Regan (1989) provide summaries]. Whether the OPs recorded in frontal scalp regions are spread by volume conduction from the retina has apparently not yet been settled, but the OPs seen in the posterior scalp regions almost certainly are generated in the brain (Whittaker and Siegfried, 1983). An apparent difference in the frequency content of these cortical OPs (high gamma band, near 100 Hz) and the visual GBR of Figure 4 (mid–gamma band, near 50 Hz) remains to be explained.

In discussing the retinal OPs, Dowling (1987) states they are produced by neuronal activity in several of the retinal layers, and specifically excludes the retinal b-wave generator as a possible source. His conclusion is important because the retinal b-wave is generated, in lower animals at least, when the excess extracellular potassium ion produced during neuronal synaptic activities is transported to the vitreous surface of the retina within the cytoplasm of the Muller cell, the major glial cell in the retina. Assuming that similar physiological mechanisms also produce the cortical OPs, and that it is legitimate to extrapolate Dowling's conclusion to the brain as a whole, it would appear unlikely that brain glia are involved in generating the gamma band rhythms that interest us.

2. My search of the literature has not yet uncovered an unequivocal example of the human visual GBR of Figure 4B. However, Regan can be said to have discovered it when he stimulated his subjects with light flickered at different rates and named the increased EEG energy present in the 30- to 50-Hz region a "high frequency system" (Regan, 1968, 1989). The visual SSR in Figure 1 is an example of what he found; it is probable that these SSRs develop when, at very short interstimulus intervals, the GBR wavelets seen in Figure 10.4B lie on top of one other.

As for the equivalent animal flash-evoked GBR, see Figure 3 in the chapter by Steriade et al. in this volume, which was recorded from the visual cortex of an unanesthetized cat. Its duration, about 150 ms as displayed, resembles that of the human response and its late wavelets resemble the cat cortical stripe response in being enhanced by stimulation of the reticular formation (see Gray et al., this volume).

3. In fish, Bullock et al. (1990) recently described 15- to 25-Hz oscillations in the retina, optic nerve, and midbrain that are approximately time-locked to the moment an omitted flash stimulus was due. Figure 5D shows examples of these low–gamma band (or high betaband?) oscillations; each one indexes a stimulus not presented and shows how readily the simple repetition of a stimulus can reorganize a collection of neurons and change its output. Bullock et al. propose that the emitted fish rhythms represent new equilibria reached between the excitatory and inhibitory consequences of each flash. However this may be, the objective sign of the newly created state of affairs is a burst of rhythmic oscillations initiated within the retina and at brain stem levels of this cold-blooded vertebrate animal.

Evidently, induced rhythms are to be found throughout the vertebrate phylum, in widespread regions of the nervous system, following many types of stimuli, and under a surprising variety of behavioral states. Simple facts about them remain to be discovered: for instance, do gamma band oscillations in the cat optic nerve reveal that the cat retina, like the fish retina, stores a history of its recent stimulation; and does the fish forebrain, like the cat cortex, emit gamma band oscillations when stripes move in front of the eyes? And beyond such mere facts, where are the concepts that will assemble them into meaningful generalizations about brain function?

Summary

1. During the process of comparing the near-40 Hz brain oscillations associated with cat and human visual stimulation, the following dichotomies and contrasts were introduced and discussed:

- spontaneous rhythms versus induced (stimulus-dependent) rhythms
- induced GBRs that are precisely time-locked to a stimulus (i.e., evoked by them) versus, the gamma band oscillations that are not.
- gamma band versus, 10 Hz-band rhythms
- oscillations in various frequency bands associated with visual, auditory, and tactile stimuli
- induced rhythms in fish versus those in mammals (rabbit, cat, man)
- oscillations that are drug-sensitive (halothane) versus those that are not
- neuronal versus glial contributions to oscillatory phenomena

2. The analysis yields two conclusions:

- visual stimuli induce several kinds of gamma band (25–110-Hz) oscillations. One of these, a response to flash in cat and man, and called here the GBR, is a burst of several wavelets that appears immediately after stimulus onset and is precisely time-locked to it. Another, recorded with microelectrodes in the cat cortex, is induced only by patterned stimuli (e.g., stripes); its latency is long and the oscillations are not precisely time-locked to the stimulus. The text and the appended Glossary differentiate these two from each other and from several other induced gamma band rhythms that are described and discussed.

- the various oscillatory phenomena considered call to mind an old generalization about the EEG, namely, whenever a vertebrate brain emits a new rhythm, or stops producing an old one, or does both of these things, its owner, if wide awake, is probably analyzing a stimulus or preparing to execute a behavioral response. From this point of view each different oscillation extracted from an induced visual response can be thought of as marking the onset and duration of some physiological process we would like to understand. Without question, many such processes run concurrently in different places (e.g., retina and cortex) and in overlapping post-stimulus time windows; modern methods should make it possible to identify how many of these mark the beginning or end of some interesting "cognitive" event and to localize the brain structures that generate them.

Glossary: Definitions of the Gamma Family of Brain Rhythms

Gamma Rhythm: the EEG in the (approximately) 25- to 110-Hz frequency band, normally spontaneously generated.

Gamma band (or **gamma-band** or **gammaband**) **oscillation** (or **rhythm**): Oscillations in the 25- to 110-Hz frequency band that are induced by stimuli; that is, the stimuli trigger or modulate the oscillation but do not provide its rhythm. Gamma band oscillations can be low (25–35 Hz), mid (36–59) or high (60– 110) in frequency content and they vary in duration. The olfactory and visual phenomena studied by Freeman, Gray, Singer, Eckhorn, and their colleagues, called "gamma oscillations" by some, are all induced gamma band rhythms (or oscillations).

The gamma band response (GBR): an induced gamma band rhythm that is also time-locked to the stimulus; synonymous with evoked gamma band response. **Time-locked alpha**: an induced alpha band rhythm that is also time-locked to a single visual stimulus; synonymous with evoked alpha response.

Emitted rhythm: a rhythmic event that is time-locked to a stimulus that has not been presented. Emitted rhythms can be alpha band, gamma band, etc. in frequency content, and include examples from man and cat (the Başar group), and from fish (Bullock et al.). Synonymous with omitted stimulus potential, missing stimulus response, expectation wave, and other terms.

References

Bartel P, Blom M, Robinson E, VanderMeyden C, Sommers DeK, Becker P (1990): Effects of chlorpromazine on pattern and flash ERGs and VEPs compared to oxazepam and to placebo in normal subjects *Electroencephalogr Clin Neurophysiol* 77:330–339

Başar E (1980): *EEG–Brain Dynamics.* New York: Elsevier

Başar E, Başar-Eroglu C, Roschke J, Schutt A (1989): The EEG is a quasi-deterministic signal anticipating sensory-cognitive tasks. In: *Brain Dynamics: Progress and Perspectives*, Başar E, Bullock TH, eds. Berlin: Springer, pp 43–71

Başar-Eroglu C, Başar E (1991): A compound P300-40 Hz response of the cat hippocampus. *Int J Neurosci* 60:227–237

Brazier MAB (1960): Long-persisting electrical traces in the brain of man and their possible relationship to higher nervous activity. In: *The Moscow Colloquium on Electroencephalography of Higher Nervous Activity*, Jasper HH, Smirnov GD, eds. The EEG Journal, Montreal, pp 347–358

Bressler SL, (1990): The gamma wave: a cortical information carrier? *Trends Neurosci* 13:161–162

Brown DD, Shallop JK (1982): A clinically useful 500 Hz evoked response. *Nicolet Potentials* 1:9–12

Bullock TH, Hofmann MF, Nahm FK, New JG, Prechtl JC (1990): Event-related potentials in the retina and optic tectum of fish. *J Neurophysiol* 64:903–914

Cracco RQ, and Cracco JB (1978): Visual evoked potential in man: early oscillatory potentials. *Electroencephalogr Clin Neurophysiol* 45:731–739

Dowling JE (1987): *The Retina.* Cambridge, MA: Harvard University

Eckhorn R, Bauer R, Jordan W, Brosch M, Kruse W, Munk M, Reitboeok HJ (1988): Coherent oscillations: a mechanism of feature linking in the visual cortex? *Biol Cybern* 60(2):121–130

Eckhorn R, Reitboeok HJ, Dicke P, Arndt M, Kruse W (1990): Feature linking across cortical maps via synchronization. In: *Proceedings International Conference on Parallel Processing in Neural Systems and Computers*, Eckmiller R, ed. Amsterdam: Elsevier, pp 1–4

Engel AK, Konig P, Gray CM, Singer W (1990): Stimulus-dependent neuronal oscillations in cat visual cortex: Inter-columnar interaction as determined by cross-correlation analysis. *Eur J Neurosci* 2:558–606

Galambos R, Makeig S (1988): Dynamic changes in steady-state potentials. In: *Dynamics of Sensory and Cognitive Processing of the Brain*, Başar E, ed. Berlin: Springer, pp 102–122

Galambos R, Makeig, S, Talmachoff P (1981): A 40 Hz auditory potential recorded from the human scalp. *Proc Natl Acad Sci USA*, 78(4):2643–2647

Jerger JF, Chmiel R, Frost JD, Coker N (1986): Effect of sleep on the auditory steady state evoked potential. *Ear Hear* 7(4):240–245

Kankkunen A, Rosenhall U (1985): Comparison between thresholds obtained with pure-tone audiometry and the 40-Hz middle latency response. *Scand Audiol*, 14:99–104

Kergoat H, Lovasik JV (1990): The effects of altered vascular perfusion pressure on the white flash scotopic ERG and oscillatory potentials in man. *Electroencephalogr Clin Neurophysiol* 76:306–322

Linden RD, Campbell KB, Hamel G, Picton T (1985): Human auditory steady state evoked potentials during sleep. *Ear Hear* 6:167–174

Makeig S (1990): A dramatic increase m the auditory middle latency response at very slow rates. In: *Psychological Brain Research*, Brunia CM, Gaillard AK, Kok A, eds. Tillburg, the Netherlands: Tilburg University Press, pp 56–60

Makeig S, Galambos R (1989a): The CERP: event-related perturbations in steady-state responses. In: *Brain Dynamics: Progress and Perspectives*, Başar E, Bullock TH, eds. Berlin: Spinger, pp 375–400

Makeig S, Galambos R (1989b): The auditory 40 Hz-band evoked response lasts 150 ms and increases in size at slow rates. *Soc Neurosci Abst* 15:113

Picton TW, Vajsar J, Rodriguez R, Campbell KB (1987): Reliability estimates for steady-state evoked potentials. *Electroencephalogr Clin Neurophysiol* 68:119–131

Rees A, Green GGR, Kay RH (1986): Steady-state evoked responses to sinusoidally amplitude-modulated sounds recorded in man. *Hear Res* 23:123–133

Regan D (1968): A high frequency mechanism which underlies visual evoked potentials. *Electroencephalogr Clin Neurophysiol* 25:231–237

Regan D (1989): *Human Brain Electrophysiology.* New York: Elsevier

Rohrbaugh JW, Varner JL, Paige SR, Eckhart MJ, Ellingson RJ (1990): Auditory and visual event-related perturbations in the 40 Hz auditory steady-state response. *Electroencephalogr Clin Neurophysiol* 76:148–164

Stapells DR, Galambos R, Costello JA, Makeig S (1988): Inconsistency of auditory middle latency and steady-state responses in infants. *Electroencephalogr Clin Neurophysiol* 71:289–295

Stapells DR, Linden RD, Suffield JB, Hamel C, Picton TW, (1984): Human auditory steady state potentials. *Ear Hear* 5(2):105–114

Stapells DR, Makeig S, Galambos R (1987): Auditory steady-state responses: threshold predictions using phase coherence. *Electroencephalogr Clin Neurophysiol* 67: 260–270

Thornton C, Catley DM, Jordan C, Lehane JR, Royston D, Jones JG (1983): Enflurane anaesthesia causes graded changes in the brainstem and early cortical auditory evoked response in man. *Br J Anaesth* 55:479–486

Whittaker SG, Siegfried JB (1983): Origin of wavelets in the visual evoked potential. *Electroencephalogr Clin Neurophysiol* 55:91–101

Human Visual Evoked Potentials: Induced Rhythms or Separable Components?

GEORGE R. MANGUN

The nervous system displays a variety of rhythmic behaviors that include such diverse and interesting phenomena as the oscillatory activity of olfactory bulb neurons and the high amplitude electroencephalogram (EEG) recordable from the human scalp. These spontaneous or "ongoing" rhythms have been considered in detail (reviewed in Bąsar, 1980). Similarly, steady-state evoked responses elicited by the repetitive, rapid presentation of stimuli have also been systematically studied (reviewed in Regan, 1989). In contrast, however, rhythmic brain activity induced by a nonoscillating external (or internal) stimulus has received considerably less attention.

The present volume considers "induced" neural rhythms and examines them from various perspectives, including the cellular, network, and systems levels. This chapter considers the neural bases of the sequential positive and negative fluctuations present in the averaged evoked potentials recorded from the human scalp in response to a transient visual stimulus. The question is whether or not certain of these apparently rhythmic fluctuations might represent a stimulus-induced brain rhythm. As detailed below, only a subset of the averaged evoked visual responses are considered; that is, the "longer latency" potentials observed between 70 and 300 ms latency. The potentials in this latency range are of particular interest because in addition to being indices of visual sensory processing in the human brain, they are also known to be modulated by visuospatial selective attention (e.g., Eason, 1981; Harter et al., 1982; Hillyard and Muente, 1984; Mangun and Hillyard, 1988, 1990, 1991; Mangun et al., in press; Neville and Lawson, 1987; Rugg et al. 1987). Thus, elucidating the neural bases of these potentials is essential for understanding the mechanisms by which higher brain centers control afferent signals in order to achieve an early neural filtering of relevant and irrelevant sensory events.

Visual Evoked Potentials

In response to a briefly flashed visual stimulus, a characteristic series of voltage fluctuations can be recorded over the human occipital scalp. These visual evoked potentials (VEPs) are small relative to the ongoing EEG and must be visualized using signal averaging. The voltage fluctuations that compose the averaged VEP include both high frequency waves (oscillatory potentials;

50–100 Hz) (Harding and Rubenstein, 1980; Whittaker and Sigfried, 1983) and slower frequency, higher amplitude waves (sensory-evoked slow waves; about 10 Hz) (e.g., Allison et al., 1977; Hackley et al., 1990). The high frequency oscillatory potentials are typically observed when the signal has been bandpass filtered to remove frequencies below 50 Hz (Fig. 1). Under such conditions, it can be seen that these oscillations have latencies of onset as

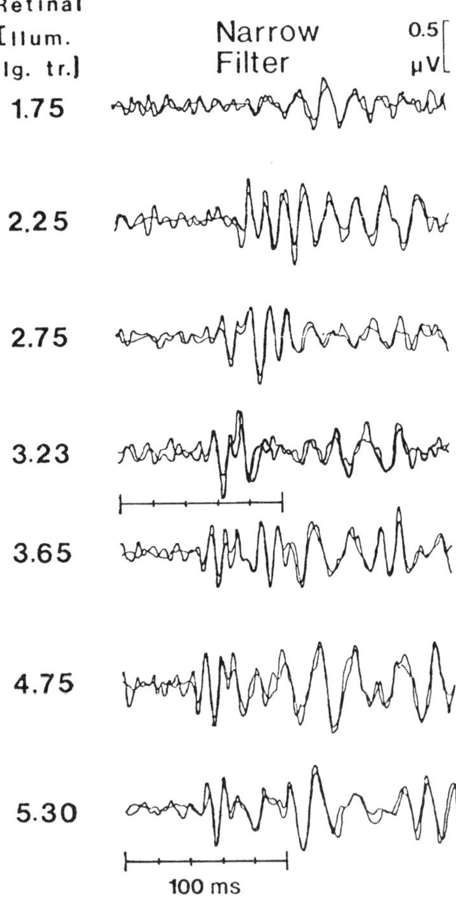

Figure 1. Visual ERPs recorded from O_z (referred to C_z) in a single subject in response to 25° unpatterned flash delivered to the right eye at different stimulus intensities. The recordings were filtered using a narrow, high frequency bandpass (60–200 Hz). Oscillatory potentials are evident as rhythmic voltage fluctuations occurring at a frequency of about 65–75 Hz. Stimulus onset is at the beginning of the trace. Positive polarity is plotted up. Modified with permission of Elsevier Science Publishers from Whittaker and Siegfried, *Electroencephalogr Clin Neurophysiol* 55:91–101, 1983.

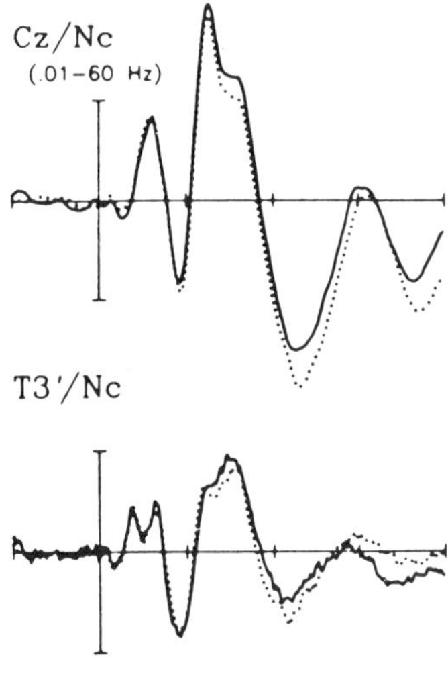

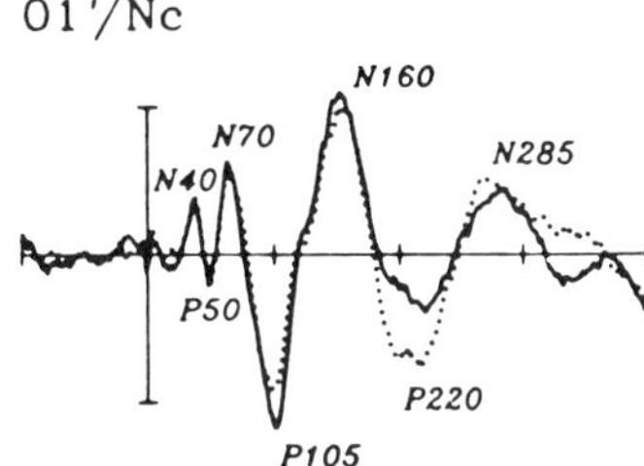

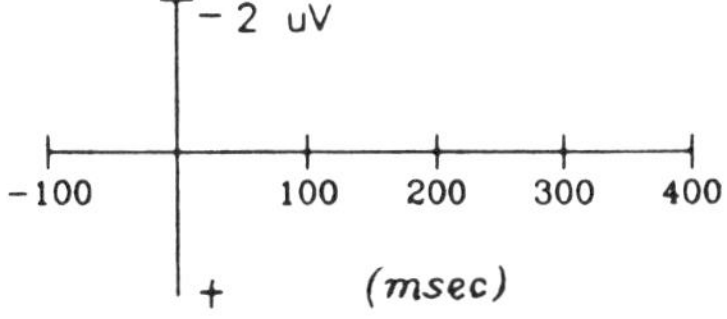

Figure 2. Grand average sensory-evoked slow potentials recorded from midline central (C_z), left temporal (T_3), and left occipital (O_1) scalp sites in a cross-modal attention experiment. The recordings were filtered with a wide band-pass of 1–300 Hz. Stimuli were large, high intensity flashes delivered to the right visual field. Over the occipital scalp in particular, a rhythmic series of high amplitude deflections can be seen between 50 and 300 ms latency that are referred to in the text as slow waves. The earliest of the major slow wave deflections is the P105 (P1) peak, and is followed by the N160 (N1), P220 (P2), and N285 (N2) deflections. Preceding the P1 peak are a series of lower amplitude deflections that may or may not be related to the oscillatory potentials shown in Fig. 1. Positive polarity is plotted downward. Modified with permission of The Society for Psychophysiological Research from Hackley et al., *Psychophysiol.*, 27:195–208, 1990.

short as 25 to 35 ms. In contrast, the major slow waves onset significantly later (Fig. 2).

The first major sensory-evoked slow wave of the VEP typically begins in the 70 to 90-ms range as a prominent, reliably elicited deflection that is sometimes referred to as the P100 or P1 (Fig. 2). The flash-evoked P1 wave is usually of maximal amplitude over lateral occipital scalp sites contralateral to the visual field of stimulation, and reaches peak amplitude at between 90 and 140 ms poststimulus (Mangun and Hillyard, 1988). The P1 peak is followed by a series of deflections that can be labeled N1, P2, and N2 to indicate their positive or negative polarities and successive appearance in the VEP waveform. The P1-N1-P2-N2 sequence results in a rhythmic waveform with a frequency of about 10 Hz. It is the rhythmic character of these longer latency "slow waves" that will be considered in this chapter.

Two contrasting interpretations can be put forth regarding the neural bases of the P1-N1-P2-N2 sequence. One view is to consider the successive positive and negative peaks as a single rhythm induced by the sensory stimulus, and to ask how it is related to other rhythmic activity in the nervous system. From this perspective, the hypothesis is that an anatomically distinct group of cortical neurons are induced by the stimulus to oscillate in their firing or postsynaptic activity, thereby producing a sequence of rhythmic voltage deflections at the scalp. The alternative view is to treat each slow wave deflection as a separate "component," each of which reflecting, in whole or part, the activity of a distinct and anatomically separate neuronal population. In this context a VEP deflection that was, for example, generated by the postsynaptic depolarization of striate cortical neurons due to thalamic input, could be considered a separate component, with respect to other VEP deflections generated by activity in the thalamus or extrastriate cortex.

The component approach to the investigation of the generator(s) of evoked responses has tended to dominate, and indeed has contributed much to our understanding of evoked potential generators. In particular, considerable success has been achieved in the identification of the neuronal generators within the ascending auditory pathway that contribute to the various peaks in the auditory brain stem response (Buchwald, 1983; Moller et al., 1981; Scherg and Von Cramen, 1985), as well as the midlatency and long-latency slow waves of the auditory evoked potential (see Celesia, 1976; Naatanen and Picton, 1987; Scherg et al., 1989).

Interestingly, however, similar attempts to identify the generators of the VEP have been somewhat less successful. In particular, no visual equivalent of the well described auditory brain stem response has been identified, although some attempts have been made to relate oscillatory potentials to subcortical structures (Cracco and Cracco, 1978; Harding and Rubenstein, 1985; Whittaker and Siegfried, 1983). Most studies of the generators of VEPs have tried to relate the sensory-evoked slow waves of the VEP to sources in the visual cortex. For example, in their "cruciform model" of visual cortex, Jeffreys and Axford (1972a, 1972b) described how stimulus-induced changes in VEP peaks could be related to the anatomy of visual cortex. They reported that two early VEP deflections, which they termed CI (65–80 ms) and CII (90–100 ms), were probably generated in striate and extrastriate visual cortex, respectively. A similar pattern of results and conclusions was obtained by Biersdorf (1974).

Subsequent studies using multichannel recording and topographic mapping have also shown that some early VEP peaks (60–140 ms) have scalp topographies that are consistent with generators in striate cortex, with later peaks being generated in extrastriate cortex (Butler et al., 1987; Darcey et al., 1980a, 1980b; see also Maier et al., 1986). Similarly, current source density (CSD) analysis of scalp potential fields elicited by flashed stimuli have arrived at similar conclusions as to the generators of the early VEPs (Srebro, 1985, 1987, 1990). Thus, to date models of the physiological bases of VEPs have tended to favor a component view, and much effort has been directed toward the identification of the neural sites at which individual VEPs are generated. However, the majority of these models have only considered the deflections occurring in the latency range of about 60 to 140 ms, whereas, as noted previously, the major P1-N1-P2-N2 slow wave sequence covers the time period from 70 to 300 ms.

So far, I have not indicated the relationship of the aforementioned early VEPs (i.e., CI or CII, etc.) to the P1-N1-P2-N2 sequence of interest here. The relationship has been somewhat unclear because different investigators have used a variety of stimulus and recording parameters as well as varied nomenclature in the naming of VEP deflections. Nonetheless, recent evidence (Mangun et al., 1990) indicates that the peak referred to here as the P1 is probably the CII peak of Jeffreys and Axford (1972b), that which they indicated was of extrastriate origin. Their CI peak, on the other hand, is most likely the negative deflection that sometimes precedes the P1 for upper field stimuli (Bodis-Wollner et al., 1989; Hackley et al., 1990). Thus, only the first deflection of the prominent P1-N1-P2-N2 slow wave sequence has been effectively modeled. It remains possible, therefore, that the voltage fluctuations in this sequence represent an induced rhythm that is triggered in visual cortex following the initial activation of striate cortex. This possibility is investigated in the next section using multichannel recording and topographic current source density mapping of the brain activity corresponding to the P1-N1-P2-N2 sequence.

Topographic Analysis of Scalp Current Density

The data presented below are from an attention study. However, it is not the goal of the present data analysis to consider the results of the attentional manipulations; those results have been presented elsewhere (Mangun et al., 1990, in press). Instead, a portion of the data will be considered from the perspective of the neural bases of the sensory-evoked slow waves. Indeed, only VEPs that were elicited by ignored stimuli will be considered, thus eliminating the possible confounding influence of attention-related electrical activity on the scalp topographies of the sensory-evoked waves (for reviews of attention effects on VEPs see, Harter and Aine, 1984; Mangun and Hillyard, 1990).

The logic of the present analysis is to use topographical mapping to determine whether single or multiple, anatomically distinct neural generators give rise the P1-N1-P2-N2 sequence of the VEP. Similar scalp topographies for each of these deflections would be consistent with the notion that a discrete neuronal population was responsible for the generation of the entire VEP sequence over this time range. Thus, the rhythmic appearance of the VEP waveform in the 70- to 300-ms range might indicate the rhythmic discharge of a population of cortical neurons that was induced, or triggered by the occurrence of a transient visual stimulus. In contrast, if the current source density (CSD) topographies in the time range of each deflection differed significantly from one another, this would argue that multiple neuronal populations contributed to the generation of these VEP peaks. Moreover, such a result would suggest that the rhythmic appearance of the slow potentials resulted from the time course of activation of the generators involved, and not from an induced rhythm at all.

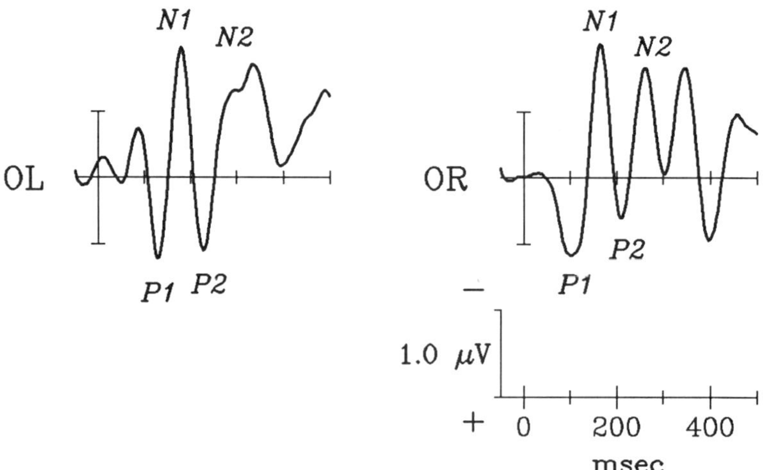

Figure 3. Visual VEPs elicited by upper left visual field stimuli when ignored. Traces are grand-averages over eight subjects and were recorded from lateral left (OL) and right (OR) occipital scalp sites. The prominent sensory-evoked slow wave sequence P1, N1, P2, and N2 is visible at both contralateral (OR) and ipsilateral (OL) scalp sites. This sequence of deflections occurs with a frequency of about 10 Hz. Note that the sequence of deflections over ipsilateral scalp is delayed by 10–15 ms with respect to those over contralateral scalp. Stimulus onset is at time zero, and positive polarity is plotted downward.

The VEPs were recorded from eight healthy right-handed persons (aged 18–30 yr). The subjects viewed vertically oriented white bars flashed for 67 ms, one at a time, to the four lateral octants of the visual field (only the VEPs to the upper field stimulus were examined here). The center of the bar stimuli were located 5.8° lateral to the vertical meridian and 3.5° from the horizontal meridian. The bars were 3.75° in height and 1.75° in width. The luminance of the flashed white bars was 0.34 candela per meter squared. The interstimulus intervals of the flashed bars varied at random between 250 and 550 ms (rectangular distribution). VEPs were recorded (0.01–100-Hz bandpass; 250-Hz digitization) from 30 scalp sites while the subjects directed their attention (but not their eyes) exclusively to one of the four visual field locations; the other locations were ignored. Their task was to detect infrequent target bars (shorter) embedded in the stream of stimuli occurring at the attended location. Eye fixation was maintained on a central point on the video screen and was verified with electrooculographic (EOG) and infrared corneal reflectance methods.

To investigate the physiological basis of the P1-N1-P2-N2 sequence of the VEP, scalp CSD topographies were calculated. CSD is the second spatial derivative of the voltage recorded from multiple locations across the scalp. The resultant CSD derivations provide information about currents flowing out of and into the skull, is reference independent, and favors local cortical activity as compared to distantly generated currents (Nunez, 1981, 1990). The approach used to interpolate and calculate the CSD was the spherical spline method (Perrin et al., 1987).

Figures 3 and 4 show the VEP waveforms elicited by the upper left- and right-field stimuli. These VEPs were recorded from lateral left and right occipital scalp locations. The prominent P1-N1-P2-N2 sequence is visible at each

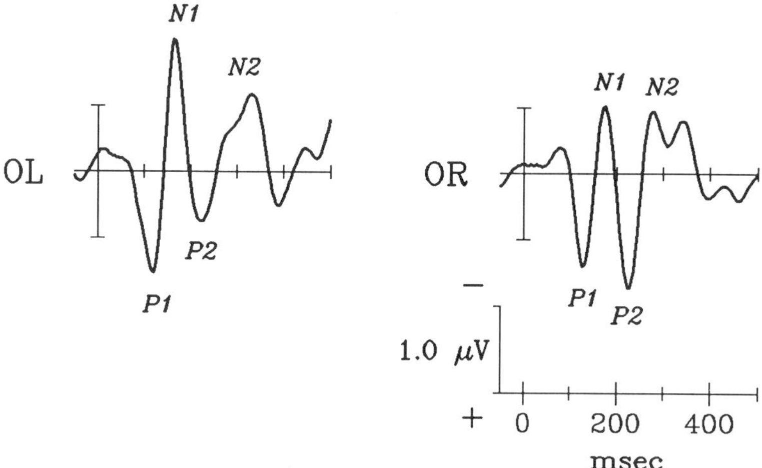

Figure 4. Same as Fig. 3 for right visual field stimuli.

scalp site in both figures. These rhythmic positive, negative fluctuations have a frequency of about 10 Hz. This rhythmicity can often be observed to continue with reduced amplitude for hundreds of ms past the N2 peak (not shown in figures). Scalp CSD topographies were calculated at latencies corresponding to the peak amplitude of each deflection and are shown in Figures 5 and 6.

In accordance with the anatomical projection of the visual pathways, the CSD topographies elicited by the left-field stimuli tended to show maximal source-sink activity over the contralateral right hemisphere (Fig. 5). Similarly,

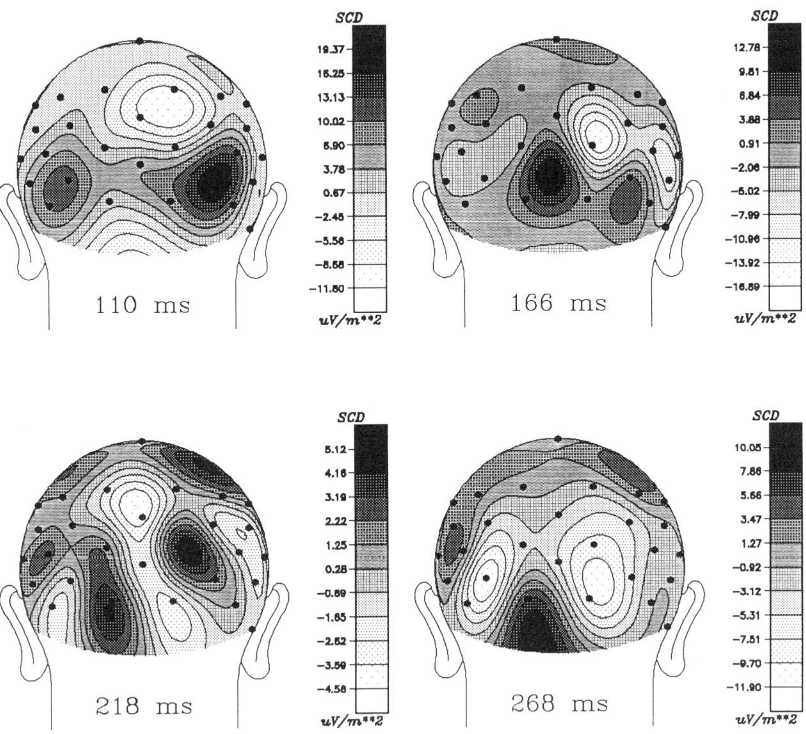

Figure 5. Topographic current source density maps at four time points corresponding to the peaks of the P1 (110 ms), N1 (166 ms), P2 (218 ms), and N2 (268 ms) deflections of the visual evoked potential to upper left field stimuli. Each map is separately scaled to cover the range from maximum to minimum value for that map. The units of measure are microvolts per square meter and are proportional to current density. Areas of outward, positive current flow (sources) are darker shades, whereas areas of inward, negative current flow (sinks) are lighter shades. Electrode locations are indicated by the black dots. The maps were derived using a spherical spline interpolation algorithm.

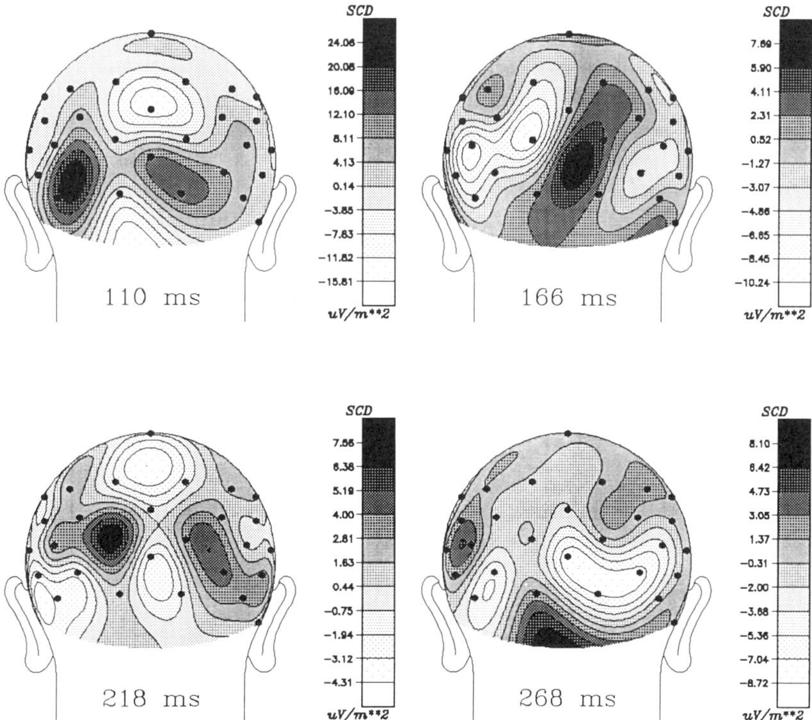

Figure 6. Same as Fig. 5 for right visual field stimuli.

right-field stimuli evoked maximal current densities over the left hemisphere (Fig. 6). The CSD distributions for each of the time points plotted are quite different. The CSD topography of the P1 peak (110 ms) shows a strong current source located over the lateral occipital cortex; a weaker current sink is situated in a dorsomedial orientation. The location of the P1 current source is at scalp sites that overlie the extrastriate visual cortex (Mangun et al., in press) and is in line with the extrastriate generator proposed for the CII peak of Jeffreys and Axford (1972b). In sharp contrast, the scalp CSD topography of the Subsequent N1 deflection (166 ms) is very different from that of the P1. At the time of the N1 deflection, a strong current sink is located over contralateral parieto-occipital scalp regions with a corresponding current source located very low on the midline. Thus, the source-sink configurations for the P1 and N1 peaks are located over different regions of the scalp and have different source-sink orientations.

The scalp CSD topographies in the time range of the later P2 (218 ms) and N2 (268 ms) deflections are somewhat more complicated, as would be expected from the greater likelihood of activation of additional visual areas with increasing time after the stimulus. However, examination of the most prominent current sources and sinks indicate patterns of activation that are quite different from the earlier peaks. The major current sources and sinks associated with the P2 peak are a lateral occipital source and midline parietal sink. This configuration is more medial and parietal and has a more narrow scalp distribution than that of the P1 deflection. The subsequent N2 peak was associated with a right occipital sink that was larger for left-field stimuli but could be observed for both left- and right-field stimuli; it is difficult to assign a complementary current source to this prominent sink; however, there is a small current source visible over right parietal regions that may be associated. This pattern appears to reflect the activation of a right hemisphere process that was elicited by both left- and right-field stimuli at about 268 ms latency. This asymmetry can be seen in the waveforms presented in Figures 3 and 4 as a double-peaked response in the latency range of 250 to 320 ms. The first peak (corresponding to the topographic map at 268 ms) is of greater amplitude for both the left- and right-field stimuli over the right hemisphere site. In contrast, the later peak (approx. 320 ms; not mapped here) appears to be contralaterally larger for both stimuli.

Discussion

The intent of this chapter has been to consider the rhythmic appearance of the slow waves of the visual evoked brain potential and to ask whether these deflections represent an induced rhythm, or instead, the sequential activation of anatomically distinct neural generators engaged in the processing of visual–sensory information. The hypothesis has been that an induced rhythm should be defined as the rhythmic discharge of an anatomically discrete population of neurons. Such activity, if synchronously activated and tightly time-locked to the inducing stimulus, would produce a rhythmic waveform at the scalp. Since an induced rhythm so defined represents the activity of a relatively localized and unchanging neuronal population, it should produce stable topographical patterns of activity over the scalp throughout its time course of activation. The data set presented here shows that the scalp topographies of current sources and sinks corresponding to the major slow wave deflections of the VEP are quite different. This result indicates that several anatomically distinct neural populations contribute to the major slow waves of the VEP between 70 and 300 ms latency. Thus, the present conclusion favors a component-based rather than induced-rhythm view of the P1-N1-P2-N2 sequence.

Such a conclusion is in line based on previous work aimed at elucidating the generators of VEP components (e.g., Darcey et al., 1980a, 1980b). The present results of scalp CSD mapping also fit well with ongoing work in my laboratory that asks a similar question by modeling the neural generators of these VEP components using inverse dipole localization methods. The view that the VEP waveform is composed of the activation of successive neuronal populations in the ascending visual pathways is no doubt correct and can be related to information from single unit recordings in animals (e.g., Robinson and Rugg, 1988). It is most likely not the case, however, that each voltage deflection in the VEP waveform (e.g., P1 or N1, etc.) necessarily reflects the activity of a discrete neuronal population involved in a specific visual computation. Although such may be the case for certain VEP waves, in many instances it is likely that several distinct neuronal populations contribute with greater or lesser weight to a particular VEP deflection (Naatenen and Picton, 1987; Nunez, 1990). Likewise, the activity of a given neuronal population may contribute to more than one VEP peak (e.g., Simpson et al., in press). Nonetheless, for many VEP components, relating specific peaks to identifiable anatomical structures can provide tractable models of the underlying physiological responses.

Precisely why the P1-N1-P2-N2 sequence appears to occur with a frequency near 10 Hz remains unanswered by these analyses. Is there some relationship between the 8- to 12-Hz alpha rhythm and the tendency for the VEP slow waves to display an alphalike frequency? Remond and Leserve (1967) used a spatiotemporal mapping technique combined with alpha-locked stimulus presentation to consider whether the rhythmic VEP fluctuations were a type of time-locked alpha rhythm. Their conclusion was that the VEP rhythms were not merely triggered alpha bursts. Indeed, they were able to show that although there were strong similarities in the frequency of the two phenomena, the two did not represent the same underlying activity. Başar and colleagues (see Başar, 1980, 1988) have investigated the relationships between EEG and evoked responses in animals and humans and described the dependence of VEPs on preceding EEG amplitude and phase. They have reported both the enhancement of alpha band activity following a stimulus and the reduction of ongoing alpha rhythms. Such combined EEG-evoked potential studies are vital for obtaining insights as to why the sensory-evoked slow waves of the visual VEPs occur with a marked alpha band rhythmicity even though they apparently represent the sequential activation of separate neuronal generators.

The present discussion has been purposely restricted to the sensory-evoked slow waves generated in visual cortex. Thus, the present data do not address the extent to which induced rhythms may be triggered in human visual cortex by a flash stimulus on a trial-by-trial basis. That is, if rhythmic oscillations of visual cortical neurons occurred, but were not tightly time-locked to the stimulus, then the averaging process would tend to eliminate such responses. Indeed, given the recent findings of rhythms induced in cat visual cortex following light stimulation (Gray et al., 1989; Gray and Singer, 1989; see also chapters by Gray and Singer in this volume), such responses may well prove to exist in the human cortex as well. Thus, it must be emphasized that the present conclusions are made only with respect to the sensory-evoked slow waves of the VEP.

Also not considered in the preceding discussion has been the high frequency oscillatory potentials recorded from the human scalp following a visual stimulus (Cracco and Cracco, 1978; Harding and Rubenstein, 1985; Whittaker and Siegfried, 1983). As noted earlier, these OPs are best visualized in records bandpass filtered so as to attenuate the slower, higher amplitude P1-N1-P2-N2 sequence. When such filtering is applied, the OPs are seen as a rhythmic series of wavelets occurring with a frequency that varies between about 50 and 100 Hz and an onset latency of between 25 and 35 ms. The amplitudes of these OPs are small relative to the later sensory-evoked slow waves, but the time-locked response patterns of OPs are quite stable for a given individual, as evidenced by the fact that they can be visualized using signal averaging (Fig. 1).

The human visually evoked OPs may represent a different type of response that could also be studied and modeled, as have been the longer latency slow waves here and in other work (e.g., Darcey et al., 1980a, 1980b; Simpson et al., in press). The fact that the P1, N1, P2, and N2 components most probably reflect the activation of separate neuronal populations does not tell us whether a similar model holds for the OPs. Indeed, the OPs bear intriguing similarity to the 40-Hz oscillations recorded from the human scalp in response to auditory stimulation (Galambos, this volume). Thus, one line of experimental investigation requiring attention is the study of the high frequency oscillatory responses elicited by visual stimuli in human subjects in order to determine whether they reflect the sequential activation of generators in the ascending visual pathways or are instead a visually induced brain rhythm.

Summary

The sensory-evoked P1-N1-P2-N2 sequence (70–300 ms latency) of the averaged VEP in humans has a characteristic frequency of about 10 Hz. These "slow waves" of the VEP are stimulus induced, and therefore are to be distinguished from spontaneous or stimulus-driven rhythms. The neural bases of this VEP sequence remains unclear. Are these deflections actually individual "components" that reflect the sequential activation of neuronal populations in the ascending sensory pathways, or instead, rhythmic oscillations of visual neurons triggered by the stimulus? Current density analyses combined with scalp topographic mapping reveal that each peak in the P1-N1-P2-N2 sequence can be related to a distinct and different distribution of currents over the scalp. Such results are in line with the notion that each of these deflections reflect the activation of anatomically distinct visual cortical areas following the presentation of a visual stimulus. Further research must ask similar questions about other visually evoked phenomena such as the high frequency oscillatory potentials (50–100 Hz) also present in the human VEP.

Acknowledgments. This research was performed with the collaboration of Dr. Steven Hillyard and Dr. Jonathan Hansen at the University of California, San Diego, and was supported by grants from the NIMH, NINDS, and the McDonnell–Pew Foundation. Special thanks to Paul Krewsky for programming involved in the preparation of the topographical maps and to Dr. Kimberly Mangun for helpful comments and critiques of this chapter.

References

Allison T, Matsumiya, Y, Goff GD, Goff WR (1977): The scalp topography of human visual evoked potentials. *Electroencephalogr Clin Neurophysiol* 42:185–197

Başar E (1980): *EEG–Brain Dynamics: Relation Between EEG and Brain Evoked Potentials.* New York: Elsevier/North-Holland

Başar E (1988): EEG-dynamics and evoked potentials in sensory and cognitive processing by the brain. In: *Sensory and Cognitive Processing by the Brain*, Başar E, ed. Berlin: Springer–Verlag

Biersdorf WR (1974): Cortical evoked responses from stimulation of various regions of the visual field. *Docum Ophthal Proc (XIth ISCERG Symposium)* 3:249–259

Bodis-Wollner I, Mylin L, Frkovic S (1989): The topography of the N70 component of the visual evoked potential in humans. In: *Topographic Brain Mapping of EEG and Evoked Potentials*, Maurer K, ed. Berlin: Springer–Verlag.

Buchwald JS (1983): Generators. In: *Bases of Auditory Brain-Stem Evoked Responses*, Moore EJ, ed. New York: Grune and Stratton

Butler SR, Georgiou GA, Glass A, Hancox RJ, Hopper JM, Smith KRH (1987): Cortical generators of the CI component of the pattern-onset visual evoked potential. *Electroencephalogr Clin Neurophysiol* 68:256–267

Celesia GG (1976): Organization of auditory cortical areas in man. *Brain* 99:403–414

Cracco RQ, and Cracco JB (1978): Visual evoked potentials in man: early oscillatory potentials. *Electroencephalogr Clin Neurophysiol* 45:731–739

Darcey TM, Ary JP, and Fender DH (1980a): Spatio-temporal visually evoked scalp potentials in response to partial-field patterned stimulation. *Electroencephalogr Clin Neurophysiol* 50:348–355

Darcey TM, Ary JP, Fender DH (1980b): Methods for localization of electrical sources in the human brain. In: *Motivation, Motor and Sensory Processes, Progress in Brain Research*, vol 54, Kornhuber HH, Deeke L, eds. Elsevier, Amsterdam: pp 128–134

Eason RG (1981): Visual evoked potentials correlates of early neural filtering during selective attention. *Bull Psychonom Soc* 18:203–206

Gray CM, Singer W (1989): Stimulus-specific neuronal oscillations in orientation columns of cat visual cortex. *Proc Natl Acad Sci USA* 86:1698–1702

Gray CM, Koenig P, Engel AK, Singer W (1989): Oscillatory responses in cat visual cortex exhibit inter-columnar synchronization which reflects global stimulus properties. *Nature* 338:334–337

Hackley SA, Woldorff M, Hillyard SA (1990): Cross-modal selective attention effects on retinal, myogenic, brainstem and cerebral evoked potentials. *Psychophysiology* 27:195–208

Harding GFA, Rubenstein MP (1980): The scalp topography of the human visually evoked subcortical potential. *Invest Ophthalmol Vis Sci* 19:318–321

Harter MR, Aine CJ (1984): Brain mechanisms of visual selective attention. In: *Varieties of Attention*, Parasuraman R, Davies DR, eds. New York: Academic Press, pp 293–322

Harter MR, Aine CJ, Schroeder C (1982): Hemispheric differences in the neural processing of stimulus location and type: effects of selective attention on visual evoked potentials. *Neuropsychologia* 20:421–438

Hillyard SA, Muente TF (1984): Selective attention to color and location: An analysis with event-related brain potentials. *Perception & Psychophysics* 36:185–198

Jeffreys DA, Axford JG (1972a): Source locations of pattern-specific components of human visual evoked potentials I. Component of striate cortical origin. *Exp. Brain Res* 16:1–21

Jeffreys DA, Axford JG (1972b): Source locations of pattern-specific components of human visual evoked potentials II. Component of extrastriate cortical origin. *Exp Brain Res* 16:22–40

Maier J, Dagnelie G, Spekreijse H, Van Dijk BW (1986): Principle component analysis for source locations of VEPs in man. *Vision Res* 27:165–177

Mangun GR, Hansen, JC, Hillyard SA (1990): Visual selective attention to spatial location: Event-related brain potential and current density analyses. *Soc Neurosci Abst* 16:578

Mangun, GR, Hillyard SA (1988): Spatial gradients of visual attention: Behavioral and electrophysiological evidence. *Electroencephalogr Clin Neurophysiol* 70:417–428

Mangun GR, Hillyard SA (1990): Electrophysiological studies of visual selective attention in humans. In: *The Neurobiological Foundations of Higher Cognitive Function*, Scheibel A, Weschler A, eds. New York: Guilford Press, pp 271–295

Mangun GR, Hillyard SA (1991): Modulations of sensory-evoked brain potentials indicate changes in perceptual processing during visual-spatial priming. *Journal of Experimental Psychology: Human Perception and Performance* 17:1057–1074

Mangun GR, Hillyard SA, Luck SJ (in press): Electrocortical substrates of visual selective attention. In: *Attention and Performance XIV*, Meyer D, Kornblum S, eds. Hillsdale, NJ: Erlbaum.

Moller AR, Jannetta PJ, Bennett M, Moller MB (1981): Intracranially recorded responses from human auditory nerve: new insights into the origin of brainstem evoked potentials. *Electroencephalogr Clin Neurophysiol* 52:18–27

Naatenen R, Picton TW (1987): The N1 wave of the human electric and magnetic response to sound: a review and an analysis of the component structure. *Psychophysiology* 24:375–425

Neville HJ, Lawson D (1987): Attention to central and peripheral visual space in a movement detection task: an event-related potential and behavioral study. I. Normal hearing adults. *Brain Res* 405:253–267

Nunez PL (1981): *Electric Fields of the Brain: The Neurophysics of EEG.* New York: Oxford University Press

Nunez PL (1990): Localization of brain activity with EEG. In: *Magnetoencephalography: Comparison with Electroencephalography and Clinical Applications*, Sato S, ed. New York: Raven Press.

Perrin F, Pernier J, Betrand O, Giard MH, Enchallier JF (1987): Mapping of scalp potentials by surface spline interpolation. *Electroencephalogr Clin Neurophysiol* 66: 75–81

Regan D (1989): *Human Brain Electrophysiology: Evoked Potentials and Evoked Magnetic Fields in Science and Medicine.* New York: Elsevier

Remond A, Leseve N (1967): Variations in average visual evoked potentials as a function of alpha rhythm phase. In: *The Evoked Potentials*, Cobb W, Morocutti C, eds. Amsterdam: Elsevier

Robinson DL, Rugg MD (1988): Latencies of visually responsive neurons in various regions of the rhesus monkey brain and their relation to human visual responses. *Biol Psychol* 26:111–116

Rugg MD, Milner AD, Lines CR, Phalp R (1987): Modulation of visual event-related potentials by spatial and non-spatial visual selective attention. *Neuropsychologia* 25:85–89

Scherg M, Von Cramen D (1985): A new interpretation of the generators of BAEP waves I–V: results of a spatio-temporal dipole model. *Electroencephalogr Clin Neurophysiol* 62:290–299

Scherg M, Vajsar J, Picton, TW (1989): A source analysis of the late human auditory evoked potentials. *J Cogn Neurosci* 1:336–355

Simpson GV, Scherg M, Ritter W, Vaughan Jr, HG (1990): Localization and temporal activity functions of brain sources generating the human visual ERP. In: *Psychophysiological Brain Research*, 1:99–105 Brunia CHM, Gaillard AWK, Kok A, eds. Tilburg, the Netherlands: Tilburg University Press

Srebro R (1985): Localization of visual evoked cortical activity in humans. *J Physiol* 360:233–246

Srebro R (1987): The topography of scalp potentials evoked by pattern pulse stimuli. *Vis Res* 27:901–914

Srebro R (1990): Localization of visually evoked cortical activity using magnetic resonance imaging and computerized tomography. *Vis Res* 30:351–358

Whittaker SG, Siegfried JB (1983): Origin of wavelets in the visual evoked potential. *Electroencephalogr Clin Neurophysiol* 55:91–101

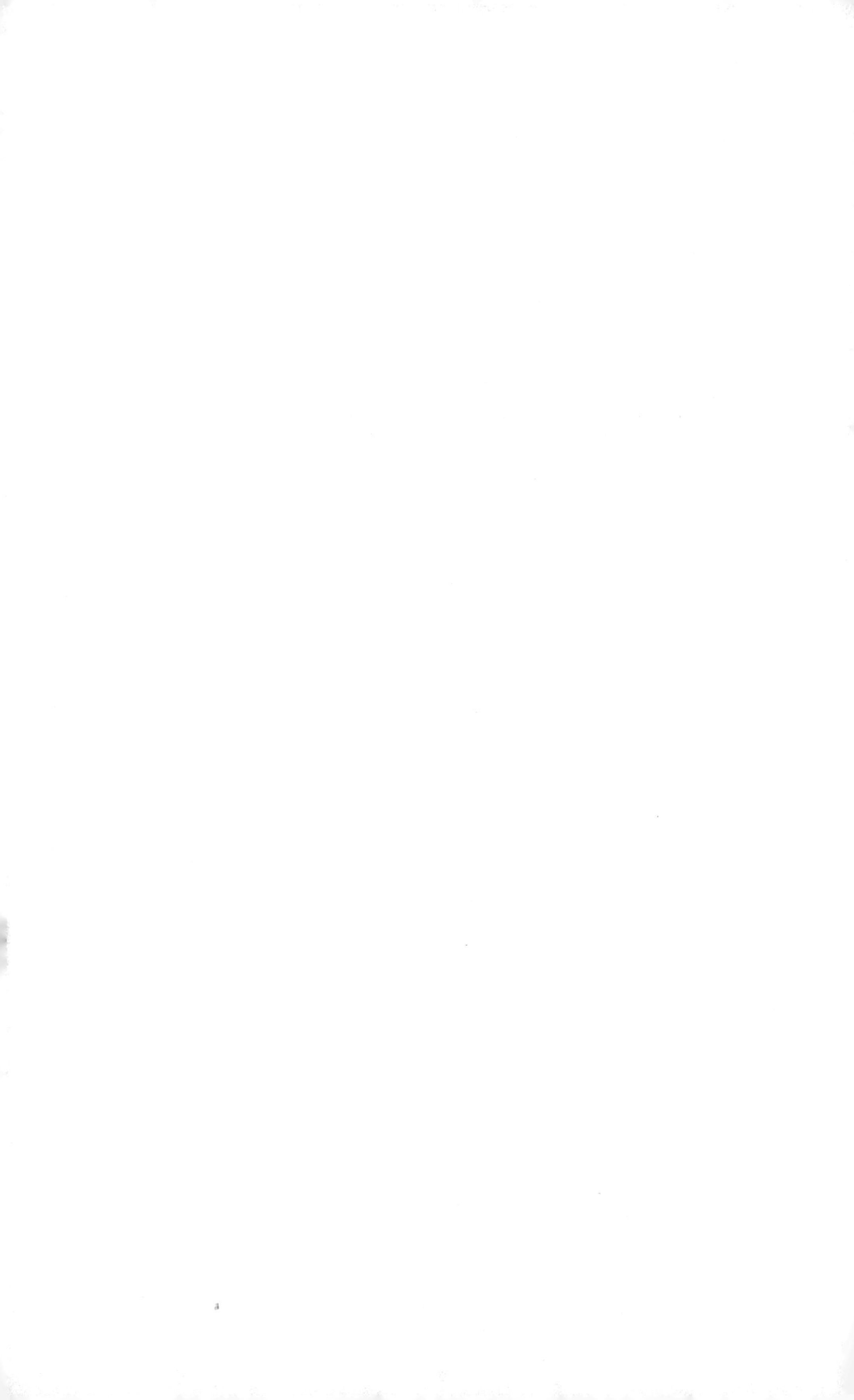

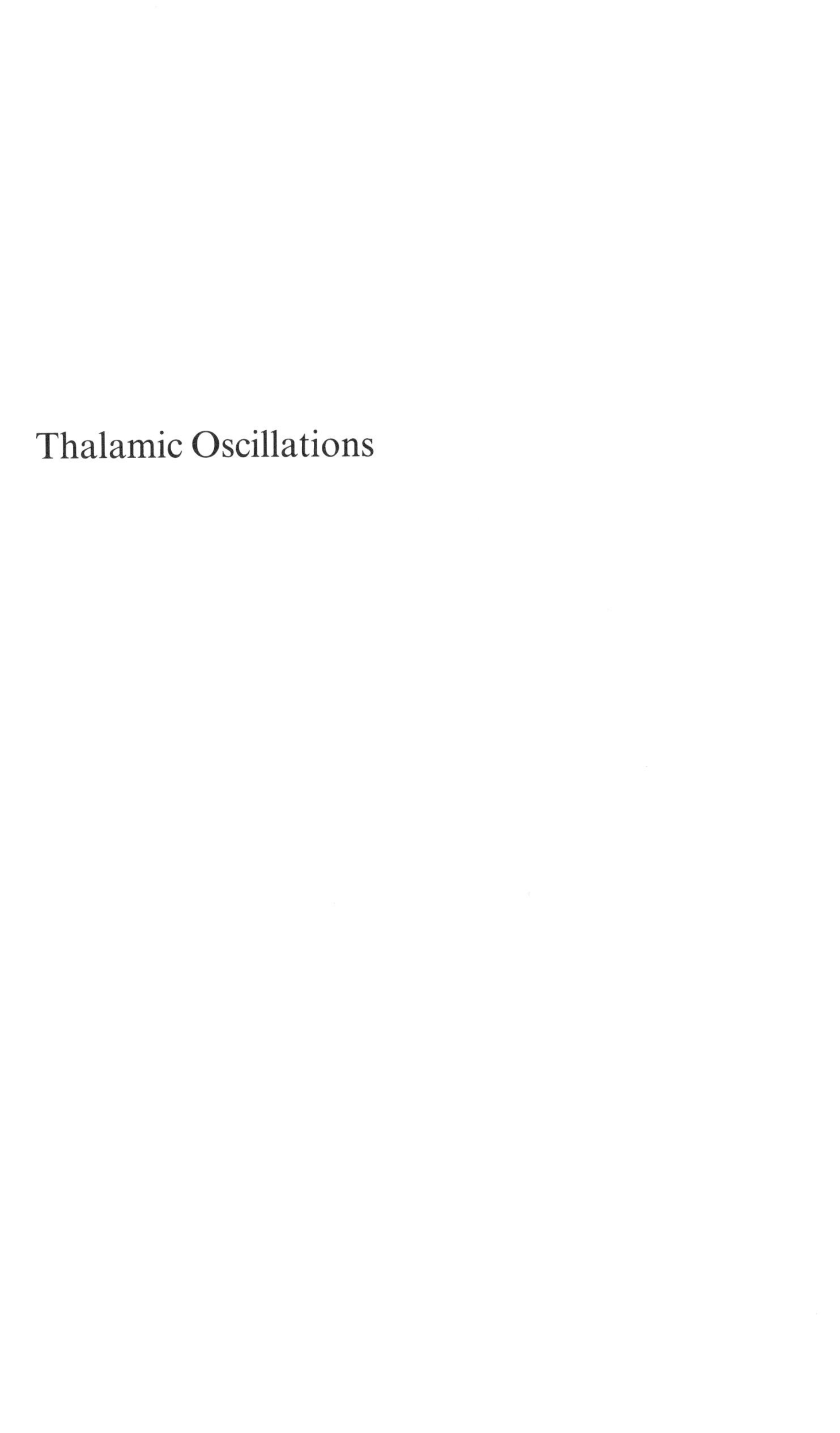

Thalamic Oscillations

Network Properties of the Thalamic Clock: Role of Oscillatory Behavior in Mood Disorders

György Buzsáki

Rhythmic oscillations of neuronal populations are present at several levels of the central nervous system. Rhythmicity can occur in the central nervous system because some neurons have ionic conductances organized to endow them with autorhythmicity and because these "pacemaker" neurons are in connections with ensembles of neurons that respond preferentially to inputs at certain frequencies (cf. Llinás, 1988). Alternatively, rhythmic patterns may occur as an emergent property of network activity of neurons, none of which is capable of maintaining oscillatory behavior in isolation (Andersen and Andersson, 1968; Traub et al., 1989).

One of the most prominent rhythm-generator structures of the mammalian central nervous system is the thalamus (Steriade and Deschenes, 1984) . Understanding the mechanism of population oscillation and its afferent control is a key to revealing the integrative function of the thalamus. The goal of this chapter is to review the collective behavior of thalamic cell populations and their afferent control systems and relate them to the behavior of the organism in physiological states and disease.

The Thalamic Clock

In humans, bilaterally synchronous, rhythmic neocortical electroencephalogram (EEG) patterns occur under physiological conditions such as sleep spindles, occipital alpha and somatosensory mu rhythms, and in disease such as spike-and-wave discharges in patients with petit mal epilepsy. Although some earlier works supported the view that rhythmic patterns are generated in the neocortex, a general consensus today is that neocortical rhythmicity is due to the oscillatory behavior of the intrathalamic or thalamocortical circuitry (see also chapter by Steriade). The different frequencies of the various neocortical rhythms have been hypothesized to derive from a division at the neocortical level due to the periodic refractoriness of neocortical neurons brought about by enhanced recurrent inhibition (Gloor and Fariello, 1988).

The pacemaker hypothesis of thalamic oscillation

Two recent discoveries advanced our understanding of the thalamic oscillation. First, thalamic neurons were found to possess a low-threshold Ca^{2+}

spike mechanism that allows them to burst rebound spikes when a hyperpolarized cell is quickly released from inhibition (cf. Steriade and Llinás, 1988). Second, selective damage of the GABAergic reticular nucleus of the thalamus (RT) (Fig. 1) or isolation of RT from the other thalamic nuclei was shown to abolish thalamic and neocortical rhythmic patterns in the cat (Steriade et al., 1985, 1987) and the rat (Buzsáki et al., 1988a). These and other

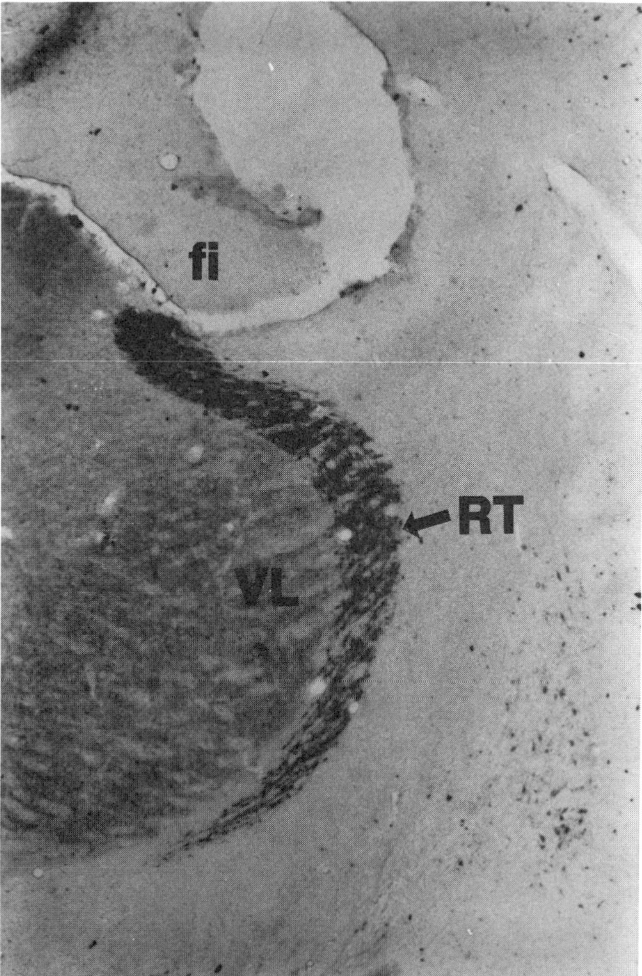

Figure 1. Parvalbumin-immunoreactivity in the thalamus. Parvalbumin is present in fast-firing GABA cells. Note the high density of immunoreactive cells in RT and the dense puncta of axon terminals and absence of immunoreactive neurons in the relay nuclei of the thalamus. VL, ventrolateral nucleus of thalamus; fi, fimbria of hippocampus.

findings led Steriade (see Chapter 13) to suggest a true "pacemaker" model of thalamic rhythms. The two major assumptions of this model are that 1) the RT nucleus "is the pacemaker of spindle rhythmicity" (Steriade and Llinás, 1988, p. 702 and 2) "hyperporarizations ... are imposed onto thalamocortical cells by inhibitory neuronal pools with pacemaker oscillatory properties" (Steriade and Llinás, 1988, p. 695). In the pacemaker model GABAergic RT cells phasically hyperpolarize their thalamocortical target neurons and, in the absence of other depolarizing inputs, voltage- and time-dependent rebound spikes occur in a phase-locked manner in these cells because of the deinactivation of low-threshold calcium channels (Jahnsen and Llinas, 1984a, 1984b).

A network model of thalamic oscillation: a new hypothesis

A key issue to be elucidated in the pacemaker model is how the individual RT neurons become synchronized to provide a phase-locked output. Since recent reports suggest that RT neurons also possess low-threshold Ca^{2+} spikes *in vitro* (McCormick and Prince, 1986), it was proposed that collective synchrony within the exclusively GABAergic population of RT is brought about by mutual hyperpolarization-rebound spike sequences (Steriade et al., 1987). Some previous observations and our recent findings argue against this explanation, however. First, RT neurons are depolarized, rather than hyperpolarized, during barbiturate spindles in the cat (Steriade and Llinás, 1988) and in the rat (Shosaku et al., 1989). Second, neurons in the RT nucleus fire repetitive spikes of similar amplitude and not bursts of decreasing amplitude (lack of calcium spikes?) in the awake rat, in contrast to the characteristic decrescendo discharge patterns of thalamocortical cells (Buzsaki et al., 1988a). Third, lasting oscillations in RT cells have not been demonstrated *in vitro*. And finally, recurrent excitation of RT cells from thalamocortical neurons appears essential for the initiation and maintenance of thalamic oscillation (see below).

In our recent experiments we examined two major issues. First, are the thalamocortical neurons actively involved in the network oscillation or do they simply follow the command input of the RT, as suggested by the pacemaker model? Second, can the neocortical rhythmic patterns with various frequencies be explained by alteration of the thalamic clock frequency? Most of our experiments were carried out in Fischer 344 rats because they display very high voltage spindles (HVS) with easily detectable spike-and-wave components (Buzsáki, 1991; Buzsáki et al., 1988a, 1988b; 1989, 1990, 1991). Multisite recording of neuronal activity and local microinjections of drugs were employed in the freely moving animal.

Recording of unit activity at multiple thalamic sites during HVS is shown in Figure 2. Thalamocortical neurons discharged dominantly during the spike components of the epidurally recorded HVS and there was not a simple relationship between the amplitude of the spike components of HVS and the synchrony of multiple unit discharges at a given electrode location. Popula-

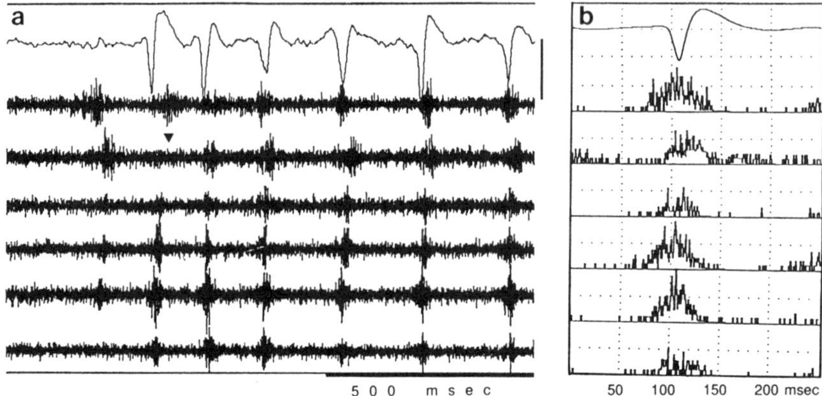

Figure 2. Recruitment of the thalamic neuronal network during HVS. **A:** Simultaneously recorded subpopulations of neurons in the ventrolateral nucleus (unit traces 1–4) and posterior nucleus (traces 5, 6) of the thalamus. The recording electrodes were spaced at 250 μm in the sagittal axis. **Uppermost trace:** Epidural recording from above the sensorimotor cortex. Note the initial jitter and subsequent phase-locking of unit firing with the spike components of HVS. Population bursting may have been initiated by neurons of the first unit trace. Omission of population burst in unit trace 2 is marked by arrowhead. Note also that rhythmic thalamic population bursts preceded the neocortical EEG change. Calibrations: 1 mV (EEG), 400 μV (unit). **B:** Cross correlation histograms of HVS and unit activity from all six channels. Reprinted from Buzsaki (1991) with permission of Pergamon Press.

tion bursts were usually initiated by neurons at one or two locations and neurons at other locations were recruited into the rhythmic population events several cycles later. Often, omissions of population bursts were observed at one or several locations during the HVS, but reoccurring bursts emerged at the time of the overall population synchrony (Fig. 2). These findings suggested that collective behavior of large neuronal aggregates is a better predictor of the neocortical patterns than unit activity recorded only at any single thalamic site. This observation was confirmed by recording from isolated single neurons.

Single thalamocortical cells often displayed bursts of several spikes of decreasing amplitude during HVS, reflecting the occurrence of low-threshold calcium spikes (Fig. 3), whereas mainly single spikes were observed during movement and during immobility periods without HVS. In contrast to multiple unit activity, individual thalamic neurons rarely fired rhythmically. Before the onset of neocortically recorded HVS, most cells decreased their overall firing rates. Rhythmic discharges for two to five consecutive cycles of HVS were observed occasionally, followed by long periods of silence. When present, however, unit discharges occurred phase-locked to the spike component of HVS. In contrast, individual RT neurons fired rhythmically and spike discharges of 1 to 10 spikes of equal amplitude occurred predominantly during

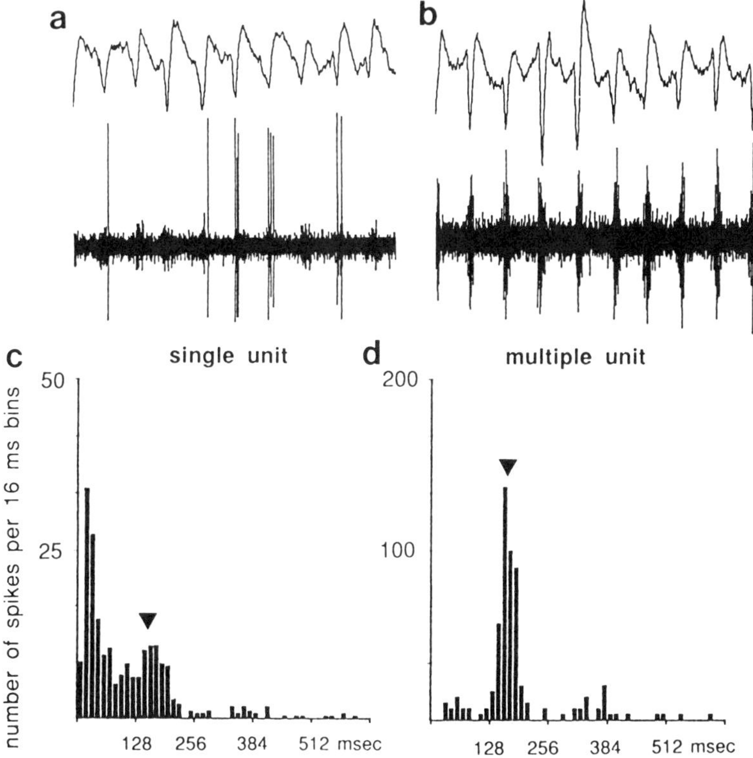

Figure 3. Relationship between individual and population behavior of thalamic neurons (VL nucleus) during HVS. **A:** Neocortical EEG and action potentials of a typical single VL neuron. Note phase-locking of the cell-firing to the spike component of HVS and its low level of rhythmicity. **B:** Neocortical HVS and multiple unit activity in VL. Note phase-locking and high level of rhythmicity. **C** and **D:** Interspike interval histograms of units shown in A and B, respectively. The arrowheads indicate the peak of the EEG spike component intervals of HVS recorded simultaneously (not shown). Note the small peak for the single cell (C) and the sharp peak for multiple unit activity (D). Reprinted from Buzsaki (1991) with permission of Pergamon Press.

the wave components of HVS (Buzsáki et al., 1988a). These findings suggest that rhythmic population synchrony in the thalamus is a collective property of neurons.

Intraperitoneal or intrathalamic injection of the noncompetitive *N*-methyl-D-aspartate (NMDA) antagonist ketamine substantially decreased the frequency of HVS, without changing its morphology or amplitude characteristics. The frequency of HVS showed a continuous decrease with postinjection time and could be as slow as 1.6/sec. Larger doses completely eliminated HVS. To evaluate the involvement of NMDA mechanisms in thalamic oscillation further we tested the effects of the specific NMDA antagonist AP-5 as well as the effects of NMDA itself. Similar to ketamine, bilateral injections of

AP-5 into the ventrobasal (motor) nuclei of the thalamus significantly decreased the frequency of neocortical HVS (Fig. 4). Soon after the injection the predrug HVS of 6 to 8/sec were interspersed with HVS of 3 to 4/sec. Eventually the frequency of HVS could be as low as 2/sec. Occasionally, spike-and-waves of 6 to 8/sec were superimposed on the very slow HVS. Unilateral injection of AP-5 into the thalamus dramatically reduced the amplitude of the HVS on the side of the AP-5 injection compared to the side injected with vehicle only. Intrathalamic NMDA infusion, on the other hand, increased the amplitude of the spike components of HVS. Recently we have seen similar effects with another glutamate receptor blocker, CNQX. Intracortical injections of any of these drugs failed to alter either the frequency or the amplitude of HVS.

Based on these observations we suggest that 1) thalamic rhythmicity is an emerging property of the thalamo–RT network, a feature not predictable from the behavior of individual neurons, and 2) the frequency of network oscillation (2–12/sec) is regulated by the interplay between two major classes of voltage-dependent conductances: the low-threshold calcium channels and the high-threshold NMDA channels. Our network hypothesis of thalamic rhythm generation encompasses the major features of the pacemaker model as well as accounts for the observations not compatible with the pacemaker hypothesis (Fig. 5). In essence, we propose that thalamic rhythms are brought about by a collective, mutual cooperation of thalamocortical and RT neurons, none of which is endowed with pacemaker properties. We envision the sequences of events as follows. Thalamic oscillation starts by the bursting discharge of spatially segregated thalamocortical cells (initiator neurons) within a relatively restricted time window (e.g., Fig. 2). Their converging output on RT cells will result in depolarization and discharge of these latter cells. In turn, the high frequency and synchronous output of these RT neurons will hyperpolarize a larger population of their thalamocortical target neurons (few-to-many divergence). The hyperpolarizing events may then induce rebound bursting in some of the affected neurons. These initial events have a dual consequence on the RT–thalamus network. First, the RT-induced hyperpolarizing effects will be spatially distributed and second, the synchrony of rebound burst discharges of thalamocortical neurons will substantially increase. These events in turn will recruit more RT neurons to fire in the same phase, and secondarily a larger population of thalamocortical cells will be affected in a time-locked manner during the subsequent cycles. The recruitment continues until a large number of RT and thalamocortical neurons will be involved in the cyclic oscillation or some external events interfere with further recruitment.

The network model also shares features with the "facultative pacemaker" hypothesis of thalamic oscillation since "no particular area serves as a general pacemaker" (Andersen and Anderson, 1968), but without the assumption of mutual recurrent excitation of thalamocortical neurons. We suggest that mutual connectivity between the GABAergic RT cells and thalamocortical neu-

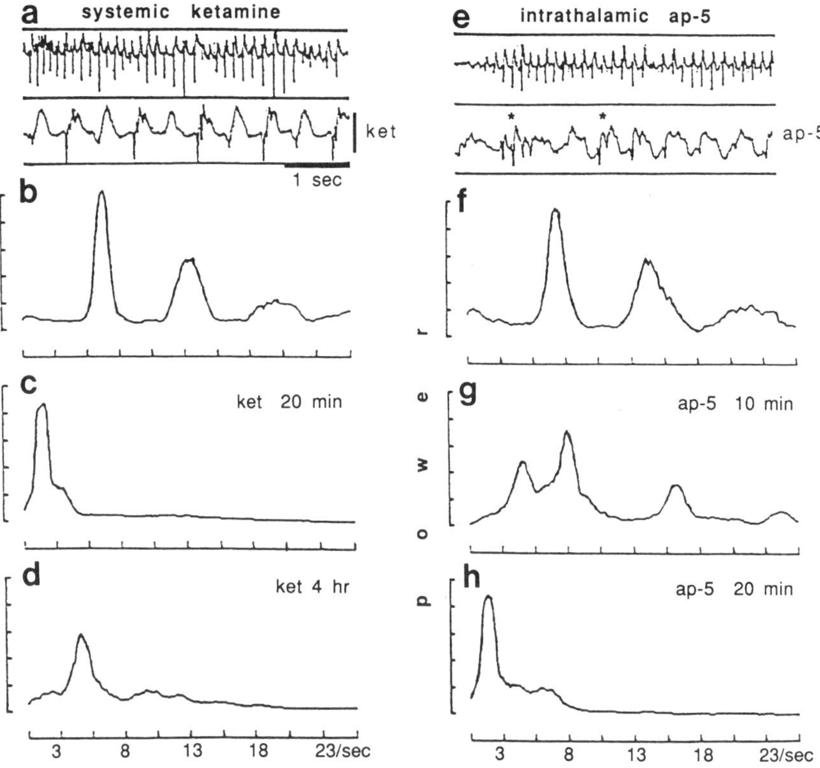

Figure 4. Effect of blocking the NMDA receptors on the frequency of thalamic oscillation. **A:** EEG samples of HVS recorded from above the sensorimotor cortex before (*above*) and after intraperitoneal administration of ketamine. Note slow (about 2/sec) spike-and-wave pattern after ketamine. The rat was pretreated with xylazine to increase the incidence of HVS. **B**, **C**, and **D:** Power spectra obtained before (B), 20 min (C), and 4 hr (D) after ketamine administration. Between 25 min and 4 hr postketamine no rhythmic patterns were present. The 4 to 5/s peak at 4 hr reflects the emergence of HVS coinciding with the recovery from anesthesia. **E.** Neocortical EEG samples of HVS before and after bilateral microinjection (0.5 μl) of AP-5 into the RT/VL region of the thalamus. Note the slow (2/s) rhythmicity after ap-5. Asterisks indicate mixtures of HVS at 7 and 2/s. **F**, **G**, **H:** Power spectra of EEG obtained before (F), 10 min (G), and 20 min (H) after AP-5 microinjection. Note the emergence of a power peak at about 3 to 4/s after 10 min (G) and the dominance of 2/s rhythmicity later (H). Ordinates: arbitrary units. Reprinted from Buzsaki (1991) with permission of Pergamon Press.

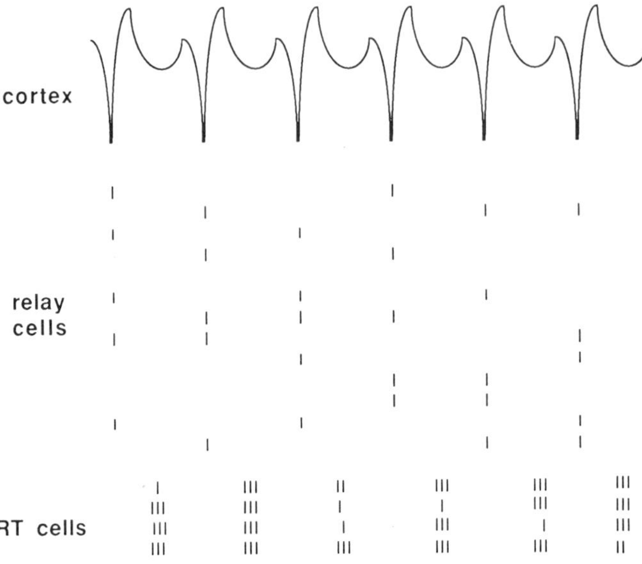

Figure 5. Diagram of the hypothesized network-generated rythmicity n the thalamus. Neither the relay cells nor RT neurons are endowed with intrinsic rhythmicity. RT cells are firing rhythmically at HVS frequency because they are excited by a converging and relatively constant population of thalamocortical relay cells. Relay cells are not rhythmic but when they discharge their action potentials are phase-locked to the population rhythmicity. Discharge of relay neurons are brought about by RT-induced hyperpolarizations and consequent rebound, low-threshold calcium spike activation.

rons, low-threshold rebound spikes, and the above-outlined network rules are the necessary and sufficient requirements of rhythmic population synchrony in the thalamus.

The distinction between the pacemaker and network models becomes essential when it comes to the examination of the afferent control and the mechanisms of frequency regulation of thalamic oscillation. Naturally, in the pacemaker model frequency changes are determined by the ionic mechanisms of putative pacemaker neurons (i.e., RT cells). In our experiments reduction of thalamic network excitability by NMDA blockers decreased the number of participating neurons in HVS and increased the intervals between successive population bursts. The very low density of NMDA binding in the RT nucleus and the moderately high density in the relay nuclei of the thalamus (Monaghan and Cotman, 1985) suggest that the likely targets of the NMDA channel blockers are the thalamocortical cells.

In addition to the low-threshold calcium conductance, presumed intradendritic recordings in thalamic cells *in vitro* (Jahnsen and Llinás, 1984a,

1984b) have also revealed a depolarization-dependent, high-threshold Ca^{2+} conductance. This conductance triggers all-or-none depolarizing responses that are followed by the activation of a Ca^{2+}-dependent K^{+}-mediated afterhyperpolarization. The length of the afterhyperpolarization is crucial in the regulation of the refractoriness of the neuron and in the timing of reexcitation. We hypothesized (Buzsaki, 1990) that release from hyperpolarization and rebound depolarization of some thalamocortical neurons during the low-threshold calcium spike is of sufficient magnitude and duration to remove the Mg^{2+}-blockade of the NMDA channels (Collingridge et al., 1983). Opening of the NMDA channels would facilitate depolarization and shorten the duration of the afterhyperpolarization. We suggest that the balance between NMDA-mediated depolarization and the Ca^{2+}- and voltage-dependent K^{+}-mediated afterhyperpolarization determines the reexcitability of individual thalamocortical cells and thereby the frequency of population rhythmicity. It remains to be clarified if NMDA receptors are involved only in excessive synchrony such as HVS-associated bursts or they also play a role in physiological oscillations, such as sleep spindles.

In summary, our research indicates that 1) thalamic rhythmicity is an emerging property of the relay nuclei–RT network and 2) the frequency and magnitude of the oscillation are regulated by the interplay between two major classes of voltage-dependent conductances: the low-threshold calcium channels and the high-threshold NMDA channels.

Afferent Control of Thalamic Oscillation

To understand the physiological functions of thalamic oscillations and to explain their role in disease, it is essential to reveal the afferent mechanisms that effectively control the kinetics of ionic conductances of the neurons involved and thereby regulate the emergence of rhythmic oscillations. The frequent association of neocortical rhythmic EEG patterns with drowsiness and sleep and the virtual absence of slow rhythmic patterns during high vigilance states led to the suggestion that a key function of the ascending activating systems is to block thalamic oscillations (Moruzzi and Magoun, 1949; Steriade and Deschenes, 1984; McCormick, 1989; Steriade and Buzsaki, 1990). As discussed above, thalamocortical neuronal population is assumed to oscillate rhythmically when low-threshold calcium channels in thalamocortical cells are deinactivated and RT neurons fire rhythmically. Any condition that interferes with these requirements is regarded as antioscillatory. The role of cholinergic, noradrenergic, and other ascending afferents in suppressing thalamic rhythmicity has been reviewed extensively (Buzsaki et al., 1988a; 1990; McCormick, 1989; Steriade and Buzsaki, 1990). The present viewpoint in this field can be briefly summarized by suggesting that the more the thalamocortical system is isolated from the ascending cholinergic and aminergic activating systems, the higher the probability of the emergence of oscillation in the thalamocortical system (cf. McCormick, 1989).

In contrast to this general belief are the observations that thalamic oscillations underlying generalized neocortical spike-and-wave discharges in petit mal epilepsy occur frequently in the quiet awake state and light sleep rather than deep stages of sleep (Gloor and Fariello, 1988). Parkinsonian tremor, another rhythmic pattern due to thalamic oscillation, is present during rest, may be increased by anxiety, and disappears during sleep. Rhythmic occipital alpha waves also disappear with sleep (Andersen and Anderson, 1968). Finally, sleep spindles dominate light sleep and gradually decrease and become mixed with irregular slow waves with deepening stages of sleep (Steriade and Deschenes, 1984). Based on these observations we can argue that a certain level of activation (i.e., release of a certain amount of neurotransmitter from the terminals of the ascending activating systems) is actually necessary for thalamic oscillation to ensue. We have recently identified two such burst- and oscillation-promoting systems: the alpha-2 adrenoceptor-mediated noradrenergic/adrenergic projection (Buzsaki et al., 1991) and the GABAergic thalamopetal inputs from the extrapyramidal system (Buzsaki et al., 1989).

Alpha-2 adrenergic facilitation of thalamic oscillation

Interference with the catecholamine system with alpha-1 antagonist and alpha-2 agonist drugs have been shown to increase the incidence of HVS in the rat and the monkey (Fig. 6) and the drug-induced effects have generally been interpreted as releasing the thalamus from its noradrenergic antioscillatory control (Micheletti et al., 1987). Our recent experiments with intrathalamic infusion of noradrenergic drugs suggest that the norepinephrine/epinephrine projection to the thalamus exerts both antioscillatory and oscillation-promoting effects, depending on the target receptors (Buzsaki et al., 1991).

The alpha-2 agonists, clonidine and xylazine, increased the incidence and average duration of HVS in a dose-dependent manner when these drugs were directly injected into the thalamus (Fig. 7), but not when the injections were made into the corpus callosum or the hippocampus. The specificity of clonidine on alpha-2 receptors was indicated by the observation that when the alpha-2 antagonist yohimbine was injected before clonidine, the HVS-inducing effect of clonidine was abolished. In order to dissociate between presynaptic and postsynaptic effects of the drugs the catecholaminergic system was damaged by the neurotoxin, 6-hydroxydopamine (6-OHDA). Despite the nearly complete depletion of catecholaminergic terminals in the thalamus by the 6-OHDA treatment, intrathalamic injection of the apha-2 agonists continued to increase the incidence of neocortical HVS. In another experiment the density of alpha-2 receptors was downregulated by chronic administration of the tricyclic antidepressive drug, amitriptyline. Following the chronic treatment (3 weeks) the HVS-inducing effect of alpha-2 agonists was significantly reduced.

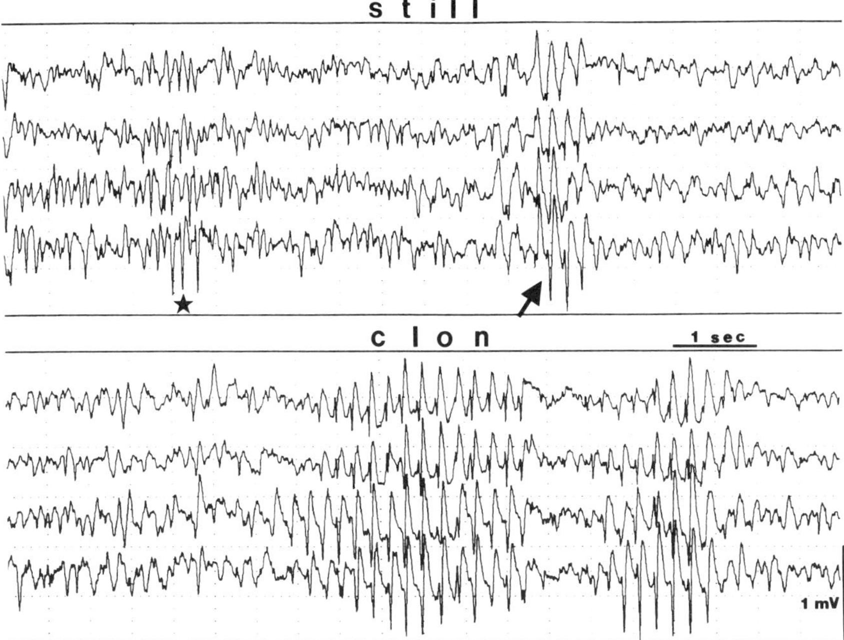

Figure 6. Epidurally recorded EEG activity from the left (traces 1, 3) and right (traces 2, 4) sensorimotor area in a 24-year-old rhesus monkey (male). **Upper record:** Awake immobility (still). In the absence of eye and head movements rhythmic bursts at 10–14/s (*star*) was the most dominant pattern in this aged animal. Occasionally, short bursts of high voltage spike-and-wave patterns (*arrow*), reminiscent of HVS in aged rats, were also present (<4/hr). In contrast to HVS in rats (7–9/s), frequency of monkey spike-and-wave bursts was 3–5/s. **Lower record:** Induction of long bursts of spike-and-wave spindles by intramuscular injection of clonidine (clon; 0.05 mg/kg). Similar to rat, clonidine powerfully increased the incidence of high voltage spike-and-wave patterns in the monkey. (Buzsáki, Horvath, Gage and Amaral, unpublished observations.)

These new findings suggest that the major action of alpha-2 agonists is exerted postsynaptically on thalamic neurons, since thalamic administration of alpha-2 agonists was equally effective after neurotoxic destruction of catecholaminergic afferents to the thalamus. We suggest that, similar to the alpha-2 effects of norepinephrine on the locus coeruleus neurons and peripheral ganglion cells (Aghajanian and Vandermaelen, 1982; Akasu et al., 1985), norepinephrine released from the noradrenergic and adrenergic terminals will increase membrane K^+ conductance via alpha-2 receptors located on the thalamocortical relay neurons. Since such an action of norepinephrine will hyperpolarize the target cells, it therefore will facilitate low-threshold Ca^{2+} spike discharges in thalamocortical neurons and consequently rhythmic oscillation at the network level. The alpha-2 receptor-mediated action of nor-

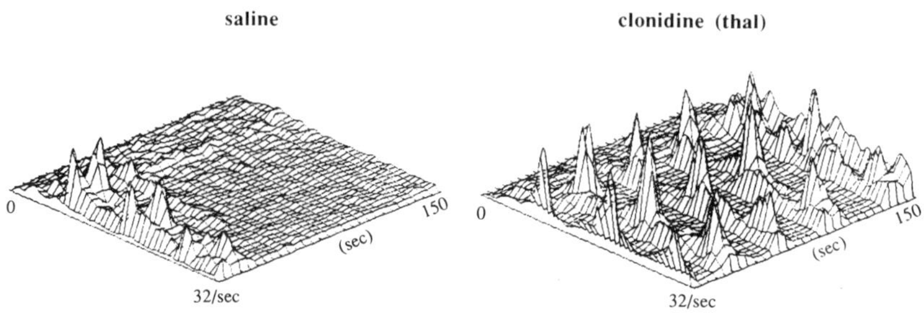

Figure 7. Spectral display of the EEG in a Fischer 344 rat after bilateral saline (*left*) and after bilateral clonidine microinjections directly into the ventrobasal thalamus. 150-s exerts (from front to back) from 30 min sessions were chosen here for illustration. Note the high incidence of HVS after clonidine as evidenced here by the amplitude peaks at about 8/s and the harmonic frequences. Reprinted from Buzsaki et al. (1991) with permission of Elsevier.

epinephrine must compete with the antiburst effects of the neurotransmitter exerted via the alpha-1 and beta receptors (McCormick, 1989; McCormick and Prince, 1988). We hypothesize that the overall action of norepinephrine in the thalamus depends on the combination of the relative density and affinity of postsynaptic alpha-1 and alpha-2 receptors and on the amount of norepinephrine released.

During high aroused states locus coeruleus cells will release large amounts of norepinephrine (Aston-Jones and Bloom, 1981) and the dominant action of the drug will be expressed via the alpha-1 and possibly beta receptors. This neurotransmitter action, together with parallel effects from other thalamopetal activating afferents, will result in fast responsivity of relay neurons (sodium spikes) and high fidelity transfer of information through the thalamus to the neocortex (McCormick, 1989; Steriade and Buzsaki, 1990). During low vigilant states, drowsiness, and light sleep the amount of released norepinephrine decreases and its main action will be expressed via the postsynaptic alpha-2 receptors. Provided that other thalamopetal afferent activity also decreases (e.g., cholinergic; Buzsaki et al., 1988a) oscillation may occur in the thalamus. Finally, in deep stages of slow wave sleep only a negligible amount of norepinephrine is released (Aston-Jones et al., 1981) and the irregular population-burst activity of neocortical neurons may interfere with thalamic oscillation by feeding back random corticothalamic impulses (Buzsaki, 1991).

Extrapyramidal control of thalamic oscillation

It has been long known that dopamine deficiency leads to oscillating behavior of thalamic neurons in Parkinson's disease but the mechanisms of how alterations of the dopaminergic system promotes rhythmic bursting activity of thalamic neurons have not yet been revealed. Recently, we have suggested a possible functional circuitry for the extrapyramidal control of thalamic rhythms in Parkinsonian tremor and petit mal epilepsy (Buzsaki et al., 1989).

Briefly, we hypothesized the existence of active burst-promoting inputs to the thalamus, operating with inhibition and involving the GABAergic afferents from the pars reticulata of substantia nigra (PrSN), entopeduncular nucleus, and the pallidum. Sustained hyperpolarization of the thalamocortical neurons, provided by these GABAergic inputs, will facilitate the opening of the low-threshold calcium channels and promote population synchrony of these thalamocortical neurons. The major inputs of the PrSN, entopeduncular nucleus, and pallidum are the GABAergic efferents from the neostriatum (caudate putamen). In turn, operation of the neostriatal circuitry is under the control of dopaminergic afferents arising from the pars compacta of the substantial nigra (PcSN). We hypothesized that the sustained level of firing of the dopaminergic neurons in the PcSN provides a steady inhibitory striatal output, thereby inhibiting the GABAergic PrSN-thalamic, entopedunculothalamic and pallido thalamic circuitries, with consequent disinhibition of the thalamocortical neurons. On the other hand, diminution of the inhibitory output level of the striatum will disinhibit the GABAergic cells of the PrSN/entopeduncular nucleus/pallidum and increased hyperpolarization of thalamic neurons by these inputs will promote burst firing and oscillation in the thalamic network.

In support of the model, we have demonstrated that intrastriatal injections of the dopamine-blocker major tranquillizers increased the incidence of HVS and associated tremor of the vibrissae (Buzsaki et al., 1989). In addition, age-related deterioration of the aminergic and cholinergic systems have been shown to increase the incidence of thalamic oscillation in the rat (Buzsaki et al., 1988b; 1990c), monkey (Fig. 6), and humans (Riekkinen et al., 1990).

The Role of Thalamic Oscillations in Mood Disorders: A Hypothesis

Antidopaminergic drugs used in the treatment of psychotic diseases not infrequently induce parkinsonian symptoms, with tremor as a major feature (Simpson et al., 1981). Another important side effect of neuroleptic drugs is a prominent increase of rhythmic theta and delta waves in the neocortex (Itil and Soldatos, 1980). Conversely, pharmacological normalization of excessive thalamic synchrony in petit mal patients occasionally results in acute psychosis (Roger et al., 1968). In our F344 rat model chlorpromazine, acepromazine, and haloperidol powerfully increased the incidence and the duration of individual HVS.

Another clinical observation supporting the importance of neuronal oscillation in mood disorders is the statistically increased incidence of depression in Parkinsonian patients (Celesia and Wanamaker, 1972). More importantly, electroconvulsive therapy in Parkinson's patients with major depression not only improved the depressed mood but also tremor and other aspects of the motor impairment (cf. Asnis, 1977; Douyon et al., 1989). In this context it is important to emphasize that before the introduction of L-DOPA therapy, tricyclic antidepressants were used successfully in the treatment of parkinsonism in the 1950s. A possible causal relationship between increased thalamic oscillation and depression is also supported by our observations that the antidepressant drugs amytriptylene and desmethylimipramine reduced the incidence of HVS in the rat (Buzsaki et al., 1990b).

Depression is strongly associated with sleep disturbance (Gillin and Borbély, 1985). Depressed patient have increased amounts of light sleep with spindles relative to deep delta sleep (Gillin 1983). Experimental sleep manipulation can turn depression off and on. Total sleep deprivation alleviates depression in about half of the patients with endogenous depression and this dramatic clinical improvement can be reversed by sleep itself (Gillin, 1983). In extreme cases as little as 1 to 10 min of sleep may be sufficient to reverse completely the antidepressant effects of sleep deprivation (Roy-Byrne et al., 1984).

Unfortunately, little emphasis has been placed on analyzing the incidence of oscillatory events (e.g., sleep spindles) in sleep studies in general and in sleep deprivation experiments in particular. The observation that extremely short naps are sufficient to reset depressive mood argues against the role of delta sleep and/or paradoxical phase of sleep as the trigger for the induction of depression. We suggest that during short naps the occurrence of thalamic oscillation underlying sleep spindles, the dominant form of light sleep stages, are causal to the consequently occurring depressive mood. Oscillation is the only thalamic operation when large numbers of neurons fire Ca^{2+} spikes. Calcium influx, on the other hand, may be essential to trigger biochemical events capable of inducing long-term modification of synaptic efficacy. Even if future research fails to demonstrate a direct link between excessive thalamic oscillation and mood disorders, experimental exploration of neuronal mechanisms of rhythmic phenomena is still warranted, since spindles and other rhythmic events may be a sensitive neurological marker for the diagnosis, prognosis, and effectiveness of drug treatment in affective disorders.

As summarized above, thalamic oscillation and associated rhythmic bursts in the neocortex require a modal change of the firing pattern of thalamic and neocortical cells. The continuous, fast sodium spikes of information-processing states are converted into burst–pause patterns of calcium spikes underlying population oscillatory behavior. The intracellular influx of calcium is crucial for triggering biochemical mechanisms that may induce long-lasting changes in the neurons and thereby affect the network operations of neuronal systems. The biochemical changes underlying thalamic oscillation and their alteration in disease may therefore exert a durable effect on the collective behavior of neurons.

Acknowledgments. The research described here was supported by NINDS-NS27058, the ADRDA, and the Whitehall Foundation.

References

Aghajanian GK, Vandermaelen CP (1982): Alpha$_2$-adrenoceptor-mediated hyperpolarization of locus coeruleus neurons: intracellular studies in vivo. *Science* 215: 1394–1396

Akasu T, Gallagher JP, Nakamura T, Shinnick-Gallagher P, Yoshimura M (1985): Noradrenaline hyperpolarization and depolarization in cat vesical parasympathetic neurones. *J Physiol* 361:165–184

Anderson P, Anderson SA (1968): *Physiological basis of the Alpha Rhythm*. New York: Appleton-Century Crofts.

Asnis G (1977): Parkinson's disease, depression and ECT: a critical review and case study. *Am J Psychiatry* 134:191–195

Aston-Jones G, Bloom FE (1981): Activity of norepi-nephrine-containing neurons in behaving rats anticipates fluctuations in the sleep-waking cycle. *J Neurosci* 1:876–886

Buzsáki G (1991): The thalamic clock: emergent network properties. *Neuroscience* 41:351–364

Buzsáki G, Bickford RG, Ponomareff G, Thal LJ, Mandel R, Gage FH (1988a): Nucleus basalis and thalamic control of neocortical activity in the freely moving rat. *J Neurosci* 8:4007–4026

Buzsáki G, Bickford RG, Armstrong DM, Ponomareff G, Chen KS, Ruiz R, Thal LJ, Gage FH (1988b): Electrical activity in the neocortex of freely moving young and aged rats. *Neuroscience* 26:735–744

Buzsáki G, Kennedy B, Solt VB, Ziegler M (1991): Noradrenergic control of thalamic oscillation: the role of alpha-2 receptors. *Eur J Neurosci* 3:222–229

Buzsáki G, Laszlovszky I, Lajtha A, Vadasz C (1990): Spike-and-wave neocortical patterns in rats: genetic and aminergic control. *Neuroscience* 38:323–333

Buzsáki G, Smith A, Berger S, Fisher LJ, Gage FH (1989): Parkinsonian tremor and petit mal epilepsy: hypothesis of a common pacemaker. *Neuroscience* 36:1–14

Celesia GG, Wanamake WM (1972): Psychiatric disturbances in Parkinson's disease. *Dis Nerv Syst* 33:577–583

Collingridge GL, Kehl SJ, McLennan H (1983): Excitatory amino acids in synaptic transmission in the Schaffer collateral-commissural pathway of the rat hippocampus. *J Physiol* 334:33–46

Douyon R, Serby M, Klutscho B, Rotrosen J (1989): ECT and Parkinson's disease revisited: a "naturalistic" study. *Am J Psychiat* 146:1451–1455

Gillin JC (1983): The sleep therapies of depression (1983) *Prog Neuro-Psychopharmacol and Biol Psychiat* 7:351–364

Gillin JC, Borbély AA (1985): Sleep: a neurobiological window on affective disorders. *Trends Neurosci* 8:537–539

Gloor P, Fariello RG (1988): Generalized epilepsy: some of its cellular mechanisms differ from those of focal epilepsy. *Trends Neurosci* 11:63–68

Itil TM, Soldatos C (1980): Epileptogenic side effects of psychotropic drugs. *JAMA* 244:1460–1463

Jahnsen J, Llinás R (1984a): Electrophysiological properties of guinea pig thalamic neurones: an in vitro study. *J Physiol* 349:205–226

Jahnsen J, Llinás R (1984b): Ionic basis for the electroresponsiveness and oscillatory properties of guinea pig thalamic neurones *in vitro*. *J Physiol* 349:227–247

Llinás RR (1988): The intrinsic electrophysiological properties of mammalian neurons: insight into central nervous system function. *Science* 242:1654–1664

McCormick DA, Prince DA (1986): Acetylcholine induces burst firing in thalamic reticular neurones by activating a potassium conductance. *Nature* 319:402–405

McCormick DA (1989): Cholinergic and noradrenergic modulation of thalomocortical processing. *Trends Neurosci.* 12:215–221

McCormick DA, Prince DA (1988): Noradrenergic modulation of firing pattern in guinea pig and cat thalamic neurons, in vitro. *J Neurophysiol* 59:978–996

Micheletti G, Warter J-M, Marescaux C, Depaulis A, Tranchant C, Rumbach L, Vergnes M (1987): Effects of drugs affecting noradrenergic neurotransmission in rats with spontaneous petit mal-like seizures. *Eur J Pharmacol* 135:397–402

Monaghan DT, Cotman CW (1985): Distribution of *N*-methyl-D-aspartate-sensitive L[^{3}H]glutamate binding sites in rat brain. *J Neurosci* 5:2909–2919

Moruzzi G, Magoun HW (1949): Brain stem reticular formation and activation of EEG. *Electroencephalogr Clin Neurophysiol* 1:455–473

Riekkinen P, Buzsaki G, Riekkineni P, Jr, Soininen H, Partanen J (1990): The cholinergic system and EEG slow waves. *Electroencephalogr Clin Neurophysiol* (in press)

Roger J, Grangeon H, Grey J (1968): Incidences psychiatriques et psychologiques du traitement par l'ethosuximide chez les epileptiques. *Encephale* 57:407–438

Roy-Byrne PP, Uhde TW, Post RM (1984): Antidepressant effects of one night's sleep deprivation: Clinical and theoretical implications. In: Post R, Ballenger J, eds. *Neurobiology of Mood Disorders.* Baltimore: Williams and Wilkins, pp 817–835

Shosaku A, Kayama Y, Sumimoto I, Sugitani M, Iwama K (1989): Analysis of recurrent inhibitory circuit in rat thalamus: neurophysiology of the thalamic reticular nucleus. *Prog Neurobiol* 32:77–102

Simpson GM, Pi EH, Sramek JJ (1981): Adverse effects of antipsychotic drugs. *Drugs* 21:138–151

Steriade M, Buzsaki G (1990): Parallel activation of the thalamus and neocortex. In: *Brain cholinergic systems*, Steriade M, Biesold D, eds. Oxford: Oxford University Press

Steriade M, Deschenes M (1984): The thalamus as a neuronal oscillator. *Brain Res Rev* 8:1–63

Steriade M, Deschenes M, Domich L, Mulle C (1985): Abolition of spindle oscillation in thalamic neurons disconnected from nucleus reticularis thalami. *J Neurophysiol* 54:1473–1497

Steriade M, Domich L, Oakson G, Deschenes M (1987): The deafferented reticular thalamic nucleus generates spindle rhythmicity. *J. Neurophysiol* 57:260–273

Steriade M, Llinás RR (1988): The functional states of the thalamus and the associated neuronal interplay. *Physiol Rev* 68:649–741

Traub RD, Miles R, Wong RKS (1989): Model of rhythmic population oscillation in the hippocampal slice. *Science* 243:1319–1325

Mesopontine Cholinergic Systems Suppress Slow Rhythms and Induce Fast Oscillations in Thalamocortical Circuits

MIRCEA STERIADE, ROBERTO CURRÓ DOSSI, and DENIS PARÉ

The terms *synchronization* and *desynchronization* have been coined for high-amplitude and slow (<15 Hz) oscillations occurring synchronously in widespread brain territories during light sleep, as opposed to low-amplitude and fast (>20 Hz) waves during arousal and sleep with dreaming episodes. This dichotomy, used because of its heuristic value, simplifies a more complex reality. Indeed, sequences of fast oscillations may occur with much higher amplitudes than those of background activity during states of increased vigilance. This phenomenon was first observed by Bremer et al. (1960), who emphasized that a flattening of the cortical electroencephalogram (EEG) on brain stem reticular stimulation (Moruzzi and Magoun, 1949) is not the only effect of this now classical experimental way of mimicking awakening. Instead, a clear-cut enhancement in amplitude of spontaneous rhythms and their acceleration up to 40 to 45 Hz was seen on cortical EEG, simultaneously with the ocular syndrome of arousal, regardless of the frequency of stimulation applied to the brainstem core (see Fig. 5C–D in Bremer et al., 1960).

This indicates that the EEG counterpart of an increase in the vigilance level should not be regarded as merely consisting of "negative" events, namely, the disruption of relatively slow EEG oscillations (spindles and delta waves) that occur during sleep. In addition to this process of desynchronization, the EEG picture reflecting arousal behavior also includes the appearance of clear-cut oscillations above 20 Hz.

In this chapter we present evidence that the cholinergic afferents to the thalamus and neocortex are effective in suppressing slow EEG rhythms, and that fast oscillations can be generated in the cerebral cortex by mesopontine cholinergic systems driving thalamocortical neurons.

Suppression of Slow Oscillations by Mesopontine and Basal Forebrain Cholinergic Systems

There are two major types of low-frequency oscillations during EEG-synchronized sleep: spindles and delta waves.

Blockage of spindles

Spindles are waves between 7 and 14 Hz, grouped in sequences that last for 1.5 to 3 s and recur every 5 to 10 s. Spindling is the epitome of EEG synchronization at sleep onset, a landmark of the transition from waking to sleep. The occurrence of spindle waves is associated with blockade of afferent information and unconsciousness. The obliteration of synaptic transmission in the thalamus deprives the cortex from the necessary input to elaborate a response. This deafferentation is a prerequisite for falling asleep.

Spindle waves appear in thalamocortical cells as rhythmic hyperpolarizations, each lasting for 70 to 150 ms and often leading to postinhibitory rebound bursts (Fig. 1A). The high-frequency bursts result from an intrinsic property of thalamic cells, deinactivated by the membrane hyperpolarization during periods of EEG-synchronized sleep (Steriade and Llinás, 1988). These bursts are transferred to the cortex where they elicit excitatory postsynaptic potentials (EPSPs) in the frequency range of spindles. As any EEG oscillation that is recordable with rather gross electrodes inserted in the brain or placed over the scalp, spindles require, in addition to special intrinsic properties of thalamic neurons, a synchronizing device that unites different elements of the ensemble.

The thalamic origin of spindles is definitely established, as they can be

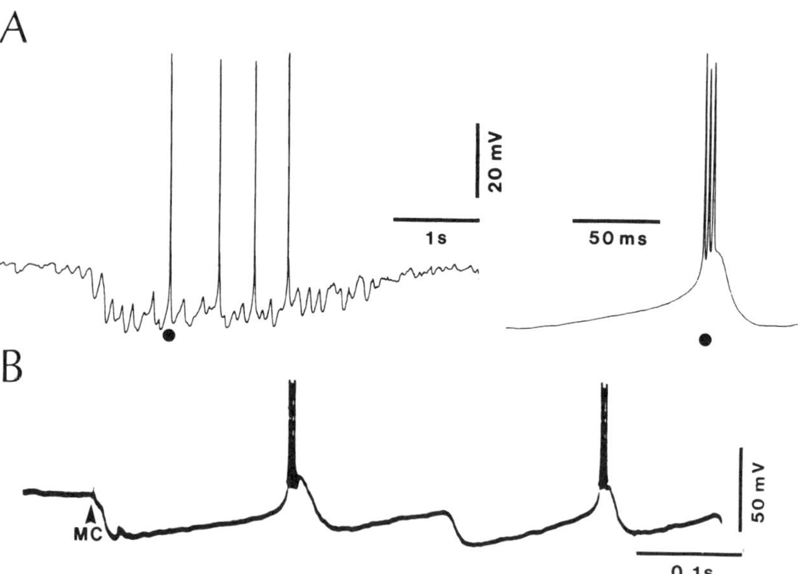

Figure 1. Spontaneous and cortically evoked spindle oscillations in intracellularly recorded thalamocortical neurons of the cat. **A:** intralaminar centrolateral neuron. **Left:** Spontaneous spindle sequence consisting of cyclic hyperpolarizations occasionally leading to postinhibitory rebound bursts. The burst marked by dot is expanded at right. **B:** Ventrolateral cell. Stimulation (*arrowhead*) of motor cortex (MC) elicited a spindle sequence with the same characteristics as those of spontaneously occurring ones. A, unpublished data by Curró Dossi and Steriade; B, modified from Steriade (1984).

recorded in the thalamus after complete decortication, high brain stem transection, and even more radical procedures (for details, see Steriade et al., 1990c). Spindles appear as rhythmic (7–14 Hz) spike barrages superimposed on a depolarizing envelope in GABAergic reticular thalamic (RE) cells, whereas an inverse image (cyclic hyperpolarizations) is seen in thalamocortical neurons (Steriade and Deschênes, 1988). This reciprocal picture suggests that RE cells impose rhythmic inhibitory postsynaptic potentials (IPSPs) onto thalamocortical neurons. The evidence that RE neurons are pacemakers of spindle oscillations can be summarized as follows: 1) spindles are abolished in thalamic territories disconnected from the RE nucleus (Steriade et al., 1985), and 2) spindles are preserved in the RE nucleus isolated from its thalamic and cortical inputs (Steriade et al., 1987a).

Similar wave forms and rhythmicity characterize spontaneously occurring spindles and spindlelike oscillations triggered by cortical stimulation (Fig. 1A, B). The difference between the powerful spindle sequences induced by cortical stimuli and the much less evident oscillations evoked by prethalamic stimulation is probably due to the direct access of corticothalamic pathways to the spindle pacemaker, the RE nucleus.

It has long been known that brain stem reticular stimulation blocks spindle oscillations. This is a major aspect of the EEG desynchronization. The mechanism of spindle suppression during natural arousal and rapid eye movement (REM) sleep or upon stimulation of mesopontine cholinergic nuclei is a muscarinic-mediated hyperpolarization of RE cells (Fig. 2A), associated with a marked increase in membrane conductance (Hu et al., 1989). This effect decouples the dendrodendritic network of RE nucleus in cat and monkey, which has been implicated in the genesis of spindle oscillations. As a consequence of spindles' blockade at the very site of their genesis, the spindle-related inhibitory oscillations of thalamocortical cells are suppressed (Fig. 2B).

In addition to the mesopontine-RE cholinergic projections (Paré et al., 1988), a basal forebrain (BF) input to the rostral pole of the RE nuclear complex has been identified in cat and monkey (Steriade et al., 1987b; Parent et al., 1988). Because the BF–RE axons arise in a minority ($<25\%$) of cholinergic BF cells, we suggested that this projection is mainly GABAergic. Our proposal found support in studies using the anterograde and retrograde transport of BF axons to the rostral pole of RE nucleus, combined with the GABA immunoreactivity of BF–RE neurons in the rat (Asanuma, 1989; Asanuma and Porter, 1990). Either cholinergic or GABAergic, the BF neurons exert a strong inhibition on their RE target neurons, with the consequence of inhibiting the spindle pacemaker. In agreement with this, it has been observed that in aged rats, with shrunken cholinergic BF cells, the incidence of spindles is enhanced (Buzsáki et al., 1988a). Also, a diminution in firing rate of BF cells is reliably followed by spindles in thalamocortical circuits (Buzsáki et al., 1988b).

Stimulation of mesopontine cholinergic nuclei also suppresses low-frequency hyperpolarizing oscillations in anterior thalamic (AT) cells (Fig.

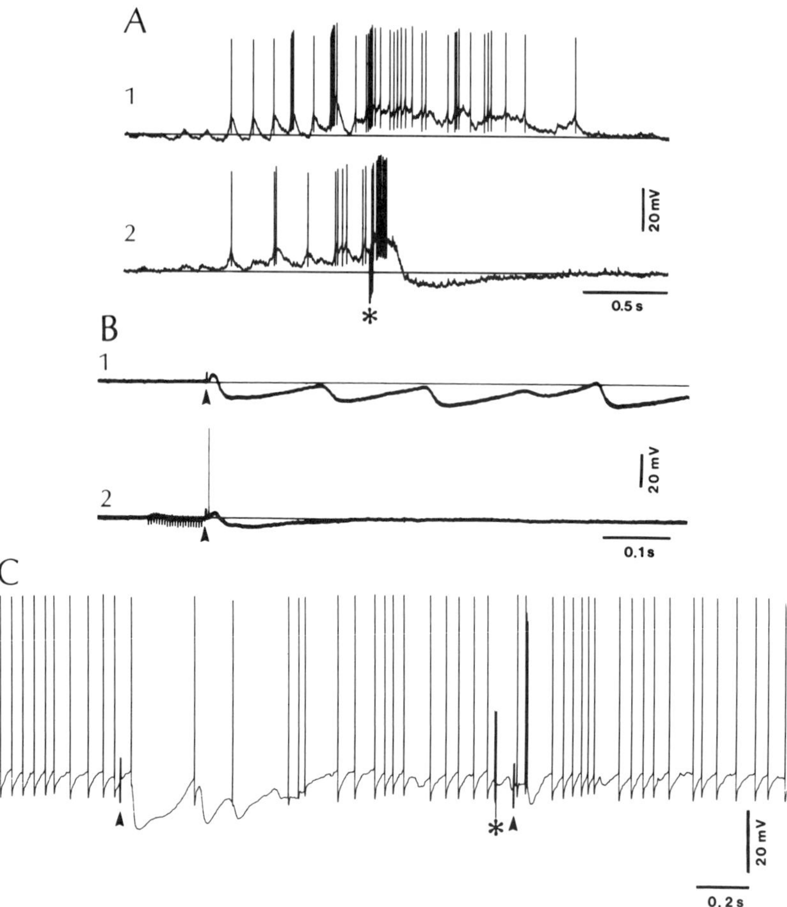

Figure 2. Blockage of spontaneous and evoked low-frequency oscillations in cat's thalamic cells by stimulation of mesopontine cholinergic nuclei. Intracellular recordings. **A:** Neuron recorded in the perigeniculate (PG) sector of RE nuclear complex. Spontaneous spindle oscillation. 1, a complete spindle sequence; 2, a spindle sequence abbreviated by stimulating (*asterisk*) the peribrachial area of the pedunculopontine nucleus. **B:** Thalamocortical neuron in the ventrolateral nucleus. 1, spindle sequence elicited by motor cortex stimulation (*arrowhead*); 2, the effect of a preceding pulse-train to the midbrain reticular formation; note facilitation of cortically evoked antidromic spike, preservation of a first hyperpolarizing component, and suppression of rhythmic spindle oscillations. **C:** Thalamocortical cell in anteromedial nucleus. Cyclic hyperpolarizations elicited by retrosplenial cortical stimulus (*arrowhead*) and their blockage by a preceding pulse-train to the laterodorsal tegmental nucleus (*asterisk*); see comments in text. A, modified from Hu et al. (1989); B, modified from Steriade and Deschênes (1988); C, unpublished data by Curró Dossi, Paré, and Steriade.

2C). Since the AT nuclear group is naturally devoid of inputs from the RE nucleus (Steriade et al., 1984; Velayos et al., 1989), the progenitors of AT cells' hyperpolarizations are GABAergic local interneurons. Our observation raises intriguing questions concerning the mechanisms underlying cyclic oscillations in AT cells and their suppression by mesopontine cholinergic stimulation. Note, first, that *spontaneous* spindle-related hyperpolarizations were never seen in AT cells, as opposed to other dorsal thalamic neurons that receive RE afferents. This supports similar findings obtained in our laboratory by Mulle et al. (1985) and Paré et al. (1987). The latter study also reported that cingular cortex stimulation elicited spindlelike (8–12 Hz) field potentials in the intralaminar centrolateral thalamic nucleus that is densely innervated by RE axons, whereas the same stimulus triggered focal waves with lower amplitudes and significantly lower frequency (5–6 Hz) in AT nuclei (see Fig. 8 in Paré et al., 1987). A similar result at the intracellular level is shown in Fig. 2C: the control sequence of cortically elicited IPSPs in the AT cell consists of waves at 5 to 6 Hz, within the frequency range of theta rhythm. The cortically induced oscillatory waves at 5 to 6 Hz in the limbic AT nuclear group may be explained by at least two nonexclusive factors: 1) excitation of AT relay cells and/or interneurons, with subsequent cyclic inhibition-rebound sequences in a hypothetical intranuclear recurrent inhibitory circuit; however, no study using intracellular staining is yet available in AT relay cells and it was found that recurrent collaterals of thalamocortical axons are lacking in most dorsal thalamic nuclei where this method has been employed (for details, see Steriade et al., 1990c), and 2) cingular cortex stimulation may elicit a series of inhibitory oscillations at the site of stimulation (or through circuitous pathways involving the septohippocampal system), followed by cyclic rebounds in corticothalamic neurons that would modulate in an inhibitory way AT relay neurons through the axons of local interneurons. The suppression of these rhythmic IPSPs in AT relay neurons by mesopontine cholinergic stimulation is in line with the demonstrated hyperpolarization, by acetylcholine (ACh), of morphologically identified interneurons in the lateral geniculate (LG) thalamic nucleus (McCormick and Pape, 1988).

Blockage of delta waves

Until recently, delta waves (0.5–4 Hz) were commonly thought to be exclusively generated in the cerebral cortex (Steriade et al., 1990b). However, earlier data pointed out that rhythmic slow (1–2 Hz) waves were focally recorded in the ventrolateral thalamic nucleus and were suppressed by midbrain reticular stimulation (see Fig. 7B in Steriade et al., 1971; see also below).

The mechanisms of cortical delta waves are unknown because there are no systematic intracellular studies of this EEG rhythm. Current source–density analyses and extracellular unit studies reported that delta waves are generated by vertically arranged dipoles of pyramid-shaped neurons between cortical layers II and V (cf. Steriade et al., 1990b). Recording of unitary activity by means of multiple electrodes inserted in 8 to 16 loci of all layers in rat's neocortex showed that a complete cessation of neuronal firing occurs throughout the cortex in close association with the depth-positive component of delta waves (see Fig. 1.21 in Steriade and Buzsaki, 1990). In addition to the role of long-lasting IPSPs in cortical cells, some intrinsic properties of cortical cells, such as a calcium-mediated potassium conductance, $g_{K(Ca)}$, lasting for about 200 to 500 ms (Connors et al., 1982; Schwindt et al., 1988a, 1988b), are presumably involved in the patterning of delta waves.

In the cerebral cortex, $g_{K(Ca)}$ is blocked by ACh (McCormick and Prince, 1986). This is consistent with the disappearance of delta waves as cholinergic BF neurons increase their firing rates upon arousal (Buzsaki et al., 1988b) and as the ACh output from the cerebral cortex is enhanced during EEG-desynchronized states of waking and REM sleep (Jasper and Tessier, 1971).

Two sets of recent data indicate that delta-type oscillations can be triggered in thalamic cells by a hyperpolarization within the voltage range of -65 to -85 mV, which activates an inward slow cation current, termed I_h. *In vitro*, McCormick and Pape (1990) have implicated the interplay between I_h and the transient calcium current (I_t) underlying the low-threshold spike (LTS) to account for the rhythmic recurrence of oscillations in a subpopulation of lateral geniculate neurons. *In vivo*, we have found that self-sustained delta-type oscillations, triggered by hyperpolarizing current pulses and consisting of rhythmic LTSs alternating with afterhyperpolarizations (AHPs), are present in virtually all antidromically identified ventrolateral, centrolateral, and lateroposterior thalamocortical neurons (Curro Dossi et al., 1992; Steriade et al., 1991a) (Fig. 3A).

Moreover, *spontaneous* oscillations at 1 to 2 Hz were detected when the membrane potential was hyperpolarized by about 8–10 mV, due to the surgical removal or functional inactivation of the respective cortical areas (Fig. 3B). In normal conditions, the cortical input provides a powerful depolarizing impingement on thalamic neurons during brain-activated states (waking and REM sleep) when the discharge of cortical cells is sustained. This action prevents the genesis of delta oscillation in the thalamus since the interplay between intrinsic currents (I_h and I_t) is critically dependent upon membrane hyperpolarization. During EEG-synchronized sleep, however, the high-frequency bursts of corticothalamic cells (Steriade, 1978) more effectively drive thalamic GABAergic neurons, thus producing an overwhelming hyperpolarization of thalamocortical neurons. This explains the potentiating effect of cortical pulse-trains on thalamic delta oscillation (Steriade et al., 1991a).

Cortical volleys were also effective in synchronizing simultaneously recorded thalamic cells, that were unrelated before cortical stimulation (Steriade et al., 1991a). It is probable that the RE thalamic complex, when set into action by bursts of action potentials generated by corticothalamic neurons during EEG-synchronized sleep, acts as a synchronizing device for the slow thalamic oscillations. Experiments in progress have substantiated this possibility (unpublished data).

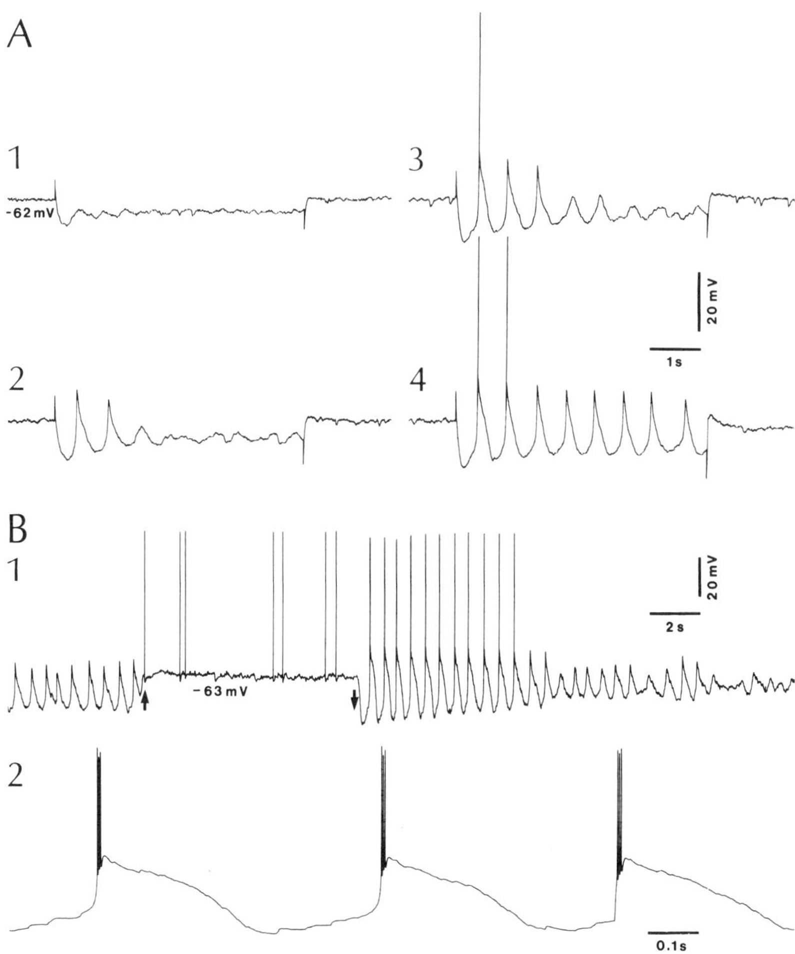

Figure 3. Slow (delta) oscillation of thalamocortical cells triggered by hyperpolarizing current pulses or occurring spontaneously. **A:** ventrolateral cell. Hyperpolarizing current pulses of 0.7 nA (in 1), 1 nA (2), 1.1 nA (3) and 1.2 nA (4) elicited an increasing number of cycles at 1.6 Hz. **B:** lateroposterior cell. At "rest", the cell oscillated spontaneously at 1.7 Hz. A 0.5 nA depolarizing current (between arrows) prevented the oscillation, and its removal set the cell back in the oscillatory mode. Three cycles after removal of depolarizing current in 1 are expanded in 2 to show high-frequency spike bursts crowning low-threshold spikes. From Steriade et al. (1991a).

Stimulation of mesopontine cholinergic nuclei prevents the delta oscillation in thalamocortical cells. Two types of effects were observed: 1) a short-lasting suppression of delta rhythm, associated with an increase in membrane conductance and abolished by mecamylamine, a nicotinic antagonist; and 2) a longer-lasting blockage, an effect that is associated with a substantial depolarization of thalamocortical cells and that can be prevented by scopolamine, a muscarinic antagonist (Steriade et al., 1991a). The depolarization seen in Figure 4 (especially in B panel) set thalamocortical cells out of the voltage range required for delta oscillation. The suppression of thalamic delta oscillation by brainstem cholinergic stimulation is associated with an EEG activation response, having a time-course similar to the blockage of delta oscillation in thalamocortical cells. This EEG response includes the appearance of a

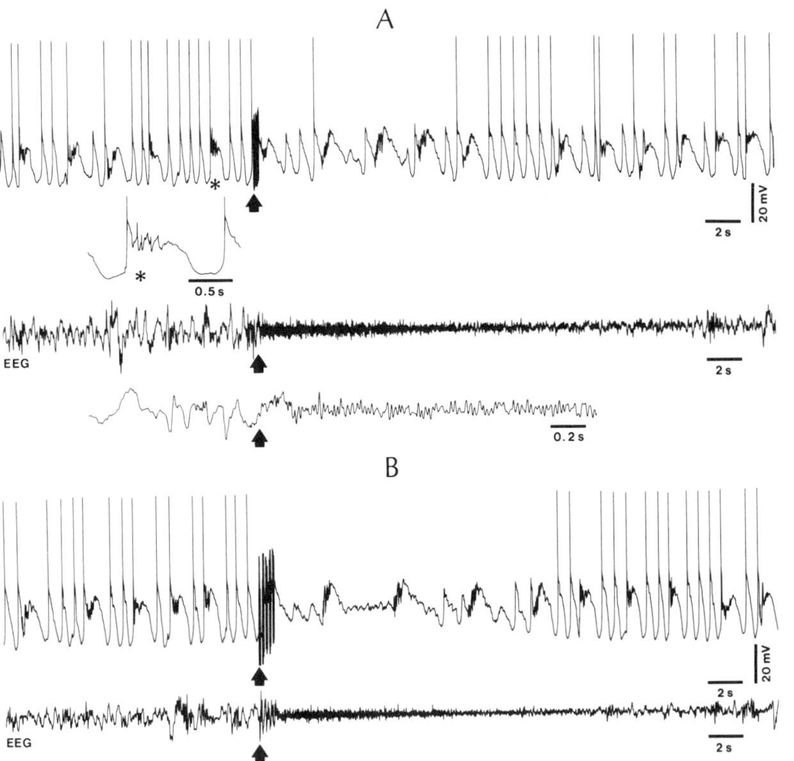

Figure 4. Intracellular recorded delta oscillation in lateroposterior thalamic cell and its suppression by brainstem peribrachial (PB) stimulation (one and five pulse-trains in A and B, respectively). Below the top (intracellular) trace, EEG cortical recording (in A, an expanded epoch of EEG trace around the PB pulse-train is also depicted to show the 40 Hz oscillation induced by PB stimulation). A sequence of fast depolarizing events in A (asterisk) is expanded and shown below. From Steriade et al. (1991a).

clear-cut fast oscillation around 40 Hz (Figure 4A) which is discussed in the following section.

Induction of Fast Oscillations in Thalamocortical Circuits by Mesopontine Cholinergic Afferents

Following Bremer's observation that EEG waves around 40 to 45 Hz can be elicited by rostral brain stem reticular stimulation (see introduction), a series of studies have investigated in more detail these fast rhythms.

Oscillations between 25 and 45 Hz of focal EEG and/or neuronal firing probability have been shown to occur spontaneously over the motor and parietal association cortices in experimental conditions qualified as hunting situations (Rougeul-Buser et al., 1983; Bouyer et al., 1987) or to be stimulus-dependent in the olfactory system (Freeman, 1975) and visual cortex where they have been implicated in cooperative interactions between remote cortical columns (Eckhorn et al., 1988; Gray and Singer, 1989; Gray et al., 1990). Moreover, the electrical stimulation of the midbrain reticular formation greatly enhanced the coherency of the fast (40–45 Hz) oscillatory responses of visual cortex cells to appropriate light stimuli (Singer, 1990). Previous data have also shown that a brief pulse-train to the midbrain peribrachial area selectively enhances the secondary component of the flash-evoked cortical response and transforms it into a distinct, fast (80 Hz) afterdischarge; this effect was not due to concomitant changes of the primary deflection (Fig. 5; Steriade et al., 1968). It was repeatedly proposed that, whereas the initial cortical response to a sensory stimulus reflects the transmission of information to the cerebral cortex, later events (particularly the fast afterdischarge) reflect activities related to intracortical processing, perhaps to early storage. Indeed, the fast afterdischarge was selectively enhanced during high levels of alertness, increased during conditioning more than the primary component, and was correlated with the subjective experience of rhythmic afterimages after a flash of light (see Steriade, 1968, for a review).

The fast oscillations discussed above are supposed to involve special synchronizing mechanisms so that they can be recorded with rather gross electrodes not only from the cortical surface and depth, as in the animal experiments mentioned above, but also over the human scalp during complex tasks (Sheer, 1984).

One of the possible mechanisms responsible for the fast cortical oscillations was revealed in slice experiments performed by Llinás et al. (1991). They showed that sparsely spinous interneurons recorded in layer 4 of guinea pig frontal cortex exhibit narrow-frequency (35–45 Hz) oscillations upon a depolarization of the membrane. The oscillation was shown to result from the activation of a voltage-dependent, persistent sodium conductance and a delayed rectifier.

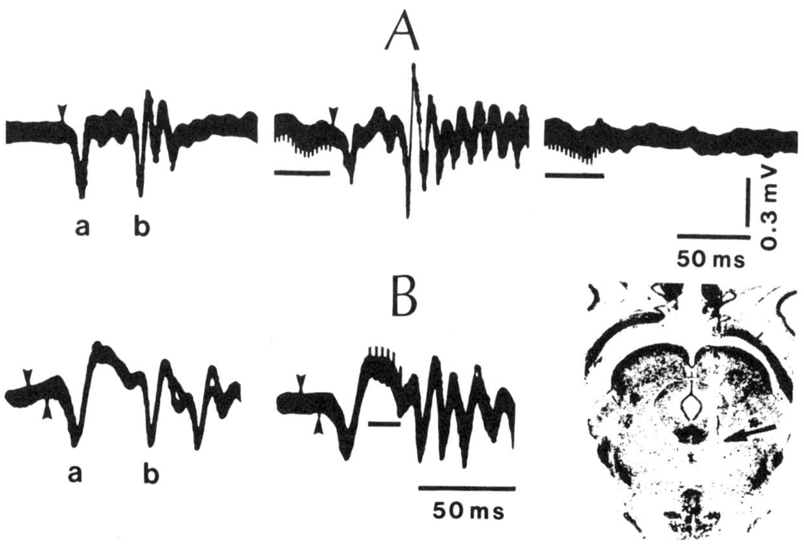

Figure 5. Potentiation of flash-evoked fast (80 Hz) cortical afterdischarge by stimulating the midbrain peribrachial area in cat. Recording of field potentials at the surface of the visual cortex. 1-ms and 10-ms flashes are indicated by single and double arrowheads in **A** and **B**, respectively. Midbrain reticular stimulation (350 Hz, *horizontal line*) was delivered just before the testing flash (A; midbrain pulse-train alone at right) or after the initial (a) flash-evoked deflection, before the b component (**B**). Note midbrain-induced selective potentiation of b component consisting of 80 Hz waves. Modified from Steriade et al. (1968).

The synchronizing mechanisms of this oscillatory process is not, however, elucidated. Whether or not thalamocortical neurons are capable of displaying such a fast oscillation was also unknown. The transmitters used by ascending brain stem reticular influxes generating or enhancing the oscillations at 40 to 80 Hz have not yet been revealed. Although the conditioning potentiating stimulation in Figure 5 was applied to the peribrachial area (that later on was demonstrated to be a major cholinergic cell group), as a rule, stimulation of the brain stem core was applied to the rostral midbrain where there are virtually no cholinergic cells; the chemical codes of neurons in that mesencephalic area are not disclosed. However, it is possible that the ascending cholinergic axons were activated by stimulation of those more rostral sites.

We report here the results of recent experiments dealing with the fast oscillations of intracellularly recorded thalamocortical neurons and with the potentiation of fast oscillations by brain stem–thalamic cholinergic systems acting on muscarinic receptors.

Subpopulations of antidromically identified thalamocortical neurons in the ventroanterior–ventrolateral complex and rostral intralaminar centrolateral nucleus have been found to display spontaneous fast prepotentials (FPPs), leading to full action potentials at slightly depolarized levels, in the frequency range of 25 to 45 Hz. In some of these cells, depolarizing current pulses triggered oscillatory events within the same frequency range (Steriade et al., 1991b). The two thalamocortical neurons illustrated in Figure 6 displayed FPPs, sometimes leading to full spikes. The autocorrelogram of FPPs in the ventrolateral cell (panel A) shows multiple peaks, demonstrating an oscillation in the 40-Hz frequency. The centrolateral cell (panel B) exhibited FPPs that occasionally boosted full spikes during a period of hyperpolarization, and regularly recurring full action potentials during a depolarizing episode; the autocorrelogram computed from both FPPs and action potentials indicates a rhythmicity of 28 Hz.

The origin of these FPPs could be any of the excitatory inputs impinging on thalamic neurons. The thalamic-projecting mesopontine cholinergic neurons have high firing rates (>20 Hz) and tonic discharge patterns during brain arousal, with most interspike intervals concentrated between 20 and 40 ms (Steriade et al., 1990a). It seems reasonable to hypothesize that one of the major sources of the fast oscillation in thalamocortical neurons is the aggregate of cholinergic cells at the mesopontine junction. A nonexclusive alternative is that the cholinergic input modulates the excitability of thalamocortical cells and allows other inputs to act.

The experiments described below concern the facilitation of the 40 Hz cortical EEG oscillation by stimulation of brain stem cholinergic nuclei. Since mesopontine cholinergic nuclei influence the cerebral cortex through two parallel pathways, one relayed in the thalamus and the other in the basal forebrain (Steriade and Buzsaki, 1990), and because we focused on the former circuit, the experiments were performed in animals with extensive excitotoxic (kainate-induced) lesions of basal forebrain cholinergic nuclei (see histology in Steriade et al., 1991b).

First, the peribrachial area was stimulated with a 1-s pulse train at various frequencies, ranging from 30 to 45 Hz. Each pulse induced a stimulus-locked wave on the cortical EEG. It should be mentioned that the peak at 32 Hz seen in Figure 7 at time 0, as the result of stimulating the brain stem reticular core with a 32-Hz pulse train, was superimposed on a cortical EEG background activity that already comprised fast waves around 40 Hz (left panel in Fig. 7). Scopolamine, a muscarinic antagonist, blocked the fast (32 Hz) evoked potentials as well as the spontaneous waves above 10 Hz while enhancing the waves slower than 7 Hz (right panel in Fig. 7). This experiment indicated that thalamocortical neurons are able to relay fast (>30 Hz) volleys originating in the mesopontine cholinergic neurons.

Second, in order to obtain evidence that an increase in fast EEG rhythms may outlast the stimulation of brain stem cholinergic nuclei, we stimulated the peribrachial area with three brief (0.1 s) pulse trains at 300 Hz. This parameter of stimulation was found particularly effective to induce a long-lasting (>20 s), muscarinic-mediated depolarization in thalamocortical neurons, associated with an increase in the apparent membrane input resistance

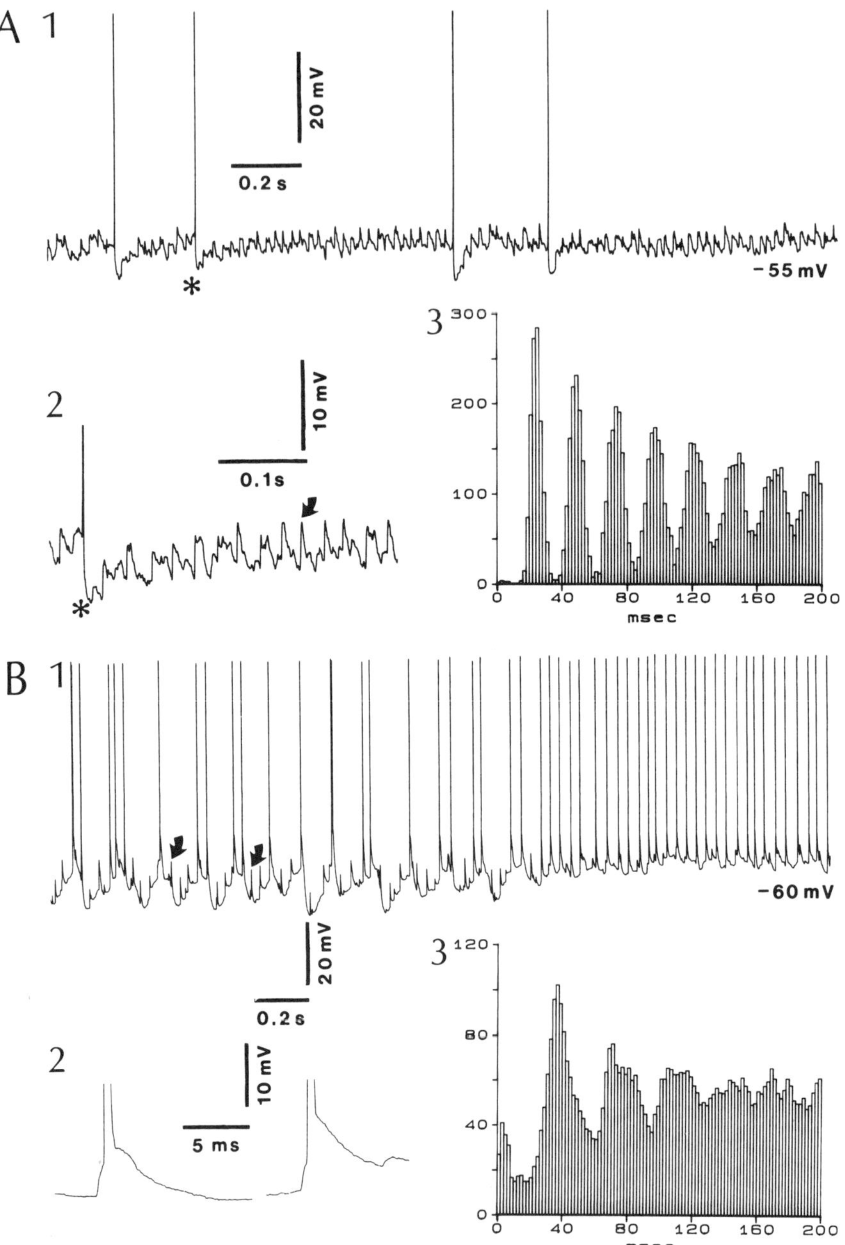

Figure 6. Fast (30–40 Hz), rhythmically recurring fast prepotentials (FPPs) in cat's thalamocortical neurons. Resting membrane potential is indicated at right in both cells. **A:** ventrolateral thalamic cell. An FPP is marked by arrow in panel 2 representing the enlarged portion depicted with asterisk in panel 1. In 3, autocorrelogram computed with resolution of 2 ms over a time range of 200 ms, indicating multiple peaks recurring with a frequency of about 40 Hz. **B:** Centrolateral cell. In 1, shift from a hyperpolarizing episode to a tonically depolarized epoch. During membrane hyperpolarization, regularly occurring FPPs (*arrows*), occasionally boosting full action potentials (see two of them in panel 2; spikes truncated). In 3, autocorrelogram computed from both FPPs and full action potentials, indicating a series of peaks with a frequency of about 28 Hz. Modified from Steriade et al. (1991b)

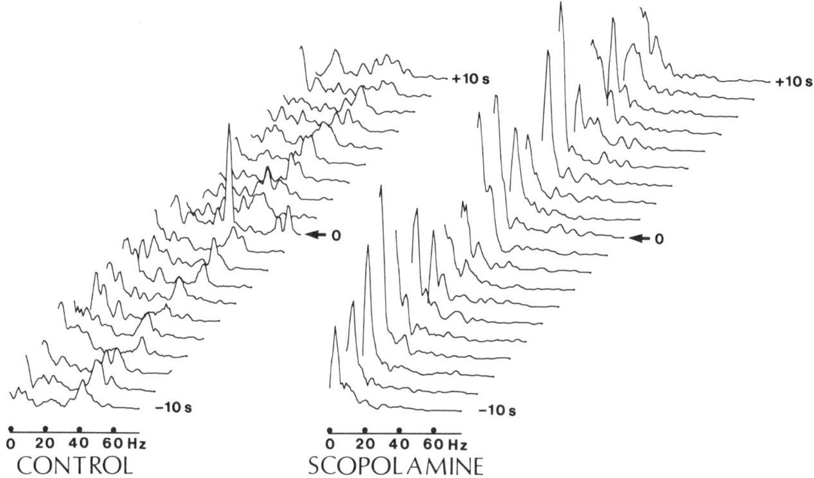

Figure 7. Spontaneous and evoked fast (30–40 Hz) EEG rhythms in cat are abolished by a muscarinic blocker, scopolamine. Evolutive power spectra established from a 20-s period; EEG record from precruciate cortical area 6. Each line corresponds to a spectral analysis of 1 s (0–75 Hz). 10 s are depicted before (−10 s to 0) and 10 s after (0 to +10 s) stimulation of the mesopontine peribrachial cholinergic area (*arrow*) with a pulse-train at 32 Hz, lasting for 1 s. Note in left panel spontaneous waves around 40 Hz and a peak at 32 Hz corresponding to the evoked waves in the cortical EEG. Both spontaneous and evoked fast waves were abolished by 0.5 mg/kg scopolamine, whereas slow (< 7 Hz) EEG rhythms were enhanced by the muscarinic antagonist.

(Curró Dossi et al., 1991). Figure 8 shows that power spectra of cortical waves around 40 Hz are doubled after brain stem peribrachial stimulation, that this potentiation outlasts brain stem stimulation by at least 10 s, and that both spontaneous 40-Hz waves and their potentiation by brain stem stimulation are abolished by scopolamine.

The present demonstration that 30- to 40-Hz oscillations take place in thalamocortical systems and are enhanced by setting into action brain stem–thalamic cholinergic projections leads us to conceive as probable that these fast cortical oscillations result from interactions in resonant cortical and thalamic networks under the facilitatory influence of the brain stem cholinergic input.

Llinás' (1990) hypothesis proposed that the 40-Hz oscillations in sparsely spinous (inhibitory) cortical interneurons would trigger IPSPs in other cortical cells, including corticothalamic neurons in layer 6, with the consequence of rhythmic 40-Hz volleys in the corticothalamic pathway driving both reticular thalamic and thalamocortical cells, thus leading to a 40-Hz EPSP–IPSP rebound sequence that reenters the cortex.

Our data support the possibility that thalamocortical cells are part of the resonant loop. During the aroused state, when 40-Hz rhythms are expected to

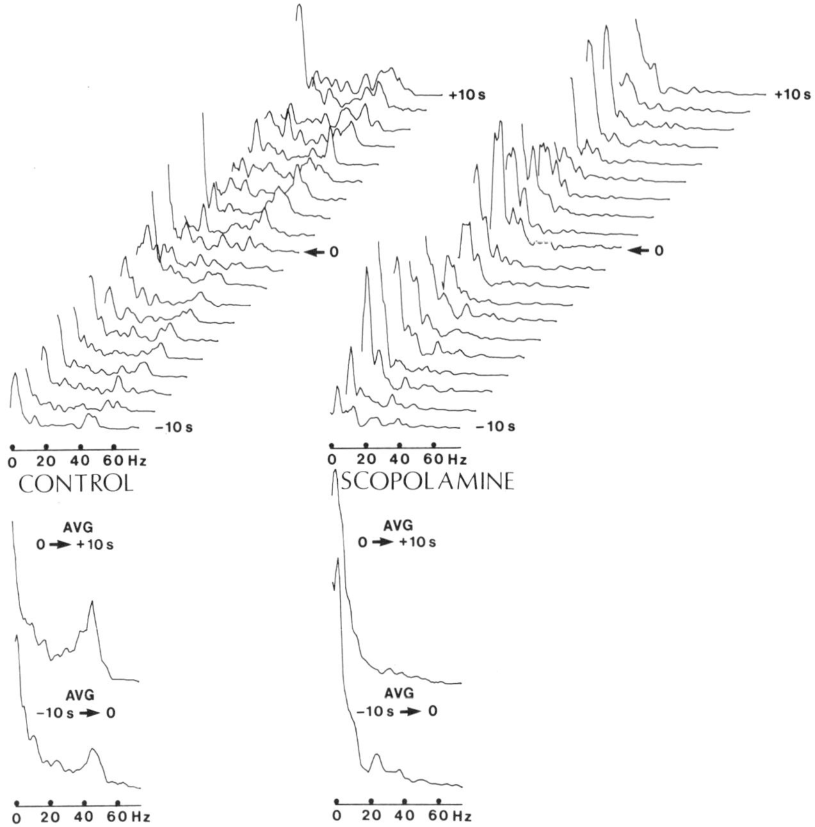

Figure 8. Potentiation of 40-Hz EEG waves in cat by stimulation of brain stem cholinergic peribrachial area and abolition of this fast rhythm by scopolamine. **Top:** Same graphical arrangement as in the preceding figure. Stimulation (at 0, *arrow*) consisted of a 0.1-s train of 300-Hz pulses. **Bottom:** Averaged power spectra (AVG) 10 s before (−10 s to 0) and after (0 to +10 s) peribrachial stimulation. Note enhancement of 40-Hz waves after stimulation during the control period and abolition of 40 Hz waves after administration of scopolamine (0.5 mg/kg). Modified from Steriade et al. (1991b).

occur with the highest probability and when thalamocortical neurons discharge tonically because of their sustained depolarization, the inhibitory input from the reticular thalamic nucleus just sculptures the tonic discharge. Then, rhythmic trains of single spikes would be transmitted to the cortex. The relay of the corticothalamic input through the reticular thalamic neurons may not even be necessary since, at 30 to 50 Hz, cortical stimulation leads to a dramatic increase of EPSPs in directly related thalamic cells (Lindström and Wrobel, 1970). There is, then, a built-in frequency amplification in the corticothalamic circuit leading to a four- to eight fold increase of the afferent input.

The present demonstration of fast oscillations in centrolateral thalamic cells is important because of the widespread neocortical distribution of rostral intralaminar thalamic axons (Jones, 1985). This would explain the fact that 40-Hz oscillations have been found by various authors in a series of distant and functionally different cortices, from the premotor to the associational somatosensory, auditory, and visual areas. This virtually ubiquitous presence of 40-Hz oscillations over the neocortex then makes probable that the significance of such fast rhythms transcends the function of associative mechanisms between columns in particular sensory receiving areas.

Acknowledgments. This work was supported by the Medical Research Council of Canada (grant MT-3689). RCD is a postdoctoral fellow, on leave of absence from the University of Padova (Italy).

References

Asanuma C (1989): Axonal arborizations of a magnocellular basal nucleus input, and their relations to the neurons in the reticular thalamic nucleus of rats. *Proc Natl Acad Sci USA* 86:4746–4750

Asanuma C, Porter LL (1990): Light and electron microscopic evidence for a GABAergic projection from the caudal basal forebrain to the thalamic reticular nucleus in rats. *J Comp Neurol* 302:159–172

Bouyer JJ, Montaron MF, Vahnée JM, Albert MP, Rougeul A (1987): Anatomical localization of cortical beta rhythms in cat. *Neuroscience* 22:863–869

Bremer F, Stoupel N, Van Reeth PC (1960): Nouvelles recherches sur la facilitation et l'inhibition des potentiels évoqués corticaux dans l'éveil réticulaire. *Arch Ital Biol* 98:229–247

Buzsáki G, Bickford RG, Armstrong RM, Ponomareff G, Chen KS, Ruiz R, Thal LJ, Gage FH (1988a): Electrical activity in the neocortex of freely moving young and aged rats. *Neuroscience* 26:735–744

Buzsáki G, Bickford RG, Ponomareff G, Thal, LJ, Mandel R, Gage FH (1988b): Nucleus basalis and thalamic control of neocortical activity in the freely moving rat. *J Neurosci* 8:4007–4026

Connors B, Gutnick MJ, Prince DA (1982): Electrophysiological properties of neocortical neurons in vitro. *J Neurophysiol* 48:1302–1320

Curró Dossi R, Nuñez A, Steriade M (1992) Electrophysiology of a slow (0.5–4 Hz) oscillation of cat thalamocortical neurons *in vivo*. *J Physiol (Lond)* 447:215–234

Curró Dossi R, Paré D, Steriade M (1991): Short-lasting nicotinic and long-lasting muscarinic depolarizing responses of thalamocortical neurons to stimulation of mesopontine cholinergic nuclei. *J Neurophysiol* 65:393–406

Freeman WJ (1975): *Mass Action in the Nervous System*. New York: Academic Press

Gray CM, Engel KA, Konig P, Singer W (1990) : Stimulus-dependent neuronal oscillations in cat visual cortex: receptive field properties and feature dependence. *Eur J Neurosci* 2:607–619

Gray CM, Singer W (1989): Stimulus-specific neuronal oscillations in orientation columns of cat visual cortex. *Proc Natl Acad Sci USA* 86:1698–1702

Hu B, Steriade M, Deschênes M (1989): The effects of brainstem peribrachial stimulation on reticular thalamic neurons. *Neuroscience* 31:1–12

Jasper HH, Tessier J (1971): Acetylcholine liberation from cerebral cortex during paradoxical (REM) sleep. *Science* 172:601–602

Jones EG (1985): *The Thalamus*. New York: Plenum Press

Lindström S, Wrobel A (1990): Frequency dependent corticofugal excitation of principal cells in the cat's dorsal lateral geniculate nucleus. *Exp Brain Res* 79:313–318

Llinás RR (1990): Intrinsic electrical properties of mammalian neurons and CNS function. In: *Fidia Research Foundation Neurosciences Award Lectures*. New York: Raven Press, pp 173–192

Llinás, R, Grace, A, Yarom Y (1991): *In vitro* neurons in mammalian cortical layer 4 exhibit intrinsic oscillatory activity in the 10 to 50 Hz frequency. *Proc Natl Acad Sci USA* 88:897–901

McCormick DA, Pape HC (1988): Acetylcholine inhibits identified interneurones in the cat lateral geniculate nucleus. *Nature* 334:246–248

McCormick DA, Pape HC (1990): Properties of a hyperpolarization activated cation current, I_h, and its role in rhythmic oscillations in thalamic relay neurons. *J Physiol (Lond)* 431:291–318

McCormick DA, Prince DA (1986): Mechanisms of action of acetylcholine in the guinea pig cerebral cortex, in vitro. *J Physiol (Lond)* 375:169–194

Moruzzi G, Magoun HW (1949): Brain stem reticular stimulation and activation of the EEG. *Electroencephalogr Clin Neurophysiol* 1:455–473

Mulle C, Steriade M, Deschênes M (1985): Absence of spindle oscillations in the cat anterior thalamic nuclei. *Brain Res* 334:169–171

Paré D, Smith Y, Parent A, Steriade M (1988): Projections of brainstem core cholinergic and non-cholinergic neurons of cat to intralaminar and reticular thalamic nuclei. *Neuroscience* 25:69–86

Paré D, Steriade M, Deschênes M, Oakson G (1987): Physiological properties of anterior thalamic nuclei, a group devoid of inputs from the reticular thalamic nucleus. *J Neurophysiol* 57:1669–1685

Parent A, Paré D, Smith Y, Steriade M (1988): Basal forebrain cholinergic and noncholinergic projections to the thalamus and brainstem in cats and monkeys. *J Comp Neurol* 277:281–301

Rougeul-Buser A, Bouyer JJ, Montaron MF, Buser P (1983): Patterns of activities in the ventrobasal thalamus and somatic cortex SI during behavioral immobility in the awake cat: focal waking rhythms. *Exp Brain Res* 7 (Suppl):69–87

Schwindt PC, Spain WJ, Foehring RC, Chubb MC, Crill WE (1988a): Slow conductances in neurons from cat sensorimotor cortex in vitro and their role in slow excitability changes. *J Neurophysiol* 59:450–467

Schwindt PC, Spain WJ, Foehring RC, Stafstrom CE, Chubb MC, Crill WE (1988b): Multiple potassium conductances and their functions in neurons from cat sensorimotor cortex in vitro. *J Neurophysiol* 59:424–449

Sheer D (1984): Focused arousal, 40 Hz EEG, and dysfunction. In: *Selfregulation of the Brain and Behavior*, Ebert T, ed. Berlin: Springer–Verlag, pp 64–84

Singer W (1990): Role of acetylcholine in use-dependent plasticity of the visual cortex. In: *Brain Cholinergic Systems*, Steriade M, Biesold D, eds. Oxford: Oxford University Press, pp 314–336

Steriade M (1968): The flash-evoked afterdischarge. *Brain Res* 9:169–212

Steriade M (1984): The excitatory-inhibitory response sequence in thalamic and neocortical cells: state-related changes and regulatory system. In: *Dynamic Aspects of Neocortical Function*, Edelman GM, Gall WE, Cowan WM, eds. New York: Wiley-Interscience, pp 105–157

Steriade M, Apostol V, Oakson G (1971): Control of unitary activities in cerebellothalamic pathways during wakefulness and synchronized sleep. *J Neurophysiol* 34: 384–413

Steriade M, Belekhova M, Apostol V (1968): Reticular potentiation of cortical flash-evoked afterdischarge. *Brain Res* 11:276–280

Steriade M, Buzsaki G (1990): Parallel activation of thalamic and cortical neurons by brainstem and basal forebrain cholinergic systems. In: *Brain Cholinergic Systems*, Steriade M, Biesold D, eds. Oxford: Oxford University Press, pp 3–62

Steriade M, Curró Dossi R, Nuñez A (1991a): Network modulation of a slow intrinsic oscillation of cat thalamocortical neurons implicated in sleep delta waves: cortically induced synchronization and brainstem cholinergic suppression. *J. Neurosci* 11:3200–3217

Steriade M, Curro Dossi R, Paré D, Oakson G (1991b): Potentiation of 40 Hz activities in thalamocortical systems by stimulating mesopontine cholinergic nuclei. *Proc Natl Acad Sci USA* 88:4396–4400

Steriade M, Datta S, Paré D, Oakson G, Curro Dossi R (1990a): Neuronal activities in brain-stem cholinergic nuclei related to tonic activation processes in thalamocortical systems. *J Neurosci* 10:2527–2545

Steriade M, Deschênes M (1988): Intrathalamic and brainstem-thalamic networks involved in resting and alert states. In: *Cellular Thalamic Mechanisms*, Bentivoglio M, Spreafico R, eds. Amsterdam: Elsevier, pp 37–62

Steriade M, Deschênes M, Domich L, Mulle C (1985): Abolition of spindle oscillations in thalamic neurons disconnected from nucleus reticularis thalami. *J Neurophysiol* 54:1473–1497

Steriade M, Domich L, Oakson G, Deschênes M (1987a): The deafferented reticular thalamic nucleus generates spindle rhythmicity. *J Neurophysiol* 57:260–273

Steriade M, Gloor P, Llinás RR, Lopes da Silva FH, Mesulam MM (1990b): Basic mechanisms of cerebral rhythmic activities. *Electroencephalogr Clin Neurophysiol* 76:481–508

Steriade M, Jones EG, Llinás RR (1990c): *Thalamic Oscillations and Signaling.* New York: Wiley-Interscience

Steriade M, Llinás RR (1988): The functional states of the thalamus and the associated neuronal interplay. *Physiol Rev* 68:649–742

Steriade M, Parent A, Hada J (1984): Thalamic projections of nucleus reticularis thalami of cat: a study using retrograde transport of horseradish peroxidase and double fluorescent tracers. *J Comp Neurol* 229:531–547

Steriade M, Parent A, Paré D, Smith Y (1987b): Cholinergic and non-cholinergic neurons of cat basal forebrain project to reticular and mediodorsal thalamic nuclei. *Brain Res* 408:372–376

Velayos JL, Jiménez-Castellanos J, Reinoso-Suarez F (1989): Topographical organization of the projections from the reticular thalamic nucleus to the intralaminar and medial thalamic nuclei in the cat. *J Comp Neurol* 279:457–469

Oscillations in CNS Neurons: A Possible Role for Cortical Interneurons in the Generation of 40-Hz Oscillations

Rodolfo R. Llinás

Despite unprecedented success, modern neuroscience continues to face many cardinal issues in relation to the overall nature of brain function. Among such quandaries, that of the essentially intrinsic or extrinsic organization of nervous system activity must be considered fundamental. A general approach to this problem was proposed by Immanuel Kant (1781) in relation to cognition, which he deemed to be an innate or "a prioristic" property. The opposite approach was taken by William James (1890), who viewed cognition as extrinsic in nature.

From this perspective, Sherrington (1906) enlarged the Jamesian concept to encompass the function of the nervous system, which he considered to be fundamentally reflexive, whereas the opposite view, that of a self-referential brain organization, was taken by Graham Brown (1911).

In modern terms this question may ultimately concern the relative significance of the intrinsic or autorhythmic behavior displayed by neurons compared to the significance of activity evoked by extero- or interoceptive stimuli. This issue has remained moot for lack of experimental evidence for the existence of significant autorhythmic activity, especially in mammalian neurons. Recently, however, electrophysiological findings have provided ample evidence of autorhythmic behavior with which central neurons can generate oscillatory changes in their membrane potential. These membrane potential oscillations promote neuronal firing, gate synaptic input, or do both when either constructive or destructive resonance occurs between intrinsic and incoming activity (cf. Llinás, 1988).

With the above in mind, I will take a cellular approach to the issues raised in this book; that is, the 40-Hz activation in the cerebral cortex (Gray et al., 1989) and its possible importance in global brain function. Indeed, recent experimental evidence indicates that cortical interneurons can generate autorhythmic activity at close to 40 Hz. We have proposed, therefore, that this intrinsic property may contribute significantly to the cortical 40-Hz activity (Llinás and Grace, 1989; Llinás et al., 1991; Walton et al., 1990). Before addressing that issue, the question of autorhythmicity in mammalian central neurons will be briefly reviewed.

Oscillations in Mammalian Central Nervous System (CNS) Neurons

Over the last decade, the study of the electrical activity of mammalian neurons *in vitro* has provided a wealth of information regarding the voltage-, ligand-, and second messenger-dependent ionic mechanisms underlying membrane oscillations (Grillner, 1986; Llinás, 1988). Because of the simplified nature of brain slices and other "reduced" *in vitro* preparations, these studies have yielded only a partial picture of the oscillatory properties of neuronal ensembles. Nevertheless, these studies have provided a first step toward understanding rhythmic network activity *in vivo* (cf. Steriade et al., 1990a, 1990b).

Inferior olivary neurons: threshold and subthreshold oscillations

In vitro experiments have demonstrated that mammalian inferior olivary (IO) neurons have a set of ionic conductances that promote single-cell oscillatory electrical activity (Benardo and Foster, 1986; Llinás and Yarom, 1981a, 1981b, 1986). The firing of IO cells is characterized by an initial fast-rising action potential (a somatic sodium spike), followed by a 10 to 15-ms afterdepolarization generated by a powerful calcium-dependent dendritic spike (Fig. 1A). This broad plateau is followed by the activation of a calcium-dependent potassium conductance ($g_{K(Ca)}$), which generates a long afterhyperpolarization (AHP) that shunts most synaptic input and silences the spike-generating activity.

As expected from the fact that the AHP is generated by the activation of a $g_{K(Ca)}$, the amount of calcium entering the dendrites during the afterdepolarization modulates the duration of the afterhyperpolarization. Following this AHP, the membrane potential demonstrates an active rebound as shown in the spontaneously generated spikes in Figure 1B. The rebound (Fig. 1B, arrow) is generated by the deinactivation of a somatic low-threshold calcium conductance (Llinás and Yarom, 1981a) similar to that generated by the *T* channels in other systems (Nowycky et al., 1986). Thus, if the dendritic calcium action potential is narrow, the duration of the AHP will be short, the low-threshold calcium conductance deinactivation may be incomplete, and the rebound response will have a low amplitude. This point is central to understanding the oscillatory properties of IO cells as it indicates that calcium entry determines the cycle time and the robustness of this neuronal oscillator. For example, compare the first and last spikes in Figure 1B.

In addition to spike oscillations, subthreshold membrane potential oscillations may be recorded intracellularly *in vitro* (Fig. 1C). These spontaneous oscillations are close to sinusoidal and represent an emerging property of the IO neuronal ensemble. Their frequency is independent of the electroresponsive state of any individual neuron. Indeed, direct activation of the recorded cell does not alter the oscillation frequency (Benardo and Foster, 1986; Llinás and Yarom, 1986), whereas electrical activation of the cellular ensemble alters the oscillation quite effectively.

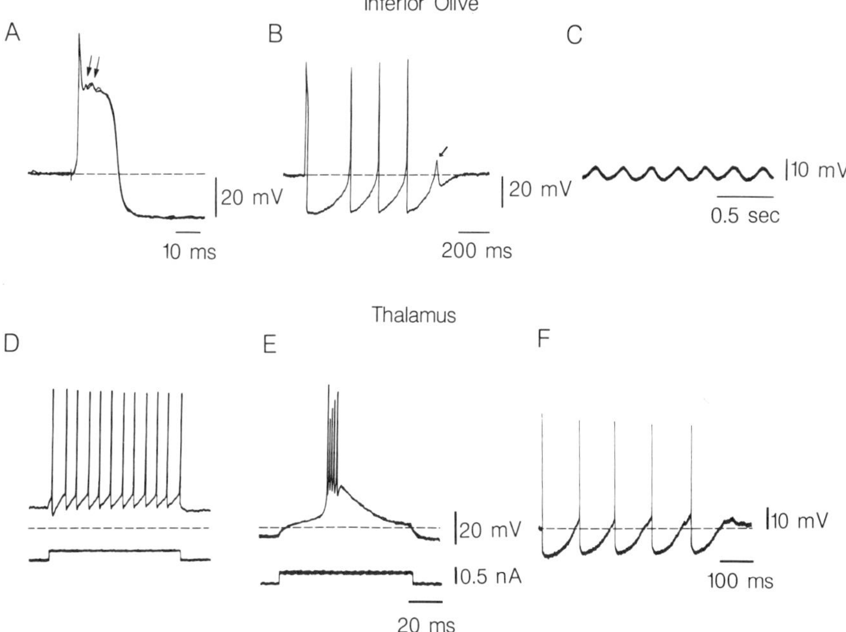

Figure 1. Oscillatory properties of CNS nuclear cells. **A–C:** Oscillatory properties of I.O. neurons recorded *in vitro.* **A:** Antidromically activated action potentials recorded intracellularly. Initial fast depolarization followed by an afterdepolarization and afterhyperpolarization can be seen. Arrows mark firing of axon. **B:** Spontaneous burst of spikes. The initial spike is followed by three action potentials and a subthreshold rebound indicated by an arrow. Note that the threshold for the rebound response is negative to the resting membrane potential. **C:** Spontaneous oscillatory potentials in inferior olivary cells. Oscillatory potentials occurring at close to resting potential, having a peak-to-peak average of approximately 8 mV and a peak-to-peak frequency of approximately 5 Hz *in vitro.* **D–F.** Oscillatory properties of thalamic cells. **D:** A depolarizing current pulse produces a train of action potentials if superimposed on a slightly depolarized membrane potential level. **E:** The cell was directly stimulated while being hyperpolarized by a constant current injection. The outward current pulse, which had the same amplitude as those in D, now triggers an all-or-none burst of spikes. **F:** Depolarization of a thalamic neuron from rest triggered self-maintained oscillation at 9 Hz. A modified from Llinás and Yarom (1981a); B & C modified from Llinás and Yarom (1986); C and D modified from Jahnsen and Llinás (1984a); E modified from Jahnsen and Llinás (1984b).

The electrical properties outlined above provide IO neurons with the ability to resonate at two distinct frequencies, one ranging from 3 to 6 Hz, the other from 9 to 12 Hz. These two frequencies reflect, respectively, the predominantly dendritic or somatic distribution of the calcium electroresponsiveness of these cells, as determined by the resting membrane potential level. In a slightly depolarized cell the firing frequency will be dominated by the calcium entering during the dendritic spike which, in turn, governs the size and duration of the AHP. At more hyperpolarized levels, however, active invasion of the dendrites is reduced and the firing frequency is dominated by the deinactivating rebound somatic calcium conductance (Llinás and Yarom, 1986).

Experiments carried out *in vivo* indicate that intrinsic properties, such as those giving rise to membrane oscillations, are essential to the organization of the timing properties of motor execution that characterizes the cerebellar control of motor coordination (Llinás and Sasaki, 1989).

Thalamic neuron oscillations: two modes of firing

In contrast to the rather stereotypical membrane oscillations of IO cells, thalamic cells may oscillate or may fire tonically. In the latter mode they resemble other CNS neurons in that their firing frequency is proportional to membrane depolarization.

Thalamic neurons can fire at high frequencies, as shown in Figure 1D, because their dendritic calcium conductance is not large, making the AHP smaller than in the IO. However, when thalamic cells are hyperpolarized as in Figure 1E, a short, phasic burst of spikes is generated. This burst is activated by a low-threshold calcium spike comparable to that in the IO (Jahnsen and Llinás, 1984b). These two types of electrical behavior allow thalamic cells to switch from a tonic to a phasic firing pattern by modulation of thc membrane potential.

In addition to the ability to fire in two distinct modes, thalamic cells fire at one of two preferred frequencies: near 6 Hz or near 10 Hz. The ionic mechanisms underlying thalamic neuron oscillatory behavior are in some aspects quite similar to those encountered in IO cells. However, in addition to having rather limited dendritic calcium-dependent excitability, thalamic cells display an early potassium conductance (*A* current) similar to that described in invertebrate neurons (Connor and Stevens, 1971; Hagiwara et al., 1961). This particular conductance allows oscillatory single cell responses near 6 Hz at negative membrane potentials. When depolarized, the activation of a persistent sodium conductance, similar to that seen in Purkinje cells (Llinás and Sugimori, 1980), dominates neuronal excitability and triggers fast sodium-dependent spikes at close to 10 Hz (Fig. 1F).

The point of interest here is that the switching of firing modes in thalamic neurons can trigger macroscopic changes in functional states as dramatic as the difference between somnolence and arousal (Llinás and Pare, 1991).

The entorhinal stellate cells of layer II: subthreshold oscillations and theta rhythmicity

The layer II stellate cells in the entorhinal cortex (ECIIsc) are the origin of the perforant path (Ramon y Cajal, 1904) and their activation is essential to the generation of the theta rhythm (Alonso and Llinás, 1989). These cells are characterized by intrinsic subthreshold oscillations; however, in contrast to oscillations in the IO and thalamus, ECIIsc oscillations are generated by the sequential activation of voltage-dependent sodium and potassium conductances rather than calcium and potassium conductances. Increasing membrane depolarization generates maintained sinusoidal-like subthreshold oscillations whose frequency is independent of the membrane potential level (Alonso and Llinás, 1989). These oscillations have a dominant frequency between 5 and 12 Hz, close to the 4- to 12-Hz theta frequencies (Bland, 1986). The oscillations in Figure 2B have a dominant frequency of 8 Hz as determined from the autocorrelogram (inset). These rhythmic activations were eliminated by superfusion with 1 μM TTX (Fig. 2B, bottom trace) (Alonso and Llinás, 1989). In another cell the dominant frequency was 10 Hz (Fig. 2C) and blocking the calcium channels by addition of $Cd2^{2+}$ to the superfusate did not eliminate the oscillations (Fig. 2C), but did reduce their dominant frequency from 10 to 8 Hz (Fig. 2C, inset) (Alonso and Llinás, 1989).

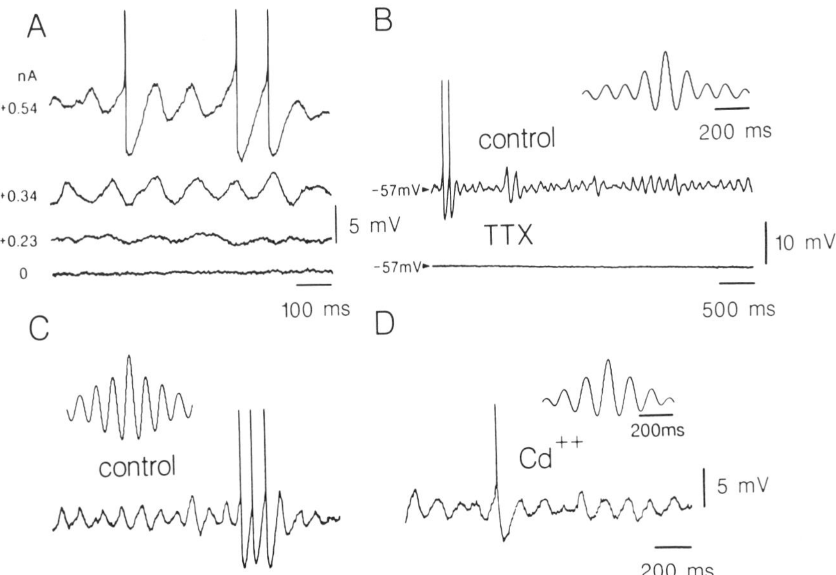

Figure 2. Electrophysiological properties of EC layer II stellate cells. **A:** Subthreshold voltage oscillations for three levels of constant current injection. The oscillatory activity became most apparent with current injection of +0.34 nA (mean membrane potential, −57 mV). **B:** The autocorrelogram illustrates the rhythmic character of the voltage oscillation at a dominant frequency of 8 Hz. Note that this oscillatory activity was abolished by bath application of TTX (1 μM). **C:** In another cell the dominant oscillatory frequency was 10 Hz. **D:** The amplitude of the subthreshold oscillations were insensitive to superfusion with Cd^{2+}, but the dominant frequency was reduced to 8 Hz. Modified from Alonso and Llinás (1989).

Neocortical interneurons: two types of subthreshold oscillations

Subthreshold membrane potential oscillations have been recorded from layer IV neocortical interneurons *in vitro* (Llinás and Grace, 1989; Llinás et al., 1991; Walton et al., 1990). Oscillations were present at the resting membrane potential in about half of the neurons recorded and were elicited by depolarization in the other cells. Two types of layer IV interneurons were identified according to the characteristics of their subthreshold oscillations: broad frequency oscillators and narrow frequency oscillators (Llinás et al., 1991).

Broad frequency oscillators. In these cells injection of low-amplitude current pulses elicited a burst of action potentials followed by irregular single-spike firing (Fig. 3A). As in the ECII stellate cells, the oscillations were generated by the sequential activation of voltage-gated sodium and potassium conductances. Accordingly, soon after addition of TTX to the superfusate (Fig. 3B) the fast action potentials activation decreased in frequency and the subthreshold oscillations were completely blocked. Later, the action potentials were also blocked (Fig. 3C). The oscillatory frequency of these cells was sensitive to membrane potential levels as shown in Figure 3D, E. As the membrane was depolarized the oscillatory frequency increased (Fig. 3D). This is also shown in Figure 3E where the dominant frequency (determined from autocorrelograms) at nine membrane potential levels is plotted as a function of membrane potential level. Note that the range of oscillations is 10 to 40 Hz.

Narrow frequency oscillations. In the second type of interneuron the frequency of the subthreshold oscillations was independent of the membrane potential. Subthreshold oscillations were rarely observed at the resting membrane potential, but were invariably evoked by membrane depolarization (Fig. 3F). Single oscillatory bursts usually lasted 22 to 28 ms and had an average amplitude of 5.9 ± 2.1 mV (Llinás et al., 1991). These cells demonstrated a clear persistent sodium-dependent plateau potential upon which subthreshold oscillations were generated. The average frequency at 37°C was 44.7 ± 4.64 Hz, as determined from autocorrelograms such as that in the inset in Figure 3F. In this type of cell a depolarizing pulse delivered during the subthreshold oscillation increased the likelihood that the oscillation reached spike threshold. The spiking occurred at the peak of the oscillation potentials and, as opposed to the broad-range oscillators, the membrane depolarization did not alter their oscillatory frequency.

Intracellular staining with Lucifer yellow or horseradish peroxidase (HRP) has shown that these cells belong to the sparsely spinous group of cortical neurons (Llinás and Grace, 1989; Llinás et al., 1991) and their axonal projection fields are consistent with their classification as cortical inhibitory interneurons (Jones and Baughman, 1988).

Neuronal oscillations and synaptic plasticity

So far I have discussed five types of neurons in the CNS that show intrinsic oscillation and have briefly reviewed the ionic mechanisms responsible for

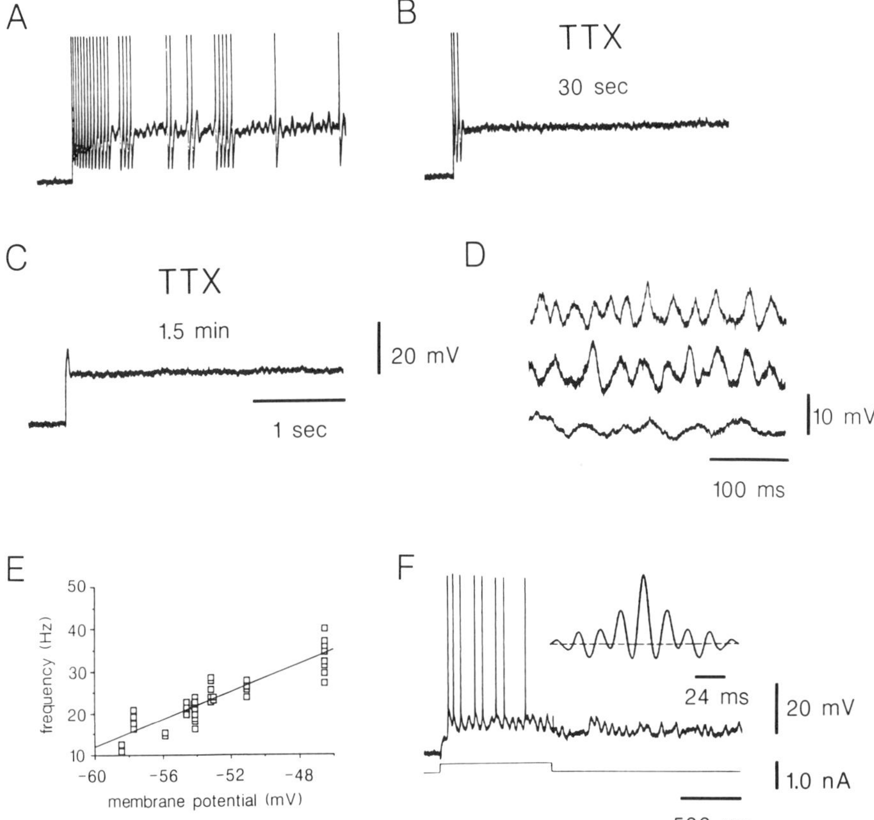

Figure 3. Oscillatory properties of layer II neurons in the entorhinal cortex. **A–E:** Properties of broad-band oscillating neurons. **A:** Firing response of the cells to a prolonged depolarizing current injection (0.6 nA). A burst of action potentials was followed by subthreshold oscillations accompanied by sporadic firing. Note the presence of large afterhyperpolarizations of approximately 10–15 mV. **B:** 30 s after bath administration of TTX. **C:** 1.5 min after administration of TTX. **D:** The relationship between membrane potential and spike generation is illustrated for three levels of depolarization. **E:** Plot of membrane potential versus the frequency of oscillation showing a range of 10–40 Hz. **F:** Narrow-band oscillating neurons. Subthreshold oscillation at approximately 42 Hz generated by a depolarizing current pulse. The autocorrelogram shows a 24-ms peak-to-peak interval. Modified from Llinás et al. (1991).

their rhythmicity. In considering the possible role of these oscillations in network function, there is the intriguing possibility that membrane potential oscillations may be important in neuronal plasticity. The ECIIsc's are of particular interest in this respect as they demonstrate long-term potentiation (LTP) that seems to be controlled in a non-Hebbian manner by subthreshold oscillation.

Non-Hebbian LTP was demonstrated in experiments where intracellular conditioning stimulation (20-s, 100-ms subthreshold depolarizing current pulses delivered at 5 Hz) was delivered (Fig. 4B). Test white matter stimuli of the same amplitude as that eliciting the control EPSPs (Fig. 4) were given at regular intervals after the intracellular postsynaptic conditioning. Intracellularly induced increases in synaptic strength, as determined by EPSP amplitude, were seen within 30 s of the intracellular stimulation (Fig. 4C). The enhanced EPSP reached firing threshold 30 s after the conditioning pulses and could be maintained for several hours (Figs. 4D, E).

Afferent stimulation as well as direct subthreshold rhythmic depolarization elicited LTP in ECIIsc (Alonso et al., 1990). Indeed, theta-pattern (Larson et al., 1986) afferent stimulation resulted in clear-cut Hebbian LTP, which was *N*-methyl-D-aspartate (NMDA)-dependent (Bliss and Lomo, 1973). Administration of DL-2-amino-5-phosphonov-alerate (APV) before extracellular or subthreshold direct stimulation prevented potentiation, indicating that the activation of NMDA receptors is necessary for the induction of both "Hebbian" and "non-Hebbian" LTP in the ECIIsc. Both types of LTP were induced and expressed by a selective increase in the NMDA-mediated component of the EPSP, suggesting that the enhancement of synaptic transmission during intracellularly induced LTP seems to be a purely postsynaptic process (Alonso et al., 1990).

The finding that LTP in the EC occurred in Hebbian as well as non-Hebbian paradigms raised the question of a role for LTP in CNS function other than memory. More specifically, the fact that rhythmic conditioning induced Hebbian and non-Hebbian LTP in a given cell and used the same mechanisms indicates that LTP may serve to enhance resonance in rhythmically firing networks. In the context of our present discussion, non-Hebbian LTP may be considered as another parameter in the generation of functional conjunction, since such potentiation should facilitate temporal linkage.

Discussion

Role of 40-Hz oscillation in CNS function

CNS neurons represent a diverse collection of elements having distinctive morphologies, connections, and physiological properties. As reviewed above, one of the many properties that may differ among neurons is their ability to oscillate at particular frequencies and to serve as pacemakers. Relevant to this book is the finding of rhythmic oscillatory potentials within a given cortical column in the visual cortex (Gray et al., 1989). These oscillations are well correlated with single unit activity within the column and are believed to serve as an associative mechanism in the temporal domain via synchronized oscillatory rhythmicity (Gray et al., 1989). This temporal association, or "binding," has been demonstrated using cross correlation between columns (Gray et al., 1989, 1990).

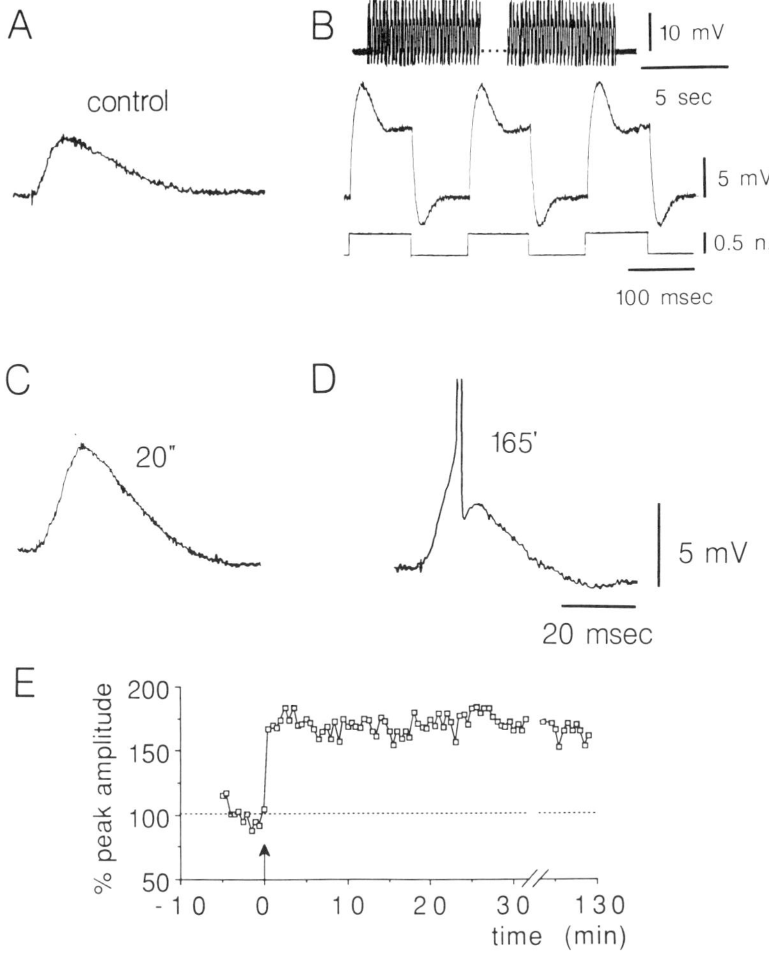

Figure 4. Time course of LTP of EPSPs induced by postsynaptic subthreshold rhythmic membrane depolarizations. **A:** Control EPSP. **B:** The characteristics of the postsynaptic stimulation. Note the powerful delayed rectification in the upper trace was broken to illustrate the beginning and end of the 30-s stimulus train. **C**, **D:** These EPSPs were recorded at the times indicated after rhythmic depolarization of the cell as shown in B. **E:** Normalized peak EPSP amplitudes during the potentiation as a function of time. Arrow indicates time of postsynaptic stimulation. Modified from Alonso et al. (1990).

However, the neuronal source of this high frequency oscillation has not been resolved. Recently it was proposed that the thalamus serves a linking function allowing conjunction by coherent resonance between different cortical regions (Llinás, 1990). This view has been strengthened by the finding that thalamic projection neurons fire at 30 to 40 Hz following activation of brainstem cholinergic inputs (Steriade, personal communication).

Our findings indicate that at least two classes of cortical interneurons are capable of subthreshold oscillatory rhythms at frequencies similar to those found in the "activated" cortical column (Gray, 1989). Of these, the broad frequency oscillators increase their frequency with membrane depolarization. This tendency may allow "coherent resonance" to occur, which may facilitate phase-locking of the oscillations in these neurons, depending on the excitatory synaptic activity in layer IV.

The findings described above suggests that these inhibitory interneurons may play a role in cortical associative processing as outlined previously (Llinás, 1990). According to that hypothesis (Fig. 5): 1) The thalamus would activate in addition to the well known excitatory input to all cortical layers (Colonnier, 1967), layer IV inhibitory interneurons that, when sufficiently depolarized, would oscillate at close to 40 Hz (Fig. 5, #1). This 40-Hz oscillation would occur when "the adequate physiological stimulus" is presented, as the magnitude of synaptic input to a particular cortical column is largest under such conditions (Gray and Singer, 1989); 2) The inhibitory interneurons would elicit IPSPs in other cortical neurons, including the pyramidal cells of layer VI (Fig. 5, #2) superimposed on the specific excitatory activity generated in the cortex by the incoming thalamic activity; 3) The rhythmic inhibition of pyramidal cell activity would be generated by these IPSPs at 40 Hz (or a harmonic frequency), producing the rhythmicity observed in the visual cortex (Gray et al., 1989). In fact, Ferster's study has clearly demonstrated 40-Hz IPSPs in visual cortex pyramidal cells during physiological stimulation of the visual system (Ferster, 1988).

An intriguing functional possibility is that this cortical oscillation may transmit 40-Hz excitation to both the nucleus reticularis thalami (NRT) (Fig. 5, #3), the intrinsic inhibitory neurons of the thalamus, and the projection thalamic neurons (Fig. 5, #4) (Llinás, 1990). This input would then establish a resonance state in the thalamocortical system via feedback through the layer IV interneurons (Fig. 5 box). The combination of intrinsic oscillations and resonance in the cortico-thalamocortical circuit may then constitute the basis for the 40-Hz rhythm recorded at the cortex (Llinás, 1990). Although Gray et al. (1989) have not observed 40-Hz oscillation in the thalamus, Bouyer et al. (1987) have demonstrated such activity at thalamic sites.

This rhythmic 40-Hz firing of pyramidal neurons would lead to synchronization across the cortical columns to which the active pyramidal cells projects, and downward (via layer VI pyramidal cells) to the thalamus. This descending 40-Hz rhythmic volley, by activating thalamic projection neurons and the thalamic reticularis neurons, which themselves may have intrinsic

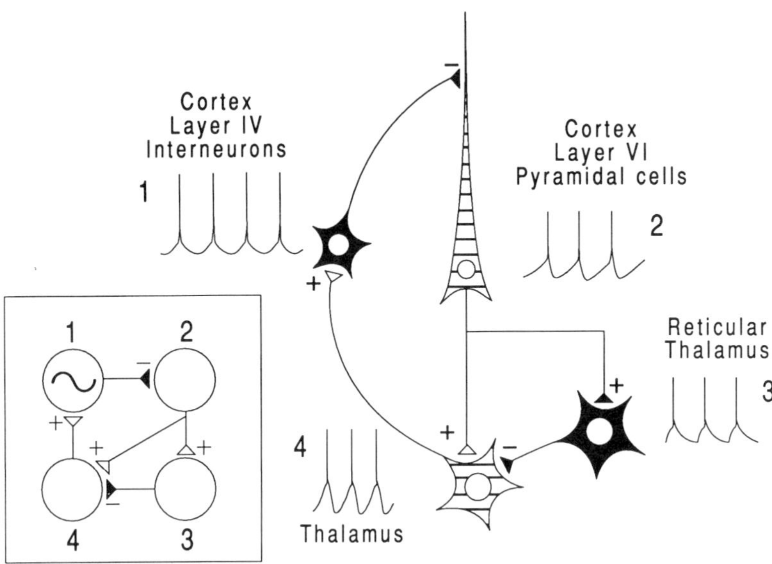

Figure 5. Diagram of a hypothetical cortico-thalamocortical circuit capable of oscillating at 40 Hz. The thalamus would activate the layer IV interneurons which oscillate intrinsically near 40 Hz (#1), are inhibitory on cortical pyramidal cells (#2), and modulate their background activity at 40 Hz. Pyramidal cells elicit synchronous monosynaptic EPSPs in nucleus reticularis (#3) and projection (#4) thalamic neurons. The reticularis neurons produce a disynaptic IPSP on the projection neurons; thus, these cells receive an EPSP–IPSP sequence at -Hz (see text). The diagram in the box delineates the circuit showing the cortical interneuron as the principal oscillator and the other neurons as resonance elements in the circuit. Intrinsic oscillation at 40 Hz may also be present in the reticularis and projection thalamic neurons.

oscillatory properties in the 40-Hz range, would result, by resonance, in the generation of a 40-Hz EPSP–IPSP sequence in the thalamus (Fig. 5, #4). It must be emphasized that in awake animals reticularis neurons generate continuous trains of spikes (Steriade et al., 1986). In agreement with these findings, oscillations due to the activation of rebound calcium spike were never seen in activated (depolarized) reticularis thalamic neurons *in vitro* (Llinás and Geijo-Barrientos, 1989), as the low-threshold conductance is inactivated at such membrane potentials.

From a functional viewpoint, rapid firing in the reticularis neurons can generate short-lasting inhibitory synaptic potentials (in the 40-Hz range) in thalamic projection neurons. Slower IPSPs are more likely to generate the spike bursts produced by rebound calicum responses. In fact, when in the activated state, thalamic projection neurons do respond with rebound oscillations in the range of 40-Hz following short IPSP-like current injection *in vitro* (Yarom and Llinás, 1990). However, this 40-Hz oscillation is not subserved by the low threshold calcium conductance responsible for the slower oscillation. This finding indicates that the electrophysiological properties necessary to support 40-Hz resonance are present in thalamic cells.

According to this view, the 40-Hz activation, having been initiated in the cortex and reorganized in the thalamus under the modulation of the brain stem, would then reenter the cortex, completing a cortico-thalamocortical resonant loop. Two events are then assumed to take place in the thalamocortical system: 1) specific activation of the cortex, relating to the nature of the sensory signal transmitted via the thalamus, and 2) an oscillatory event allowing coherence between cortical areas responding to an "adequate peripheral stimulus" at the thalamic level as the 40-Hz activity returns to the thalamus. However, since the oscillatory states range in frequency (Gray et al., 1989), it is possible that several resonant conditions may be simultaneously supported by the thalamocortical loop, allowing several coherent patterns to coexist as separate vectors. In principle, such a conjunctive functional state could serve to bind the diverse components that constitute a given sensory input into the cognitive experiences that underlie our view of the external world.

In short then, I am quite definitely of the view that the organization of the CNS is fundamentally intrinsic. From this perspective brain activity is essentially determined by the functional scaffolding required for generating an internal image consistent with external reality. Such scaffolding, which implements the coordinate transformations that characterize brain activity, seems to be inscribed by the intrinsic properties of its neurons and their connectivity.

Summary

The intrinsic electrical properties of several types of mammalian central neurons are described in relation to circuit oscillations. The ionic mechanisms responsible for such neuronal oscillations are delineated for the inferior olive, the thalamus, the entorhinal cortex, and neocortical interneurons. Two major ionic mechanisms are involved 1) a calcium-dependent depolarization–calcium-dependent potassium hyperpolarization sequence that is responsible for oscillations at low frequencies, and 2) a persistent sodium-dependent depolarization–calcium-dependent potassium hyperpolarization sequence that generates oscillations in the 7- to 10-Hz range as observed in the entorhinal cortex and the 40-Hz rhythm of the neocortical sensory areas.

The proposal is made that neuronal oscillations serve as elements 1) in a timing or pacemaker circuit, or 2) by allowing synchronization of neuronal activity leading to coherence. This last possibility is considered in relation to the issue of temporal conjunction in relation to the 40-Hz cortical rhythmicity. It is proposed that such 40-Hz cortical oscillation is a thalamo-cortico thalamic property in which inhibitory interneurons in layer IV of the cortex may serve as an important entrainment mechanism for this oscillation.

Acknowledgments. This research was supported by Grants from the National Institutes of Neurological Disorders and Stroke NINCDS 13742.

References

Alonso A, deCurtis M, and Llinás, R (1990): Postsynaptic Hebbian and Non-Hebbian Long-term Potentiation of Synaptic Efficacy in the Entorhinal Cortex in slices and in the Isolated adult Guinea-Pig brain. *PNAS* 87:9280–9284.

Alonso A, Llinás, R (1989): Subthreshold Na-dependent theta-like rhythmicity in stellate cells of entorhinal cortex layer II. *Nature* (*Lond*) 342:175–177

Benardo LS, Foster RE (1986): Oscillatory behavior in inferior olive neurons: mechanism, modulation, cell aggregates. *Brain Res Bull* 17:773–784

Bland BH (1986): The physiology and pharmacology of hippocampal formation theta rhythms. *Prog Neurobiol* 26:1–54

Bliss TV, and Lomo T (1973): Long-lasting potentiation of synaptic transmission in the dentate area of the anaesthetized rabbit following stimulation of the perforant path. *J Physiol* (*Lond*) 232:331–356

Bouyer JJ, Montaron F, Vahneed JM, Albert MP, Rougeul A (1987): Anatomical localization of cortical beta rhythms in cat. *Neuroscience* 22:863–869

Brown GT (1911): The intrinsic factors in the act of progression in the mammal. *Proc R Soc B* 84:308–319

Colonnier M (1967): The fine structural arrangement of the cortex. *Arch Neurol* 16: 651–657

Connor JA, Stevens CF (1971): Voltage clamp studies of a transient outward membrane current in gastropod neural somata. *J Physiol* 213:21–30

Ferster D (1988): Spatially opponent excitation and inhibition in simple cells of the cat visual cortex. *J Neurosci* 8:1172–1180

Gray CM, Engel AK, Konig P, Singer W (1990): Stimulus-dependent neuronal oscillations in cat visual cortex: receptive field properties and feature dependence. *Eur J Neurosci* 2:607–619

Gray CM, Konig P, Engel AK, Singer W (1989): Oscillatory responses in cat visual cortex exhibit inter-columnar synchronization which reflects global stimulus properties. *Nature* 338:334–337

Gray CM, Singer W (1989): Stimulus-specific neuronal oscillations in orientation columns of cat visual cortex. *Proc Natl Acad Sci* 86:1698–1702

Grillner S (1985): Motor acts in vertebrates. *Science* 228:143–149

Hagiwara S, Kusano K, Saito N (1961): Membrane changes of *Onchidium* nerve cell in potassium-rich media. *J Physiol* 155:470–489

Jahnsen H, Llinás, R (1984a): Electrophysiological properties of guinea-pig thalamic neurones: an in vitro study. *J Physiol* (*Lond*) 349:205–226

Jahnsen H, Llinás R (1984b): Ionic basis for the electro responsiveness and oscillatory properties of guinea-pig thalamic neurons in-vitro. *J Physiol* (*Lond*) 349:227–248

James W (1890): *Principles of Psychology*. New York: Repro. Dover, 1950 ed

Jones KA, Baughman RW (1988): NMDA- and non-NMDA-receptor components of excitatory synaptic potentials recorded from cells in layer V of rat visual cortex. *J Neurosci* 8:3522–3534

Kant E (1781): *Critique of Pure Reason*. Garden City: Doubleday & Company, Inc., 1966 ed

Larson J, Wong D, Lynch G (1986): Induction of synaptic potentiation in hippocampus by patterned stimulation involves two events. *Science* 232:985–988

Llinás R (1988): The intrinsic electrophysiological properties of mammalian neurons: insights into central nervous system function. *Science* 242:1654–1664

Llinás R (1990): Intrinsic electrical properties of mammalian neurons and CNS function. In: *Fidia Research Foundation Neuroscience Award Lectures*. New York: Raven Press

Llinás R, Geijo-Barrientos E (1989): In vitro studies of mammalian thalamic and reticularic thalamic neurons. In: *Cellular Thalamic Mechanisms*, Bentivoglio M, Spreafico R, eds. Amsterdam: Elsevier

Llinás R, Grace AA (1989): Intrinsic 40 Hz oscillatory properties of layer IV neurons in guinea pig cerebral cortex in vitro. *Soc Neurosci Abst* 15:660

Llinás R, Pare D. Of Dreaming and Wakefulness. *Neuroscience* 44:3 521–535, 1991.

Llinás RR, Grace AA, Yarom Y (1991): *In vitro* neurons in mammalian cortical layer 4 exhibit intrinsic oscillatory activity in the 10- to 50-Hz frequency range. *PNAS* 88:897–901

Llinás R, Sasaki K (1989): The functional organization of the olivo-cerebellar system as examined by multiple Purkinje cell recordings. *European J Neuroscience* 1:587–602

Llinás R, Sugimori M (1980): Electrophysiological properties of in vitro Purkinje cell somata in mammalian cerebellar slices. *J Physiol* (*Lond*) 305:171–195

Llinás R, Yarom Y (1981a): Electrophysiology of mammalian inferior olivary neurones in vitro. Different types of voltage-dependent ionic conductances. *J Physiol* (*Lond*) 315:549–567

Llinás R, Yarom Y (1981b): Properties and distribution of ionic conductances generating electroresponsiveness of mammalian inferior olivary neurones *in vitro*. *J Physiol* (*Lond*) 315:569–584

Llinás R, Yarom Y (1986): Oscillatory properties of guinea-pig inferior olivary neurons and their pharmacological modulation: an in vitro study. *J Physiol* (*Lond*) 376:163–182

Nowycky MC, Fox AP, Tsien RW (1985): Three types of neuronal calcium channel with different calcium agonist sensitivity. *Nature* 316:440–443

Ramon y Cajal S (1904): *Histologie du Systeme Nerveux de l'Homme et des Vertebrés*. Madrid: Instituto Ramon y Cajal

Sherrington C (1906): *The Integrative Action of the Nervous System*. New Haven: Yale University Press

Steriade M, Domich L, Oakson G (1986): Reticularis thalamic neurons revisited: activity changes during shifts in states of vigilance. *J Neurosci* 6:68–81

Steriade M, Gloor P, Llinás RR, Lopes da Silva F, Mesulam MM (1990a): Basic

Mechanisms of Cerebral Rhythmic Activities. *Electroencephalogr Clin Neurophysiol* 76:481–508

Steriade M, Jones EG, Llinás RR (1990b): *Thalamic Oscillations and Signalling.* New York: John Wiley & Sons

Walton KD, Yarom Y, Llinás R (1990): Intrinsic subthreshold 10–50 Hz membrane oscillations in interneurons in the fourth layer of the frontal cortex. *Neurosci Soc Abst* 16:1134

Yarom Y, Llinás R (1990): Intracellular autostimulation of *in vitro* guinea-pig thalamic neurons (TH) utilizing a hardware bio-electric re-entry system. *Soc Neurosci Abst* 16:955

Cellular and Subcellular Mechanisms Based on Invertebrate and Simple Systems

Modification of Oscillator Function by Electrical Coupling to Nonoscillatory Neurons

Eve Marder, L.F. Abbott, Thomas B. Kepler, Scott L. Hooper

Neurons with intrinsic oscillatory properties are known to be present in all nervous systems studied to date. Indeed, it is now clear that many neurons not only fire rapid action potentials, either spontaneously or in response to synaptic inputs or sensory stimuli, but also display slowly varying voltage- and time-dependent conductances that allow them to burst rhythmically or to generate slow plateau potentials (Llinás, 1988; Jacklet, 1989). Induced rhythms have been defined in this volume (see introductory chapter) as oscillations that are triggered or altered by an external influence that itself is not necessarily oscillatory. Despite our growing realization that oscillatory processes and slowly activating and/or inactivating voltage-dependent processes are likely to play critical roles in the generation of rhythmic motor activity, as well as in higher order sensory processes, remarkably little is known about the ways in which networks that contain oscillatory elements function. Likewise, little is understood concerning how network interactions modulate the properties of their oscillatory elements. In this chapter we review some recent experimental studies in the stomatogastric nervous system of crustaceans as well as some theoretical studies motivated by these experimental findings that shed light on how neurons that are electrically coupled to oscillatory neurons can shape the frequency and waveform of the oscillations.

The Pyloric Network Pacemaker Neurons

Central to the activity of the pyloric network of the stomatogastric ganglion (STG) are three electrically coupled neurons. These are the single anterior burster (AB) neuron, and the two pyloric dilator (PD) neurons. Figure 1A shows simultaneous intracellular recordings from an AB and a PD neuron, and illustrates that these neurons synchronously depolarize and fire bursts of action potentials and then hyperpolarize and become silent during interburst intervals. It has long been appreciated that these neurons provide a critical pacemaking function for the pyloric rhythm (Maynard, 1972; Maynard and Selverston, 1975). Interestingly, it is now clear that the AB and PD neurons differ greatly in many important respects (Marder, 1984; Marder and Eisen, 1984a, 1984b). This chapter describes the separate roles that the membrane properties of the AB and PD neurons play in the control of the frequency and burst durations of the neurons of this small pacemaker network.

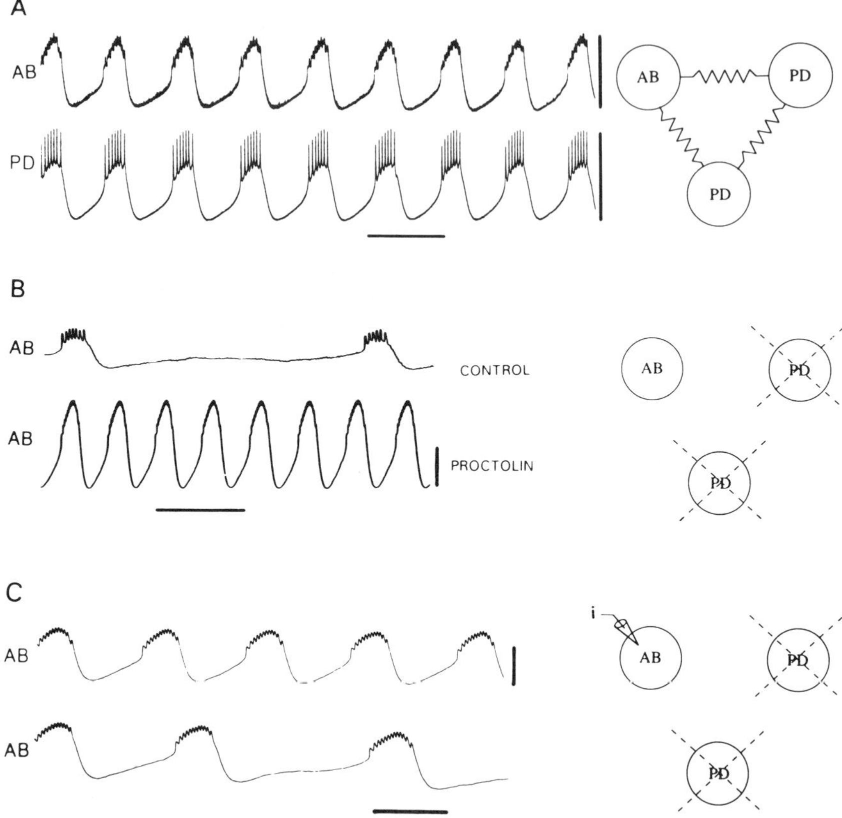

Figure 1. A: The AB cell and PD neurons are electrically coupled. Simultaneous intracellular recordings of an AB and a PD neuron. During normal network function these cells fire synchronous rhythmic bursts of action potentials. Action potentials in AB are truncated by the cable properties of the cell, and are therefore seen as attenuated ripples on the top of the slow wave. Time bar, 1 s, vertical bars, 20 mV. **B:** The peptide proctolin has a dramatic effect on the frequency of an isolated AB neuron, in this case increasing its frequency by a factor of seven. Time bar, 1 s, vertical bar, 10 mV. Modified from Hooper and Marder, 1987. **C:** The frequency of the AB can be changed by injecting current into the cell. When this is done the period is modified due to a change in the interburst interval but the burst durations remain unchanged. In this figure the upper trace shows control recordings whereas the lower trace shows a slower rhythm caused by the injection of hyperpolarizing current. Time bar, 1 s, vertical bar 15 mV. In the network schematics shown with each figure, electrical synapses are denoted by resistor symbols, and killed cells are shown with dashed crossbars.

The AB neuron is a Modulated Oscillator

The properties of the "isolated" AB have been studied by killing the PD neurons and the single ventricular dilator (VD) neuron by filling the neurons to be killed with the dye Lucifer yellow and illuminating the preparation (Miller and Selverston, 1979; Marder and Eisen, 1984; Flamm and Harris-Warrick, 1986; Hooper and Marder, 1987; Harris-Warrick and Flamm, 1987; Bal et al., 1988). The AB neuron has been termed a conditional oscillator (e.g., Bal et al., 1988), because its cycle frequency and the amplitude of its membrane potential oscillations are modulated by many substances that are released into the neuropil of the STG (Marder and Eisen, 1984a; Flamm and Harris-Warrick, 1986; Hooper and Marder, 1987; Marder and Meyrand, 1989). If all inputs to the STG are removed, the AB neuron may stop entirely (Nagy and Miller, 1987) or may burst at low frequency (<0.3 Hz) (Hooper and Marder, 1987). However, if modulatory inputs to the STG are left attached, or if any of a variety of substances is placed in the bath, the AB neuron will generate large amplitude, high frequency membrane potential oscillations and bursts of action potentials. Figure 1B shows the response of an isolated AB neuron to one of these modulatory substances, the pentapeptide proctolin (Hooper and Marder, 1987). Peptide application increases the amplitude of the slow membrane potential oscillations as well as markedly increasing their frequency. Note in this example that the frequency of the AB neuron went from about 0.3 Hz to about 2.1 Hz, and that almost all of the frequency increase was associated with a decrease in the interburst interval.

The isolated AB neuron responds to injected current in a manner characteristic of many bursting neurons, and this is shown in Figure 1C. As the AB neuron is hyperpolarized, its burst duration remains constant, and the interburst interval increases.

The PD Neurons

The two PD neurons are electrically coupled to the AB neuron and ordinarily burst synchronously with it. When the AB neuron is killed and the PD neurons are studied in isolation from the AB and other neurons of the pyloric network (Marder and Eisen, 1984a, 1984b; Flamm and Harris-Warrick, 1986; Hooper and Marder, 1987; Bal et al., 1988), it becomes clear that the PD neurons are quite different from the AB neuron. In the absence of modulatory inputs the PD neurons show no intrinsic bursting or oscillatory behavior, but fire action potentials tonically. In the presence of some modulatory substances or inputs from anterior ganglia, PD neurons isolated from the other STG neurons can show slow, irregular plateau potentials that are significantly longer in duration and period than those of the isolated AB neuron, or those of the PD neurons in the intact network during pyloric activity.

Not only do the PD neurons differ from the AB neurons in terms of their electrical activity, they also do so in their response to a number of modulatory substances. Bursting in the AB neuron is activated by serotonin, dopamine, muscarinic agonists, proctolin, and octopamine (Marder and Eisen, 1984a; Flamm and Harris-Warrick, 1986; Harris-Warrick and Flamm, 1987; Hooper and Marder, 1987; Marder and Meyrand, 1989). However, the PD neurons are inhibited by dopamine (Marder and Eisen, 1984a; Flamm and Harris-Warrick, 1986), are not responsive to proctolin (Hooper and Marder, 1987), and are only serotonin responsive under certain conditions (Johnson et al., 1990).

The PD Neurons Modify the Frequency of the AB Neuron

The PD neurons play an important role in modifying the frequency of the AB neuron, to which they are electrically coupled. This effect is seen most dramatically in the experiment reported by Hooper and Marder (1987) in which the effects of proctolin were studied on both the intact pyloric network and on each of its neurons in isolation. Proctolin application to the intact pyloric network increased the pyloric frequency to about 1 Hz, but no faster. If the network was either inactive or slowly cycling, proctolin increased the frequency of the pyloric rhythm. If the network was already rapidly active, little or no effect of proctolin on the pyloric rhythm frequency was seen. [The same result was later found when an identified proctolin-containing neuron was stimulated (Nusbaum and Marder, 1989)]. In this same study Hooper and Marder (1987) found that the isolated AB neuron in proctolin generated bursts at about 2 Hz (Fig. 1B), whereas the isolated PD neurons did not respond to proctolin. Thus, in the presence of proctolin, the frequency of the AB neuron in the network is lower than when the AB neuron is isolated. One explanation

Figure 2. Effect of electrical coupling on oscillator frequency. **A:** The pyloric cycle frequency recorded in the presence of proctolin of networks containing the neurons listed under each bar. Networks consisting of the AB, VD, and two PDs cycled at about 1 Hz, while reduced networks cycled faster. Modified from Hooper and Marder, 1987. **B:** Effect of coupling conductance on cycle frequency for a model oscillator. In the left panel the cycle of oscillator (a) is dominated by a hyperpolarized phase whereas that of oscillator (b) shown in the right panel is dominated by a depolarized phase. In both cases the oscillating cell is coupled to a passive, hyperpolarized neuron (c). Moving down the figure the strength of the electrical coupling is increased and the effect on cycle frequency can be seen. These results are summarized in the graph of period versus coupling strength, g, at the bottom of each panel. As the coupling conductance g is increased neuron (a) slows down while neuron (b) first speeds up and then slows down. This result shows that the effect of electrical coupling depends on the nature of the oscillator. Reprinted with permission from Kepler et al. (1990): The effect of electrical coupling on the frequency of model neuronal oscillators. *Science* 248:84, copyright 1990 by AAAS. ▶

for this is that the two PD neurons and the single VD neuron to which the AB neurons are electrically coupled decrease the frequency of the AB neuron. To test this idea, Hooper and Marder (1987) sequentially deleted these three neurons and measured the frequency in proctolin of the reduced networks (Fig. 2A). Note that as the network is decreased in size, the frequency of the remaining subnetworks increases.

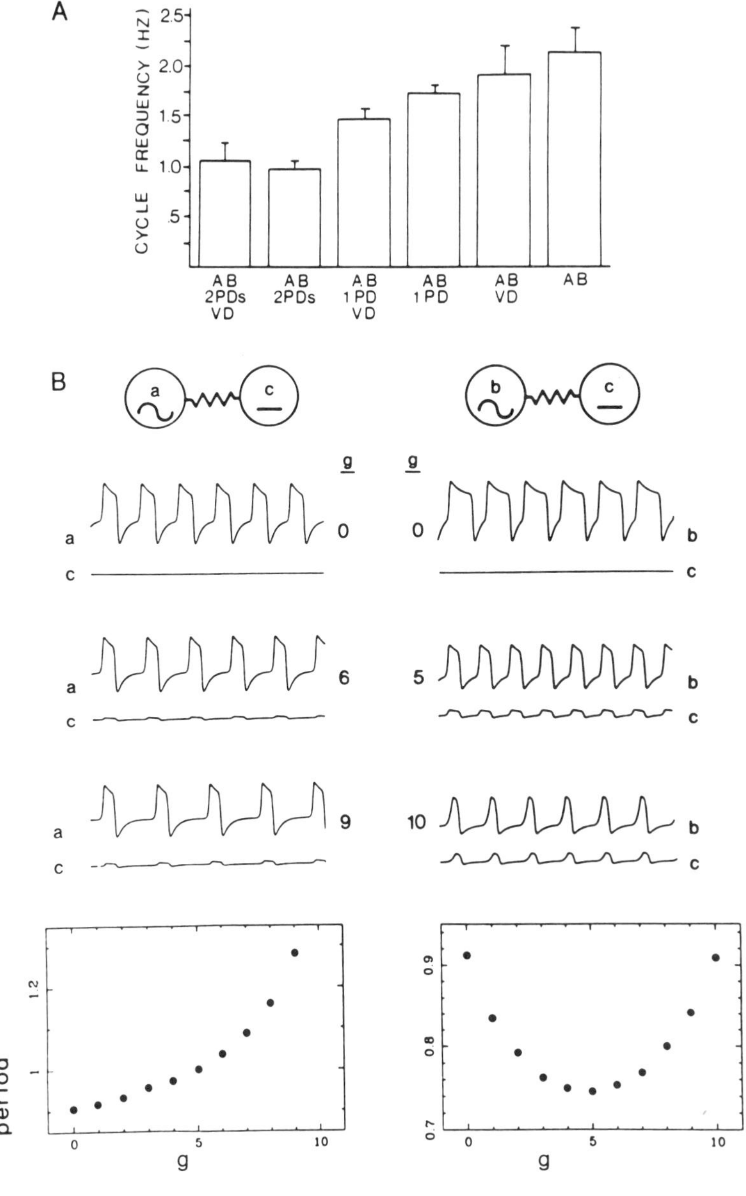

To determine the generality of the finding that electrically coupled neurons tend to slow down oscillatory neurons, we built several different mathematical models to represent the two-cell network consisting of the bursting AB neuron and the nonbursting but electrically excitable PD neuron. To our surprise we found that the effect of the nonbursting neuron depended critically on the waveform of the oscillator (Fig. 2B) (Kepler et al., 1990). Kepler et al. (1990) constructed simple oscillators using modified FitzHugh (1961) equations, and coupled these to a silent neuron. The strength of the electrical coupling between these neurons was then varied. When the oscillator had the property that the inward current phase of the burst was longer than the outward current phase, increasing the strength of the coupling to a hyperpolarized second neuron decreased the frequency of the oscillator. However, when the oscillator had an outward current phase that was longer than the inward current phase, the reverse occurred, and the oscillator increased in frequency as the coupling was increased (Fig. 2B) (Kepler et al., 1990). These effects can be understood qualitatively by noting that electrical coupling to a passive, hyperpolarized cell provides an additional outward current to the oscillating cell. This added current tends to accelerate portions of the cycle dominated by outward currents and retard those during which the current is inward. Thus, when the inward current phase of the cycle is long relative to the outward current phase, the coupled cell will slow down the oscillator. When the outward current phase is long relative to the inward current phase, the coupled cell will speed up the oscillator. Under conditions when the coupled cell is depolarized, these relations will be inverted. This qualitative picture is supported by more quantitative analyses presented in Kepler et al. (1990).

To ensure that this result was not a consequence of the form of the models used to describe these neurons, we used a more complex oscillator model constructed to mimic an AB-like oscillator (Epstein and Marder, 1990) that is based on equations describing individual membrane currents. Again, in this model, simulations showed that the waveform of the oscillator was critical to understanding the effect of the electrically coupled element on the oscillator frequency (Kepler et al., 1990).

The implications of this result for neurobiological networks are clear. Many neuromodulatory substances are known to change the duration of the plateau phase of bursts and action potentials. As either inward or outward currents important in burst generation are modulated (Jacklet, 1989; Llinás, 1988), the effect of any electrically coupled neurons on the frequency of the bursting neuron may also change.

The PD Neurons Control the Shape of the AB Neuron Burst

In addition to influencing the frequency of the AB neuron burst, PD neurons also profoundly change the character of that burst. This can be seen by comparing the effect of hyperpolarizing the AB neuron when it is isolated, to the effect of hyperpolarizing the AB neuron when it is still coupled to the PD neurons. When the isolated AB neuron is hyperpolarized (Fig. 1C) the interburst interval increases, but the burst duration is approximately constant. This is also shown in Figure 3A. However, when the same experiment is done in the network, an entirely different result is seen. Now, as the cell is hyperpolarized, the interburst interval and the burst duration both increase, so that

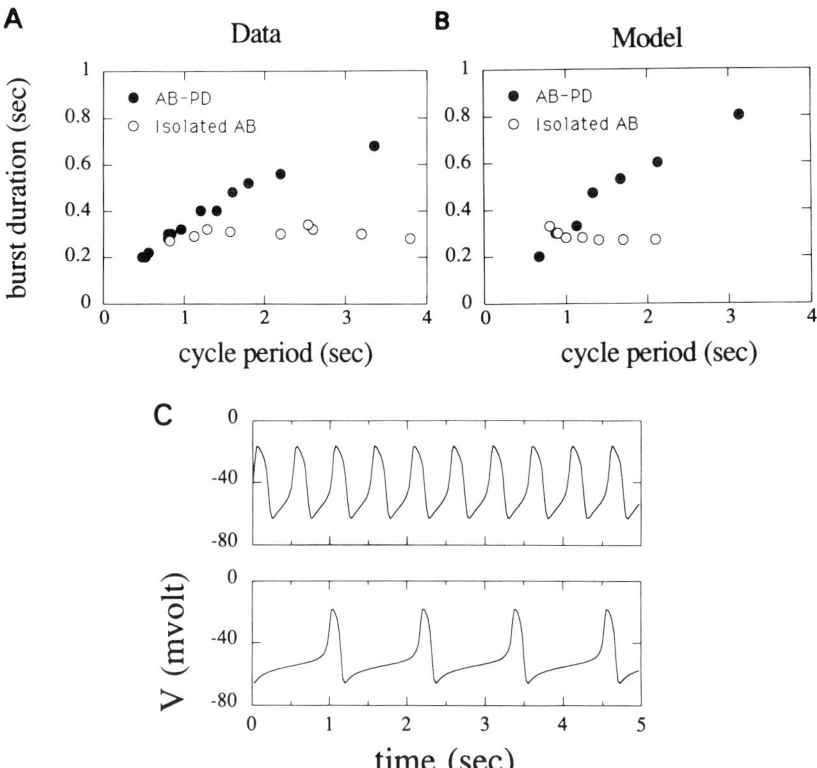

Figure 3. The PD neuron modifies the burst properties of the AB neuron. **A:** Burst duration as a function of cycle frequency for the AB/PD network and an isolated AB cell. For the isolated AB cell (*open circles*) the burst duration does not change as the period is modified by current injection. However, when the AB is coupled to the PD cells (*filled circles*) the burst duration increases approximately linearly as the period is increased. As a result the coupled system exhibits approximately constant duty cycle oscillations. Data from preparations of *Panulirus interruptus.* **B:** Burst duration versus cycle period for the model cells. The open circles show that the isolated AB produces oscillations with a fixed burst duration, whereas the filled circles show that coupling to the model PD cell produces oscillations of constant duty cycle in which the burst duration increases with the cycle period. **C:** The behavior of an isolated model AB cell. As in the real cell, the model AB burst duration does not change when the cycle period is modified by injected current.

the AB–PD network maintains an approximately constant duty cycle (Fig. 3A). Thus, the electrically coupled PD neurons have transformed the character of the AB neuron's burst. In an attempt to understand this transformation, we have written mathematical models to represent both the AB and PD neurons (Abbott et al., 1991).

The AB neuron is represented by a simple oscillator model (Abbott et al., 1991) that mimics the behavior of the isolated AB neuron (Fig. 1C). The slowly varying voltage-dependent conductances of the AB cell that are responsible for its rhythmic bursting are modeled by a single variable obeying a first-order, nonlinear, voltage-dependent equation. The model duplicates quite well the effect of injected current on both the frequency and amplitude of AB oscillations. The oscillating waveform of a model AB cell at two different frequencies is shown in Figure 3B. This simple model does not include action potentials but instead models only the "slow wave" part of the AB oscillations. Like the real AB cell, the model AB maintains a constant burst duration as its frequency is varied (compare Fig. 3C with Fig. 1C and also the open circles in Figs. 3A, B).

The model PD cell is in some respects similar to the AB model but it lacks the slow current variable that causes oscillations in the model AB. Instead the model includes a slowly varying, voltage-dependent outward current that plays a key role in regulating burst duration when the AB and PD cells are coupled to each other. This outward current is activated by depolarization. The maximal conductance of this current slowly increases when the cell is depolarized and decreases even more slowly when the cell is hyperpolarized. Under normal conditions the stable state of the isolated model PD cell is tonic depolarization. By modifying the parameters associated with the slowly varying current the model PD can be made to oscillate slowly.

When the model AB cell is electrically coupled to the model PD, the PD cell is driven by the AB into rhythmic oscillations. The PD decreases the frequency of the AB–PD bursts and prolongs their duration (compared to the isolated AB). When the AB is depolarized with injected current, the maximal conductance of the slowly varying current of the PD increases because the AB neuron's intrinsic constant burst duration causes it initially to spend most of its cycle in the depolarized state. As the slowly varying current increases over several cycles, it will truncate successive bursts more, until an equilibrium is reached. This equilibrium is attained when the ratio of the burst duration to the interburst interval matches the ratio of the rate of decrease of the maximal conductance of the slow current to its rate of increase (Abbott et al., 1991).

If however the AB neuron is hyperpolarized by current injection, its intrinsic constant burst duration causes the AB–PD complex initially to be predominantly hyperpolarized. Under these conditions, the maximal conductance of the slow current decreases. As it does so, the AB–PD bursts slowly increase in duration, until the same equilibrium condition is met. The equilibrium condition is determined by the ratio of the rates of increase and decrease of the slow current. In the example shown here (Fig. 3B) this ratio is two, resulting in a constant duty cycle of one-third.

The implications of this finding for pattern generation in the pyloric network are direct. The AB and PD neurons inhibit the remaining neurons of the pyloric network, that are thus forced to fire out of phase with the pacemaker unit. As the pacemaker ensemble maintains an approximately constant duty cycle during the full pyloric rhythm, this will facilitate generation of pyloric rhythms with approximately constant phase relationships over a substantial frequency range (Abbott et al., 1991).

Summary

We have used simple mathematical models to explore the properties of small networks consisting of bursting pacemaker neurons and nonbursting neurons that are electrically coupled to the pacemaker neuron. Our studies have focused on the ways in which electrical coupling to nonoscillatory (or slowly oscillatory) neurons modifies both the frequency and the pattern of the oscillations. This work is motivated by experimental results obtained from the STG of decapod crustaceans. The pacemaker AB neuron of the pyloric network fires at a different frequency when isolated than when it is part of the network. Model studies have shown that electrical coupling to other neurons can either increase or decrease the frequency of pacemaker, in a manner that is totally predictable given a description of the waveform of the oscillator. When isolated, the AB cell produces bursts of a duration that is independent of frequency. However, in the network the AB burst duration increases as the period is increased, resulting in a constant duty cycle (fixed ratio of burst duration to cycle period). We constructed a model pacemaker that generates constant duration bursts at various frequencies to show that a model network can generate constant duty cycle oscillations as a consequence of the electrical coupling between a fast bursting neuron and a nonbursting neuron with a slowly activating and inactivating conductance. These studies show clearly how networks containing oscillators can produce outputs quite different from the properties of the oscillators that drive them.

Acknowledgments. This work was supported by research grants from the National Institutes of Health and National Institute of Mental Health, the Department of Energy (EM and LFA), and postdoctoral fellowships (Individual and Institutional Research Service Awards) from the National Institutes of Health.

References

Abbott LF, Marder E, Hooper SL (1991): Oscillating networks: control of burst duration by electrically coupled neurons. *Neural Computation* 3:487–497

Bal T, Nagy F, Moulins M (1988): The pyloric central pattern generator in crustacea: a set of conditional neuronal oscillators. *J Comp Physiol* 163:715–727

Epstein IR, Marder E (1990): Modulation of a conditional neural oscillator: A model describing the action of multiple modulatory substances. *Bio Cyber* 63:25–34

Fitzhugh R (1961): Impulses and physiological state in theoretical models of nerve membrane. *Biophys J* 55:847–881

Flamm RE, Harris-Warrick RM (1986): Aminergic modulation in the lobster stomatogastric ganglion. II. Target neurons of dopamine, octopamine, and serotonin within the pyloric circuit. *J Neurophysiol* 55:866–881

Harris-Warrick RM, Flamm RE (1987): Multiple mechanisms of bursting in a conditional bursting neuron. *J Neurosci* 7:2113–2128

Hooper SL, Marder E (1987): Modulation of a central pattern generator by the peptide, proctolin. *J Neurosci.* 7:2097–2112

Jacklet J, ed. (1989): *Cellular and Neuronal Oscillators.* New York: Marcel Dekker, Inc

Johnson BR, Peck JH, Harris-Warrick RM (1990): Elevated temperature alters the ionic dependence of amine-induced oscillations in a conditional burster neuron. *Soc Neurosci Abst* 16:855

Kepler, TB, Marder E, Abbott LF (1990): The effect of electrical coupling on the frequency of model neuronal oscillators. *Science* 248:83–85

Llinás RR (1988): The intrinsic electrophysiological properties of mammalian neurons: insights into central nervous system function. *Science* 242:1654–1664

Marder E (1984): Roles for electrical coupling as revealed by selective neuronal deletions. *J Exp Biol* 112:147–167

Marder E, Eisen JS (1984a): Electrically coupled pacemaker neurons respond differently to the same physiological inputs and neurotransmitters. *J Neurophysiol* 51:1362–1373

Marder E, Eisen JS (1984b): Transmitter identification of pyloric neurons: electrically coupled neurons use different transmitters. *J Neurophysiol* 51:1345–1361

Marder E, Meyrand PM (1989): Chemical modulation of oscillatory neural circuits. In: Jacklet J, ed. *Cellular and Neuronal Oscillators.* New York: Marcel Dekker, Inc, pp 317–338

Maynard DM (1972): Simpler networks. *Ann NY Acad Sci* 193:59–72

Maynard DM, Selverston AI (1975): Organization of the stomatogastric ganglion of the spiny lobster. IV. The pyloric system. *J Comp Physiol* 100:161–182

Miller JP, Selverston AI (1979): Rapid killing of single neurons by irradiation of intracellularly injected dye. *Science* 206:702–704

Nagy F, Miller JP (1987): Pyloric pattern generation in *Panulims interruptus* is terminated by blockade of activity through the stomatogastric nerve. In: *The Crustacean Stomatogastric System,* Selverston AI, Moulins M, eds. Heidelberg: Springer–Verlag, pp 136–139

Nusbaum MP, Marder E (1989): A modulatory proctolin-containing neuron (MPN). II. State-dependent modulation of rhythmic motor activity. *J Neurosci* 9:1600–1607

Biological Timing: Circadian Oscillations, Cell Division, and Pulsatile Secretion

FELIX STRUMWASSER

The term "rhythms" in biology refers to a wide range of phenomena that have one feature in common, the process or variable of interest oscillates with time. There are numerous examples of biological processes that oscillate, some in a sustained fashion and some with damping. Common examples of such biological processes are the heart beat, respiration, and the sleep–waking cycle, processes readily monitored without invasive or sophisticated procedures. Heart beat and respiration, as well as flagellar rotation in bacteria, are in the middle range of biological oscillations (arbitrarily rates of ≈ 0.1 to 300 Hz). Sleep–waking and annual cycles (migration, hibernation) are in the low to very low frequency range (10^{-5} to 10^{-8} Hz). There are some biological processes that are driven by external stimuli that operate at very high frequencies ($> 10^4$ Hz), such as the membrane ion currents due to the resonance of stereocilia on hair cells in the inner ear, and these are probably the highest biological frequencies that cells, as intact structures, can generate. The wide range of such biological oscillations, some 12 orders of magnitude, suggests that very different mechanisms must be at work to cover such a range.

This chapter deals with three examples in the low to moderate frequency range: circadian (24-hr) oscillations, the cell division cycle ($\approx$30-min period), and pulsatile secretion of endocrine cells (minutes to hours). Each of these examples of biological timing falls into the broader categorization of "induced" rhythms, as defined earlier in this book. The mitotic cycles in eggs are normally triggered by fertilization and the oscillatory nature of the response is endogenous to the egg. Both circadian oscillation and endocrine pulsatile secretion are also examples of induced rhythms for it is not necessary for the external stimulus to be periodic to release or modulate an oscillatory response. This chapter gives a brief overview of the three processes and emphasizes what is currently known about biochemical mechanisms for the circadian and cell division cycles.

Circadian Oscillators

Circadian oscillators are widespread

Circadian cycles of activity are commonplace in multicellular animals and unicellular eukaryotes as are circadian cycles of photosynthesis, petal movements, and streaming in plant cells. The observable outputs of circadian clocks even include emission of light as in the bioluminescent rhythm in the dinoflagellate *Gonyaulax*. All of these cycles must be measured under free-running conditions (i.e., the absence of a light–dark or temperature cycle) in order to be sure that they are not "reflex" responses to such stimuli. Circadian cycles are endogenous oscillations that are genetically determined. They can be entrained by a variety of environmental stimuli of which light and temperature are the most reliable entrainers, in that order.

Circadian oscillators as clocks

Circadian oscillators are daily "clocks" for many organisms, because the organism can use the oscillation, which is precise enough, to measure time of day. One of the dramatic examples of such time of day measurement is in bird navigation. Starlings and other migratory birds will take a flight direction, when released, that is related to the phase of their circadian oscillation. Thus, it is possible to entrain birds on a light–dark schedule that is reversed (180° out of phase) with the normal solar day, and show that their initial flight direction is reversed also, compared with controls.

Discrete localization of circadian structures

In animals with nervous systems (which originates in *Cnidarians*), circadian oscillators can be localized to discrete structures in the brain or central ganglia. There are, however, examples of circadian oscillations in isolated non-nervous organs, such as the testis–seminal ducts complex of the gypsy moth (Giebultowicz et al., 1989). In mammals the suprachiasmatic nuclei (SCN), a small bilateral medial nucleus at the base of the hypothalamus above the optic chiasm, is necessary for the circadian cycles of locomotion, sleep, drinking behavior, body temperature, and hormone release patterns. In passerine birds (sparrows), the pineal is essential for the expression of circadian locomotion (perch–hopping). In cockroaches, the optic lobes contain a circadian oscillator and in a marine mollusk, *Aplysia*, the oscillators are actually located in the two eyes. In certain arthropods there is a circadian efferent control of retinal sensitivity (reviewed by Fleissner and Fleissner, 1988). One generalization that emerges from the diversity of animals that have been investigated is that circadian oscillators are either present in light-detecting organs or are not too far removed from photic input.

The strongest argument that discrete structures can control circadian timing comes from transplant experiments. In pinealectomized sparrows that are arhythmic, pineal transplants in the anterior chamber of the eye restore rhythmicity with the phase of the donor pineal. In hamsters that have bilateral lesions of the SCN and are arhythmic, transplants of neonatal mutant SCN at the base of the third ventricle will restore rhythmicity as well as the specific period of the mutant donor SCN (Ralph et al., 1990).

Ontogeny of circadian oscillators and environmental influences

In rodents, it has been possible to determine when circadian oscillations start in the central nervous system (CNS) of the developing animal. Circadian oscillations start in the SCN before retinal afferents to the SCN have developed. Using ^{14}C-labeled 2-deoxyglucose as a metabolic label to mark "active" cells, the SCN are found to begin oscillating at postnatal day 1 (Fuchs and Moore, 1980). There was no evidence for circadian oscillations in the SCN 1 to 2 days before birth. The retinohypothalamic tract does not develop and innervate the SCN until postnatal days 3 to 4.

If lizards and mice are raised in non-24-hr environments (20- and 28-hr light cycles), there are no permanent effects on the period of the free-running circadian locomotor ryhthm, compared with controls. However, in cockroaches the situation is different (Barrett and Page, 1989). As a result of 22-hr light cycles, the free-running circadian period was significantly shorter, by almost an hour, from controls (period $= 23.7 \pm 0.2$ hr). With 26-hr light cycles, the free-running period was about 0.6 hr greater than normal. These effects were not reversible in the adults after exposure to 24-hr light cycles. As more organisms are examined, it could turn out that there is fine-tuning of the period of the innate oscillator by the environmental period. It would appear to be adaptive to bring the innate oscillator as close to the planetary daily period so that entrainment, as seasons change, can be rapid.

Entrainment of circadian oscillators

Clocks are of no use unless they can be adjusted to local time. Animals may cross several time zones if they are migrating (fish, birds, whales). As the seasons change, in latitudes away from the equator, the times of sunrise and sunset change. Mechanisms have evolved, probably from when circadian oscillators first appeared, to allow these biological clocks to be reset every day with sunrise and/or sunset and environmental temperature. Such a process is termed "entrainment."

In the laboratory, the response of an organism's circadian system to entraining stimuli can be best described by a phase-response curve (PRC). In a PRC, the magnitude and direction of phase shift induced by a fixed perturbing stimulus, such as a fixed intensity and duration of light, is plotted as a function of the phase in the circadian cycle at which the perturbation is presented. Johnson (1990) has compiled from the literature about 340 PRCs in an atlas. In a wide variety of organisms, the overall shape of the PRC is remarkably similar. Phase advances to light are most prominent in the early subjective day (i.e., during the organism's active phase) whereas phase delays are prominent in the middle of the subjective night (i.e., the organism's inactive period). In *Aplysia*, the PRCs to light and serotonin in the isolated eye are almost mirror images of each other, emphasizing that within the same organ there may be different PRCs for different inputs to the circadian system. A similar situation is present in the SCN, studied in the isolated brain slice, with regard to PRCs generated by cyclic 5′, 3′, adenosine monophosphate (cAMP) and cyclic 5′, 3′ guanosine monophosphate (cGMP) (Prosser et al., 1989). In the isolated *Bulla* eye it has been possible to demonstrate that phase shifts of the circadian oscillator can be initiated by depolarizing or hyperpolarizing a single output neuron (McMahon and Block, 1987). Such output neurons, those with axons in the optic nerve, are known to be electrically coupled.

Temperature compensation of circadian oscillators

In poikilotherms, biological clocks would be useless as timing devices if they responded passively, as biochemical machines, to environmental temperature changes. Temperature compensation (i.e., temperature independence) of the period of the circadian oscillation appears to be a universal property of circadian systems, that have been examined to date, with Q_{10} values typically between 0.9 and 1.1. Pittendrigh (1954) was the first researcher to demonstrate temperature compensation in any organism, using the fruit fly *Drosophila*. Recently, there are reports of temperature compensation of the period of certain ultradian oscillations (e.g., the tyrosine aminotransferase activity in *Euglena*, which has a period of 4–5 hr) (Balzer et al., 1989).

Integration of physiological Processes by circadian systems

Whereas historically it was clear that certain organismic behaviors are markedly under circadian control, it is now clear that there is an "inner day" organizing most if not all physiological functions. In mammals there is an array of hormonal outputs that are linked to circadian time: growth hormone is secreted during the onset of slow wave sleep, cortisol secretion begins to rise before waking, and prolactin secretion occurs between these two phase points. The evidence that there is a circadian orchestration of hormonal secretion is not limited to mammals but appears among the invertebrates as well. Eclosion hormone is secreted in a distinct window of circadian time in moths and is the final command for eclosion of the adult from its cocoon.

Mechanisms of circadian oscillators

There have been three approaches to determining the mechanisms generating approximately 24-hr oscillations. These three approaches are:

1. the use and analysis of mutations to alter phase and period
2. the use of pharmacological agents to interfere with the rhythm
3. biochemical approaches involving the expression of genes and/or synthesis of proteins during the cycle.

Mutations that alter period. The most well characterized mutants are *per* in the fruit fly *Drososphila* (Hall and Kyriacou, 1990) and *frq* in the bread mould

Neurospora (Dunlap, 1990). Both of these mutations alter the period of the clock. As an example, *per*^{s} is a mutant with a short period (18–20 hr), *per*^{1} is a mutation with a long period (27–28 hr), and *per*^{0} is arhythmic. The difficulty with any mutation is understanding the mechanism of the phenotype. The *per* gene has been cloned and sequenced. There is, in the middle of the inferred protein, a repeating threonine–glycine theme. By analogy to a similar serine–glycine repeating theme in a vertebrate proteoglycan "serglycin" it has been suggested that *per* may be glycosylated (glycosaminoglycan side chains on the threonine residues). Thus, *per* appears to code for a proteoglycan, such proteins being normally but not exclusively extracellular. In experiments on electrical coupling between salivary gland cells from the various *per* mutants, a correlation has appeared. The *per*^{s} mutant has stronger electrical coupling than the wild type, whereas *per*^{1} has weaker coupling. One view of the *per* phenotype is that it influences circadian period by controlling the strength of gap-junction coupling between independent oscillator cells. Since the *per* transcript (mRNA) and protein (in photoreceptor nuclei, putative glial cells, and certain brain neurons) fluctuate with a circadian rhythm, another view suggests that *per* may itself be part of the clock machinery (Zerr et al., 1990). This hypothesis will be strengthened only when it can be demonstrated in an expression system that *per* and/or other genes can transfer rhythmic characteristics to a system in which a circadian oscillation is absent.

Pharmacological agents. Some insights have been obtained using pharmacological agents whose actions are known to be relatively specific. The period can be lengthened by chronic use of a reversible protein synthesis inhibitor in the unicellular eukaryote *Euglena*, whereas short pulses cause phase shifts whose amplitude and direction are functions of the phase at which the agent is applied. Thus, one can generate PRCs with pulses of protein synthesis inhibitors. Transcriptional inhibitors (Actinomycin D) suppress circadian oscillation in many but not all systems. The circadian rhythm of streaming in the unicellular alga *Acetabularia* is insensitive to Actinomycin D, although the drug is known to inhibit transcription in that system. X rays suppress the circadian oscillation in the isolated eye of *Aplysia* in a selective manner, not interfering with phototransduction or the synchrony of the pacemaker compound action potentials, which is mediated by gap junctions. Other agents, which are thought to increase intracellular Ca^{2+}, such as Li^+, La^{3+}, and caffeine, all increase circadian period in a dose-dependent fashion. One agent, creatinine, shortens circadian period in the dinoflagellate *Gonyaulax*.

The above pharmacological studies, with translational and transcriptional inhibitors, suggest that ongoing protein synthesis is essential for normal functioning of the circadian clock and that in most but not all systems, ongoing transcription appears to be required also. As more comparative pharmacological studies are performed in a variety of unicellular eukaryotes, it should be possible to construct whether the basic mechanisms of circadian oscillation are similar in all these forms or whether, early in evolution, a number of different mechanisms arose. The ease with which period can be changed by a number of agents, including even amino acids, suggests that whereas the circadian period may be temperature-compensated, the clock may not be compensated for anything else. In other words, the clock is part of the biochemical machinery in a cell and depends on buffering of the internal milieu by mechanisms that are outside the direct control of the clock.

Genes and proteins. A circadian system at the single cell level has at least three different subsystems (Strumwasser, 1967):

1. the oscillator
2. input to the oscillator
3. output from the oscillator

Studies on the biochemistry of the oscillator have involved quantitating the ≈ 1000 proteins synthesized by the isolated eye of *Aplysia* during a 2-hr pulse of radiolabeled amino acid at six time points in the circadian cycle. The most interesting protein to emerge from these studies is the circadian sawtooth oscillator protein, an acidic protein of molecular weight 42 kD (Strumwasser, 1989). This protein incorporates an increasing amount of ^{35}S-methionine linearly between CT 2 and CT 22 (CT 0 = start of subjective day), even though the labeling period is fixed at 2 hr. Between CT 22 and CT 26 (2 hr into cycle 2), the protein is incorporating low levels of radioactivity again (Fig. 1). The behavior of this protein can be described as a sawtooth oscillator protein since it accumulates radioactivity linearly with time and "resets" to a low level approximately every 24 hr. In other words, one can read time of day by the level of the newly synthesized protein. It is quite possible that proteins such as this are involved in generating the circadian oscillation. Later we will see that the behavior of the protein "cyclin" during cell division has similar properties.

Most of the remaining knowledge in the biochemical field has come from experiments on inputs to the oscillator. Thus, it is known that in the isolated eye of *Aplysia*, second messengers such as cAMP and cGMP can substitute for serotonin and light, respectively, in generating phase shifts. Furthermore, it has been found that different acidic proteins are synthesized as a result of phase shifting by serotonin or light. Serotonin induces the synthesis of a 34-kD protein whereas light (or cGMP or high K^+) induces the synthesis of a 30- and 31-kD protein (Yeung and Eskin, 1987; Raju et al., 1990). Light (or cGMP or high K^+) causes a decrease in the synthesis of a 42-kD protein.

The quantitation of gene transcripts during the circadian cycle has only recently begun. Loros et al. (1989) have recently developed a subtractive cDNA protocol to enrich for probes that detect morning-specific versus evening-specific mRNAs in *Neurospora.* Using this approach they have shown that there are at least two clock-controlled genes that are expressed primarily in the morning phase of the circadian rhythm. Using this subtractive tech-

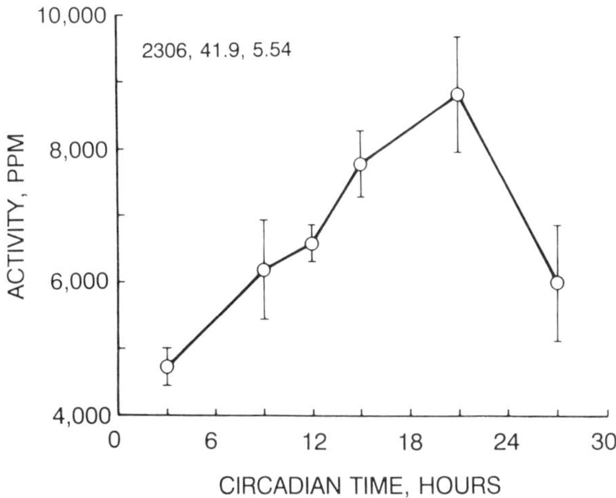

Figure 1. The incorporation of ^{35}S-methionine into the circadian sawtooth oscillator protein (spot 2306) as a function of circadian time. The ordinate ("activity") is given in parts per million of counts in spot 2306 (apparent m.w. 41.9 pI 5.54) divided by total counts in all of the spots on the two-dimensional (2-D) gel autoradiogram. Error bars are standard deviation of the mean. Each of the six time points had four experiments, except CT 20-22, which had six experiments. In each experiment four eyes were incubated with ^{35}S-methionine (150 μCi/ml) for 2 hr at 15°C. After rinses, eyes were homogenized and electrophoresed on an isoelectric focusing (IEF) tube gel (pH 3–10 ampholytes). Subsequently, the proteins in the IEF gel were electrophoresed on a 12.5% polyacrylamide slab gel. Analysis of the 2-D gel autoradiograms was accomplished with PDQUEST (Protein Databases Inc.).

nique they could not find evidence for clock-controlled evening genes. The subtractive cDNA protocol is limited by the necessity to use a 100- to 1000-fold excess of driver cDNA. In this type of protocol "low level" mRNA changes (e.g., tenfold) would be selected against and this may underestimate the total number of clock-controlled genes. Nevertheless, it is surprising to find that in *Neurospora* only two all-or-none type clock-controlled genes could be found with this methodology. In the dinoflagellate *Gonyaulax*, the luciferin binding protein (LBP) is synthesized with a circadian cycle and is an essential step for the bioluminescent rhythm. The present evidence indicates that the mRNA transcripts do not vary over the 24-hr period, suggesting that the cyclical synthesis of LBP is handled at the translational level (Morse et al., 1990).

In summary, investigations into the biochemical basis of the circadian oscillation are in their infancy. Much more needs to be learned about the genes and proteins that are expressed during a circadian cycle before common patterns between different phyla will reveal what has been conserved in the course of evolution.

Cell Division Cycle

Oscillations of a protein kinase control cell division

It has become apparent in the last several years, from studies of developing eggs of favorable organisms (*Xenopus*, the surf clam *Spisula*, and sea urchins), that cell division is an oscillatory event (Murray and Kirschner, 1989). The two states of the cell cycle are mitosis and interphase (cell at rest). In the *Xenopus* egg, fertilization initiates a series of 12 nearly synchronous cell divisions, the early embryonic cell cycle, with clocklike regularity ($\approx$30-min period). One of the important cytoplasmic factors initiating cell division is maturation promoting factor (MPF). MPF was discovered by injecting cytoplasm from mature eggs into immature oocytes, which induced meiosis. MPF is a protein kinase (an enzyme that phosphorylates proteins) that can phosphorylate histone H1. The catalytic subunit of MPF is thought to be a 34-kD protein ($p34^{cdc2}$), homologous with the product of the important fission yeast cell division cycle control gene, *cdc2*. MPF itself oscillates with the cell cycle, increasing as cells enter mitosis and falling as cells enter interphase. MPF oscillation does not appear to get significant feedback from the machinery of mitosis itself or the nucleus because the cortical contractions of the *Xenopus* and sea urchin eggs still proceed, with the same periodicity, after colchicine block of microtubule assembly or enucleation and centriole removal.

A second protein, cyclin, behaves as a sawtooth oscillator

During interphase of the early embryonic cell cycle, a second important protein is synthesized and accumulates and then disappears at the end of mitosis. This protein, termed cyclin, has a 56-kD molecular weight and was first discovered in clam (*Spisula*) eggs. It is known now that there are at least two cyclins (cyclin A and B), and that cyclin A peaks earlier than B (Fig. 2) in the *Xenopus* cell cycle (Minshull et al., 1990). Cyclin synthesis appears to be constant but the degradative mechanism is cyclic. In cell-free systems it has been possible to demonstrate that cyclin plays a direct role in the cell cycle. In such cell-free systems, it is possible to deplete endogenous mRNAs with ribonuclease and demonstrate that cyclin is the only protein synthesized when exogenous cyclin mRNA is added. The cell cycle, under these conditions, could only proceed when cyclin could be synthesized. If endogenous cyclin B mRNA, in the cell-free extract, is destroyed specifically by antisense oligonucleotide and endogenous RNAase H, then the cell cycle is arrested in interphase (Minshull et al., 1989). The state of the field, at this moment, is that the two proteins controlling the cell cycle, cyclin and MPF, are associated physically with one another. How cyclin activates MPF remains to be fully worked out. There is reasonable evidence that MPF is activated by dephosphorylation (Gautier et al., 1989).

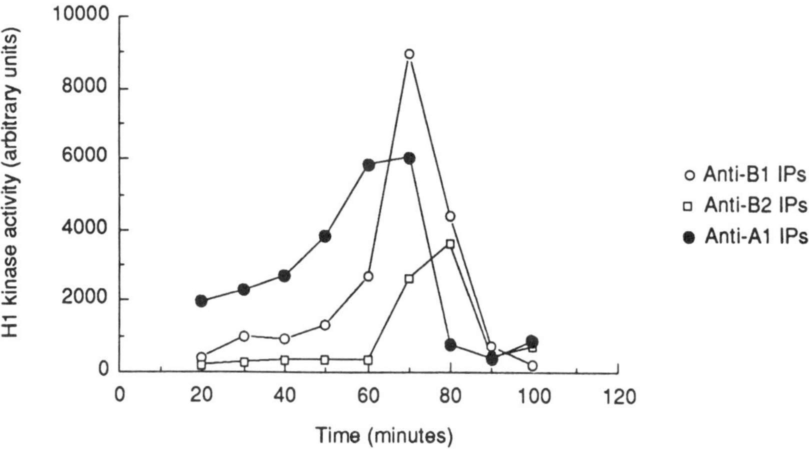

Figure 2. The temporal variation of A- and B-type cyclin associated *cdc2* kinase activity in *Xenopus*. A cell-free extract of *Xenopus* eggs and sperm nuclei were sampled at 10-min intervals for phosphorylation studies. Histone H1 kinase activity was measured after immunoprecipitation (IP) of the cell-free extract, with anti-cyclin antibodies (anti-B1, anti-B2, anti-A1) as described in Minshull et al. (1990). Reprinted with permission of IRL Press of Oxford University Press from Minshull et al. (1990): The A- and B-type cyclin associated *cdc2* kinases in *Xenopus* turn on and of at different times in the cell cycle. *EMBO J* 9:2865–2875.

In summary, the timing of the cell division cycle, at least in early embryogenesis, appears to be driven by one protein, cyclin. Cyclin accumulates steadily during interphase and this accumulation is a necessary prerequisite for mitosis. During mitosis, cyclin is rapidly degraded. MPF, a protein kinase, is activated at some threshold level of cyclin. It appears to be the important effector in the cell that initiates nuclear breakdown, chromosome condensation, spindle assembly, and cyclin degradation by phosphorylating a number of different proteins. There is an association between cyclin and MPF and activation of MPF appears to be related to its dephosphorylation. The biochemical events of the cell division cycle may be instructive and a model for research on circadian oscillators.

Pulsatile Secretion

Hormone secretion is pulsatile, not steady

If the secretion of almost any hormone is examined in unanesthetized vertebrates (including man) over a long time period without specific external stimuli, it turns out to be pulsatile (episodic) rather than steady or slowly varying.

Perhaps the earliest hint of the pulsatile nature of hormone secretion was the measurement of growth hormone (GH) secretion in humans (Hunter and Rigal, 1966). These studies involved taking blood samples at hourly intervals while healthy children and adolescents were in bed. GH plasma levels were not steady but rather fluctuated in a pulsatile manner. GH levels rose some 3 to 4 hr after meals but there were also a significant number of peaks before meals. During sleep GH levels were high. In more recent studies on fasting humans, there is a clear ultradian rhythm of GH secretion with about 6 to 10 pulses of GH per 24-hr period (Ho et al., 1988). Fasting over 5 days increases the pulsatile frequency by about 70%.

Target tissue response is optimal at the natural hormone frequency

In rats, the ultradian rhythm of GH has a frequency of about 7 to 8 pulses per 24 hr. It is natural to inquire whether growth depends on this temporal patterning of GH secretion over the course of a day. It is quite remarkable that the growth of a hypophysectomized rat is best when exogenous GH is delivered in periodic pulses rather than as a single bolus, even though the total GH delivered in any 24-hr period is the same. Thus, rats grow best when GH is delivered at nine pulses/day versus three pulses/day or a single large pulse per day (Isaksson et al., 1986).

Pulsatility in hormones is a general phenomenon and likely has early evolutionary origins

As a result of improvements in the sensitivity of hormone assays, it is rather routine, in vertebrates, to take small blood samples by an indwelling cannula at time intervals as short as a few minutes over the course of 1 or more days. These measurements have led to the discovery that most hormone release is pulsatile or ultradian (e.g., oxytocin, ACTH, TSH, GnRH, LH, β-endorphin, α-MSH, insulin) (Leng, 1988). The frequencies vary for the different hormones. In humans, TSH pulsatile secretion occurs at rates between 9.9 and 11.4 pulses per day, about twice the basal pulsatile rate of GH (Brabant et al., 1990). The pulsatile rate of luteinizing hormone–releasing hormone (LHRH) neurons, controlling luteinizing hormone (LH) release from the pituitary, in the mediobasal hypothalamus of the ovariectomized rhesus monkey, is about 1 pulse per hour (Knobil, 1987). It is important to realize that even in much simpler forms, periodic signalling is used. During a starvation stimulus, the amoeba, *Dictyostelium*, stops growing and emits cAMP pulses at about 10-min intervals, which induces the aggregation response (Gerisch, 1987).

The significance of periodic signaling

The growth results due to exogenous GH described above suggest that target tissue responses are most likely tuned to the natural frequency of the pulsatile or ultradian release. Goldbeter (1988) suggests that periodic signaling overcomes desensitization of receptors. Although this may be one important factor, it is likely that there are other considerations in target tissue responsiveness. Some of the long time intervals involved in pulsatile release (hours) suggest that membrane receptor properties are not the only limiting factors. It is not unlikely that the crescendo of second messenger and phosphorylation cascades within a target cell, in response to a hormone, is followed by activation of the genome and subsequent modulation of the membrane. These steps take time and probably are important rate-limiting steps.

Acknowledgments. I thank Dr. Neal Cornell and Ms. Jackie Vogel for their helpful comments on an earlier draft of the manuscript. The research described in Figure 1 was performed with grants from the NIH (MH41223) and NSF (BNS-9010115).

References

Balzer I, Neuhaus-Steinmetz U, Hardeland R (1989): Temperature compensation in an ultradian rhythm of tyrosine aminotransferase activity in *Euglena gracilis* Klebs. *Experientia* 45:476–477

Barrett RK, Page TL (1989): Effects of light on circadian pacemaker development. I. The freerunning period. *J Comp Physiol A* 165:41–49

Brabant G, Prank K, Ranft U, Schuermeyer T, Wagner TO, Hauser H, Kummer B, Feistner H, Hesch RD, von zur Muhlen A (1990): Physiological regulation of circadian and pulsatile thyrotropin secretion in normal man and woman. *J Clin Endocrinol Metab* 70:403–409

Dunlap JC (1990): Closely watched clocks: Molecular analysis of circadian rhythms in *Neurospora* and *Drosophila*. *TIG* 6:159–165

Fleissner G, Fleissner G (1988): *Efferent Control of Visual Sensitivity in Arthropod Eyes: With Emphasis on Circadian Rhythms.* Stuttgart: Gustav Fischer

Fuchs JL, Moore RY (1980): Development of circadian rhythmicity and light responsiveness in the rat suparachiasmatic nucleus: a study using the 2-deoxy[1-^{14}C]-glucose method. *Proc Natl Acad Sci USA* 77:1204–1208

Gautier J, Matsukawa T, Nurse P, Maller J (1989): Dephosphorylation and activation of *Xenopus* p34^{cdc2} protein kinase during the cell cycle. *Nature* 339:626–629

Gerisch G (1987): Cyclic AMP and other signals controlling cell development and differentiation in *Dictyostelium*. *Annu Rev Biochem* 56:853–879

Giebultowicz JM, Riemann JG, Raina AK, Ridgway RL (1989): Circadian system controlling release of sperm in the insect testes. *Science* 245:1098–1100

Goldbeter A (1988): Periodic signaling as an optimal mode of intercellular communication. *NIPS* 3:103–105

Hall JC, Kiriacou CP (1990): Genetics of biological rhythms in *Drosophila*. In: *Advances in Insect Physiology*, Evans PD, Wigglesworth VB, eds. New York: Academic Press, pp 221–298

Ho KY, Veldhuis JD, Johnson ML, Furlanetto R, Evans WS, Alberti KGMM, Thorner MO (1988): Fasting enhances growth hormone secretion and amplifies the complex rhythms of growth hormone secretion in man. *J Clin Invest* 81:968–975

Hunter WM, Rigal WM (1966): The diurnal pattern of plasma growth hormone concentration in children and adults. *J. Endocrinol* 34:147–153

Isaksson OGP, Jansson J-O, Clark RG, Robinson I (1986): Significance of the secretory pattern of growth hormone. *NIPS* 1:44–47

Johnson C (1990): *An Atlas of phase response curves for Circadian and Circatidal Rhythms.* Vanderbilt University: Dept. of Biology

Knobil E (1987): A hypothalamic pulse generator governs mammalian reproduction. *NIPS* 2:42–43

Leng G (1988): *Pulsatility in Neuroendocrine Systems.* Boca Raton, FL: CRC Press

Loros JJ, Denome SA, Dunlap JC (1989): Molecular cloning of genes under the control of the circadian clock in *Neurospora. Science* 243:385–388

McMahon DG, Block GD (1987): The *Bulla* ocular circadian pacemaker I. Pacemaker neuron membrane potential controls phase through a calcium-dependent mechanism. *J Comp Physiol A* 161:335–346

Minshull J, Blow JJ, Hunt T (1989): Translation of cyclin mRNA is necessary for extracts of activated *Xenopus* eggs to enter mitosis. *Cell* 56:947–956

Minshull J, Golsteyn R, Hill CS, Hunt T (1990): The A- and B-type cyclin associated cdc2 kinases in *Xenopus* turn on and off at different times in the cell cycle. *EMBO J* 9:2865–2875

Morse DS, Fritz L, Hastings JW (1990): What is the clock? Translational regulation of circadian bioluminescence. *TIBS* 15:262–265

Murray AW, Kirschner MW (1989): Dominoes and clocks: The union of two views of the cell cycle. *Science* 246:614–621

Pittendrigh CS (1954): On temperature independence in the clock system controlling emergence time in *Drosophila. Proc Natl Acad Sci USA* 40:1018–1029

Prosser RA, McArthur AJ, Gillette MU (1989): cGMP induces phase shifts of a mammalian circadian pacemaker at night, in antiphase to cAMP effects. *Proc Natl Acad Sci USA* 86:6812–6815

Raju U, Yeung SJ, Eskin A (1990): Involvement of proteins in light resetting ocular circadian oscillator of *Aplysia. Am J Physiol* 258:R256–R262

Ralph MR, Foster RG, Davis FC, Menaker M (1990): Transplanted suprachiasmatic nucleus determines circadian period. *Science* 247:975–978

Strumwasser F (1967): Neurophysiological aspects of rhythms. In: *The Neurosciences: An Intensive Study Program*, Quarton GC, Melnechuk T, Schmitt FO, New York: Rockefeller University Press, pp 516–528

Strumwasser F (1989): A short history of the second messenger concept in neurons and lessons from long lasting changes in two neuronal systems producing afterdischarge and circadian oscillations. *J Physiol (Paris)* 83:246–254

Yeung SJ, Eskin A (1987): Involvement of a specific protein in the regulation of a circadian rhythm in *Aplysia* eye. *Proc Natl Acad Sci USA* 84:279–283

Zerr DM, Hall JC, Rosbash M, Siwicki KK (1990): Circadian fluctuations of *period* protein immunoreactivity in the CNS and visual system of *Drosophila. J Neurosci* 10:2749–2762

Comparison of Electrical Oscillations in Neurons with Induced or Spontaneous Cellular Rhythms due to Biochemical Regulation

ALBERT GOLDBETER

Biological rhythms can be classified broadly into different categories, according to the way in which they occur. Thus, they can arise spontaneously in a given set of experimental conditions, as exemplified by rhythmic activity in nodal tissues of the heart, or they can be driven by some external periodic process. In the latter case, the biological rhythm is generally entrained in a certain range at the frequency of the forcing stimulus. Oscillations can also occur as a result of a change in external conditions that brings about the transition from a stable steady state to an oscillatory regime. The latter situations relate to different sorts of induced rhythms; indeed (see the introductory chapter by Bullock), induced rhythms are either triggered from silence or modulated from an ongoing rhythm by an external event, transient or sustained.

Both the spontaneous and induced rhythms thus defined are *endogenous*, that is, they result from the regulatory properties of the biological system rather than from the periodic nature of its environment. This is in contrast with *exogenous* rhythms, which merely reflect the passive linking of cellular processes to some external periodicity. The difference between induced and spontaneous rhythms is less significant, even for induced rhythms that correspond to the transition from a stable steady state to sustained oscillations: besides the admittedly important distinction that the first require to be triggered while the second need not, there is no fundamental difference between the two kinds of phenomena; induced and spontaneous rhythms can indeed originate from common mechanisms and occur in closely related conditions.

Endogenous oscillations are widespread in neurons or muscle cells, which are electrically excitable, but they also occur in other cell types. This chapter draws a parallel between neuronal oscillations, which represent the central theme of this book, and the rhythms that occur in a number of cells as a result of biochemical regulation rather than electrical excitability. The comparison of the two types of oscillations allows us to draw some general conclusions on rhythmic behavior at the cellular level. Moreover, knowledge gained from the study of spontaneous or induced biochemical oscillations might provide useful insights into the occurrence of analogous rhythms in the brain.

The Three Best Known Examples of Biochemical Rhythms

To begin, it is desirable to start by delineating the meaning of the term "biochemical" in the present context. All cellular rhythms could, of course, eventually be described in terms of a biochemical mechanism. It is useful, however, to distinguish, on the one hand, rhythms of an electrical or, rather, electrochemical nature that are based on electrical impedance changes and membrane processes as in nerve or muscle cells, and on the other hand, biochemical rhythms that originate from the regulation of enzyme activity, receptor–enzyme interactions, or transport processes in which voltage-dependent controls do not play a primary role. Of the latter biochemical rhythms, three well characterized examples will be considered here. Each illustrates properties that will be compared with corresponding aspects of neuronal oscillations. Further details and references can be found in a recent monograph (Goldbeter, 1990) and in several reviews devoted, respectively, to biochemical rhythms (Hess and Boiteux, 1971; Goldbeter and Caplan, 1976), to a comparison of rhythms in electrically excitable and nonexcitable cells (Berridge and Rapp, 1979), and to the more recently discovered phenomenon of Ca^{2+} oscillations (Berridge and Galione, 1988; Cuthbertson, 1989; Jacob, 1990).

Glycolytic oscillations

When a glycolytic substrate is injected at a constant rate into a suspension of yeast cells or into yeast extracts, sustained oscillations develop with a period of the order of several minutes (Hess and Boiteux, 1971; Goldbeter and Caplan, 1976). The most interesting aspect of these oscillations is that they occur in well defined conditions, within a range bounded by two critical values of the substrate input. The period of the rhythm decreases while the amplitude goes through a maximum, as the substrate injection rate increases. The origin of the oscillations can be traced back to one of the enzymatic reactions of the glycolytic system, namely, that catalyzed by phosphofructokinase.

Relay and oscillations of cyclic AMP (cAMP) in *Dictyostelium* amoebae

After starvation, cells of the slime mold *Dictyostelium discoideum* aggregate in waves by a chemotactic response to cAMP signals emitted by centers, with a periodicity of 5 to 10 min (Gerisch et al., 1979; Devreotes, 1982). The rhythmic synthesis of cAMP that underlies wavelike aggregation also occurs in cell suspensions (Gerisch and Wick, 1975). Whereas aggregation centers emit periodic cAMP pulses in an autonomous manner, other cells are capable of relaying suprathreshold cAMP signals; this relay property reflects the excitability of the cAMP signaling system in *Dictyostelium*.

Signal-induced Ca^{2+} oscillations

Intracellular Ca^{2+} oscillations occur in a variety of cells, with periods ranging from seconds to minutes, either spontaneously or as a result of stimulation by an external signal such as a hormone or a neurotransmitter (for recent reviews, see Berridge and Galione, 1988; Cuthbertson, 1989; Jacob, 1990). Ca^{2+} oscillations are clearly those that most resemble induced rhythms of the brain, since they generally occur as a result of external stimulation, with a frequency that increases with the magnitude of the stimulus.

Comparison of Biochemical and Neuronal Rhythms

Mechanism

Common to the three biochemical rhythms discussed above and to neuronal oscillations is the primary role played by positive feedback in the molecular mechanism of periodic behavior.

An endogenous rhythm can be viewed as the repetitive alternance of an ascending phase, often due to self-amplification associated with such a positive feedback, and a decreasing phase in which the former process is superseded by some limiting factor. Thus, the instability that leads to glycolytic oscillations originates from the activation of phosphofructokinase by one of its reaction products, ADP (Fig. 1A) while the decreasing phase is brought about mainly by the limiting supply of substrate.

In *Dictyostelium*, binding of extracellular cAMP to a membrane receptor enhances the synthesis of cAMP, which in turn leads to the release of more cAMP into the extracellular medium (Fig. 1B). Oscillations result from the coupling of this positive feedback with the limiting counterpoise provided by receptor desensitization.

As to Ca^{2+} oscillations, they involve the cycling of Ca^{2+} ions between the cytosol and an intracellular store (Berridge and Galione, 1988). Here again, regulation of the transport process provides the positive feedback responsible for oscillations (Fig. 1C): over a period, the Ca^{2+} content of the store progressively builds up until it abruptly discharges into the cytosol in a process activated by cytosolic Ca^{2+}.

In these three systems, oscillations involve a seesaw relationship between two variables: substrate and product in the case of glycolytic oscillations, active receptor and cAMP in *Dictyostelium*, and intravesicular and cytosolic Ca^{2+} in signal-induced Ca^{2+} oscillations (Martiel and Goldbeter, 1987; Goldbeter, 1990; Goldbeter et al., 1990). In each case, the first variable (X) accumulates at a nearly constant pace until the second variable (Y), which exerts the positive feedback, increases autocatalytically at the expense of X, which drops in an abrupt manner. This produces a spike in Y that repeats itself once variable X has replenished up to a sufficient level and Y has again reached the threshold where autocatalysis becomes significant.

A

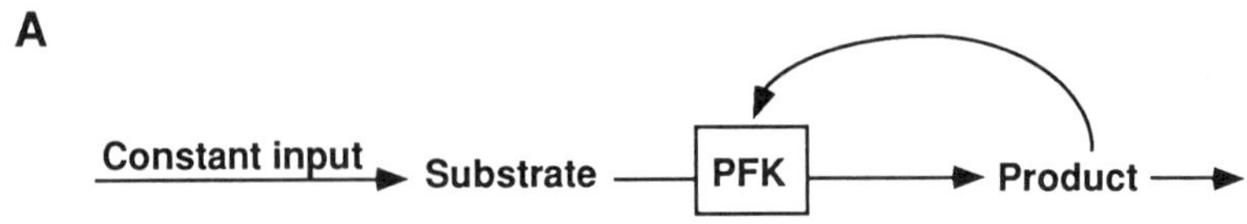

B

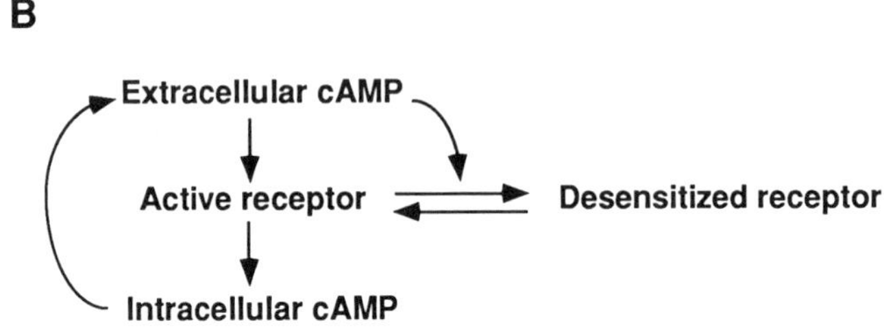

C

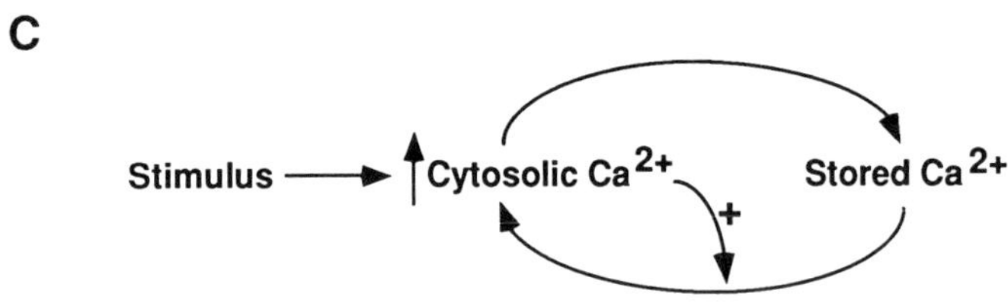

D

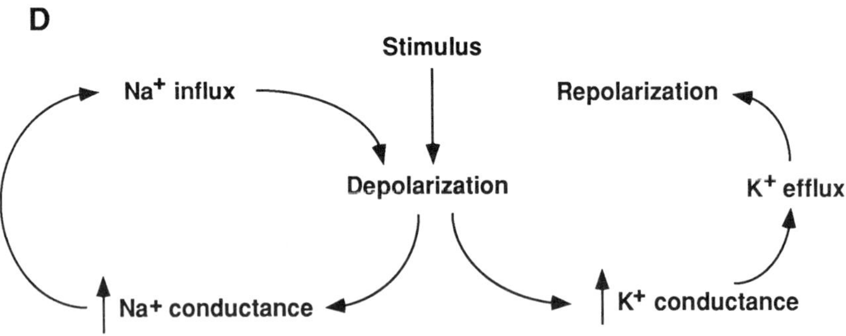

Figure 1. Schematic mechanisms of biochemical and neuronal oscillations (see text for further details). **A**: Glycolytic oscillations result from the positive feedback exterted by a reaction product on phosphofructokinase (PFK) whose substrate is supplied at a constant rate. **B**: Cyclic AMP (cAMP) oscillations in the slime mold *Dictyostelium discoideum* result from the positive feedback exerted by extracellular cAMP on its intracellular synthesis, in the presence of receptor desensitization. **C**: Signal-induced Ca^{+} oscillations originate from the Ca^{2+}-induced release of Ca^{2+} from an intracellular pool into the cytosol (the triggering role of inositol 1,4,5-trisphosphate is not represented). **D**: Mechanism of generation of an action potential in the giant squid axon, based on the voltage-dependent changes in Na^{+} and K^{+} conductances; in the presence of an appropriate depolarizing stimulus the process becomes repetitive, giving rise to a neuronal rhythm.

Such alternating phases find direct correspondences in the ionic mechanisms responsible for neuronal rhythms. Thus, in the simplest case illustrated by the squid axon (Huxley, 1959; Guttman et al., 1980), the sequential activation of an inward current carried by Na^+ ions and an outward current carried by K^+ ions repetitively generates an action potential. Self-amplification originates here from the positive feedback loop that governs Na^+ influx during depolarization (Fig. 1D), whereas repolarization follows from inactivation of the Na^+ conductance and from the efflux of K^+ ions initiated at the height of the depolarization phase. Many more currents are involved in bursting neurones (Adams and Benson, 1985, 1989) but, *mutatis mutandis*, the type of voltage-dependent oscillatory mechanism found in the squid remains unchanged.

Induction of rhythmic behavior

In neurons, all that is required for the onset of rhythmic activity is often a depolarizing stimulus. Such a situation is well illustrated in the simple case of the squid axon where the membrane, initially in a resting state, is induced to fire rhythmically by application of a steady depolarizing current (Huxley, 1959; Guttman et al., 1980). Such a stimulus brings the membrane above the self-excitation threshold and thereby induces the neural rhythm.

There exists the possibility, however, that already in the absence of external stimulation the membrane is unable to reach a resting state because the latter is unstable at the given extracellular ionic concentrations. Then, rhythmic behavior develops spontaneously and the cell behaves as pacemaker; such is the case for the bursting *R15* neuron of *Aplysia* (Adams and Benson, 1985).

The factors that induce rhythmic behavior in biochemical systems can take different forms. Much as in the neural situation, their effect is to change the conditions in such a manner that the system is brought across the self-excitation threshold beyond which repetitive spiking occurs. Thus, in glycolysis, oscillations start once the steady state becomes unstable owing to the increase in product associated with a sufficient rise in substrate input. As to *Dictyostelium*, no rhythm-inducing factor is needed, given that cAMP oscillations appear spontaneously in the course of development (see below).

The situation closest to induced neural rhythms is that of signal-induced Ca^{2+} oscillations. There, indeed, an external stimulus elicits the synthesis of inositol 1,4,5-trisphosphate (IP_3) and the subsequent release of a certain amount of Ca^{2+} from an IP_3-sensitive intracellular store; the resulting elevation of cytosolic Ca^{2+} destabilizes the steady state and thereby triggers the cycling of Ca^{2+} between the cytosol and an IP_3-insensitive store. Once again, it is a rise in the variable responsible for the positive feedback—here, cytosolic Ca^{2+}—that brings about the transition from a stable, resting state into sustained oscillations (Goldbeter et al., 1990; Dupont et al., 1991). For a similar reason, the rhythm can be induced by merely raising the level of Ca^{2+} in the extracellular medium. Induction of the rhythm by external stimulation also occurs in an alternative mechanism (Meyer and Stryer, 1988) that relies on another type of positive feedback; in that model, the cross activation of IP_3 synthesis and Ca^{2+} release into the cytosol leads to concomitant oscillations of Ca^{2+} and IP_3.

Range of oscillations

Another point common to biochemical and neural rhythms is that both types of oscillations occur in well defined conditions, generally over a finite range of the control parameter. Thus, glycolytic oscillations occur when the substrate input is in a range bounded by two critical values. Similarly, signal-induced Ca^{2+} oscillations occur when the external stimulus is in an appropriate range; when the stimulus is absent or below that range, there is a stable, low level of cytosolic Ca^{2+} whereas a stable, elevated level of cytosolic Ca^{2+} is established when stimulation becomes too high.

In neurons, a similar range of oscillations, bounded by two critical values of the control parameter, has been observed in experiments and/or in Hodgkin–Huxley-type models when varying the applied current (Rinzel, 1985), the extracellular K^+ or Na^+ concentrations (Aihara and Matsumoto, 1982), or the maximum conductances of these ions (Holden and Yoda, 1981).

Ontogenesis

How rhythmic behavior appears in the course of development is well illustrated by the example of cAMP oscillations in *Dictyostelium* cells. During the hours that follow starvation, the amoebae first become capable of relaying suprathreshold cAMP pulses before generating these signals autonomously in a periodic manner (Gerisch et al., 1979). The theoretical analysis of a model for the cAMP signaling system shows how the sequence of developmental transitions from no relay to relay and from relay to oscillations can result from a continuous increase in the level of cAMP receptor or in the activity of enzymes involved in cAMP signaling, namely, adenylate cyclase or phosphodiesterase (Goldbeter and Segel, 1980; Goldbeter, 1990).

In neurons, likewise, rhythmic behavior could originate during development from the continuous build-up of some component of the oscillatory mechanism, such as an ionic channel within the membrane (Holden and Yoda, 1981). Alternatively, the ontogenesis of some neural rhythms could be ascribed to the appearance of inhibitory or excitatory connections between neurons when the rhythm appears to be a network (Selverston and Moulins, 1985) rather than a cellular property.

Phase plane analysis and the link between excitable and oscillatory behavior

A most revealing approach that illustrates well the common properties of biochemical and neural rhythms is provided by phase plane analysis. This approach works best for two-variable systems although it can, in certain conditions, be applied to three-variable systems as well (see below). Because of the usefulness of phase plane analysis, a primary goal of theoretical studies of rhythmic phenomena has always been to obtain a description of the oscillatory system in terms of only two variables.

Let us return to the two variables X and Y defined above: Y denotes the variable that undergoes a self-amplifying increase in the course of oscillations whereas X denotes the limiting variable that acts as a counterpoise to this process. The phase plane approach relies on the study of nullclines, which are the loci in the (X, Y) plane in which X or Y do not vary—these loci thus correspond to the curves obtained from the equations $dX/dt = 0$ and $dY/dt = 0$. A recurrent result in the theoretical study of oscillating systems is that the Y nullcline possesses an "S" or "N" shape, depending on the choice of axes. When the steady state, which is the intersection of the two nullclines, is located on the central branch of the Y nullcline, in a region of sufficiently steep slope, it is unstable and the system evolves to a closed curve in the phase plane—a limit cycle—that surrounds the unstable steady state and corresponds to sustained oscillations (Fig. 2A).

Starting from a low initial value corresponding to a stable steady state, an increase in the rhythm-inducing factor, which plays the role of the control or bifurcation parameter, can trigger oscillations once it passes a critical, threshold value. Just before the onset of rhythmic behavior, the steady state is stable but excitable as the system can amplify suprathreshold perturbations in a pulsatory manner before returning to the resting state (Fig. 2A, dashed line).

Phase plane analysis further makes clear how the increase in the control parameter (e.g., the intensity of the applied depolarizing current in the neuronal case or the substrate input in glycolysis) first triggers rhythmic behavior and later suppresses it when a higher, critical value is reached.

The main virtue of phase plane analysis is therefore to explain the existence of a finite range for the occurrence of oscillations, and to show that excitable and oscillatory behavior arise in closely related conditions and originate from a common underlying mechanism operating in adjacent regions of the parameter space.

Such a link between excitability and oscillations is one of the most conspicuous properties of neurons, and was first demonstrated by phase plane analysis in the classical work of Fitzhugh (1961), who further provided an explanation for the existence of a sharp threshold for excitability and for the fact that the excitable response is characterized by both a relative and an absolute refractory period.

Later studies in terms of Hodgkin–Huxley equations aimed at reducing the number of variables initially considered (these four variables are the membrane potential V, the activation variables m and n for the Na^+ and K^+ currents, respectively, and the inactivation variable h for the Na^+ current). Thus, Rinzel (1985) proposed to describe the dynamics of a simple nerve membrane in terms of only two variables, namely, the potential V and a recovery variable W that takes into account the variation of n and h.

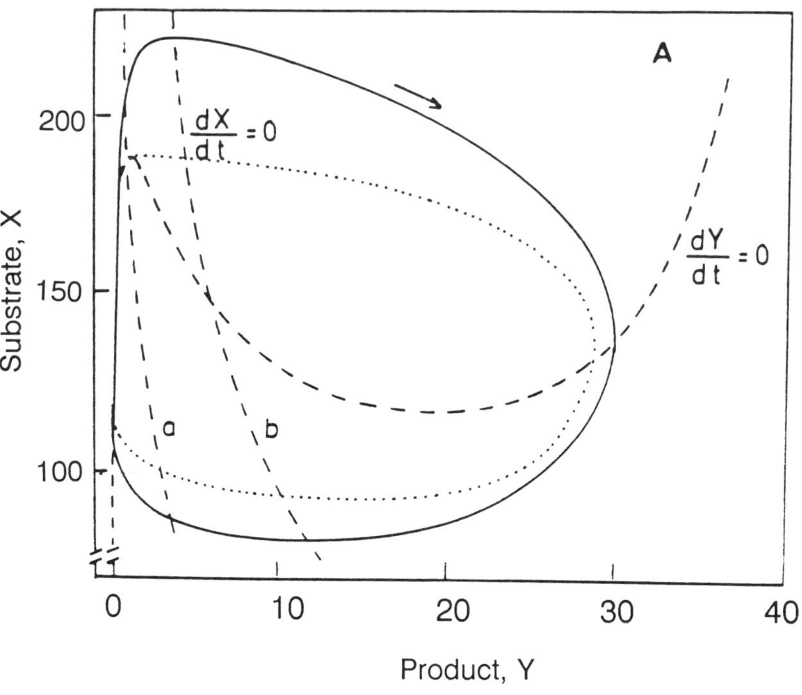
A
200
150
100
Substrate, X
$\frac{dX}{dt} = 0$
$\frac{dY}{dt} = 0$
a
b
0
10
20
30
40
Product, Y

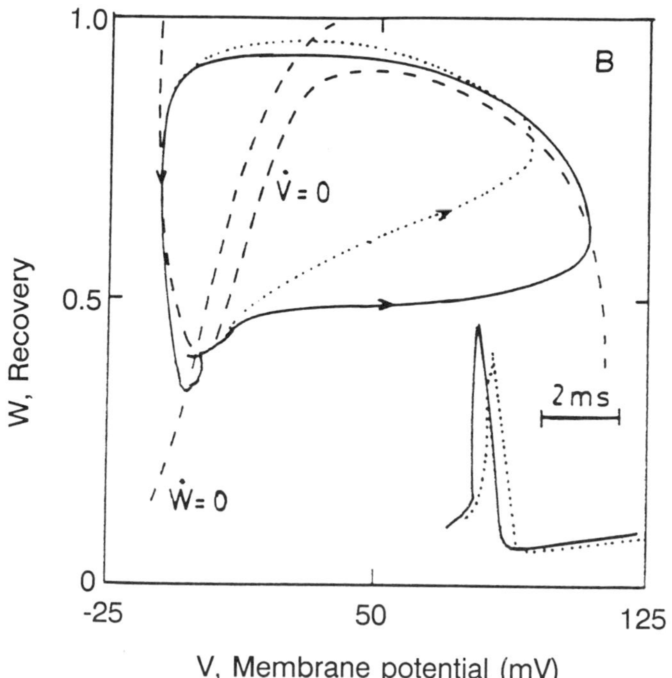
1.0
0.5
0
B
$\dot{V} = 0$
$\dot{W} = 0$
2 ms
W, Recovery
-25
50
125
V, Membrane potential (mV)

The significant point is that here also the $dV/dt = 0$ nullcline possesses an "S" (or "N") shape (see Fig. 2B); when the steady state lies on the middle branch of that nullcline, it is unstable and a limit cycle surrounding it is established. Again, excitability rather than oscillations occurs when the steady state lies in the immediate vicinity of the instability domain. In these conditions, a slight, transient depolarization will induce a single action potential (Fig. 2B, dotted line). If, however, the depolarizing stimulus is maintained, a stable rhythm will occur (Fig. 2B, solid line).

Another situation, sometimes encountered in neural systems (see, e.g., Aihara and Matsumoto, 1982; Rinzel, 1985), is that of hard excitation (Minorsky, 1962), where a stable limit cycle is separated from a stable steady state by an unstable limit cycle. In such conditions, the transition from the resting state to the rhythm can be induced by a transient, suprathreshold perturbation; in other words, the stimulus need not be maintained for oscillations to be sustained.

Multiple oscillations

A prediction based on phase plane analysis is that some biochemical or neuronal systems, initially in a stable resting state, undergo one type of oscillations when subjected to an increase in the control parameter, and another type of rhythmic behavior, unrelated to the first one, when subjected to a decrease in that parameter. The condition for the occurrence of such multiple modes of rhythmic behavior is that the nullcline, which previously showed but a single domain of negative slope, should possess two such domains.

Models with such characteristics have been constructed for biochemical oscillations (Goldbeter and Moran, 1988) or neuronal activity (Rose and Hindmarsh, 1985). Multiple oscillations have in fact been observed in neurobiology. Thalamic neurons indeed display the capability of firing at two distinct frequencies, according to the stimulation that they receive. When the thalamic cell is in a stable resting state, a slight depolarization will induce oscillations at a 10-Hz frequency, whereas a slight hyperpolarization will induce rhythmic behavior at a 6-Hz frequency (Jahnsen and Llinás, 1984;

◀ **Figure 2.** Phase plane dynamics in a model for glycolytic oscillations (**A**) and in a simplified, two-variable model of neuronal oscillations based on Hodgkin–Huxley equations. In each panel, the nullclines (*dashed lines*) of the two variables of the model are shown, together with the limit cycle (*solid line*) corresponding to sustained oscillations, and with a trajectory (*dotted line*) corresponding to excitable behavior. Excitability and oscillations are linked as they occur in closely related conditions, depending on whether the steady state that lies at the intersection of the two nullclines is stable or not; the two situations give rise to the nullclines marked (a) and (b) for variable Y in Fig. 2A (although the two situations are also illustrated in Fig. 2B, only one nullcline is shown there for variable W). Fig. 2B is redrawn, with permission, from Rinzel (1985).

Llinás, 1988). A more recent theoretical study (Rose and Hindmarsh, 1989) accounts for rhythmic properties of thalamic neurons in terms of equations of the Hodgkin–Huxley type.

Bursting

The kind of periodic behavior in which trains of high-frequency spikes are separated by phases of quiescence and recur at regular intervals is known as bursting. Such rhythmic behavior is characteristic of many neurons, for example, *R15* in *Aplysia* (Adams and Benson, 1985, 1989) or hippocampus cells in the brain (Johnston and Brown, 1984); the phenomenon involves a larger number of currents and ionic species—including Ca^{2+}—than in the giant axon of the squid.

To account for bursting oscillations, a model must contain at least three variables, in contrast to simple oscillations of the limit cycle type, which require only two variables. Phase plane analysis, however, can still be resorted to when one of the three variables is treated as a slowly varying parameter. Analyses of that kind have successfully shed light on the origin of bursting in a model for membrane potential oscillations in pancreatic β-cells (Rinzel, 1987) as well as in a multiply regulated biochemical model (Decroly and Goldbeter, 1987). In particular, this approach explains the transition from simple periodic oscillations to bursting, while the use of one-dimensional maps allows us to account for the transition from a bursting pattern with n spikes per period to a pattern with $(n + 1)$ spikes.

Bistability and birhythmicity

A characteristic property of nonlinear systems, shared by the nerve membrane and by regulated biochemical reactions, is that they often admit multiple, coexisting states in a given set of conditions. Besides the above-mentioned phenomenon of hard excitation in which a stable steady state coexists with a stable rhythm, the best known and most common type of such a multiplicity is certainly that of two coexisting, stable steady states, a phenomenon generally referred to as "bistability" (strictly speaking, however, bistability refers to the coexistence of two stable states of any kind, i.e., stationary in time, periodic, or even chaotic; for further discussion and examples, see Decroly and Goldbeter, 1982; Goldbeter, 1990).

Bistability often occurs in conditions close to those that produce rhythmic behavior. The phenomenon has been observed experimentally, and accounted for by theoretical models, both in biochemical reactions and in electrically excitable systems including neurons (see, e.g., Aihara and Matsumoto, 1982; Rinzel, 1985) and cardiac cells (Gadsby and Wit, 1981).

There exists a rhythmic counterpart to bistability: in a given set of conditions, two stable, distinct rhythms may indeed coexist. This phenomenon, called "birhythmicity" (Decroly and Goldbeter, 1982), differs from the multiple oscillations considered earlier where the two different rhythms occurred in distinct conditions. The coexistence between two (and even more) different, stable rhythms has been described in several biochemical models (Decroly and Goldbeter, 1982; Markus and Hess, 1984; Goldbeter, 1990). Birhythmicity is a property that has not yet been observed in neuronal systems, although appropriate conditions are likely to be met in thalamic cells. It would allow a neuron to switch reversibly between two rhythms characterized by different amplitudes and frequencies upon suitable, transient stimulation.

Chaos

Aperiodic oscillations, known as chaos, are characterized both by their irregular nature and by their sensitivity to initial conditions. Such phenomena have been observed experimentally and theoretically in biochemical and neuronal systems, as well as in other fields of biology (for recent reviews, see Olsen and Degn 1985; Holden, 1986; Glass and Mackey, 1988). Chaos often occurs when an oscillatory system fails to be entrained by a periodically varying parameter; alternatively, chaos is said to be autonomous when it occurs in the absence of periodic forcing. Analyses of the electroencephalogram (EEG) have suggested that the brain could sometimes operate in a chaotic rather than periodic manner (Babloyantz and Destexhe, 1986; Skarda and Freeman, 1987; Roschke and Başar, 1988; Rapp et al., 1989). It should be remembered, however, that such measurements represent a macroscopic average of the activity of a huge number of cells that are likely to be heterogeneous in their excitable and oscillatory properties. Autonomous chaos has also been reported to occur at the level of a single neuron (Holden et al., 1982).

Biochemical models show that autonomous chaos can result from the interplay between two endogenous oscillatory mechanisms present within the same cellular system. The best example is provided by cAMP oscillations in *Dictyostelium* which, for some parameter values, are chaotic (Martiel and Goldbeter, 1985). Such a result could account for the aperiodic nature of aggregation in the *Fr17* mutant of the slime mold (Durston, 1974). Studies of this mutant in cell suspensions showed regular rather than chaotic oscillations (Goldbeter and Wurster, 1989). One reason might be that the mutant cells had evolved toward the domain of periodic behavior, which is much larger than the domain of chaos in parameter space. Alternatively, the presence of a certain proportion of cells oscillating periodically could destroy the chaotic properties of other cells present within the mixed suspension.

The latter conjecture has recently been verified in a theoretical model for cAMP signaling in *Dictyostelium*. This analysis indicates that a tiny proportion of periodic cells suffices to suppress chaos in suspensions where cells are strongly coupled through extracellular cAMP (Halloy et al., 1990; Li et al., 1992). These results could bear on the possible suppression of chaos by periodic oscillations in other biological systems (e.g., in neuronal populations). The latter are also subjected to strong coupling through several factors such as synaptic connections and the extracellular ionic concentrations that govern the cellular membrane potential. Thus, whereas the spatial heterogeneity of oscillatory properties may, as noted above, contribute to disturb periodic behavior and lead to some form of spatiotemporal chaos, the coupling between chaotic and periodic cells may also bring about the suppression of aperiodic oscillations. Although this might account for the occurrence of more regular modes of periodic behavior in the brain, a different mechanism should probably be invoked to explain the coherent oscillations that have been observed in the cortex as a result of specific sensory stimulation (Eckhorn et al., 1988; Gray and Singer, 1989; Gray et al., 1989).

Concluding Remarks

Even if they are not, by far, as widespread as rhythms of electrical origin in nerve and muscle cells, the occurrence of rhythmic phenomena in a number of biochemical and nonneural cellular systems clearly indicates that oscillations are not an exclusive property of electrically excitable membranes such as those of neurons or cardiac cells. The above comparison has shown, however, that there exists a profound unity between biochemical and electrical rhythms.

As other endogenous biological oscillations, the two kinds of rhythms represent temporal dissipative structures that occur in the form of limit cycles beyond a critical point of instability of a nonequilibrium steady state (Nicolis and Prigogine, 1977). Beyond this common thermodynamic framework, further convergences bear on the underlying mechanism, which often involves positive feedback of one kind or another, on the existence of a finite domain over which a parameter (or stimulus) can induce rhythmic behavior, and on the ontogenesis of oscillations which can appear in the course of development as a result of the continuous increase in some molecular component of the rhythm-generating mechanism. Another common point is that the core of the oscillatory mechanism can often be described in terms of two variables (for limit cycle oscillations) or three (for bursting or chaos).

That the two types of rhythms might sometimes be coupled in a given cell is exemplified in the heart, where spontaneous or induced oscillations in cytosolic Ca^{2+}, described above, can serve as a pacemaker mechanism initiating rhythmic activity in cardiac cells (Tsien et al., 1979). Likewise, in neurons, cytosolic Ca^{2+} oscillations can give rise to oscillatory membrane currents (Kuba and Takeshita, 1981).

From the known examples discussed above, it would seem that the variety of oscillatory mechanisms at the cellular level is greater for biochemical rhythms than for neuronal ones: only the currents and ionic species involved may change for the latter in different cells or organisms, but the basic mechanism of neural rhythms always remains that of an interplay between several voltage-dependent conductances arranged in time so that repolarization follows the explosive depolarization phase of the action potential. Rhythmic activity arising from activating or inhibitory connections between cells in a neuronal circuit provide, however, a distinctive mechanism for generating rhythmic behavior at the supracellular level (Selverston and Moulins, 1985).

Phase plane analysis provides a unifying framework that demonstrates the necessary link between excitable and oscillatory behavior in biochemical as well as neural systems. Similar phase portraits are obtained regardless of the physicochemical nature of the variables and the molecular details of the underlying mechanisms. Besides simple periodic behavior, complex oscillatory phenomena such as bursting, chaos, multiple oscillations, and birhythmicity can also occur in all these systems; the latter phenomenon, however, has not yet been demonstrated experimentally in neurobiology or in biochemistry.

A further link between biochemical and neural oscillations regards their physiological function. In both cases, it appears that rhythmic behavior allows for the frequency encoding of signals in intercellular communication (Rapp, 1987; Li and Goldbeter, 1989; Goldbeter, 1990). Thus, in *Dictyostelium*, the amount of cAMP synthesized in response to pulses of cAMP depends on the frequency of the pulsatile signal (Li and Goldbeter, 1990). Likewise, Ca^{2+} oscillations, whose period varies according to the magnitude of the stimulus, could be encoded in terms of their frequency through protein phosphorylation by a Ca^{2+}-activated protein kinase (Berridge and Galione, 1988; Goldbeter et al., 1990). In neurons as well, the response of a target cell often depends on the frequency of the incoming action potentials, which is in turn dictated by the intensity of stimulation. Some of the clearest examples of frequency encoding in neurobiology relate to secretory processes (Cazalis et al., 1985; Whim and Lloyd, 1989). Other instances may arise in the coherent oscillatory response of the cortex to specific stimuli (Eckhorn et al., 1988; Gray and Singer, 1989; Gray et al., 1989).

Another well known example of frequency encoded signal arises in endocrinology (Knobil, 1980). Thus, in the rhesus monkey, gonadotropin-releasing hormone (GnRH) signals must be released by the hypothalamus in a pulsatile manner, at the appropriate frequency close to one pulse per hour, to induce successfully the release of gonadotropin hormones by target cells in the pituitary. A most intriguing question is that of the cellular mechanisms underlying the generation of slow electrical oscillations of a period of the order of an hour, responsible for the periodic generation of the GnRH signal. Recent results (Y.X. Li and A. Goldbeter, in preparation) indicate that such slower rhythmic activity in the brain could involve the reversible, covalent modification of ion channels. When incorporating into a model for bursting (Rinzel, 1987) the assumption that a potassium conductance is activated through phosphorylation by a calcium-dependent protein kinase, slow rhythms of a period of up to an hour or more can be readily generated by assuming that the inactivation of the channel by dephosphorylation proceeds in a sufficiently slow manner, owing to the reduced rate of the phosphatase. This approach shows how the coupling of electrical excitability with biochemical regulatory mechanisms could give rise to slow neuronal oscillations.

Acknowledgments. This work was supported by the Belgian National Incentive Program for Fundamental Research in the Life Sciences (Convention BIO/08) launched by the Science Programming Policy Unit of the Prime Minister's Office (SPPS).

References

Adams WB, Benson JA (1985): The generation and modulation of endogenous rhythmicity in the *Aplysia* bursting pacemaker neurone R15. *Prog Biophys Mol Biol* 46:1–49

Adams WB, Benson JA (1989): Rhythmic neuronal burst generation: experiment and theory. In: *Cell to Cell Signalling: From Experiments to Theoretical Models*, Goldbeter A, ed. London: Academic Press, pp 29–45

Aihara K, Matsumoto G (1982): Temporally coherent organization and instabilities in squid giant axon. *J Theor Biol* 95:697–720

Babloyantz A, Destexhe A (1986): Low-dimensional chaos in an instance of epilepsy. *Proc Natl Acad Sci USA* 83:3513–3517

Berridge MJ, Galione A (1988): Cytosolic calcium oscillators. *FASEB J* 2:3074–3082

Berridge MJ, Rapp PE (1979): A comparative survey of the function, mechanism and control of cellular oscillations. *J Exp Biol* 81:217–279

Cazalis M, Dayanithi G, Nordmann JJ (1985): The role of patterned burst and interburst interval on the excitation-coupling mechanism in the isolated rat neural lobe. *J Physiol* 369:45–60

Cuthbertson KSR (1989): Intracellular calcium oscillators. In: *Cell to Cell Signalling: From Experiments to Theoretical Models*, Goldbeter A, ed. London: Academic Press, pp 435–447.

Decroly O, Goldbeter A (1982): Birhythmicity, chaos, and other patterns of temporal self-organization in a multiply regulated biochemical system. *Proc Natl Acad Sci USA* 79:6917–6921

Decroly O, Goldbeter A (1987): From simple to complex oscillatory behaviour: analysis of bursting in a multiply regulated biochemical system. *J Theor Biol* 124:219–250

Devreotes PN (1982): Chemotaxis. In: *The Development of Dictyostelium discoideum*, Loomis WF, ed. New York: Academic Press, pp 117–168

Dupont G, Berridge M J, Goldbeter A (1991): Signal-induced Ca^{2+} oscillations: Properties of a model based on Ca^{2+}-induced Ca^{2+} release. *Cell Calcium* 12:73–85

Durston AJ (1974): Pacemaker mutants of *Dictyostelium discoideum*. *Dev Biol* 38:308–319

Eckhorn R, Bauer R, Jordan W, Brosch M, Kruse W, Munk M, Reitboeck HJ (1988): Coherent oscillations: a mechanism of feature linking in the visual cortex? Multiple electrode and correlation analyses in the cat. *Biol Cybern* 60:121–130

Fitzhugh R (1961): Impulses and physiological states in theoretical models of nerve membranes. *Biophys J* 1:445–466

Gadsby DC, Wit AL (1981): Electrophysiologic characteristics of cardiac cells and the genesis of cardiac arrhythmias. In: *Cardiac Pharmacology*. New York: Academic Press, pp 229–274

Gerisch G, Malchow D, Roos W, Wick U (1979): Oscillations of cyclic nucleotide concentrations in relation to the excitability of *Dictyostelium* cells. *J Exp Biol* 81: 33–47

Gerisch G, Wick U (1975): Intracellular oscillations and release of cyclic AMP from *Dictyostelium* cells. *Biochem Biophys Res Commun* 65: 364–370

Glass L, Mackey MC (1988): *From Clocks to Chaos: The Rhythms of Life*. Princeton: Princeton University Press

Goldbeter A (1990): *Rythmes et chaos dans les systèmes biochimiques et cellulaires*. Masson: Paris. (An English translation is to be published by Cambridge University Press under the title *Rhythms and chaos in biochemical and cellular systems*)

Goldbeter A, Caplan SR (1976): Oscillatory enzymes. *Annu Rev Biophys Bioeng* 5: 449–476

Goldbeter A, Dupont G, Berridge MJ (1990): Minimal model for signal-induced Ca^{2+} oscillations and for their frequency encoding through protein phosphorylation. *Proc Natl Acad Sci USA* 87: 1461–1465

Goldbeter A, Moran F (1988): Dynamics of a biochemical system with multiple oscillatory domains as a clue for multiple modes of neuronal oscillations. *Eur Biophys J* 15: 277–287

Goldbeter A, Segel LA (1980): Control of developmental transitions in the cyclic AMP signaling system of *Dictyostelium discoideum*. *Differentiation* 17: 127–135

Goldbeter A, Wurster B (1989): Regular oscillations in suspensions of a putatively chaotic mutant of *Dictyostelium discoideum*. *Experientia* 45: 363–365

Gray CM, König P, Engel AK, Singer W (1989): Oscillatory responses in cat visual cortex exhibit inter-columnar synchronization which reflects global stimulus properties. *Nature* 338: 334–337

Gray CM, Singer W (1989): Stimulus-specific neuronal oscillations in orientation columns of cat visual cortex. *Proc Natl Acad Sci USA* 86: 1698–1702

Guttman R, Lewis S, Rinzel J (1980): Control of repetitive firing in squid axon membrane as a model for a neuroneoscillator. *J Physiol (Lond)* 305: 377–395

Halloy J, Li YX, Martiel JL, Wurster B, Goldbeter A (1990): Coupling chaotic and periodic cells results in a period-doubling route to chaos in a model for cAMP oscillations in *Dictyostelium* suspensions. *Phys Lett A* 151: 33–36 and 159: 442

Hess B, Boiteux A (1971): Oscillatory phenomena in biochemistry. *Annu Rev Biochem* 40: 237–258

Holden AV, Ed. (1986) *Chaos*. Manchester: Manchester University Press

Holden AV, Winlow W, Haydon PG (1982): The induction of periodic and chaotic activity in a molluscan neurone. *Biol Cybern* 43: 169–173

Holden AV, Yoda M (1981): Ionic channels density of an excitable membrane can act as bifurcation parameter. *Biol Cybern* 42: 29–38

Huxley AH (1959): Ion movements during nerve activity. *Ann NY Acad Sci* 81: 221–246

Jacob R (1990): Calcium oscillations in electrically non-excitable cells. *Biochim Biophys Acta* 1052: 427–438

Jahnsen H, Llinás R (1984): Ionic basis for the electroresponsiveness and oscillatory properties of guinea-pig thalamic neurones in vitro. *J Physiol (Lond)* 349: 227–247

Johnston D, Brown TH (1984): Mechanism of neuronal burst generation. In: *Electrophysiology of Epilepsy*. New York: Academic Press, pp 277–301

Knobil E (1980): The neuroendocrine control of the menstrual cycle. *Rec Prog Horm Res* 36: 53–88

Kuba K, Takeshita S (1981): Simulation of intracellular Ca^{2+} oscillation in a sympathetic neurone. *J Theor Biol* 93:1009–1031

Li YX, Goldbeter A (1989): Frequency specificity in intercellular communication: The influence of patterns of periodic signaling on target cell responsiveness. *Biophys J* 55:125–145

Li YX, Goldbeter A (1990): Frequency encoding of pulsatile signals of cyclic AMP based on receptor desensitization in *Dictyostelium* cells. *J Theor Biol* 146:355–367

Li YX, Halloy J, Martiel JL, Wurster B, Goldbeter A (1992): Suppression of chaos by periodic oscillations in a model for cyclic AMP signalling in *Dictyostelium* cells. *Experientia* (in press)

Llinás R (1988): The intrinsic electrophysiological properties of mammalian neurons: a new insight into CNS function. *Science* 242:1654–1664

Markus M, Hess B (1984): Transitions between oscillatory modes in a glycolytic model system. *Proc Natl Acad Sci USA* 81:4394–4398

Martiel JL, Goldbeter A (1985): Autonomous chaotic behaviour of the slime mould *Dictyostelium discoideum* predicted by a model for cyclic AMP signaling. *Nature* 313:590–592

Martiel JL, Goldbeter A (1987): A model based on receptor desensitization for cyclic AMP signaling in *Dictyostelium* cells. *Biophys J* 52:807–828

Meyer T, Stryer L (1988): Molecular model for receptor-stimulated calcium spiking. *Proc Natl Acad Sci USA* 85:5051–5055

Minorsky N (1962): *Nonlinear Oscillations*. Princeton: Van Nostrand

Nicolis G, Prigogine I (1977): *Self-Organization in Nonequilibrium Systems. From Dissipative Structures to Order through Fluctuations*. New York: Wiley

Olsen LF, Degn H (1985): Chaos in biological systems. *Q Rev Biophys* 18:165–225

Rapp PE (1987): Why are so many biological systems periodic? *Prog Neurobiol* 29: 261–273

Rapp PE, Bashore TR, Martinerie JM, Albano AM, Mees AI (1989): Dynamics of brain electrical activity. *Brain Topogr* 2:99–118

Rinzel J (1985): Excitation dynamics: insights from simplified membrane models. *Fed Proc* 44:2944–2946

Rinzel J (1987): A formal classification of bursting mechanisms in excitable systems. *Lect Notes Biomath* 71:267–281

Roschke J, Başar E (1988): The EEG is not simple noise: strange attractors in intracranial structures. In: *Dynamics of Sensory and Cognitive Processing in the Brain*, Başar E, ed., *Springer Series in Brain Dynamics*. Berlin: Springer–Verlag, 1:203–216

Rose RM, Hindmarsh JL (1985): A model for a thalamic neuron. *Proc R Soc Lond B* 225:161–193

Rose RM, Hindmarsh JL (1989): The assembly of ionic currents in a thalamic neuron. III. The seven-dimensional model. *Proc R Soc Lond B* 237:313–334

Selverston AI, Moulins M (1985): Oscillatory neural networks. *Annu Rev Physiol* 47: 29–48

Skarda CA, Freeman WJ (1987): How brain makes chaos in order to make sense of the world. *Behav Brain Sci* 10:161–195

Tsien RW, Kass RL, Weingart R (1979): Cellular and subcellular mechanisms of cardiac pacemaker oscillations. *J Exp Biol* 81:205–215

Whim MD, Lloyd PE (1989): Frequency-dependent release of peptide cotransmitters from identified cholinergic motor neurons in *Aplysia Proc Natl Acad Sci USA* 86: 9034–9038

Signal Functions of Brain Electrical Rhythms and their Modulation by External Electromagnetic Fields

W. Ross Adey

In setting a rubric for this volume, Bullock has defined induced brain rhythms as "oscillations caused or modulated by stimuli or state changes that do not directly drive successive cycles." This perspective offers an opportunity to evaluate two sets of related but inverse problems. There are *tonic* responses to rhythmic stimuli, responses that extend beyond a brief epoch of rhythmic stimulation. There are also *phasic* responses to continuing rhythmic stimuli.

Their significance in brain functions has been revealed through imposition of electromagnetic (EM) fields as tools that induce brain tissue fields mimicking in varying degrees components of intrinsic brain electrical rhythms. Initial studies centered on modulation of brain ionic mechanisms (Adey, 1981a, 1981b; Bawin and Adey, 1976; Bawin et al., 1975, 1978) and behavioral responses (Gavalas et al., 1970; Gavalas-Medici and Day-Magdaleno, 1976). They were followed by investigations of developmental modifications and behavioral teratology following embryonic and fetal exposures (Delgado et al., 1982; Juutilainen et al., 1986a, 1986b; McGivern et al., 1990; Sikov et al., 1987).

These studies in brain tissue have led to the investigation of possible similar phenomena in nonnervous tissue, with the conclusion that sensitivity to weak low-frequency EM fields may be a general biological property of cells in tissue (Adey, 1988a, 1988b; 1989a, 1989b, 1989c; 1990a, 1990b, 1990c), and pointing to a private language of intrinsic tissue communication by which cells may "whisper together" in activities such as metabolic cooperation and growth regulation.

Intracellular enzymes mediating metabolic, messenger, and growth functions have been used as molecular markers of transductive coupling of EM fields in cell surface receptor mechanisms: adenylate cyclase (Luben et al., 1982; Luben and Cain, 1984), protein kinases (Byus et al., 1984), and ornithine decarboxylase (Byus et al., 1987, 1988).

Evidence for "Tissue Tuning" in Response to a Spectrum of Low-Frequency EM Fields

We focus here in some detail on release of calcium from brain tissue exposed to EM fields, since this response provided the first evidence of a sensitivity to imposed EM fields (Kaczmarek and Adey, 1973, 1974). Concurrent observations indicated that this modulation of calcium efflux occurs in narrow bands of field frequency and intensity. It should also be emphasized that the field-sensitive enzyme systems just cited are all calcium-dependent.

Initial studies of EM field effects in cerebral tissue examined modulation of Ca efflux from isolated chick cerebral cortex (Bawin and Adey, 1976; Bawin et al., 1975). Ca efflux follows a "tuning curve" across an EM field spectrum from 0 to 35 Hz, peaking in the vicinity of 16 Hz. As will be discussed, this phenomenon of a windowed frequency response has also been seen in other cellular sensitivities, including enzyme activity (Byus et al., 1984), allogeneic cytotoxicity (Lyle et al., 1983), and mitogen release (Fitzsimmons et al., 1986, 1989).

EM field intensity is another factor showing windowed interactions in calcium efflux from isolated chick cerebral hemisphere. With capacitively coupled electric fields at 16 Hz that induced tissue gradients in the range 10^{-7} V/cm, $^{45}Ca^{2+}$ efflux was reduced by as much as 15% with fields in air of 10 V/m ($p < 0.01$) and 56 V/m ($p < 0.05$), but efflux changes with fields of 5 and 100 V/m were not significant (Bawin and Adey, 1976).

Results of similar studies with isolated cat cerebral cortex also suggested a matrix of frequency and intensity windowing. Significant reduction in $^{45}Ca^{2+}$ efflux occurred at 6 Hz ($p < 0.05$) and 16 Hz ($p < 0.01$) with 56 V/m field gradients in air. Nonsignificant trends toward decreased efflux also occurred at 1, 32, and 75 Hz at this field strength. No significant effects were observed with 10 V/m at 6, 16, and 32 Hz, nor with 100 V/m fields at 6 and 16 Hz. Again, these data support a tuning curve with maximal tissue sensitivity in the vicinity of 6 and 16 Hz, and at a field amplitude between 56 and 100 V/m (Bawin and Adey, 1976).

There is evidence for frequency and intensity windowing in this modulation of cerebral Ca efflux by EM fields over a quite broad low-frequency spectrum (Blackman et al., 1985a, 1985b). Although complex, the findings suggest a series of frequency and amplitude windows. Although there was no enhanced efflux with a 42-Hz field at 30, 40, 50, or 60 V/m, a 45-Hz field caused enhanced efflux at around 40 V/m. A 50-Hz field enhanced efflux in a narrower region between 45 and 50 V/m, but 60-Hz fields enhanced efflux only at 35 and 40 V/m, intensities slightly lower than those that are effective at 50 Hz. Finally, a frequency scan for a 42.5-V/m field revealed two regions eliciting enhanced efflux, one centered at 15 Hz, and the other extending from 45 to 105 Hz.

An Experiential Stamp on Embryonic Brain Tissue: $^{45}Ca^{2+}$ Efflux Following Prenatal Exposures, 60-Hz versus 50-Hz Fields

Is there evidence of a lasting, frequency-specific effect from chronic exposure of embryonic brain tissue to environmental EM fields? And if so, can this be detected by a chemical marker?

Blackman et al. (1988) exposed fertilized domestic hen's eggs continuously during their 21-day incubation to either 50- or 60-Hz sinusoidal electric fields at an average intensity of 10 V/m. Within 1.5 days after hatching, $^{45}Ca^{2+}$ ion efflux from the brain was tested in either 50- or 60-Hz EM fields (15.9 V/m and 73 nT in a local geomagnetic field of 38 uT, 35°N). For eggs exposed to 60-Hz electric fields during incubation, the chicken brains showed a significant response to 50-Hz fields, but not to 60-Hz fields. In contrast brains exposed to 50-Hz fields during incubation were not affected by either 50- or 60- Hz fields. The investigators conclude that exposure of a developing organism to ambient fields at the U.S. power-line frequency of 60 Hz at levels typically found inside buildings can alter the response of brain tissue to field-induced calcium ion efflux.

Phasic Responses to Continuing Stimuli

Weak EM fields at electroencephalogram (EEG) frequencies can be used as a direct central nervous stimulus with a variety of experimental endpoints. They may evoke broad changes in brain states, as in shifting states from sleep to wakefulness, or in a redistribution of sleep levels.

Among the EEG concomitants of this tonic field stimulation (Bawin et al., 1973; Gavalas et al., 1970) are evoked bursts of EEG rhythms at around the field frequency (or in the case of imposed radiofrequency fields, at modulation frequencies within the EEG spectrum).

Phase Detection in Hippocampal and Midbrain Reticular Formation EEG Records

Regularity of cat hippocampal EEG wave trains during a visual task performance with delayed response has been assessed with continuous phase-and-amplitude examination (Adey and Walter, 1963), revealing a rhythmic phase modulation on wave trains that appear as a single frequency during visual discrimination. By contrast with wide excursions in frequency and amplitude that occurred in the delay period, the frequency record during discrimination showed a narrow spectrum between 5 and 6 Hz, and also clearly indicated a rhythmic frequency or phase modulation at 1 to 2 Hz on this "carrier" frequency of 5 Hz.

Also, the relative-amplitude readout frequently showed amplitude modulation at much the same frequency as the phase modulation. Since care was taken to eliminate possible interaction between amplitude and frequency modulation in the analysis, it was concluded that their occurrence simultaneously at essentially identical rates was validly detected and that they were independent of one another. Probability bounds in EEG cross-spectral analysis of records from different hippocampal regions indicated major differences in patterns of phase relations occurring in correct and incorrect responses, patterns that were consistent in different responses.

EEG Rhythm Bursts Evoked by Low-Frequency EM Fields

Imposed EM fields that mimic aspects of the EEG may be used as tools to manipulate the central processes of behavioral conditioning, and at the same time to study concurrent EEG patterns. Coupling of imposed fields to the brain is a function of field frequency.

Thus, sinusoidal low-frequency electric fields at 7 to 10 Hz, with an electric gradient in air of 10 V/m, would produce a very small tissue gradient of the order of 10^{-7} V/cm, based on simple capacitive coupling. On the other hand, for radiofrequency fields, coupling may be much stronger, since the dimensions of bodies of mammals, including man, may be a significant portion of a wavelength at the frequency of the imposed field. The body may therefore function as an efficient antenna. Thus, a 100-MHz radiofrequency field with an incident energy of 1.0 mW/cm^2 (electric gradient in air 61 V/m) would induce a tissue gradient in the body of man in the range of 10^{-2}-10^{-1} V/cm: approximately 10^6 greater than that induced by the ELF electric field. We may expect that consequences of EM field exposure in EEG patterns and behavioral states would occur more rapidly with fields inducing larger tissue gradients.

In electric fields of 2.8 V_{p-p}/m at 7 Hz, monkey hippocampal EEG records showed a slow increment in EEG spectral activity at the field frequency over a 4-hr exposure period, as compared with sham no-field exposures (Gavalas et al., 1970). Concurrent behavioral testing in these animals involved a subjective estimate of a 5-s interval. The estimate was significantly shortened in the 7-Hz field.

A related study in cats examined EEG and behavioral performance while continuously exposed to a 147-MHz radiofrequency field (incident energy 1.0 mW/cm^2), amplitude-modulated at EEG frequencies (Bawin et al., 1973). The induced brain field was in the same intensity range as the EEG measured at cellular dimensions in perineuronal fluid (10–100 V/cm). Cats were operantly trained to produce specific transient EEG rhythms in cortical and subcortical structures, following presentation of a light flash at 30-s intervals. Each animal was tested in conditioning and extinction trials. In one series, the imposed fields were modulated at the dominant frequencies of these selected EEG transient patterns and in a control group, testing was in the absence of fields. The exposed animals differed markedly from the control group in the rate of performance, accuracy (in terms of frequency bandwidth) of the reinforced patterns, and resistance to extinction (minimum of 50 days vs. 10 days).

In the same study, the specificity of the low-frequency amplitude-modulation was tested in another group of animals where spontaneous transient

EEG rhythm bursts in cortical and subcortical structures were used to trigger short epochs (20 s following every burst) of the radiofrequency field, amplitude-modulated at various EEG frequencies. The fields clearly acted as reinforcers (increasing the rate of occurrence of the spontaneous rhythm bursts) only when modulated at frequencies close to the biologically dominant frequency of the selected intrinsic EEG rhythmic episodes.

Special precautions are necessary to preclude antenna effects that might be associated with fields induced in wire leads to cerebral structures in studies of this type, since 1) they might stimulate tissue at the electrode recording site, and 2) they might contaminate EEG spectral analyses. In the monkey study cited above, visual inspection of EEG records did not reveal any obvious field components. However, spectral analysis revealed small peaks in power from some brain structures (hippocampus, amygdala, and centrum medianum) at the field frequency for epochs of predominantly incorrect responses near the end of the 4-hr run. In the cat studies, the shielded leads were also filtered (120-dB attenuation at 147 MHz). For this radiofrequency field, artifacts, due to voltages induced and rectified at the electrode–tissue contact, would be expected to appear uniformly at all electrodes, and to be present, unchanged, during the field exposure. In fact, no evidence of generalized or sustained artifacts was seen. EEG changes were anatomically localized, highly specific in terms of frequency and associated with transient patterns, with the conclusion that the tissue effects are not attributable to direct injection of field voltages via electrodes.

Minimal Duration of a Specific Frequency in Rhythmic Stimulation to Elicit Enzyme Activation

If there are specificities in EM field frequency for cell functions modulated by these exposures, is there a required minimum duration (coherence time) of exposure at a specific frequency before a response ensues? Can this requirement be assessed by an established molecular marker, such as intracellular enzyme marker? This question has been addressed in cultures of an adherent line of mouse fibroblasts (L929) exposed to an amplitude-modulated 0.9-GHz microwave field (Krause et al., 1990). The highly inducible enzyme ornithine decarboxylase (ODC) was used as a marker.

First, monolayer cultures of logarithmically growing L929 cells were exposed to unmodulated (continuous wave) 0.9-GHz microwaves, or to the same microwave signal amplitude-modulated at 60 Hz [specific absorption rate (SAR) 3 mW/g]. No enhanced ODC activity ensued with unmodulated fields, but an 8-hr (optimal) exposure to the 60-Hz modulated field enhanced ODC activity 2.1-fold.

The role of coherence time was then tested by shifting the modulation frequency from 55 to 65 Hz at user-selected intervals. Short coherence times of 0.1 and 1.0 s failed to enhance ODC activity. But epochs of 10.0 and 50.0 s enhanced ODC activity to levels seen with 60-Hz modulation; epochs of 5.0 s gave intermediate values (1.71 over control). Thus, the cells responded fully to the applied field only when the coherence time exceeded a minimum value between 5.0 and 10 s.

Whole-Body Vibration: Effects on Short-Term Memory and EEG

Aircrew and astronauts are frequently required to perform complex tasks during whole-body vibration. Manual control and visual monitoring may be disrupted by involuntary movements of the hand (McLeod and Griffin, 1986) or eye (Moseley and Griffin, 1986). As a rhythmic stimulus, whole-body vibration elicits an intense multimodal sensory barrage from surface, proprioceptive, enteroceptive, and vestibular receptors. EEG (Adey et al., 1967) and cognitive (Sherwood and Griffin, 1990) effects have been reported. Laboratory testing in man and animals uses an electrodynamic vibrator, similar to a voice-coil operated loudspeaker and driven by an oscillator that typically covers the extremely low-frequency (ELF) spectrum (nominally 0–300 Hz).

Sherwood and Griffin (1990) exposed human subjects to 16-Hz sinusoidal whole-body vibration at four magnitudes: 0, 1.0, 1.6, and 2.5 ms^{-2} rms. Subjects were tested in a short-term memory task that avoided direct mechanical action of vibration on visual and manual control. Vibration adversely affected performance, as measured by mean reaction time ($p < 0.001$) and number of attentional lapses ($p < 0.01$). They conclude that vibration disrupts central cognitive mechanisms used in processing information in short-term memory.

EEG studies in the intact monkey (*Macaca nemestrina*) and after eighth nerve section produced supportive evidence for vibration-induced modulation of brain electrical patterns (Adey et al., 1967). These monkeys were exposed to vibration over a continuous spectral sweep from 5 to 40 Hz. EEG analyses involved extensive calculations of auto- and cross-spectra, including calculations of shared amplitudes, phase angles, and coherence.

The induced EEG rhythmicity occurred at certain frequencies of whole-body vibration and had the characteristics of EEG "driving," and appeared distinguishable from superficially similar phenomena of artifactual origin. For example, autospectral density plots showed little or no evidence of EEG driving below 9 Hz, despite powerful head movements. Driving at the vibration rate was frequency selective and maximal in the range of 10 to 15 Hz. However, in many instances, maximum EEG energy peaks occurred at other than shaking frequencies, and without harmonic relationship to shaking frequencies.

Coherence calculations (a measure of linear predictability) was high between cortical and subcortical leads at EEG frequencies unrelated to concurrent vibration frequencies and absent from baseline records before and after vibration. This may imply aspects of cerebral system organization with ephemeral sharing of activity elicited by the vibratory volleys. Coherence of head and table accelerometers with cortical and subcortical leads was below significant levels at fundamental driving frequencies below 11 Hz, although significant coherence peaks appeared at other EEG frequencies. Shaking in the 11 to 17-Hz range produced many coherent relationships at fundamental driving frequencies and at harmonically related and unrelated EEG frequencies. Bilateral eighth nerve section did not abolish this driving.

Collective "Heads" with Regional EEG Spectral Signatures in Defined Behavioral Situations: Development of a Human EEG "Normative Library"

Are there common factors that would categorize EEG records from a group of subjects for a series of specified behavioral states? Our studies (Walter et al., 1967) established existence of these signatures for the first time, in test states covering a wide gamut from quiet wakefulness to extreme focusing of attention, and in the various stages of sleep. A "normative library" (a term coined in this study and subsequently gaining wide currency) of EEG data was acquired from 200 astronaut candidates. Collective and individual patterns were detected in 50 of these subjects by extensive spectral analysis and pattern recognition.

A tape recorded test protocol ensured uniformity of task presentation to all subjects. The tests included recurrent somatic, auditory, and visual stimuli and behavioral tasks at different levels of difficulty. They ranged from simple auditory vigilance tasks, with a requirement to recognize presence or absence of three tones in a series presented at 6-s intervals, to recognition of the largest of six circles in a matrix, with a 3-s test epoch in some series and a 1-s epoch in others. The 3-s task required moderate concentration but the 1-s epoch was near the limit of performance capability in many subjects.

After computation of EEG spectra for each subject over all test situations, averages were prepared for each of 50 subjects at each scalp electrode location (in a modified 10–20 configuration). These analyses used EEG epochs lasting 10 s. The average was over 12 situations, including eyes closed at rest, eyes open at rest, eyes closed during 1/s flash stimuli, and during the auditory vigilance task and the visual discriminations presented at 3- and 1-s intervals. The contours of these "lumped" spectra became the basis for comparison with the spectra for individual situations. This comparison then generated a "head" displaying, as a bar graph at each scalp location, variations (as the standard deviation of power at each frequency of the spectrum) about the mean established by the average of the 12 situations.

With 1/s flashes there was a marked increase in the power of the alpha peak in central and vertex leads, a broadening of this midspectral peak in parietal areas, and a major increase in spectral power at all frequencies, even though the low flash rate was clearly not responsible for any driving phenomenon.

The auditory vigilance task produced a pattern distinctly different from that during slow repetition of flashes or during visual discriminative performances. Vertex, parieto-occipital, and temporo-occipital leads showed distinctly bimodal spectral distributions, with separate peaks centered around 10 and 20 Hz. Thus, the most striking changes occurred in the temporo-parieto-occipital belt of cortex.

During the visual discrimination tasks, EEG spectra were distinctly different from those in either resting records or vigilance tasks. In the 3-s tests, frontal activity incremented sharply over the whole spectrum, declining gradually toward central and vertex leads, where the alpha peak noted in other tests was sharply reduced to levels below the multisituational mean. In bi-occipital leads, powers above 2 Hz were reduced below the group mean at all frequencies. Trends observed in 3-s tests were more obvious in those lasting only 1 s, but the two "heads" were similar.

ON- and OFF-Phenomena in Nonnervous Systems Associated with Intermittent EM Field Exposure

Adaptation in responses to repeated stimulus presentation is well recognized in central nervous organization, particularly in orienting responses to brief auditory or visual stimuli as an aspect of waning novelty after their initial presentation. In nonnervous systems, environmental EM fields may also elicit a transient response that wanes despite continuing field exposure. Two examples are discussed here: one involving a transient ON- response of lymphocyte protein kinases, and the other occurring as an OFF- response in activation of bone cell adenylate cyclase at the conclusion of EM field exposure.

ON-Response of Human Lymphocyte Protein Kinases to Initiation of EM Field Exposure

In all eukaryotic cells, activity of the membrane-related enzyme adenylate cyclase is essential in conversion of adenosine triphosphate to cyclic adenosine monophosphate (cAMP), releasing metabolic energy; its stripped phosphate groups activate protein kinase messenger enzymes. In addition to these cAMP-dependent protein kinases, other groups of protein kinases are functionally active without interaction with cAMP. The latter include protein kinase C, playing an essential role in regulation of cell growth and responses to chemical cancer promoters (phorbol esters) that act at cell membranes. In *Aplysia* neurons, a role for protein kinase C has been reported in regulation of transmembrane Ca movement (DeRiemer et al., 1985).

In cultures of human tonsil lymphocytes (Byus et al., 1984), activity of cAMP-dependent protein kinases remained unaltered relative to controls when exposed to a 450-MHz field (peak envelope intensity 1.0 mW/cm^2) sinusoidally amplitude-modulated at frequencies of 16 or 60 Hz for 15, 30, and 60 min. By contrast, total non–cAMP-dependent protein kinase activity fell to less than 50% of unexposed control levels after 15- and 30-min exposure, but, despite continuing field exposure, returned to control or preexposure levels at 45 and 60 min. With 60-Hz modulation, a smaller reduction (20–25%) was also restricted to exposure durations of 15 and 30 min. Unmodulated fields had no effect. In the frequency domain, reduced enzyme activity occurred with 16-, 40-, and 60-Hz modulation, but not with 3-, 6-, 80-, or 100-Hz modulation. This rapid but transient reduction in protein kinase activity is consistent with "windowing" with respect to modulation frequency and exposure duration.

Phasic Responses in Bone Cells to EM Field Exposure

Parathyroid hormone (PTH) strongly stimulates adenylate cyclase in bone cells, an essential step in regulation of bone growth and an action sensitive to low-frequency pulsed magnetic fields used in therapy of fracture non-union (Luben et al., 1982). Luben noted an inhibition of this adenylate cyclase response to PTH by as much as 90% in the presence of either of two pulsed magnetic fields (72-Hz pulse train or 15-Hz pulse bursts, burst duration 5 ms, pulse repetition rate 4 KHz, field peak intensities 8 gauss).

In cultured bone samples and in monolayer cultures of an osteoblastlike cell line (MMB-1) exposed for 48 hr, this inhibition was observed only as an OFF- response after cessation of field exposure (Luben and Cain, 1984). It may be noted that this regulatory action involves induced pericellular field components that were only in the range of 1 to 3 mV/cm at a current density approximating 1.0 μA/cm^2, or expressed in terms the rate of change of the magnetic field pulses, 0.6 μA/cm^2 per T/s (Fitton Jackson, 1985). The Hodgkin–Huxley model of nerve fiber excitation envisages a transmembrane current at threshold in the range of 1.0 mA/cm^2. Taking account of the higher impedance of this transmembrane path when compared with pericellular fluid, these induced currents would be 10^6 below a Hodgkin–Huxley excitation threshold (1.0 mA/cm^2), further suggesting that these sensitivities may have a basis in nonequilibrium thermodynamic interactions (Adey, 1990a, 1990b, 1990c).

Related studies of mineralization in embryonic bone tissue have tested a series of intermittent exposure schedules (Fitton Jackson, 1985), using protein-bound ^{45}Ca to assess its seeding in newly formed osteoid material. The 15-Hz pulse train stimulus delivered 6 hr daily for 7 days increased uptake by 40% or more, but incorporation dropped backed to control levels with prolonged exposure. By contrast, the 72-Hz single pulse train stimulus was only effective with a 9-hr ON/3hr OFF schedule; if the frequency of the single pulse train was reduced from 72 to 15 Hz, the incorporation of ^{45}Ca with both 6-hr and 9-hr ON schedules was raised 75% to 100% in comparison with controls.

Tonic Responses to Rhythmic Stimuli

We consider here neural and nonneural responses that persist beyond a period of rhythmic EM field stimulation. In neural tissue, they include persisting EEG rhythms at an imposed field frequency and neuroendocrine and neurobehavioral teratology following fetal exposure. In nonneural systems, we cite enzymatic responses in growth regulation, effects on growth regulation in cell cocultures, modulation of gap junction-mediated toxin actions, and spectral "tuning" in field-modulated enhancement and inhibition of cell growth.

Poststimulus EEG Rhythms Induced by Long-Term Pulsed Microwave Exposure and by ELF-Modulated Radiofrequency Fields

High frequency EEG rhythms have been detected in rats following termination of prolonged exposure to pulsed microwave fields. These rhythms were locked to the pulse repetition frequency (PRF) of the microwave field (Servantie et al., 1975). Rats were exposed for 10 days to a 3-GHz pulsed field (1 μs pulses, average field intensity 5 mW/cm^2, PRF 525 pulses/s). Control animals were maintained under the same environmental conditions. A sharp spectral line at the PRF was detected postexposure in occipital records. This spectral line was not detected with an unstable PRF, nor in control animals. This synchronized EEG record was intermittent, appearing for 1 to 2 min, then disappearing for several minutes.

A similarly persistent modification of EEG patterns induced by long-term EM field exposure has been reported in rabbits (Takashima et al., 1979). Rabbits were exposed for 2 hr daily for 6 weeks to radiofrequency fields at 1 to 10 MHz with 15-Hz sinusoidal modulation. EEG records were acquired with silver electrodes glued on the skull surface, with only 3 to 4-cm connecting leads protruding to the exterior. EEGs were recorded only before and after field exposure. These modulated RF fields enhanced low frequency components and reduced high frequency activity in EEG spectra. However, since the experiments were conducted under pentobarbital anesthesia, precise interpretation of specific frequency changes remains unclear. In acute experiments with 60-Hz modulation, no EEG changes were detected.

Prenatal Exposure to Low Frequency Pulsed Magnetic Fields Demasculinizes Adult Rat Scent Marking Behavior and Increases Accessory Sex Organ Weights

Periods have been delineated in early development when hormones most readily elicit long-lasting changes in sex-related behaviors (Goy and McEwen, 1980). In the rat this time of greatest susceptibility to the organizational action of gonadal steroids is during the last week of gestation and continues for 4 or 5 days after parturition. Complete masculinization of the male brain during this period is dependent on normal secretory patterns of testosterone as well as on normal ontogenetic development of the brain, especially regions that are sensitive to steroid actions, such as the amygdala and hypothalamus.

This system appears sensitive to EM field exposure (McGivern et al., 1990). Pregnant Sprague–Dawley dams were exposed to pulsed magnetic fields (15 Hz, 0.3 ms duration, peak intensity 8 gauss) for 15 min twice daily from day 15 through day 20 of gestation. No differences in litter size, number of stillborns, or body weight were observed in offspring of field-exposed dams. At 120 days of age, field-exposed male offspring exhibited significantly less scent marking behavior than controls. Accessory sex organ (prostate, epididymis, and seminal vesicles) were approximately doubled in field-exposed subjects at this age. However, circulating levels of testosterone, luteinizing hormone, and follicle-stimulating hormone as well as epididymal sperm counts were normal.

These results indicate that EM field exposure did not interfere with the hypothalamic–pituitary–gonadal axis, despite the increased gonadal organ weights, but the decreased scent-marking behavior in field-exposed animals in the presence of normal levels of circulating testosterone suggests a possible central androgen insensitivity to the activational effects of testosterone on this behavior.

Tonic Responses in Nonneural Systems to Low- Frequency Components of EM Fields

Low-frequency fields (and radiofrequency fields with low-frequency modulation) may induce either 1) transient responses to a continuing EM field stimulus, as in the example of lymphocyte protein kinases already cited, or 2) sustained responses that may last substantially beyond the period of initial stimulation. The latter situation is also exemplified by an enzyme, ODC, essential in cell growth. Beyond these categories of immediate enzymatic effects, there are other responses, most also growth-related, in which transient field exposures may exercise long-term effects on aspects of growth regulation.

Ornithine Decarboxylase Stimulation by Weak EM Fields: Responses in Cultured Liver, Skin, Ovary, and Myeloma Cells

ODC is the rate-limiting enzyme in synthesis of the polyamines spermidine and putrescine by decarboxylation of ornithine. In turn, polyamines are required in all cells for DNA synthesis and cell growth. They are also exported from the cell of origin, and have been shown to regulate activity of NMDA receptors in cerebellar neurons (Williams et al., 1991). ODC activity is high in growing cells and in cancer cells.

A 1-hr exposure of human lymphoma CEM cells to a 60-Hz EM field (10 mV/cm) produced a fivefold increase in ODC activity and a two- to threefold increase in P3 mouse myeloma cells (Byus et al., 1987). ODC activity remained elevated for several hours after the field exposure ended. Fields as weak as 0.1 V/cm produced a 30% increase in ODC activity in Reuber H35 hepatoma cells in a 1-hr exposure, but continuous exposure at 10 V/cm for 2 hr and 3 hr produced no change.

A similar study that exposed cells to an athermal 450-MHz microwave field (1.0 mW/cm^2, < 0.1°C temperature rise) sinusoidally amplitude-modulated at 16 Hz also found increased ODC activity (Byus et al., 1988). In Reuber H35 hepatoma cells, a 1-hr exposure increased ODC activity by about 50%. This increase persisted for several hours following exposure. Similar fields modulated at 60 and 100 Hz had no effect. The stimulated ODC activity in these cultured cells that followed treatment with a phorbol ester tumor promoter (tetra-decanoylphorbol acetate, TPA) was further potentiated by prior exposure to this same low-energy field. This field did not alter either basal or TPA-stimulated DNA synthesis. Two additional cell lines (Chinese hamster ovary and 294T melanoma) responded similarly.

EM Fields and Growth Regulation: Cocultures of Normal and Mutant Cells, Modulation of Gap-Junction Organization, and Modulation of Yeast Cell Growth

Available evidence points to cell membranes as the prime tissue site in transductive coupling of imposed EM fields (Adey, 1989a. 1989b, 1989c, 1990a, 1990b, 1990c), as will be discussed. We shall also examine the concept that, in their detection and coupling at cell membranes, EM fields can modulate inward and outward streams of signals that pass through the membrane (see section on cell membranes).

Outward signals, chemical and electrical, influence neighboring cells, in part through specialized protein plaques, the gap-junctions. Substances synthesized in one cell may be essential for the normal health of its neighbor (metabolic cooperation), and can pass to that cell through tiny channels (connexons, about 0.9 nm in diameter) located in the plaque of the gap junction.

Slow electrical events are also coupled through gap-junctions in neural and nonneural tissue. Loss of normal intercellular communication leads to unregulated growth (Yamasaki, 1987) in test sytems of myoblasts, keratinocytes, and fibroblasts (Newmark, 1987). Its restoration inhibits unregulated growth.

Implication of cell membrane dysfunctions in essential steps of tissue growth regulation has led to new concepts of the biology of tumor formation subsumed under the rubric of epigenetic (nongenotoxic) carcinogenesis (Butterworth and Slaga, 1987). Consistent with the generally accepted initiation–promotion model of tumor formation, initiation (transformation) of a cell by damage to nuclear DNA is envisaged as only the first step toward tumor formation. The transformed cell is indeed a cancer cell, but may remain in that condition throughout the life of the individual without tumor formation. For tumor formation to ensue, the initiated cell must be exposed repeatedly and intermittently to promoting agents, which, by definition, are generally incapable of damaging DNA as initiators. Many common chemical promoters (insecticides, PCBs, tobacco smoke condensate, phorbol esters found in croton oil, saccharin) have sites of action at cell membranes.

In the frame of multistep initiation-promotion models of carcinogenesis, there is only limited evidence that environmental EM fields act as initiators by damaging DNA stores in cell nuclei. Aberrations in lymphocyte chromosomes have been reported in radar workers exposed an average of 15 years to fields around 10 to 20 $\mu W/cm^2$ (Garaj-Vhrovac et al., 1990).

By contrast, there is considerable evidence that these fields may participate in the promotion phase by effects on mechanisms regulating cell growth. Powerful chemical promoters that act at cell membranes are enhanced by concurrent cell exposures to EM fields. These chemical cancer promoters direct inward signals from cell membranes to enzymes that regulate growth, including ODC and certain protein kinases, such as protein kinase C. DNA synthesis is increased in mammalian cells by 100-Hz pulsed magnetic fields (Takahashi et al., 1986) and by 16-Hz electric fields in bone cells (Fitzsimmons et al., 1986, 1989). They also interfere with outward signals necessary for intercellular communication, and may thus induce unregulated growth in cells that are thereby isolated. Proto-oncogenes also express proteins that interfere with gap-junction communication. Both low-frequency and radiofrequency fields with low-frequency modulation may act alone at cell membranes to modulate these growth regulating enzymes, or synergically with chemical cancer promoters (for review, see Adey, 1991b).

EM Field Influences on DNA Transcriptional Mechanisms

Exposure of endoreduplicated chromosomes of *Sciara* salivary gland cells to low-frequency EM fields has revealed qualitative and quantitative changes in polypeptide synthesis (Goodman and Henderson, 1988). Transcription autoradiograms showed that previously undetected transcription occurred after exposure of these cells to low-frequency fields with diverse waveforms, causing the appearance of polypeptides, some of which were signal-specific and some identical with heat shock proteins; and with the conclusion that these EM fields activate a limited number of genes that were either previously silent or not detectable.

Evidence of EM field effects on transcription of specific genes has come from nuclear run-off assays, which allow measures of relative rates of gene transcription as a function of the state of the cell. Phillips et al. (1991) have used this assay to assess changes in transcription of early activation genes in human T-lymphoblastoid cells exposed to a 1-gauss 60-Hz magnetic field. There was increased transcription of genes encoding for the proto-oncogenes c-*myc*, c-*fos*, c-*jun*, and protein kinase C, as a function of the nature of the exposure period (continuous vs. multiple ON/OFF periods) and of the density of the cell culture.

Epidemiological studies lend support to the concept of increased risk of brain tumors from EM field exposure, with a possible joint role for EM fields and chemical factors. Workers with 20 or more years' exposure to microwaves and to soldering fumes and/or electronic solvents have a 10-fold increased risk of astrocytomas (Thomas et al., 1987). Brain cancer odds for electrical engineers and technicians were 2.7 in a 16-state study in the years 1985–1986 (Loomis and Savitz, 1990). Electricians in Los Angeles County showed an odds ratio of 4.3 for astrocytoma over 5 years, 1980–1984 (Preston-Martin et al., 1989). New York telephone line-splicers, exposed to weak EM fields and soldering fumes, also showed a higher risk of brain tumors (Matanoski et al., 1991).

Growth Regulation in Cocultures of Normal and Mutant Fibroblasts: 60-Hz Magnetic Fields Increase Foci of Mutants Induced by a Chemical Tumor Promoter

When parental mouse embryonic fibroblasts (C3H10T1/2) were cocultured with mutant daughter cells (UV-TDTx10e) transformed by ultraviolet light (parent/daughter cell ratio around 4 : 1), unregulated mutant cell growth was inhibited by contact with parent cells (Herschman and Brankow, 1986, 1987). This equilibrium was disrupted by the cancer promoter tetradecanoylphorbol acetate (TPA). This recurrence of unregulated growth in the mutants produces defined clumps of growing cells (foci), heaped on one another and forming "tumors in a dish."

This system has offered the first evidence that EM fields affect tumor formation per se (Cain et al., 1991). Chronic intermittent exposure (4 1-hr epochs daily for 28 days) to 60-Hz sinusoidal magnetic fields (1 gauss) enhanced the number of foci formed by mutant daughter cells in cocultures with parental fibroblasts following treatment with TPA promoter. For field-exposed cultures, the number of TPA-induced foci increased by approximately 65% compared to sham-exposed cultures at all TPA concentrations tested (1–100 ng/ml, half-maximal response at 20 ng/ml). The fields alone did not induce focus formation, suggesting that EM fields in conjunction with TPA influenced communication between parental cells and transformants, with more prominent expression of the transformants.

Disruption of Intercellular Communication Through Gap-Junctions by Phorbol Esters and EM Fields

Phorbol esters and other tumor promoters disrupt transfer of chemical signals between cells (Fletcher et al., 1987b; Yotti et al., 1979). Trosko has hypothesized that gap-junctional communication involves a minimum of four systems: recognition by neighboring cells of one another through action of adhesion molecules, such as nerve cell adhesion molecules (nCAMs) in nervous tissue, functional gap-junctions, small regulatory or signaling molecules; and transducing protein receptors for these signaling molecules. Dye transfer techniques offer sensitive measures of inhibition of intercellular communication by cancer promoters (Budunova et al., 1989). In studies of progressive changes in homologous and heterologous communication at selected stages of skin carcinogenesis, there was a progressive loss of homologous, but not heterologous, communication as the neoplastic process increased (Klann et al., 1989).

Fletcher et al. (1987a) noted that blockage of entry of natural cytolytic substances, alpha-lymphotoxins (LT), and recombinant tumor necrosis factor (TNF) into Chinese hamster ovary cells depends on their ability to form gap junctions, a function varying in different strains of these cells. Fletcher found that the cancer promoter TPA opens gap-junctions to permit entry of LT, leading to a dose-dependent cell lysis. Weak EM fields (450 MHz, 1.0–1.5 mW/cm^2 incident energy) with 16-Hz sinusoidal amplitude-modulation enhanced this ability of TPA to impair gap-junction communication (Fletcher et al., 1986). Moreover, this enhanced response required the presence of 16-Hz modulation and did not occur with an unmodulated carrier wave of the same intensity.

Yeast Cell Growth Successively Enhanced and Inhibited Across a Spectral Band of Millimeter Wave Exposures

Resonant interactions with imposed EM fields in biomolecular fluids may occur in the millimeter wave and far-infrared region (Illinger, 1981). At these frequencies, the duration of collisional molecular perturbations in relation to the period of the EM field is crucial in determining the form of the dielectric response function. Since the duration of a typical collision in a molecular fluid is fixed at a given temperature and pressure, the field frequency determines whether there is a relaxation or resonance spectrum.

Grundler, Keilman and their colleagues (1983, 1984, 1991) have examined growth of yeast cells as a function of frequency in exposures to millimeter wave fields, typically centered around 41.5 GHz. Extreme care was taken to stabilize field frequency (± 1 MHz) and to eliminate temperature fluctuations. Turbidometric measures indicated a succession of peaks and troughs in cell growth as the exposure frequency was changed in small increments over the spectrum 41.5–41.9 GHz, with a periodicity of approximately 8 MHz. With microscopic measures of yeast cell growth, Grundler (1991) has detected adjacent peaks and troughs at these same spectral locations with fields as weak as 5 picowatts/cm^2.

Cerebral Actions of Static and Oscillating Magnetic Fields

Static magnetic fields and modulation of pineal melatonin and EEG

The orientation of the head with respect to the earth's geomagnetic field has been shown to influence activity of the pineal gland (Semm, 1983). In pigeons, guinea pigs, and rats firing rates of about 20% of pinealocytes respond to changes in direction and intensity of the earth's magnetic field. The pineal hormone melatonin exercises strong regulation on circadian rhythms; it also plays an essential role in somatic and sexual development, and has been implicated in regulation of normal and cancerous growth in breast, prostate, and ovarian tissues (Blask, 1990; Reiter, 1990).

Nocturnal inversion of the horizontal component of the geomagnetic field decreased synthesis and secretion of melatonin and the activity of its synthesizing enzymes (Welker et al., 1983). Studies of similar inversions of the geomagnetic field at 5-min intervals by Reiter and his colleagues (Lerchl et al., 1990) found a sharp reduction in serotonin synthesis in rats and mice. Although not measured, these investigators suggest possible modulation of melatonin synthesis by this interference with the serotonin pathway.

The EEG in man has been reported sensitive to static magnetic fields much stronger than the geomagnetic field. Using a field of 0.2 tesla (2000 gauss), von Klitzing (1989, 1991) noted increased power at frequencies of 6 to 8 Hz, confined mainly to the occipital region (leads 01/02), rarely seen in P3/P4, and never in Fz. This increment was seen when the polarity of the initial field was inverted, but remained when the field was switched back to its original polarity. Von Klitzing has modeled this phenomenon on the assumption that fluxes of electric charges are diverted from their original isotropic distribution, due to Lorenz forces exerted by the static magnetic field, producing Hall effect voltages.

Oscillating EM Field Actions on Melatonin in Animals and Man

Melatonin diurnal cycling is also sensitive to oscillating EM fields. Melatonin is produced by action of *N*-acetyltransferase (NAT) and hydroxyindole-O-methyl transferase (HIOMT) on serotonin (Deguchi and Axelrod, 1972). Chronic exposure of rats to 60-Hz electric fields reduces the normal nocturnal rise in both pineal NAT activity and melatonin concentration (Wilson et al., 1986, 1990a, 1990b).

Rats (23 days old) chronically exposed to 60-Hz electric fields simulating high-voltage power line fields showed an approximate 40% reduction in the nocturnal peak in blood melatonin levels and a delay of 1.4 hr in its occurrence. Rats 55 days old at the onset of exposure showed no significant differences in nocturnal and diurnal melatonin levels after 21 days' exposure, but within 3 days of cessation of electric field exposure, strong pineal melatonin rhythms were reestablished.

Wilson has extended these observations in studies of a melatonin urinary metabolite in human volunteers (32 female and 10 male) sleeping under electric blankets (Wilson et al., 1990a). They used either conventional or modified continuous polymer wire (CPW) blankets for 8 weeks. Overnight excretion of 6-hydroxymelatonin sulfate (6-0HMS), a stable urinary metabolite of melatonin, was used to assess pineal gland function. Subjects using the conventional blankets showed no variations in 6-0HMS excretion, either as a group or as individuals, but 7 of 28 volunteers using CPW blankets showed significant changes in their mean nighttime 6-OHMS excretion. The CPW blankets switched on and off approximately twice as fast as conventional blankets, and produced magnetic fields that were 50% stronger, leading to the conclusion that periodic exposure to pulsed DC or to low-frequency electric or magnetic fields of sufficient intensity and duration can affect pineal gland function in certain individuals.

Evidence for Joint Static/Oscillating Field Interactions in Modulation of Tissue Cation Binding: Biophysical Models

Are these effects of static magnetic fields mediated by their direct detection in brain tissue, or in peripheral sensors that modulate central functions? There is conflicting evidence supporting both options, with an indication that interactions between static and oscillating magnetic fields are involved.

Section of the optic pathways is reported to abolish pineal melatonin responses to static magnetic fields (Reuss and Olcese, 1986). On the other hand, efflux of $^{45}Ca^{2+}$ from the chick cerebral hemisphere is directly modified by static magnetic field exposure (Blackman et al., 1985b). Halving the local geomagnetic field with a Helmholtz coil rendered a previously effective 15-Hz field ineffective, and doubling the geomagnetic field caused an ineffective 30-Hz field to become an effective stimulus. These findings have focused interest on biophysical models that might relate to the ubiquitous role of calcium in transductive and enzymatic processes, as well as offering testable hypotheses that have attempted to account for resonant low-frequency phenomena.

Biophysical Models of Low-Frequency EM Field Sensitivities: Cyclotron Resonance and Ca Coordination Compound Models

In a cyclotron oscillator, charged particles are exposed to a static magnetic field and to an oscillating magnetic field at right angles to one another. The particles will move in circular orbits at right angles to the two imposed fields when the frequency of the imposed oscillating field matches the particle gyrofrequency, determined by its mass, charge, and the intensity of the static magnetic field.

Polk (1984) noted that free (unhydrated) Ca ions in the earth's geomagnetic field would exhibit cyclotron resonance frequencies around 10 Hz, and that these cyclotron currents would be as much as five orders of magnitude greater than the Faraday currents if the Ca ions exhibited nearest-neighbor coherence. This model has been extended theoretically and experimentally (Liboff, 1985; Liboff and McLeod, 1988; McLeod and Liboff, 1986; McLeod et al., 1986). Liboff noted that for a mean value for the earth's geomagnetic field of 0.5 gauss, most of the singly and doubly charged ions of biological interest have gyrofrequencies in the range of 10 to 100 Hz.

Liboff (1985) hypothesized that imposed EM fields at frequencies close to a given resonance may couple to the corresponding ionic species in such a way as to transfer energy selectively to these ions. He proposed that data from the Blackman experiments cited above may relate to cyclotron resonance in singly-ionized K^+, with secondary effects on Ca efflux. Despite its support in experimental observations, criticism of this model has been directed at its requirements for ions to be stripped of hydration shells that would presumably alter gyrofrequencies, and to presumed ion motion in the direction of the magnetic field, rather than orthogonally, as would be predicted on physical grounds.

Lednev (1991) has proposed a quite different explanation that would account for cyclotron resonancelike behavior of Ca^{2+} ions in interaction of weak magnetic fields with biological systems. An ion inside a Ca^{2+}-binding protein can be approximated by a charged oscillator. A shift in the probability of an ion transition between different states of vibrational energy occurs when there is a combination of static and alternating magnetic fields. This in turn affects the interaction of the ion with surrounding ligands. This effect is maximal when the frequency of the alternating field is equal to the cyclotron frequency of this ion or to some of its harmonics or subharmonics.

Do these sensitivities betoken intrinsic biological rhythms in the same frequency spectrum? Cerebral electric and magnetic field rhythmicity offers a ready answer, but as yet there is no clear evidence for a similar organization in nonneural tissues. In part, an answer awaits needed instrumentation with appropriate temporal and spatial resolution to measure these weak focal magnetic and electric fields in subcellular systems *in vivo*.

Functional Organization of Cellular Mechanisms in Detection of Weak Oscillating EM Fields

As already discussed, initial events in transductive coupling of weak low-frequency EM fields appear to occur at cell membranes. Cell surface events associated with the first detection of chemical and weak EM stimuli lead ultimately to coupling of signals to the cell interior. We may model this coupling as occurring through a sequence of anatomical structures or molecular domains. This structural sequence also plays a complex role in a hierarchical sequence of energetic steps. There is a cascade in major steps of the energetic sequence, with each step typically larger than that immediately preceding. Thus, cell membrane transductive coupling requires cell membrane amplification of initial weak surface stimuli.

EM fields have proved unique tools in revealing key steps in the transductive sequence. Many of these interactions are "windowed" with respect to field frequency, intensity, and duration of exposure. Windowing of these responses points to their nonlinear and nonequilibrium character, and focuses current and future research on physical substrates for these interactions (Adey, 1975, 1977, 1981a, 1981b, 1984, 1986; Lawrence and Adey, 1982; Maddox, 1986).

The first detection of weak electrochemical oscillations in pericellular fluid appears to involve the highly negatively charged tips of protein strands that pass through the lipid plasma membrane and form a glycoprotein surface layer, the glycocalyx, sensing chemical and electrical signals in surrounding fluid. This polyanionic layer attracts cations, particularly Ca^{2+} and H^{+}, and it is in the modulation of Ca^{2+} binding to these anionic surface sites that the first transductive events appear to occur. Manipulation of initial events at cell membrane receptor sites with EM fields causes a far greater increase or decrease in Ca^{2+} binding than is accounted for in events of receptor-ligand binding (Bawin and Adey, 1976; Bawin et al., 1975; Kaczmarek and Adey, 1973, 1974; Lin-Liu and Adey, 1982), and the non-equilibrium character of this altered binding is suggested by its occurrence in narrow frequency and amplitude windows.

Concepts of Cooperativity in Stimulus Amplification at Cell Membranes

At cell surfaces, energy levels of fixed charges on polyanionic terminals of glycoprotein strands are modulated by energy supplied from intracellular metabolic processes, as seen in lymphocyte receptor movements accompanying the cooperative phenomena of patching and capping (Yahara and Edelman, 1972).

Cooperativity is defined in this context as ways in which components of a macromolecule, or a system of macromolecules, act together to switch from one stable state to another (Schmitt et al., 1975). These joint actions frequently involve phase transitions, hysteresis, and avalanche effects in input–output relationships. On cell membrane surfaces, a weak trigger at one point may cause a progression of increasing energy release from ions bound to proteins along the membrane surface. In such a cooperative system, these are nonequilibrium processes, since external energy has been supplied to move at least one of its parameters far from an equilibrium state. Studies of acridine dye binding to biopolymers have shown very long relaxation times in the millisecond range (Schwarz, 1975; Schwarz and Balthasar, 1970; Schwarz and Seelig, 1968; Schwarz et al, 1970). These long relaxation times have suggested cooperative interactions that depend on coherent states between neighboring fixed charges on polymer sheets. All charge sites would then be at the same higher energy level above the ground state, thus creating a coherent domain over a significant area of the membrane surface. The model suggests that these domains might persist for a finite time until returning to ground state, releasing energy cooperatively in response to a weak trigger (see Adey, 1991a for review).

Sequence of Energetics in Cell Detection of Rhythmic Extracellular Fields: Nonlinear Models

An emergent conclusion from studies of these interactions of weak EM fields with biomolecular systems is that they reside in sensitivities to rhythmic stimuli, and not to single punctate events. Temporal integration of regularly recurring events at low frequencies, typically below 100 Hz, appears as a fundamental aspect of cell membrane organization. These sensitivities to coherent stimuli are not restricted to cerebral tissue. Their widespread occurrence in nonnervous cells and tissues suggests that this may be a general biological property.

Entrainment of Weak Coherent Stimuli in Large Pseudorandom Systems

We have reviewed EM field interactions with cells and tissues based on oscillating ELF tissue gradients between 10^{-7} and 10^{-1} V/cm. They clearly involve degrees of cooperativity many orders of magnitude greater than envisaged in thresholds described in Hodgkin–Huxley models of nerve fiber excitation, or in electric gradients in the range of 20 kV/cm needed to produce some molecular transitions, such as the helix-coil transition in ribosomal RNA (Neumann and Katchalsky, 1972).

This discrepancy appears to relate to far greater sensitivities of cellular systems to low-frequency oscillating EM fields than to imposed step functions or DC gradients that have been used in many electrochemical experiments and models to test levels of cooperativity in biological systems (Blank, 1972). Factors requiring consideration include temporal entrainment of activity in large systems of random generators by coherent oscillations far weaker than this random activity (Nicolis et al., 1973, 1974). Nicolis (1983) has examined the role of chaos in reliable information processing in simple nervous systems, as in the leech or cockroach, where complex behavioral repertoires exist in the absence of elaborate neural substrates. For example, certain nonlinear dissipative systems with just three degrees of freedom can exhibit random behavior that is analogous to that produced by explicit stochastic equations. Instead of creating new degrees of freedom with increased bandwidth or dimensionality of state space, these systems generate iterative self-similar processes that decrease resolution or expand the dynamics of trajectories in a low-dimensional state space.

The EEG as an Archetypal Model of Large Pseudorandom Systems

Self-sustained oscillations in biological systems may be modeled on the requirement for interaction of regular external perturbations with free internal oscillations, resulting in synchronization of the system to the external drives (Kaiser, 1984). A sharp frequency response results, exhibiting both frequency and intensity windows and rather irregular behavior near the entrainment region.

The observed phenomena depend on increasing levels of external driving energy. With increasing driving energy, the first shift from free internal oscillations to a self-organized state involves limit cycles, with periodic patterns developed and maintained by nonlinear processes and the influx and efflux of energy. At higher input levels, entrainment occurs, associated with sharp resonances, windows, and threshold effects. These interactions are all athermal. A further increase in external driving energy, both static and periodic, leads to sequences of period-doubling bifurcations, alternating with quasiperiodic and irregular episodes (quasiperiodicity, chaos). As a consequence, a regularly driven self-oscillating system may exhibit intrinsic chaotic behavior, even when the underlying dynamic is strongly deterministic. Finally, still higher energy inputs destabilize the system (collapse), leading to onset of propagating pulse (solitary waves or solitons). Nonlinear temporal structure is thus replaced by a nonlinear spatiotemporal structure.

Kaiser points out that systems having both periodic and chaotic states can exhibit completely different behaviors under periodic driving, and that therein lie additional possibilities for responses of large systems to imposed fields, as in the genesis of the EEG. Extreme sensitivity of chaotic systems to external driving may carry implications for differences between regular and irregular EEG patterns.

Conclusions

It is no longer a matter of speculation that biomolecular systems are responsive to low-level, low-frequency electromagnetic fields. Not only is tissue heating not the basis of these interactions, but the many instances of responses windowed with respect to field frequency and intensity set a rubric for their consideration in physical mechanisms involving long-range ordering at the atomic level (Adey, 1988a, 1988b). These interactions with biomolecular systems occur in response to a broad frequency spectrum of electromagnetic fields.

Fields in the spectrum below 100 Hz have been used as tools in identifying the sequence and energetics of events that couple chemical stimuli from cell surface receptor sites to the cell interior. Observed sensitivities involve pericellular electric gradients in the range of 10^{-1} to 10^{-7} V/cm and extracellular current densities in the range of 1 to 10 $\mu A/cm^2$. They require temporal integration of rhythmic stimuli and are not seen with single, punctate events. Transmembrane components of these fields are thus many orders of magnitude below threshold transmembrane currents described in Hodgkin–Huxley axon models around 1.0 mA/cm^2. These low-frequency sensitivities occur at cell membranes as a function of cooperative behavior and coherent states of electric charges in molecular assemblies or subsets of these assemblies. On the other hand, it is at the atomic level within these molecular systems that physical, rather than chemical, events appear to shape the flow of signals and the transmission of energy.

Radiofrequency and microwave fields at frequencies below the gigahertz region are not associated with similar sensitivities unless they are amplitude- or pulse-modulated at extremely-low-frequencies (ELF), again typically in the spectrum below 100 Hz. It is only with fields in the higher gigahertz spectrum (millimeter wave and far-infrared regions) that resonant interactions occur directly with biomolecules or portions of these molecules.

Static magnetic fields, including the earth's geomagnetic field, modulate cerebral mechanisms, ranging from calcium ion binding to diurnal melatonin synthesis and secretion by the pineal gland. There are interactions between static and oscillating magnetic fields in these cerebral mechanisms.

Recent observations have opened doors to new concepts of communication between cells as they whisper together across barriers of cell membranes. There is a temporal and an energetic sequence in this transductive coupling consistent with cell membrane ultrastructure. Regulation of cell surface chemical events by these fields indicates a major amplification of initial weak triggers associated with binding of hormones, antibodies, and neurotransmitters to their specific binding sites. Calcium ions play a key role in this stimulus amplification. Many of these responses are "windowed" with respect to field frequency and amplitude, evidence supporting long-range interactions in nonlinear, nonequilibrium processes at critical steps in transmembrane coupling.

> Now there is evidence that it is the informational aspect of biological systems that characterizes the essential view of life. And this is less reflected by the biochemical findings, but rather by a level beyond the domain of chemical reactivity, namely that of electromagnetic fields (Li, 1989).

Acknowledgments. We gratefully acknowledge support for studies in our laboratory from the U.S. Department of Energy, the U.S. Environmental Protection Agency, the U.S. Bureau of Devices and Radiological Health (FDA), the U.S. Office of Naval Research, the U.S. Veterans Administration, and the Southern California Edison Company.

References

Adey WR (1975): Effects of electromagnetic radiation on the nervous system. *Ann NY Acad Sci* 247:15–20

Adey WR (1977): Models of membranes of cerebral cells as substrates for information storage. *BioSystems* 8:163–178

Adey WR (1981a): Tissue interactions with nonionizing electromagnetic fields. *Physiol Rev* 61:435–514

Adey WR (1981b): Ionic nonequilibrium phenomena in tissue interactions with nonionizing electromagnetic fields. In: *Biological Effects of Nonionizing Radiation*, Illinger KH, ed. Washington, DC: American Chemical Society Symposium Ser. No. 157. pp 271–298

Adey WR (1984): Nonlinear, nonequilibrium aspects of electromagnetic field interactions at cell membranes. In: *Nonlinear Electro- dynamics in Biological Systems*, Adey, WR, Lawrence AF, eds. New York: Plenum. pp 3–21

Adey WR (1986): The sequence and energetics of cell membrane transductive coupling to intracellular enzymes. *Bioelectrochem Bioenerg* 15:447–456

Adey WR (1988a): Physiological signalling across cell membranes and cooperative influences of extremely low frequency electromagnetic fields. In: *Biological Coher-*

ence and Response to External Stimuli, Frohlich H, ed. Heidelberg: Springer–Verlag, pp 148–170

Adey WR (1988b): Biological effects of radio frequency electromagnetic radiation. In: *Interaction of Electromagnetic Waves with Biological Systems*, Lin JC, ed. New York: Plenum Press, pp 109–140

Adey WR (1989a): Biological effects of radio frequency electromagnetic fields. In: *Electromagnetic Interaction with Biological Systems*, Lin JC, ed. New York: Plenum, pp 109–140

Adey WR (1989b): Cell membranes, electromagnetic fields and intercellular communication. In: *Brain Dynamics*, vol. 2, Başar E, Bullock TH, eds. New York–Berlin–Heidelberg: Springer–Verlag, pp 26–42

Adey WR (1989c): The extracellular space and energetic hierarchies in electrochemical signaling between cells. In: *Charge and Field Effects in Biosystems*, vol. 2, Allen MJ, Cleary SF, Hawkridge FM, eds. New York: Plenum Press, pp 263–292

Adey WR (1990a): Nonlinear electrodynamics in cell membrane transductive coupling. In: *Membrane Transport and Information Storage*, vol. 4, Aloia RC, Curtain CC, Gordon LM, eds. Wiley-Liss: New York, pp 1–28

Adey WR (1990b): Electromagnetic fields, cell membrane amplification, and cancer promotion. In: *Extremely Low Frequency Electromagnetic Fields: The Question of Cancer*, Wilson BW, Stevens RG, Anderson LE, eds. Columbus OH: Battelle Press, pp 211–250

Adey WR (1990c): Electromagnetic fields and the essence of living systems. In: *Modern Radio Science*, Andersen JB, ed. Oxford: Oxford University Press, pp 1–36

Adey WR (1991a): Collective properties of cell membranes. In: Symposium, *Resonance and other Interactions of Electromagnetic Fields with Living Systems*, Royal Swedish Academy of Sciences, Stockholm. Ramel C, Norden B, eds. Oxford: Oxford University Press

Adey WR (1991b): Extremely low frequency magnetic fields and promotion of cancer—experimental studies. In: Symposium, *Resonance and other Interactions of Electromagnetic Fields with Living Systems*, Royal Swedish Academy of Sciences, Stockholm. Ramel C, Norden B, eds. Oxford: Oxford University Press

Adey WR, Kado RT, Walter DO (1967): Results of electroencephalograpic examinations under the influence of vibration and centrifuging in the monkey. *Electroencephalogr Clin Neurophysiol* 25 (Suppl): 228–245

Adey WR, Walter DO (1963): Application of phase detection and averaging techniques accompanying learned discriminative performance in the cat. *Exp Neurol* 7:259–281

Bawin SM, Adey WR (1976): Sensitivity of calcium binding in cerebral tissue to weak electric fields oscillating at low frequency. *Proc Natl Acad Sci USA* 73:1999–2003

Bawin SM, Adey WR, Sabbot IM (1978): Ionic factors in release of $^{45}Ca^{2+}$ from chick cerebral tissue by electromagnetic fields. *Proc Natl Acad Sci USA* 75:6314–6318

Bawin SM, Gavalas-Medici R, Adey WR (1973): Effects of modulated very high frequency fields on specific brain rhythms in cats. *Brain Res* 58:365–384

Bawin SM, Kaczmarek LK, Adey WR (1975): Effects of modulated VHF fields on the central nervous system. *Ann NY Acad Sci* 247:74–80

Blackman CF, Benane SG, House DE, Joines WT (1985a): Effects of ELF (1–120 Hz) and modulated (50Hz) RF fields on the efflux of calcium ions from brain tissue, in vitro. *Bioelectromagnetics* 6:1–12

Blackman CF, Benane SG, Rabinowitz JR, House DE, Joines WT (1985b): A role for the magnetic field in the radiation-induced efflux of calcium ions from brain tissue, in vitro. *Bioelectromagnetics* 6:327–338

Blackman CF, House DE, Benane SG, Joines WT, Spiegel RJ (1988): Effect of ambient levels of power-line-frequency electric fields on a developing vertebrate. *Bioelectromagnetics* 9:129–140

Blank M (1972): Cooperative effects in membrane reactions. *J Colloid Interface Sci* 41:97–104

Blask DE (1990): The emerging role of the pineal gland and melatonin in oncogenesis. In: *Extremely Low Frequency Electromagnetic Fields: The Question of Cancer*, Wilson BW, Stevens RG, Anderson LE, eds. Columbus, OH: Battelle Press, pp 319–336

Budunova IV, Mittelman LA, Belitska GA (1989): Identification of tumor promoters by their inhibitory effect in intercellular transfer of Lucifer yellow. *Cell Biol Toxicol* 5:77–89

Butterworth TE, Slaga TJ, eds. (1987): *Nongenotoxic Mecnanisms in Carcinogenesis.* 25th Banbury Report. New York: Cold Spring Harbor Laboratory.

Byus CV, Lundak RL, Fletcher RM, Adey WR (1984): Alterations in protein kinase activity following exposure of cultured lymphocytes to modulated microwave fields. *Bioelectromagnetics* 5:34–51

Byus CV, Pieper SE, Adey WR (1987): The effects of low-energy 60 Hz environmental electromagnetic fields upon the growth-related enzyme ornithine decarboxylase. *Carcinogenesis* 8:1385–1389

Byus CV, Kartun K, Pieper S, Adey WR (1988): Increased ornithine decarboxylase activity in cultured cells exposed to low energy modulated microwave fields and phorbol ester tumor promoters. *Cancer Res* 48:4222–4226

Cain CD, Thomas DL, Adey WR (1991): 60 Hz magnetic fields increase focus formation induced by tumor promoter in C3H10T1/2/UV-TDTx fibroblast co-culture system. Bioelectromagnetics Soc., Proc. 13th Annual Meeting, Sat Lake City. (Abstract)

Deguchi T, Axelrod J (1972): Control of circadian change of serotonin *N*-acetyltransferase in the pineal organ by the beta-adrenergic receptor. *Proc Natl Acad Sci USA* 69:2547–2550

Delgado JMR, Leal J, Monteagudo JL, Garcia MG (1982): Embryological changes induced by weak, extremely low frequency electromagnetic fields. *J Anat (Lond)* 134:533–552

DeRiemer SA, Strong JA, Albert KA, Greengard P, Kaczmarek LK (1985): Enhancement of calcium current in Aplysia neurons by phorbol ester and kinase C. *Nature (Lond)* 313:313–316

Fitton Jackson S (1985): Biophysical studies of pulsed magnetic field interaction with biological systems: part 1—biophysical interactions. In: *Interactions between Electromagnetic Fields and Cells*, Chiabrera A, Nicolini C, Schwan HP, eds. New York: Plenum Press, pp 537–545

Fitzsimmons RJ, Farley J, Adey WR, Baylink DJ (1986): Embryonic bone matrix formation is increased after exposure to a low-amplitude capacitively coupled electric field, in vitro. *Biochim Biophys Acta* 882:51–56

Fitzsimmons RJ, Farley J, Adey WR, Baylink DJ (1989): Frequency dependence of increased cell proliferation, in vitro, in exposures to a low-amplitude, low-frequency electric field: evidence for dependence on increased mitogen activity released into culture medium. *J Cell Physiol* 139:586–591

Fletcher WH, Byus CV, Walsh DA (1987a): Receptor-mediated action without occupancy: a function for cell-cell communication in ovarian follicles. In: *Requlation of Ovarian and Testicular Function*, Mahesh V, ed. *Adv Exp Med Biol* 219:299–323

Fletcher WH, Shiu WW, Haviland DA, Ware CF, Adey WR (1986): A modulated microwave field and tumor promoters similarly enhance the action of alpha-lymphotoxin (aLT). Bioelectromagnetics Soc. 8th Annual Meeting, Madison WI. Proceedings p 12 (Abstract)

Fletcher WH, Shiu WW, Ishida TA, Haviland DL, Ware CF (1987b): Resistance to the cytolytic action of lymphotoxin and tumor necrosis factor coincides witrh the presence of of gap junctions uniting cells. *J Immunol* 139:1–7

Garaj-Vrhovac V, Fucic A, Horvat D (1990): Comparison of chromosome aberration and micronucleus induction in human lymphocytes after occupational exposure to vinyl chloride monomer and microwave radiation. *Periodicum Biologorum* 92:411–416

Gavalas RJ, Walter DO, Hamer J, Adey WR (1970): Effeci;s of iow-ievel, low-frequency electric fields on EEG and behavior in *Macaca nemestrina. Brain Res* 18:491–501

Gavalas-Medici R, Day-Magdaleno SR, (1976): Extremely low frequency weak electric fields affect schedule-controlled behaviour in monkeys. *Nature* (*Lond*) 261:256–258

Goodman R, Henderson AS (1988): Exposure of salivary gland cells to low-frequency electromagnetic fields alters polypeptide synthesis. *Proc Nat Acad Sci USA* 85: 3928–3932

Goy RW, McEwen BS (1980): *Sexual Differentiation in the Rat Brain.* Cambridge, MA: MIT Press

Grundler W (1991): Experimental evidence for coherent excitations correlated with cell growth. In: Symposium Proceedings, *Coherent and Emergent Phenomena in Biomolecular Systems*, NATO Advanced Workshop, University of Arizona Halth Sciences Center, Tucson, AZ

Grundler W, Keilmann F, Putterlik V, Santo L, Strube D, Zimmermann I (1983): Nonthermal resonant action of millimeter microwaves on yeast growth. In: *Coherent Excitation in Biological Systems*, Frohlich H, Kremer F, eds. Heidelberg: Springer–Verlag, pp 25–33

Herschman HR, Brankow DW (1986): Ultraviolet irradiation transforms C3H10T1/2 cells to a unique suppressible phenotype. *Science* 234: 1385–1388

Herschman HR, Brankow DW (1987): Cell size, cell density and the nature of the tumor promoter are critical variables in the expression of a transformed phenotype (focus formation) in co- cultures of UV-TDTx and C3H10T1/2 cells. *Carcinogenesis* 8:993–998

Illinger KH, ed. (1981): *Biological Effects of Nonionizing Radiation.* American Chemical Society Symp. Ser. No. 157. Washington DC: American Chemical Society

Juutilainen J, Harri M, Saali K, Lahtinen T (1986): Effects of 100 Hz magnetic fields with various waveforms on the development of chick embryos. *Radiat Environ Biophys* 25:65–74

Juutilainen J, Sali K (1986): Development of chick embryos in 1 Hz to 100 kHz magnetic fields. *Radiat Environ Biophys* 25:135–140

Kaczmarek LK, Adey WR (1973): The efflux of $^{45}Ca^{2-}$ and ^{3}H-gamma-aminobutyric acid from cat cerebral cortex. *Brain Res.* 63:331–342

Kaczmarek LK, Adey WR (1974): Weak electric gradients change ionic and transmitter fluxes in cortex. *Brain Res* 66:537–540

Kaiser F (1984): Entrainment-quasiperiodicity-chaos-collapse: bifurcation routes of externally driven self-sustained oscillating systems. In: *Nonlinear Electrodynamics in Biological Systems*, Adey WR, Lawrence AF, eds. New York: Plenum Press

Keilmann F, Grundler W (1984): Nonthermal resonant action of millimeter microwaves on yeast growth. In: *Nonlinear Electrodynamics in Biological Systems*, Adey WR, Lawrence AF, eds. New York: Plenum Press, pp 59–64

Klann RC, Fitzgerald DJ, Piccoli C, Slaga TJ, Yamasaki H (1989): Gap-junctional intercellular communication in epidermal cell lines from selected stages of SENCAR mouse skin carcinogenesis. *Cancer Res* 439:699–706

Klitzing L von (1989): Static magnetic fields increase the power density of EEG in man. *Brain Res* 483:201–203

Klitzing L von (1991): A new electroencephalographic effect in human brain generated by static magnetic fields. *Brain Res* 540:295–296

Kravse D, Mullins JM, Litovitz T (1990): Effect of coherence time of the applied field on the bioelectromagnetic enhancement of ornithine decarboxylase activity. US Dept. Energy, Office of Energy Management, Washington DC. Annual Rev. Research on Biological Effects of 50 and 60 Hz Electric and Magnetic Fields. Proceedings, p. A40

Lawrence AF, Adey WR (1982): Nonlinear wave mechanisms in interactions between excitable tissue and electromagnetic fields. *Neurol Res* 4:115–153

Lednev VV (1991): Possible mechanisms for the influence of weak magnetic fields on biolosical systems. *Bioelectromagnetics* 12:71–76

Lerchl A, Nonaka KO, Stokkan K-A, Reiter RJ (1990): Marked rapid alterations in nocturnal pineal serotonin metabolism in mice and rats exposed to weak intermittent magnetic fields. *Biochem Biophys Res Commun* 169:102–108

Li KH (1989): In: *Electromagnetic Bio-Information*, Popp FA, Warnke U, Konig HL, Peschka W, eds. Munchen–Wien–Baltimore: Urban and Schwarzenberg. Preface to Second Edition

Liboff AR (1985): Cyclotron resonance in membrane transport. In: *Interactions between Electromagnetic Fields and Cells*, Chiabrera A, Nicolini C, Schwan HP, eds. New York: Plenum Press, pp 281–296

Liboff AR, McLeod BR (1988): Kinetics of channelized membrane ions in magnetic fields. *Bioelectromagnetics* 9:39–52

Lin-Liu S, Adey WR (1982): Low-frequency, amplitude-modulated microwave fields change calcium efflux rates from synaptosomes. *Bioelectromagnetics* 3:309–322

Loomis DP, Savitz DA (1990): Mortality from brain cancer and leukemia among electrical workers. *Br J Indust Med* 47:633–638

Luben RA, Cain CD (1984): Use of bone cell hormone responses to investigate bioelectromagnetic effects on membranes, in vitro. In: *Nonlinear Electrodynamics in Biological Systems*, Adey WR, Lawrence AF, eds. New York, Plenum Press pp 23–33

Luben RA, Cain CD, Chen M-Y, Rosen DM, Adey WR (1982): Effects of electromagnetic stimulation bone and bone cells, in vitro. *Proc Nat Acad Sci USA* 79:4180–4183

Lyle DB, Schechter P, Adey WR, Lundak RL (1983): Suppression of T lymphocyte cytotoxicity following exposure to sinusoidally ampl itude-modulated fields. *Bioelectromagnetics* 4: 281–292

Maddox J (1986): Physicists about to hijack DNA? *Nature* (*Lond*) 324:11

Matanoski G, Breysse PN, Elliott EA (1991): Electromagnetic field exposure and male breast cancer. *Lancet* 337:737

McGivern RF, Sokol RZ, Adey WR (1990): Prenatal exposure to a low- frequency electromagnetic field demasculinizes adult scent marking behavior and increases accessory sex organ weights in rats. *Teratology* 41:1–8

McLeod RW, Griffin MJ (1986): A design guide for visual display of manual taks in vibration environments. Part II. Manual. Southampton University, England. Institute of Sound and Vibration Research. Technical Report 133

McLeod BR, Liboff AR (1986): Dynamic characteristics of membrane ions in multifield configurations of low-frequencies. *Bioelectromagnetics* 7:179–189

McLeod BR, Smith SD, Liboff A, Cooksey K (1988): Marine diatoms and ELF cyclotron resonance. Bioelectromagneties Soc., Proc. 8th Annual Meeting, Madison WI. Abstract M4

Moseley MJ, Griffin MJ (1986): A design guide for visual display of manual tasks in vibration environments. Part I. Visual displays. Southampton University, England. Institute of Sound and Vibration Research. Technical Report 133

Neumann E, Katchalsky A (1972): Long-lived conformation changes induced by electric pulses in biopolymers. *Pro Natl Acad Sci USA* 69:993–997

Newmark P (1987): Oncogenes and cell growth. *Nature* (*Lond*) 327:101

Nicolis JS (1983): The role of chaos in reliable information processing. In: *Synerqetics of the Brain*, Basar E, Flohr H, Haken H, Mandell AJ, eds. Berlin: Springer–Verlag, pp 330–334

Nicolis JS, Galanos G, Protonotarios EN (1973): A frequency entrainment model with relevance to systems displaying adaptive behaviour. *Int J Control* 18: 1009–1027

Nicol is JS, Protonotarios E, Liar,os E (1974): The role of noise in "self-organizing" systems. University of Patras, Greece, Dept Electrical Engineering. Technical Report CSB-1

Phillips JL, Haggren W, Adey WR (1991): Effects of 60 Hz magnetic field exposure of specific gene transcription in CEM-CM3 human T-lymphoblastoid cells. Bioelectromagnetics Soc., Proc. 13th Annual Meeting, Salt Lake City UT. (Abstract)

Polk C (1984): Time-varying magnetic fields and DNA synthesis: magnitude of forces due to magnetic fields on surface-bound counterions. Bioelectomagnetics Soc., Proc. 6th Annual Meeting, p 77 (Abstract)

Preston-Martin S, Mack W, Henderson BE (1989): Risk factors for gliomas and meningiomas in males in Los Angeles County. *Cancer Res* 49:6137–6143

Reiter RJ (1990): Effects of light and stress on pineal function. In: *Extremely Low Frequency Electromagnetic Fields: the Question of Cancer*, Wilson BW, Stevens RG, Anderson LE, eds. Columbus, OH: Battelle Press, pp 87–108

Reuss S, Olcese J (1986): Magnetic field effects on the rat pineal gland: role of retinal activation by light. *Neurosci Lett* 64:97–101

Schmitt FO, Schneider DM, Crothers DM, eds. (1975): *Functional Linkage in Biomolecular Systems*. New York: Raven Press

Schwarz G (1975): Sharpness and kinetics of cooperative transitions. In: *Functional Linkage in Biomolecular Systems*, Schmitt FO, Schneider DM, Crothers DM, eds. New York: Raven Press, pp 32–35

Schwarz G, Balthasar W (1970): Cooperative binding of linear biopolymers, 3. Thermodynamic and kinetic analysis of the acridine orange-poly (L-glutamic acid) system. *Eur J Biochem* 12:461–467

Schwarz G, Klose S, Balthasar W (1970): Cooperative binding to linear biopolymers. 2. Thermodynamic analysis of the proflavine-poly (L–glutamic) system. *Eur J Biochem* 12:454–467

Schwarz G, Seelig J (1968): Kinetic properties and electric field effect of the helix-coil transition of poly (gamma-benzoyl L-glutamate) determined from dielectric rlaxation measurements. *Biopolymers* 6:1263–1277

Semm P (1983): Neurobiological investigations on the magnetic sensitivity of the pineal gland in rodents and pigeons. *Comp Biol Physiol* 159:619–625.

Servantie B, Servantie AM, Etienne J (1975): Synchronization of cortical neurons by a pulsed microwave field as evidenced by spectral analysis of electrocorticograms from the white rat. *Ann N Y Acad Sci* 247:82–86.

Sherwood N, Griffin MJ (1990): Effects of whole-body vibration on short-term memory. *Aviation Space Enviren Med* 61:1092–1097

Sikov MR, Rommereim DN, Beamer JL, Buschbom RL, Kaune WJ, Phillips RD (1987): Developmental studies of Hanford miniature swine exposed to 60 Hz ewlectric fields. *Bioelectromagnetics* 8:229–242

Takahashi K, Kaneko I, Date M, Fukada E (1986): Effect of pulsing electromagnetic fields on DNA synthesis in mammalian cells in culture. *Experientia* 42:185–186

Takashima S, Onaral B, Schwan HP (1979): Effects of modulated RF energy on the EEG of mammalian brains. *Rad Enviran Biophys* 16:15–27

Thomas TL, Stolley PD, Stemhagen A, Fontham ETH, Bleecker ML, Stewart PA, Hoover RN (1987): Brain tumor mortality among men with electrical and electronics jobs: a case-control study. *J Nat Cancer Inst* 79:233–238

Walter DO, Kado RT, Rhodes JM, Adey WR (1967): Electroencephalographic baselines in astronaut candidates estimated by computation and pattern recognition techniques. *Aerospace Med* 38:371–379

Welker HA, Semm P, Willig P, Willschko W, Vollrath L (1983): Effects of an artificial magnetic field on Serctionin-N-acetyltransferase activity and melatonin content of the rat pineal gland. *Exp Brain Res* 50:426–432

Williams K, Romano C, Dichter MA, Molinoff PB (1991): Modulation of the NMDA receptor by polyamines. *Life Sci* 48:469–498

Wilson BW, Anderson LE (1990a): ELF electromagnetic field effects on the pineal gland. In: *Extremely Low Frequency Electromagnetic Fields: the Question of Cancer*, Wilson BW, Stevens RG, Anderson LE, eds. Columbus, OH: Battelle Press, pp 159–186

Wilson BW, Chess EK, Anderson LE (1986): 60 Hz electric field effects on pineal melatonin rhythms: time course for onset and recovery. *Bioelectromagnetics* 7:239–242

Wilson BW, Wright CW, Morris JE, Buschbom RL, Brown DP, Miller DL, Sommers-Flannigan R, Anderson LE: Evidence for an effect of ELF electromagnetic fields on human pineal gland function. *J Pineal Res* 9:259–269

Yahara I, Edelman GM (1972): Restriction of the mobility of lymphocyte immunoglobulin receptors by concanavalin A. *Proc Natl Acad Sci USA* 69:608–612

Yamasaki H (1987): The role of cell-to-cell communication in tumor promotion. In: *Nongenotoxic Mechanisms in Carcinogenesis*, Butterworth TE, Slaga TJ, eds. 25th Banbury Report. New York: Cold Spring Harbor Laboratory, pp 297–309

Yotti L, Chang CC, Trosko JE (1979): Elimination of metabolic eooperation in Chinese hamster ovarycells by tumor promoter. *Science* 206:1089–1091

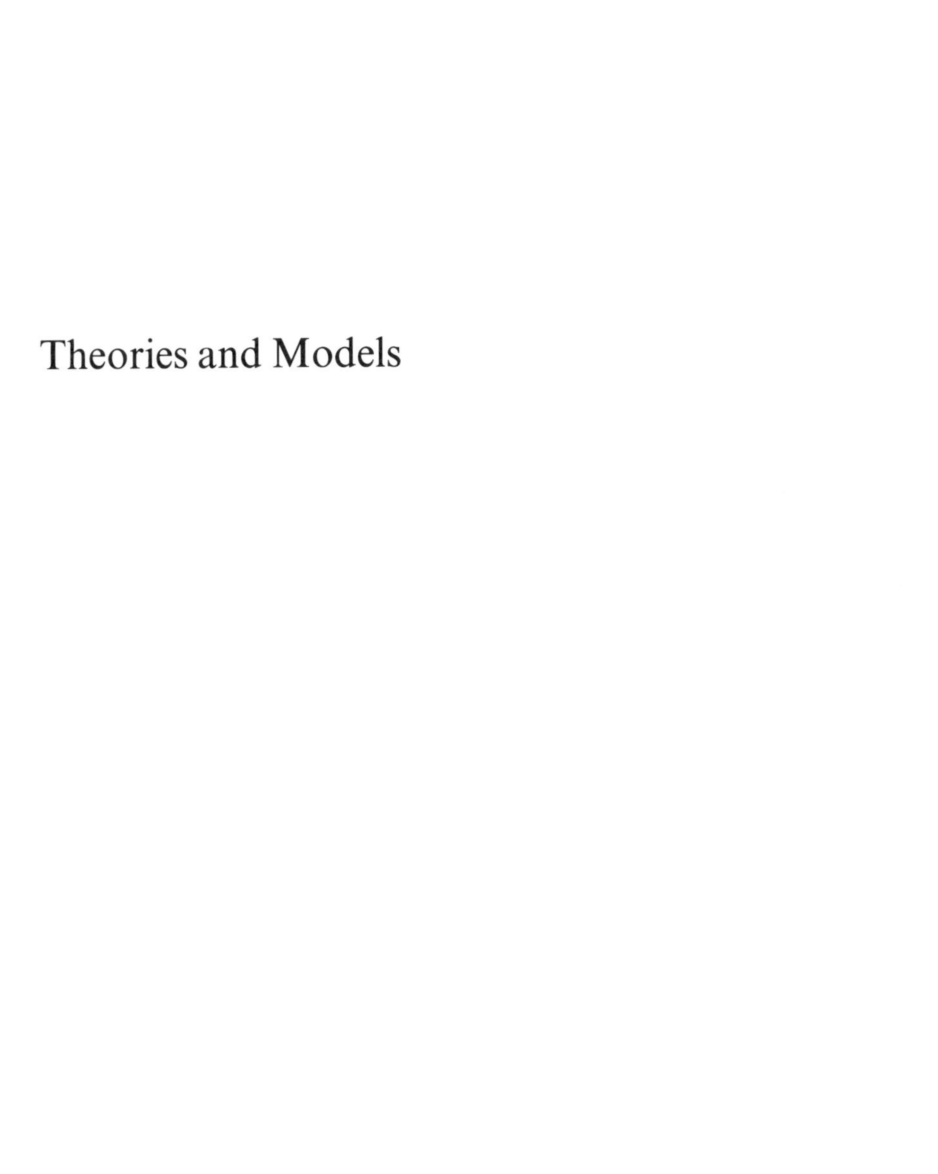

Theories and Models

Inhibitory Interneurons can Rapidly Phase-Lock Neural Populations

William W. Lytton and Terrence J. Sejnowski

The discovery of correlated trains of action potentials in the visual system (Eckhorn et al., 1988; Gray and Singer, 1989; Gray et al., 1989) has been long awaited (Sejnowski, 1986). The well-established existence of rhythms in field potentials recorded from the surface of the brain, or even the skull, would be difficult to explain if the responses of single neurons were not, under some circumstances, entrained to a common firing pattern. More surprising is the observation that neurons that are unlikely to have direct excitatory connections appear to be phase-locked; that is, they fire action potentials within a few milliseconds of each other (Gray et al., 1989). Regardless of the functional significance of these correlations, their existence requires a physical explanation. In a complex, highly nonlinear system of neurons, phase-locking can occur through a variety of mechanisms (Eckhorn et al., 1990; Kammen et al., 1990; Konig and Schillen, 1991a; 1991b; Sporns et al., 1991). One particular mechanism, explored in this chapter, is entrainment and phase-locking through a common, inhibitory interneuron. Inhibition could be effective in entraining pyramidal neurons in local circuits, as we demonstrate here with computer simulations.

Traditionally, inhibition has been viewed as a means of turning cells off. However, in the context of a dynamic network of neurons, synaptic inputs must be viewed in terms of their effects on timing of firing rather than simply on average firing rate (Perkel et al., 1964). Inhibitory mechanisms were earlier proposed by Andersen and Sears (1964) in their "inhibitory phasing theory" to explain rhythmic firing of cells in the thalamus. They postulated that an anode break mechanism might permit thalamic cells to produce repetitive bursting due to mutual inhibitory connections. Although subsequent research has modified this theory, it still appears that response to inhibition is critical in spindle generation (Steriade and Llinás, 1988). Similar inhibitory mechanisms may also occur in other brain areas. In this chapter, we will show that inhibitory interneurons could serve to phase-lock cortical pyramidal neurons (Lytton and Sejnowski, 1991).

Excitatory projections cover great distances and could provide coordinated firing between different cortical areas. Inhibitory interneurons have mainly local projections and might permit synchronization to be localized within a single column. Inhibitory interneurons could serve as control points that would allow projections from other parts of cortex to influence firing throughout a column. Excitatory postsynaptic potentials (EPSPs) can produce phase-locked spiking in a quiescent cell by providing large periodic depolarizations that cause periodic spiking. Long-lasting inhibitory postsynaptic potentials (IPSPs) can do the same if a cell shows a rebound response to the level of hyperpolarization provided. Either type of postsynaptic potential can show more subtle effects in a cell that is not quiescent but shows spontaneous firing. In this case, much smaller postsynaptic potentials can shift firing times slightly and alter the firing pattern. Spontaneous background firing appears to be the rule in the central nervous system. Therefore, we studied these more subtle timing effects of synaptic inputs.

Physiological experiments and neuronal modeling studies have both demonstrated that interneurons do not invariably reduce activity levels in postsynaptic neurons. In fact, an IPSP can be either facilitating or defacilitating. In its facilitating role, an IPSP will increase the probability of firing in response to a following EPSP. The facilitation may be due to deinactivation of sodium and calcium channels or to closing of potassium channels at the hyperpolarized membrane potential. This is closely related to the phenomenon of anode break excitation, in which a burst of firing occurs following release of a neuron from an hyperpolarizing current clamp. With slightly different timing, the direct effect of IPSP hyperpolarization or conductance change will take precedence, giving defacilitation. Similarly, an EPSP can have a defacilitating effect. The defacilitation in this case could be due to inactivation of sodium and calcium channels or to activation of potassium channels during depolarization.

Phase-locking of a spontaneously repetitively firing cell requires that an input be able to shift the time of firing in either direction. If a cell would otherwise fire too early, the input must delay the firing of the cell. If a cell would fire too late, the input must cause firing to occur sooner. Because postsynaptic potentials interact with intrinsic voltage-sensitive membrane conductances, an IPSP can speed up or slow down a cell's firing. Although the speeding up is related to anode break excitation, it is a different phenomenon since it occurs in a cell that is already firing repetitively. Where an anode break response may require large sustained hyperpolarizations, inhibitory exaltation can occur with much more modest voltage transients.

Three-Channel Model Neuron

We used a simplified compartmental model of a pyramidal neuron to show how an IPSP could entrain firing to a particular frequency (Fig. 1A). The model used three voltage-sensitive channels: a fast sodium and delayed rectifier comparable to those originally described by Hodgkin and Huxley and a potassium channel with slower kinetics that permitted slow constant firing in response to excitation. The model neuron was activated with various constant current inputs to produce regular firing from 30 to 50 Hz. After the model stabilized at the test frequency, a 40-Hz train of IPSPs was initiated in

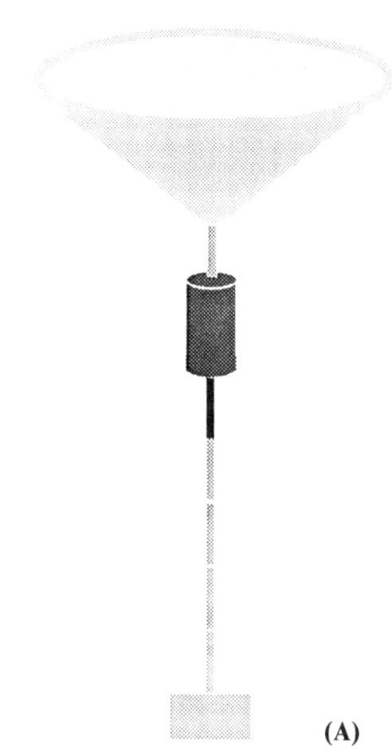

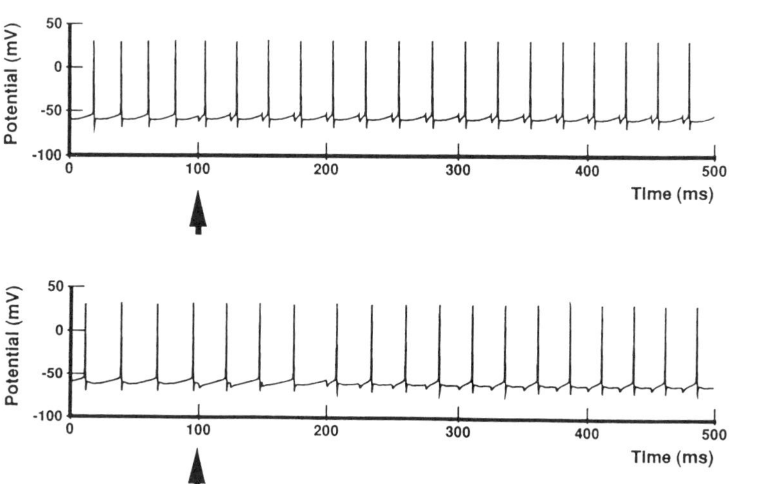

Figure 1. A: Compartment model of pyramidal neuron used a single large compartment to represent the dendritic tree, which is connected to the soma by a thinner compartment representing the proximal apical dendrite. The axon also has a large low impedance compartment as a low impedance termination. Active channels were placed in the axon initial segment (*black*) and the soma (*dark gray*).

B: Entrainment of the model neuron occurred in response to a constant frequency 40-Hz train using hyperpolarizing conductance changes with a maximum of 60 nanoSiemens (60 nS IPSPs). The IPSP train started at 100 ms (*arrows*). The bottom trace shows acceleration of firing from 35.7 Hz to 40 Hz. The top trace shows deceleration from 47.2 Hz to 40 Hz.

the proximal apical dendrite. The model entrained perfectly for initial frequencies between about 34 and 47 Hz (Fig. 1B). If the spontaneous cell firing was too low, inhibitory exaltation could be maintained for only a brief period. If the spontaneous rate was too high, firing frequency was irregular. The dependence of this mechanism on a limited range of firing rates illustrates that these inhibitory effects are of a modulatory nature and dependent on the initial state of the cell. This background firing, dependent on a particular balance between excitatory and inhibitory tone, could be subtly shifted by relatively small changes in the degree of synchrony between different inhibitory inputs.

The phase relation between the driving inhibitory cell and the model neuron was fixed, but the value depended on the initial frequency of the model neuron (Fig. 2). At lower initial frequencies, the IPSPs accelerated firing. After the IPSP, the lag in recovery of voltage-sensitive channels causes increased inward current and early firing. The precise phase relation depends on the time course of response of these voltage-sensitive channels. As seen in Figure 2, IPSPs and spikes are approximately in antiphase at these frequencies. At high initial frequencies, the IPSP inhibits firing by shunting incoming current. Therefore, the neuron fires almost immediately after the IPSP terminates. The phase lag between IPSP and spike is brief, approximately $\pi/2$.

The previous simulations showed that IPSPs can influence neuron firing in either direction: speeding up or slowing down. We therefore simulated the effect of an IPSP train on a model neuron firing irregularly, as it might in response to sustained but uncoordinated excitation due to multiple uncorrelated synaptic inputs. The amount of excitation was tuned to produce spiking in the 30- to 50-Hz range, the range for which inhibitory frequency entrainment could occur. Although the activity appeared to be fairly regular

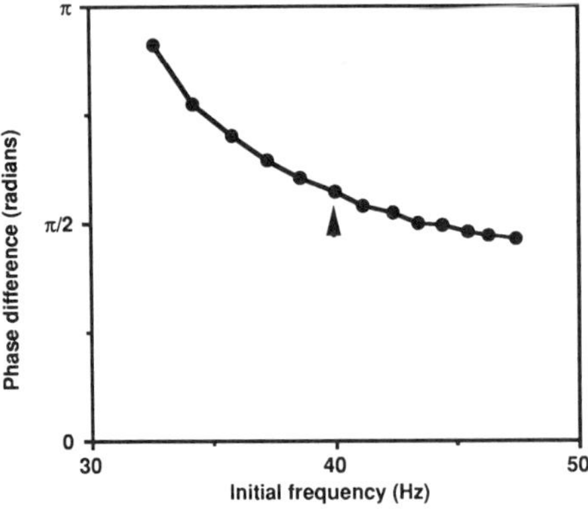

Figure 2. The final phase difference between the IPSP and postsynaptic firing varied with the initial frequency of firing of the postsynaptic cell. Phase was measured from the beginning of the IPSP to the spike.

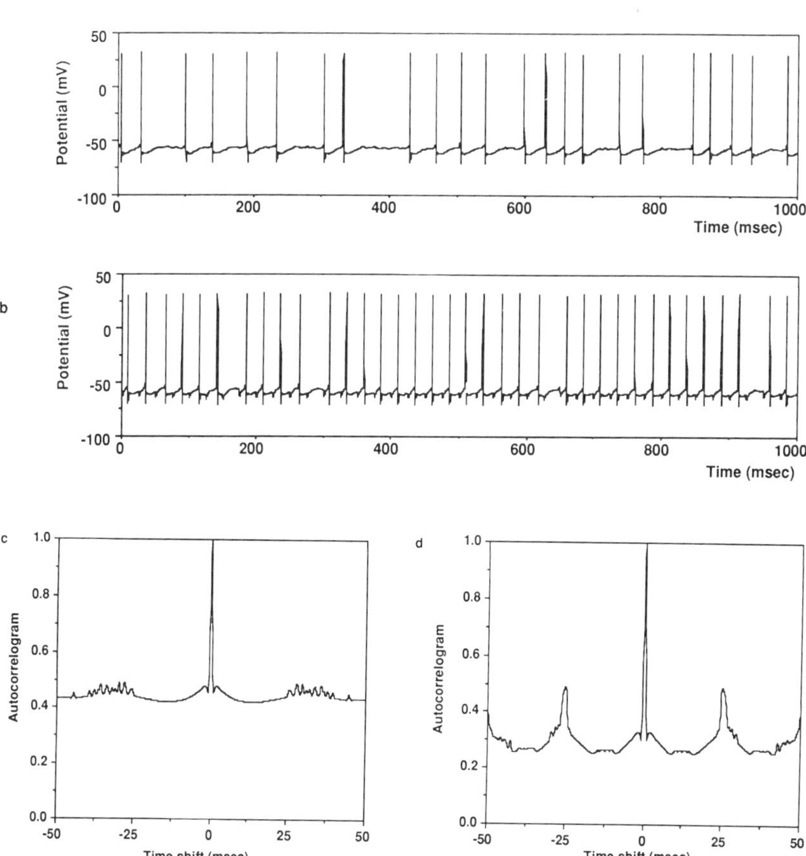

Figure 3. Phase entrainment in the model neuron with uncorrelated multisynaptic excitation of the apical dendrite. Maximal IPSP conductance was 50 nS. **A**: Slightly irregular firing is seen in the model neuron in the absence of inhibitory synaptic activity. **B**: With the regular inhibitory train, entrainment of the model neuron occurs. **C**: An autocorrelogram of 5 s of the model neuron voltage trace shown in A indicates that there is only slight correlation at 25–40 ms. **D**: An autocorrelogram of 5 s of model neuron voltage trace with IPSP train (B) shows a peak at 25 ms, indicating 40-Hz spike entrainment.

(Fig. 3A), it was uncorrelated, as shown by the absence of peaks in the autocorrelogram (Fig. 3C). When the entraining IPSP was activated, the model neuron was closely entrained (Fig. 3B, D). IPSP and spikes were approximately in antiphase.

This simulation showed that phase-locking of a model pyramidal cell was possible. The peak in the autocorrelogram showed the periodicity of firing. However, the phase relation of IPSP and spike was not entirely consistent. In

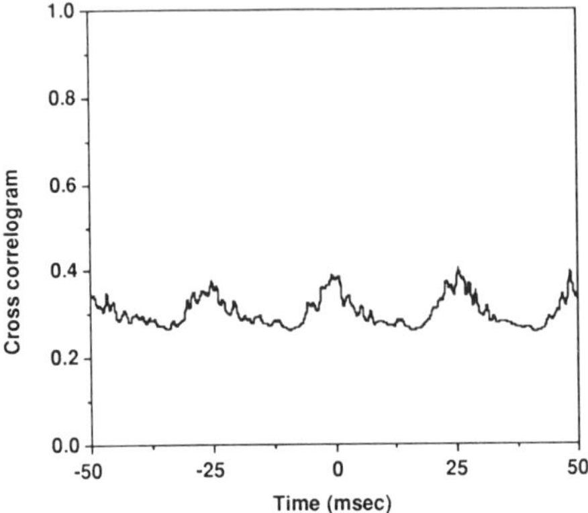

Figure 4. A cross-correlogram between two model neurons receiving identical trains of 50 nS IPSPs at 40 Hz shows a peak at 0, which indicates that the two cells are firing in synchrony. The next peak at 25 ms, shows that they share a common frequency of 40 Hz.

order to get an oscillating field potential, follower pyramidal cells would have to fire simultaneously, requiring that the phase relation between driver and followers be consistent across neurons. We therefore assessed cross-correlation between two model neurons sharing common IPSP input (Fig. 4). The peak at 0 ms the cross-correlogram indicates that both cells are firing together. The 40-Hz periodicity is evinced by the 25-ms gap between peaks. Pairwise correlations such as this in a large number of neurons would result in an oscillating population field potential.

There are a variety of interneuron types that could entrain pyramidal neurons through inhibitory phasing. Two interneurons that show distinct patterns of connectivity are basket cells and chandelier cells. Both interneurons typically synapse on 50 to 200 pyramidal neurons. Basket cells have axons extending up to 1 mm from their cell bodies whereas those of chandelier cells only extend 100 to 300 μm Basket cells synapse onto pyramidal cell bodies and proximal apical dendrites whereas chandelier cells synapse exclusively on axon initial segments. We used this latter difference to perform simulations contrasting the relative efficacy of basket cells and chandelier cells in entraining pyramidal neurons. We compared entrainment from IPSPs at the proximal apical dendrite to entrainment by IPSPs at the axon initial segment. Synapses at either location entrained the model neuron. This occurred using either shunting or inhibitory synapses and with a wide variety of parameter values including variation of specific membrane resistance, density of active channels in the soma, and presence or absence of a first node of Ranvier. With all parameters, entrainment occurred slightly more easily when the IPSP was situated in the apical dendrite. The increased conductance at the spike generation zone during the chandelier cell simulation appeared to interfere slightly with the action potential, preventing entrainment from very high or very low initial frequencies.

Recordings from current-clamped interneurons in cortical slices have shown that they give nonaccommodating spike trains at a higher frequency than is seen with pyramidal neurons. It seemed possible that phase-locking would not occur at these high rates. Therefore, we produced IPSP trains of 200 to 300 Hz and assessed their effect on a regularly firing cortical pyramidal cell. We found that the model neuron spike train entrained to subharmonics of the inhibitory interneuron firing frequency. In general, the cell would find the subharmonic closest to its initial firing rate, conditioned by the amount of ongoing excitatory input it was receiving. With IPSP frequencies that are multiples of 40 Hz for example, there was a peak in the autocorrelation at 25 ms corresponding to a frequency of 40 Hz (Fig. 5). Lesser peaks in the autocorrelogram corresponded to other integral subharmonics. In Figure 5, for

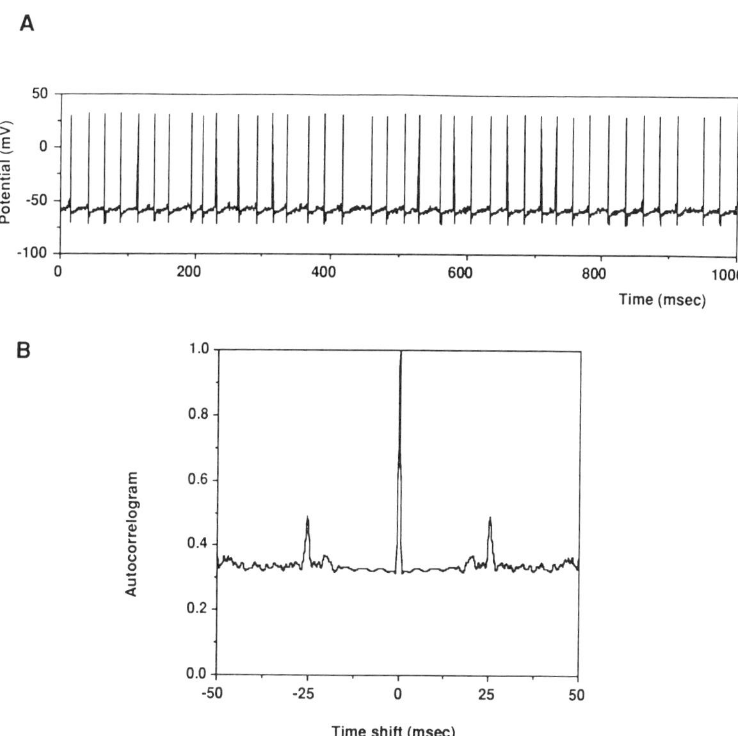

Figure 5. Higher frequency trains of inhibitory input can also produce entrainment. In this case, a 50 nS IPSP train at 200 Hz entrains a model cell receiving uncorrelated excitatory synaptic input into the apical dendrite. The membrane potential is shown above and the autocorrelogram below. There are peaks at 25 ms and 20 ms corresponding to subharmonics of 40 and 50 Hz.

example, there is a smaller peak seen at about 20 ms. This corresponds to a frequency of 50 Hz, another subharmonic of the 200-Hz driving frequency.

Eleven-Channel Model Neuron

The phase-locked firing that has been observed in visual cortex involves pyramidal neurons firing short, high-frequency bursts spaced at 20 to 30 ms, suggesting the existence of two different sets of channels operating on widely different time scales. Using a restricted set of channels, we had simulated the activity at the longer time scale in isolation. We were concerned that the complex interactions between the larger variety of voltage- and calcium-gated membrane conductances in a cortical pyramidal cell could interfere with the mechanism outlined here. Therefore, we simulated a neocortical pyramidal cell that had in its soma most of the channels that have been described in cells of this type. This included both fast and persistent sodium channels, five types of potassium channels including two that were calcium-sensitive, three types of calcium channels, and a mixed channel, the mixed cation conducting anomalous rectifier. There were also several mechanisms to permit elimination of calcium. Current injection into the model resulted in repetitive bursting behavior similar to that observed in cortical neurons that phase-lock (C. Gray, personal communication). Despite the great complexity of this model, it was still very simple relative to a neocortical pyramidal cell with its spatial distribution of active channels in the dendrites and multiplicity of intracellular second messenger systems.

We found that the mechanism of inhibitory exaltation was also present in our more complex cell, although it was due to a somewhat different mechanism. The model would also exhibit phase-locking in response to a periodic IPSP train. In order to assess how IPSP phase-locking would compare to EPSP phase-locking in this model, we designed a simulation of two pyramidal neurons, each receiving 500 very strong excitatory inputs on distal dendrites and 100 inhibitory inputs on proximal apical dendrite. These 500 excitatory inputs were meant to represent the roughly 10,000 relatively weak excitatory synapses that are found on a neocortical pyramidal cell. The locations of the synapses were chosen to correspond to the most common site of termination for these two types of projections. The two neurons started firing at different times, putting them in antiphase with respect to one another. Initially, all of the synapses onto both neurons fired randomly as individual uncorrelated Poisson processes. In separate simulations, a certain percentage of either the excitatory or inhibitory synapses were made to fire synchronously in both cells, simulating a set of shared inputs with periodic firing. With about 20% to 40% synchronization of either EPSPs or IPSPs, the two neurons shifted from firing in antiphase to firing in phase.

Although these simulations showed the efficacy of EPSP entrainment to be roughly comparable to the efficacy of IPSP entrainment expressed in percentage, consideration of absolute numbers of inputs reveals a large disparity. Since there are many more EPSP boutons than IPSP boutons on a pyramidal cell, these similar percentages indicate that many fewer synchronized inhibitory inputs produce the effect seen with a large number of synchronized excitatory inputs. As few as 40 synchronized inhibitory synapses might have as much effect as 4000 synchronized excitatory synapses. These 40 inhibitory boutons might come from as few as 5 to 10 inhibitory interneurons. The surprising efficacy of inhibitory inputs in this setting is probably due to two factors. First, the inhibitory inputs arise closer to the soma and spike generating zone. Therefore, they are less attenuated by passage down the dendrite. Second, in our paradigm, EPSPs must also influence a spontaneously firing cell by slightly altering the firing time on each cycle. Therefore, the EPSP must not only speed up the firing of the cell in a classical excitatory manner, but also slow down the firing at times by a paradoxical defacilitation. This defacilitation can occur due to the interaction of EPSPs and voltage-sensitive channels as noted above.

The significance of the correlated discharges observed in some cortical neurons remains an open question. Do these synchronized neurons form a linkage that helps the later stages of visual processing group together the common elements of a coherent pattern (von der Malsburg, 1981; Wang et al., 1990)? Are the correlated patterns of firing in the ensemble of neurons actively filtering sensory information, based on the relatively small subset of neurons that are near the threshold of firing (Sejnowski, 1981)? Or are these correlations a by-product of a nonlinear system that is prone to such "spurious" states, to be suppressed as soon as they are formed? Many more experiments will be needed to sort out these possibilities.

Acknowledgments. TJS was supported by the Howard Hughes Medical Institute and the Office of Naval Research. WWL was supported by a Physician Scientist Award from the National Institute of Aging.

References

Andersen P, Andersson SA (1968) *Physiological Basis of the Alpha Rhythm.* New York: Appleton-Century-Crofts

Andersen, P, Sears. TA (1964) The role of inhibition the the phasing of spontaneous thalamocortical discharge. *J physiol (Lond)* 173:459–480

Eckhorn R, Bauer R, Jordan W, Brosch M, Kruse W, Munk M, Reitboeck HJ (1988): Coherent oscillations: a mechanism of feature linking in the visual cortex. *Biol Cybern* 60:121–130

Eckhorn R, Reitboeck HJ, Arndt M, Dicke P (1990): Feature linking via synchronization among distributed assemblies: simulations of results from cat visual cortex. *Neur Comput* 2:293–307

Gray CM, Konig P, Engel AK, Singer W (1989): Oscillatory responses in cat visual cortex exhibit inter-columnar synchronization which reflects global stimulus properties. *Nature* 338:334–337

Gray CM, Singer W (1989): Stimulus-specific neuronal oscillations in orientation columns of cat visual cortex. *PNAS* 86:1698–1702

Kammen D, Koch C, Holmes PJ (1990): Collective oscillations in the visual cortex. In: *Neural Information Processing Systems* 2, Touretzky DS, ed. San Mateo, CA: Morgan Kaufmann, pp 76–83

Konig P, Schillen TB (1991a): Stlmulus-dependent assembly formation of oscillatory responses: II. Desynchronization. *Neur Comput* 3:167–177

Konig P, Schillen TB (1991b): Stimulus-dependent assembly formation of oscillatory responses: I. Synchronization. *Neur Comput* 3:155–166

Lytton WW, Sejnowski TJ (1991): Inhibitory interneurons may help synchronize oscillations in cortical pyramidal neurons. *J Neurophysiol* 66:1059–1079

Perkel DH, Schulman JH, Bullock TH, Moore GP, Segundo JP (1964): Pacemaker neurons: effects of regularly spaced synaptic input. *Science* 145:61–63

Sejnowski TJ (1981): Skeleton filters in the brain. In: *Parallel Models of Associative Memory*, Hinton GE, Anderson JA, eds. Hillsdale, NJ. Lawrence Erlbaum, pp 189–212

Sejnowski TJ (1986): Open questions about computation in cerebral cortex. In: *Parallel Distributed Processing: Explorations in the Microstructure of Cognition, vol.* 2: *Psychological and Biological Models*, Rumelhart DE, McClelland JL, eds. Cambridge: MIT Press, pp 372–389

Sporns O, Tononi G, Edelman GM (1991): Modeling perceptual grouping and figure-ground segregation by means of active reentrant connections. *PNAS* 88:129–133

Steriade M, Llinás R (1988): The functional states of the thalamus and the associated neuronal interplay. *Physiol Rev* 68:649–742

von der Malsburg C (1981): *The Correlation Theory of Brain Function: Internal Report 81-2*. Goettingen: Abteilung fuer Neurobiologie, MPI fuer Biophysikalische Chemie

Wang D, Buhmann J, von der Malsburg C (1990): Pattern segmentation in associative memory. *Neur Comput* 2:94–106

The Problem of Neural Integration: Induced Rhythms and Short-Term Correlations

GIULIO TONONI, OLAF SPORNS, and GERALD M. EDELMAN

Induced Rhythms

Since the beginnings of neurophysiology and electroencephalography, various rhythmic patterns of brain activity have been recorded, differing in frequency, location, and relationship to behavior or cognitive activity. Recently, the cortical frequency band around 40 Hz (gamma range) has become a focus of attention (Bressler, 1990). To be sure, this band has already been studied in the past (cf. Sheer, 1970; Sheer and Grandstaff, 1970; Basar, 1980); for instance, 40-Hz electroencephalogram (EEG) activity has been shown to be related to focused arousal (Sheer, 1976; Bouyer et al., 1981, 1987), and sensory (Galambos et al., 1981) as well as cognitive 40-Hz event-related potentials (ERPs) (Bauer and Jones, 1976; Spydell et al., 1985) have been widely examined. Rhythmic neuronal activity can show varying degrees of stimulus dependence. Ongoing background rhythms tend to be relatively independent of specific stimuli. By contrast, in stimulus-driven rhythms, temporal fluctuations of the neuronal activity are tightly locked to temporal fluctuations in the stimulus itself. What characterizes induced rhythms is that, although they are triggered by an external stimulus, their temporal structure is largely determined by interactions within the participating neuronal circuits. The possibility of reliably inducing rhythmic neuronal activity with specific and controlled stimuli greatly facilitates the experimental investigation; a good example is the olfactory system, where it has been possible to clarify the nature, origin, dynamics, and functions of fast induced rhythms in considerable detail (Freeman and Skarda, 1985). Most recently, induced rhythms around 40 Hz have been described in the visual cortex (Freeman and van Dijk, 1987) and carefully analyzed at the level of single cell and multiunit activity (Gray and Singer, 1987, 1989; Eckhorn et al., 1988; Gray et al., this volume). The ease with which visual stimuli can be manipulated, the enormous body of knowledge concerning the visual system, and the precision of the data that can be collected with cortical microelectrodes have made these results particularly interesting.

In this chapter we first briefly review these new findings. Second, we explore some of their implications for the important theoretical problem of how distinct brain events are integrated. Third, we present several computer models that reproduce and extend the experimental results. One model illustrates how the nervous system may deal with the problem of integration at various levels of organization. Another model uses the same approach to suggest a possible neural basis for perceptual grouping and figure-ground segregation, as well as for some of the so-called Gestalt laws. Finally, we discuss the problem of the effectiveness of integration and present some computer simulations in which synchronous oscillations can give rise to an elementary behavior.

Brief Review of Some Recent Findings

Orientation-selective neurons in the primary visual cortex of the cat (area 17) can show oscillatory activity when a light bar of optimal orientation, velocity, and direction of movement is passed through their receptive field (Gray and Singer, 1987, 1989). Under conditions of light anesthesia, multi-unit activity as well as the simultaneously recorded local field potential (LFP) oscillate at a frequency of about 40 to 50 Hz. Single cell recordings can also exhibit signs of oscillatory activity, but usually in a less compelling way and after some temporal averaging. Rhythmic activity is limited to a subpopulation of mostly complex cells, located in layers II and III of the primary visual cortex; it is all but absent in simple cells located in layer IV. The amplitude of the oscillations is enhanced by binocular stimulation and reduced by combined stimulation with optimal and orthogonally oriented light bars (Gray et al., 1990a). The frequency is independent of stimulus orientation, but increases slightly with stimulus velocity (Eckhorn et al., 1988; Gray et al., 1990a).

When a long light bar is moved across the receptive fields of spatially separated neurons with similar orientation and direction specificity, cross-correlation of multiunit or LFP recordings from area 17 reveals that the oscillatory responses are synchronized (Eckhorn et al., 1988; Gray et al., 1989; Engel et al., 1990). The synchronization becomes weaker if a gap is inserted into the stimulus contour and it disappears completely if two parts of the contour are moved separately and in opposite directions (Engel et al., 1991). Synchrony is established rapidly, often within 100 ms, and lasts for 50 to 500 ms. Frequency and phase of the oscillations change continuously and stochastically but stay within the range of 40 to 60 Hz and ± 3 ms, respectively (Gray et al., 1991). An independent study in cat visual cortex has confirmed the existence of neuronal oscillations and of intracolumnar as well as intercolumnar short-term correlations (Eckhorn et al., 1988). In addition, synchronization of oscillatory activity was observed between different cortical areas. During the presentation of an appropriately oriented light bar, oscillatory LFPs appeared simultaneously in columns both in area 17 and area 18, and they were coherent with near-zero phase delay. More recently, stimulus-dependent coherent oscillations have also been described between the two hemispheres and between extrastriate and striate cortical areas (Engel et al., 1991).

These findings are significant for several reasons. They stress the rhythmic nature of cortical activity in the fast frequency range at the single cell level. More generally, they demonstrate the relevance of the fine temporal structure of neuronal discharge. This had been somewhat neglected, although basic methods for analyzing temporal patterns in spike trains of neurons had already been introduced in the 1960s (Perkel et al., 1967a; 1967b; Gerstein, 1970; Moore et al., 1970), and they have been considerably refined since then (see, e.g., Abeles, 1982; Melssen and Epping, 1987; Palm et al., 1988; Bullock and McClune, 1989). In addition, these results indicate that groups of synchronously active neurons are found in the cerebral cortex, and that short-term correlations are established among them. In our view, the latter aspects have a special theoretical relevance. In fact, they lie at the heart of the theory of neuronal group selection (TNGS), proposed first in 1978 (Edelman, 1978, 1987), and they have important implications for what we consider to be a fundamental problem of neurophysiology and psychology alike, that of functional integration in the nervous system.

The Problem of Integration

That the issue of integration is central to any explanation of brain function has been recognized long ago (cf. Sherrington, 1906). The physicist Erwin Schrödinger stated it clearly when he wrote:

> Both the pathology of the brain and physiological investigations on sense perception speak unequivocally in favor of a regional separation of the sensorium into domains whose far-reaching independence is amazing because it would let us expect to find these regions associated with independent domains of the mind; *but they are not.* (Schrödinger, *Mind and Matter*, 1958, p. 142, italics ours).

In fact, the cerebral cortex of higher vertebrates can be subdivided into a number of anatomically and physiologically distinct areas. Even regions of the cortex devoted to a single sensory modality are composed of multiple, relatively well separated areas that contain neurons with distinct response properties. The primate visual cortex, for example, contains at least 17 subfields that are connected by a characteristic pattern of interareal fibers (Zeki, 1969; Van Essen, 1985; Van Essen and Maunsell, 1983; Zeki and Shipp, 1988). Increasing evidence from neuroanatomy, neurophysiology, and neuropsychology indicates that each of these areas is devoted to the analysis of specific stimulus dimensions, like form, color, and motion. The distributed character of the visual system, and of the cerebral cortex in general, poses a fundamental problem for our understanding of its overall function: How are the operations of these segregated areas integrated to provide the basis for a perceptually unified picture of the world, which is a prerequisite for adaptive and flexible behavior?

The theory of neuronal group selection and the problem of integration

A traditional solution to the problem of integration is to postulate the existence of a singular master area somewhere in the brain that keeps track of all lower level cortical maps and guides their function by controlling their interactions. There are several problems with such a hierarchical concept, including the fact that no cortical area has been identified that receives convergent cortical inputs to an extent that would make it a likely candidate for such a central or superordinate role (cf. Damasio, 1989). Instead, most cortical areas have a variety of convergent and divergent connections with other maps (Jones and Powell, 1970; Symonds and Rosenquist, 1984).

A radically different point of view states that the integration within and between cortical maps, allowing "a spatiotemporally continuous representation of objects or events" (Edelman, 1989, p. 56), is achieved through the establishment of temporal correlations (Edelman, 1978,1987). These correlations are the result of a fundamental process called "*reentry*," which has been defined as "the temporally ongoing parallel signaling between separate maps along ordered anatomical connections" (Edelman, 1989, p. 49). The notion of reentry extends well beyond those of simple feedback, feedforward, or recurrent circuits, and should not be confused with them. As Ashby (1956) has pointed out, "complex systems [such as the brain] cannot be treated as an interlaced set of more or less independent feedback circuits, but only as a whole." Reentry is inherently parallel, has a statistical nature, and is distributed, in that it can occur simultaneously within and across several different areas via multiple parallel and reciprocal connections (as seen in corticocortical, corticothalamic, and thalamocortical radiations); it can also occur via more complex arrangements linking the cortex with the hippocampus or with the basal ganglia. These connections form a powerful system that allows the correlation of processes occurring in parallel and at spatially distant locations. As shown by a computer model simulating reentry among the segregated areas of the visual cortex, reentrant interactions among multiple neuronal maps can also be critically involved in the generation of the response properties of neurons within each area, and can give rise to new properties of the overall system, such as cross-modal construction, conflict resolution, and recursive synthesis (Finkel and Edelman, 1989).

According to the theory of neuronal group selection (Edelman, 1978,1987), reentry takes places between populations of neurons, rather than between single units. Such populations of neurons, called "neuronal groups," form as the result of competitive and selective processes within cortical maps (Pearson et al., 1987), and are the basic functional units of cortical processes. Neurons within a group tend to be strongly connected and share many physiological properties. As we will see below, some of these properties, such as the tendency to discharge in a correlated way, are determined by cooperative interactions resulting from excitatory and inhibitory connections within such collectives.

Some requirements for integration

As briefly mentioned above, we consider the establishment of correlations through reentry to be a fundamental mechanism for the solution of the problem of integration. In addition, some important requirements have to be taken into account. One is that integration must take place at many different levels of organization (Sporns et al., 1991). According to the TNGS, a fundamental level is the functional integration of single cells into neuronal groups. Another level is the "linking" of the responses of neuronal groups belonging to the same (sensory) feature domain by means of reentrant connections within a single cortical area. A simple example that has been addressed both experimentally and in computer models is the integration of neuronal responses to oriented line segments forming an extended contour. Still another level is the "binding" of the responses of neuronal groups from different feature domains by means of reentry among different cortical areas. An example is the integration of neuronal responses to a particular contour with those to its direction of movement or to its color. At a higher level, the integration of perceptual and conceptual components is required to categorize objects. Furthermore, several objects can be integrated into a coherent scene and, ultimately, several modalities, thoughts, memories, and feelings are integrated into a conscious state referring to a single self. At its highest level, the problem can be stated succinctly: consciousness is one, but brain events are many. How are they integrated into a single perspective?

Recently, we have begun to address the problem of integration at early levels, the functional integration of neurons into groups and some instances of linking and binding, in a series of computer simulations (Sporns et al., 1989, 1990, 1991a, 1991b), for which the findings of Gray and Singer (1989; Gray et al., 1989) and Eckhorn et al. (1988) have provided a natural empirical starting point. Some relevant results obtained from these simulations will be summarized in the next sections. We will also show that this approach may provide a possible solution to the classical problem of perceptual grouping and figure-ground segregation.

Another requirement that any mechanism proposed for perceptual and behavioral integration must satisfy is that the integration should be accomplished, sustained, and modified on a time scale of perhaps 50 to 500 ms. These temporal constraints, as well as relevant results obtained from both experiments and computer simulations, will be briefly discussed later.

Finally, a most important requirement is to realize that the concept of integration is necessarily related to that of "*effectiveness as a whole*". We propose that, in order for a collection of elements (such as active neurons) to be considered integrated, they must interact in such a way that the effects they produce are different from those they would produce if they were active independently. Perhaps the most obvious example, although by no means the only one, is when a behavioral output or action depends on the cooperative action of distributed neuronal activities. As an illustration, we will present a computer model that shows how the integration of neuronal groups through temporal correlations may allow them to act together by producing an elementary behavior.

Computer Simulations

Neuronal groups: generation of coherent oscillatory activity

Within the few hundreds of milliseconds necessary for perceptual as well as behavioral integration, a single cell in the cortex will generally produce only a few, apparently stochastic spikes. As a consequence, a single cell is not reliable enough for the establishment of significant temporal correlations within this short period of time. Moreover, it appears that the effect of the discharge of a single cell on any given target cell is negligible. Only when a few dozen cells happen to fire together does their target change its probability of firing (cf. Abeles, 1982). These and other findings indicate that the relevant units of cortical function are neuronal groups rather than single cells. Correlated activity in a population, recorded as a multiunit activity or a local field potential, is statistically more reliable and allows the establishment of significant correlations with other groups. Moreover, since cells in a group tend to share their anatomical projections, their correlated discharge will generally be effective in modifying the probability of firing of target neurons (see below) and often of a whole target group.

In several computer simulations (Sporns et al., 1989, 1991a, 1991b), we modeled neuronal groups as collections of 40 to 160 excitatory cells and 20 to 80 inhibitory cells. In all simulations, the activity function of each cell is such that inputs arriving within a time period of a few milliseconds (the membrane time constant of the cell) are summed and thus have a cooperative effect; inputs separated by longer time intervals act independently and noncooperatively. The interactions between excitatory and inhibitory cells within a group are responsible for the generation of oscillatory activity. Furthermore, they, together with the local cooperative interactions among excitatory cells, lead to the emergence of correlated activity within the group. The activity of inhibitory cells trails that of the excitatory cells by about a quarter of the oscillation period (compare to Gray et al., this volume). As in the experimental data, the activity of a single cell often does not seem to be periodic over a short time period, whereas the activity of the whole group does (Fig. 1). Our simulations show that such coherent oscillatory behavior based on sparsely connected local populations of neurons is an inherently rich and variable phenomenon, a result that is in full accord with the experiments (Gray et al., 1991). Thus, the coherent activity of neuronal groups overcomes the intrinsic unreliability of single cells and represents a first, elementary step for establishing functionally significant correlations.

Another set of mechanisms that might generate oscillations involves the

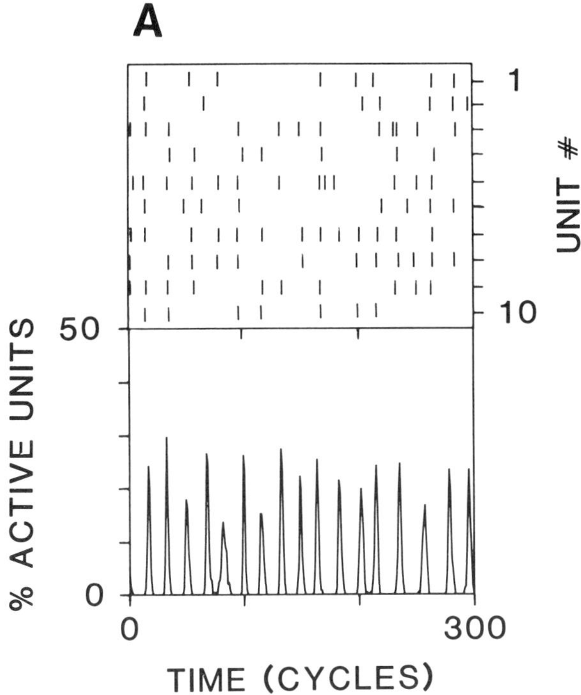

Figure 1. Single unit activity (*top*) and population activity (*bottom*) of orientation-selective units in OR responding to a simulated light bar in preferred orientation moving through the unit's receptive field. Ten orientation-selective units within the same neuronal group are recorded simultaneously (*top*) and their activity is compared to the population activity of that group (*bottom*). Only a few single units appear to discharge at regular intervals, making identification of oscillatory behavior without the use of statistical techniques difficult. The instantaneous frequency of the neuronal groups shifts significantly around 40 Hz. A varying proportion of the group's constituent units participates in each oscillation cycle. Reprinted from Sporns et al., 1989, reproduced with permission of National Academy of Sciences, USA.

intrinsic rhythmic activity of cortical or thalamic neurons (Llinás, 1990). For example, stellate cells located in layer II of the rat's entorhinal cortex show sustained subthreshold oscillatory fluctuations of their membrane potential around 40 Hz (Alonso and Llinás, 1989). Injection of a depolarizing constant current leads to oscillatory spike activity. The oscillations are generated intrinsically under participation of a sodium conductance, but independent of a calcium conductance, and might be influenced by afferent thalamic activity (Llinás, 1990). Other examples of intrinsically oscillating neocortical neurons were described by Chagnac-Amitai and Connors (1989). An open question for both experimental research and modeling is how these cellular phenomena relate to population-based oscillations as observed in the cat visual cortex. It might be predicted that the synchronization and coherency of oscillatory activity in large masses of cortical neurons will require local and global network interactions even if some neurons act as intrinsic oscillators (Bush and Douglas, 1991).

Intra-areal and interareal reentry: linking and binding

In this section, we will describe a computer model of some aspects of the visual system (Sporns et al., 1989, 1991a), which demonstrates the emergence of temporal correlations both within and between visual maps. The model consists of two areas (called OR and MO) containing neuronal groups responsive to different stimulus attributes (orientation and movement, respectively) but sharing common primary dimensions (gross topography of visual space). Each neuronal group is explicitly modeled as a local population of excitatory and inhibitory neurons (see Fig. 1). Upon external stimulation, local recurrent network interactions give rise to oscillatory activity. Groups at different positions within the separate visual maps are connected by two kinds of reentrant connections. Intra-areal reentrant connections link adjacent groups of the same stimulus specificity. In this model, there are no connections between groups of orthogonal specificity (e.g., horizontal and vertical orientations). In addition, there are interareal reentrant connections linking groups within OR and MO. These connections are divergent–convergent in both directions: groups in MO have larger receptive fields and in turn project back onto a larger region of the primary network OR. As a result of their afferent connectivity, groups in MO are selective for the direction of motion of a spatially extended stimulus contour (pattern motion); in contrast, groups in OR are only selective for the orientation and motion of short line segments (component motion). Figure 2 is a selection of movie frames showing the state of each of the model's constituent networks as it responds to a stimulus contour.

Reentrant interactions within OR give rise to temporal correlations between neighboring as well as distant groups with a near-zero phase lag. In accord with the experiments (Gray et al., 1989; Engel et al., 1990), correlations are found between units in groups that have non-overlapping receptive fields if a long, continuous moving bar is presented. These distant correlations disappear if two collinear short bars (separated by a gap) are moved separately with the same velocity. This relatively simple simulation (see also Eckhorn et al., 1989; Kammen et al., 1989; Schillen and König, 1990; Sompolinsky et al., 1990) may serve as an example of linking, the establishment of correlations among features belonging to the same feature domain (in this case, orientation).

Interareal reentrant connections give rise to temporal correlations between the two visual areas. If the model is presented with a moving contour shaped like a corner, OR responds to the orientation and precise position of the parts of the contour, but does not respond to the overall motion of the entire stimulus. By contrast, MO responds to the direction of motion of the entire corner (pattern motion), but not to the orientation and precise position of the parts of which it is composed. However, interareal reentry establishes coherent oscillations between the two maps and achieves the integration of the stimulus as a "moving corner." If the reentrant connections between MO and OR are cut, the coherency of the oscillations between the two maps disappears. Groups in OR that respond to the horizontal and vertical components of the corner also become uncorrelated. In this model, the establishment of correlations between two different stimulus attributes, orientation and motion, may serve as an example of binding. Another analogous case would be the binding of the color and the motion of an object; the available evidence suggests that in the primate visual system color and movement tend to be analyzed in separate, but reentrantly linked, channels (Zeki, 1978; Livingstone and Hubel, 1987).

According to Treisman (Treisman and Gelade, 1980; Treisman, 1988), whereas the linking of elementary features within a given domain (as in perceptual grouping and figure-ground segregation, see below) would be fast, parallel, and preattentive, the conjunction or binding of features belonging to different domains would be slower, serial, and would require attention. However, the distinction between these two stages in the integration of visual features should not be taken too strictly (cf. Nakayama and Silverman, 1986). Note that in the computer model described in this section, linking and binding result from a single mechanism, the reentrant signaling between neuronal groups. Furthermore, linking and binding are functionally interdependent; the binding of orientation and motion depends partially on local correlations (brought about by linking) within each domain, and vice versa.

Modeling perceptual grouping and figure-ground segregation

Temporal correlations as established by reentrant signaling may provide a key to the solution of a classical problem in visual perception, that of perceptual grouping and figure-ground segregation. These two processes, both of fundamental importance in perceptual organization, refer to the ability to group together elementary features into discrete objects and to segregate these objects from each other and from the background. Gestalt psychologists have extensively investigated the factors influencing grouping and the distinction between figure and ground, and have described a number of laws, such as those of similarity, continuity, proximity, and common motion (Wertheimer, 1923; Koffka, 1935; Köhler, 1947). However, their attempts to identify the underlying neural mechanisms, such as postulating the existence of isomorphic brain fields, have failed. The following quotation from one of Wolfgang Köhler's papers on Gestalt psychology illustrates these points:

> For too long the perceptual field has been treated analytically, in an artificial an unrealistic manner, as though, e.g., in visual space, individual local sensory

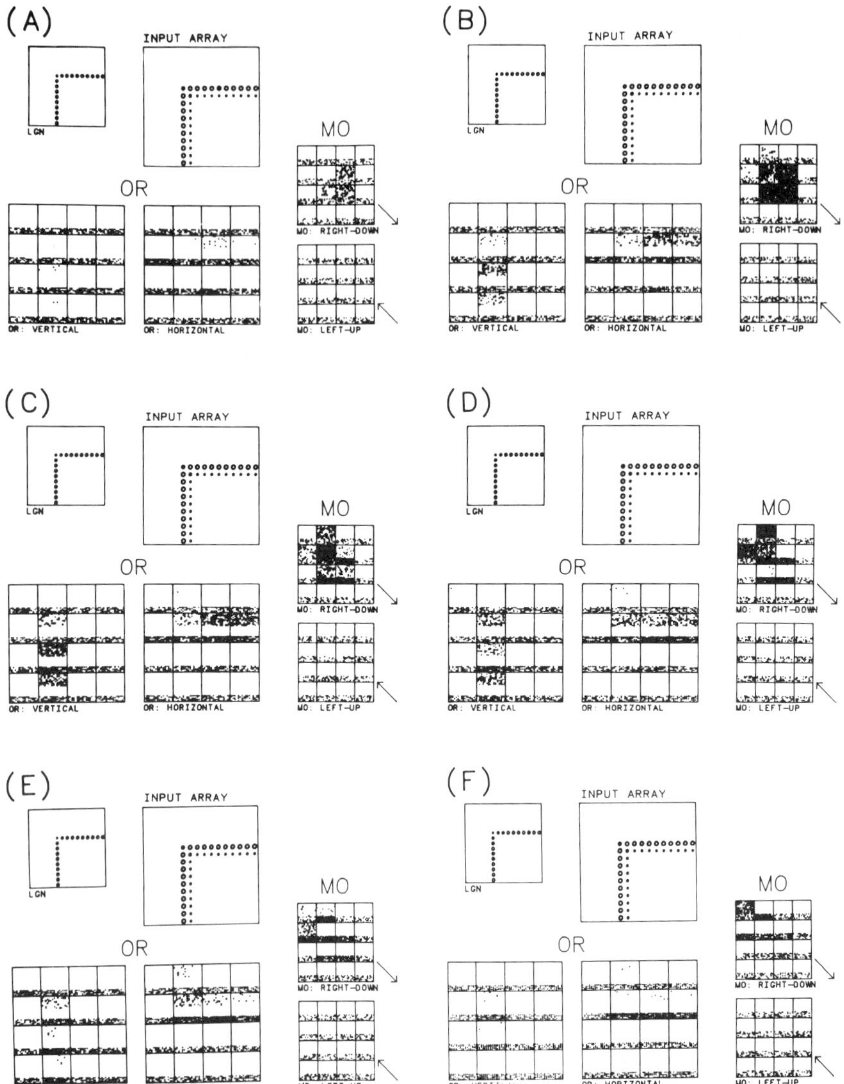

Figure 2. Six frames from a movie showing the oscillatory activity of neuronal groups responding to a stimulus contour moving in a southeast direction. Panels **A** to **F** correspond to iterations 889, 891, 892, 893, 895, and 897 of the simulation run; one iteration corresponds roughly to 1 ms. The input array (*central upper square in each panel*) shows the moving corner-shaped contour. (Movement of the stimulus contour is too slow to be noticed in this short segment of the run.) Simulated cortical area OR is split into two subparts; the box on the left of each panel (labeled "OR: VERTICAL") contains orientation-selective neuronal units responding optimally to vertical bars; the box at the lower center of each panel (labeled "OR: HORIZONTAL") contains orientation-selective neuronal units responding optimally to horizontal bars. On the right of each panel is shown the simulated cortical area MO, with two boxes contain-

> qualities were essentially determined by individual local stimuli, so that an incoherent mosaic of such qualities would have to result. Of course the phenomenal world does not look like this to anybody. We have before us patches, bounded surfaces, and things or groups of these: also we see, hear or feel events of definite form. Thus there is a concrete structuring of the whole field in its spatial and temporal extension ... If there is a multitude of local stimuli, the organism by no means reacts with separate local sensory processes for each of them. A now tremendous body of experience forces us rather to think of the sensory processes as a functionally connected continuum in which local conditions may at once acquire more than local significance. Therefore distributions, specific connections, and separations are formed and re-formed in reciprocal dynamic interaction across the whole system until the whole comes to rest. (Köhler, 1930; quoted after Henle, 1971, pp. 175–176).

In principle, perceptual grouping and figure-ground segregation could be accomplished by a number of neural mechanisms (Fig. 3). In a hierarchical model based on specialized detector units (so-called grandmother cells; Figure 3, left), an appropriately connected detector "reassembles" the elementary features and signals the presence of the figure (a kind of hierarchical strategy has been proposed, e.g., by Barlow, 1981). However, the number of detectors needed to guarantee a response for each possible object in varying positions and contexts would be prohibitively large. More recently, several modelers and theoreticians have argued that cooperative processes may play a role in figure-ground segregation (e.g., Caelli, 1985; Grossberg and Mingolla, 1985; Kienker et al., 1986), although the explanations provided by these models are not always consistent with known principles of neural function. Expressed

Figure 2 (*continued*)
ing pattern motion-selective neuronal units responding optimally to contours moving southeast (box labeled "MO: RIGHT-DOWN") and northwest (box labeled "MO: LEFT-UP"). Each of the four boxes comprising the simulated cortical areas OR and MO contains 16 neuronal groups topographically arranged in a 4 × 4 grid. In OR, only two layers of neuronal units are displayed, the orientation-selective units (in the upper half of each group) and the inhibitory units (in the lower quarter of each group); direction-selective units and their associated inhibitory units are omitted for clarity of the display. In MO, pattern-motion selective units occupy the upper two thirds and inhibitory units the lower one third of each group.

In **panel A**, motion-selective neuronal groups in MO begin to respond to the motion of the stimulus contour in a southeast direction. Their reentrant signals reaching OR facilitate the onset of correlated activity in orientation-selective neuronal groups (**panel B**). In return, the activity of motion-selective groups grows to be even more pronounced. **Panels C and D** show the oscillatory activity in both OR and MO at its peak; notice that groups in both the VERTICAL and the HORIZONTAL parts of OR are activated in a synchronous fashion. **Panels E and F** show the activity slowly dying away, restoring the initial situation. Reprinted with permission of VCH Publishers, Inc., 220 East 23rd St., New York, N.Y., 10010 from: Schuster HG, ed, *Nonlinear Dynamics and Neuronal Networks*: Sporns O, Tononi G, Edelman GM: Dynamic Interactions of Neuronal Groups and Cortical Integration, Figure 10, Page 228.

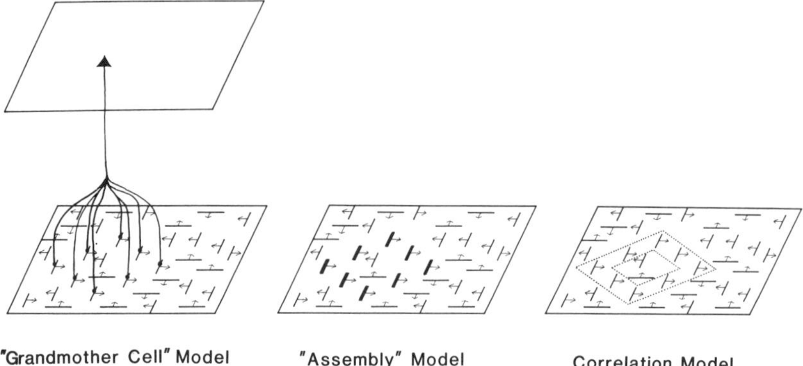

Figure 3. Different possible models of perceptual grouping and figure-ground segregation. In all three cases an identical display of moving short light bars is presented to a primary layer of direction-selective neurons. Eight of these bars move coherently to the right (the "figure," shaped like a diamond), the other bars move in random directions ("ground"). **Left**: A specialized layer of "grandmother cells," which are appropriately connected to the primary layer, detects the coherently moving object. The firing of a cell within this layer "codes" for the presence of the figure. **Middle**: Neurons within the primary layer responding to the coherently moving figure enhance their firing frequency (indicated by thick bars). Other neurons responding to the non-coherent background remain at a lower level of firing. The mean activity level of an assembly of cells "codes" for the figure. **Right**: Neurons within the primary layer responding to the coherently moving figure correlate their firing, which becomes synchronous. This temporally correlated collection of neurons is called a "cohort," the spatial extent of which is marked by the stippled line. Other neurons responding to the background are uncorrelated to neurons within the cohort and can therefore be segregated.

more directly in neural terms, a cooperative "assembly" model proposes that all those neurons that respond to a coherent figure enhance their mean activity (Singer, 1985; Fig. 3, middle). Ambiguity arises, however, if several "assemblies" responding to different objects or to an object and a coherent background have to be distinguished (Gray et al., 1990b). This would not be the case in a model based on temporal correlations (Fig. 3, right), which achieves grouping and segmentation by linking features through correlated activity among neuronal groups, made possible by intra-areal reentry. Furthermore, this possibility is now supported both by experimental results and theoretical considerations (Gray et al., 1990b).

Recently, we have extended and modified the computer model discussed in the previous section to address the problem of perceptual grouping and segmentation in vision (Sporns et al., 1991b). The model consists of an input array, four sets of elementary feature detectors, and four repertoires of orientation- and direction-selective neuronal groups. Groups of different specificities are connected only if they have overlapping receptive fields, whereas groups of similar specificities have more extended lateral connections, which fall off with distance. These assumptions are justified by anatomical and physiological observations in the visual cortex (Gilbert and Wiesel, 1989; Luhmann et al., 1990). An important feature incorporated into this extended model is rapid and reversible plasticity of synaptic efficacies. These can change on a very short time scale (in the range of tens of milliseconds, if a single iteration is taken to correspond to 1 ms). The increased efficacy of reentrant connections among correlated groups rapidly amplifies and stabilizes correlations.

The model is presented with an extended pattern composed of several bars moving coherently, embedded in a background of vertical and horizontal bars moving right, left, up, and down at random (Fig. 4). The groups responding to the bars that move in the same direction are rapidly linked by coherent oscillations (within 60–100 ms after stimulus onset), even though the lateral spread of the connections from each group is much less than the size of the object. The ability to establish specific linking (grouping) is directly related to the ability to achieve segmentation. Accordingly, there is no coherency among groups responding to elements of the figure and others responding to elements of the background; the latter include elements moving in the same direction as the figure, but placed some distance away. The model is also able to segregate a figure from a coherent background of identical texture moving in a different direction or from another, overlapping figure (Fig. 5). In addition, the model can link together the contour of a coherently moving figure, even if it is composed of both vertical and horizontal segments. All these results are strongly dependent on the presence of rapid changes in synaptic efficacy.

This computer model shows that, at least in principle, the neural basis for the integration and segregation of elementary features into objects and background might be the pattern of temporal correlations among neuronal groups. In addition, since the resulting grouping and segregation are consistent with the Gestalt laws of continuity, proximity, similarity, common orientation, and common motion, it suggests that the neural basis for these laws is to be found implicitly in the specific pattern of connectivity incorporated into the architecture and in the ensuing dynamics of short-term correlations.

Anatomical and temporal determinants of patterns of correlations. Patterns of correlations can be determined primarily by the organization of the anatomical connectivity among neuronal groups or by the fine temporal structure of their activity. In the former case, correlations would tend to arise whenever active groups are connected, either directly or through an uninterrupted chain of other active and connected groups. In the latter, correlations are established selectively among specific subsets of groups even if they are all active and connected. In general, of course, the two mechanisms that we will briefly discuss in this section will interact in variable proportions according to the circumstances.

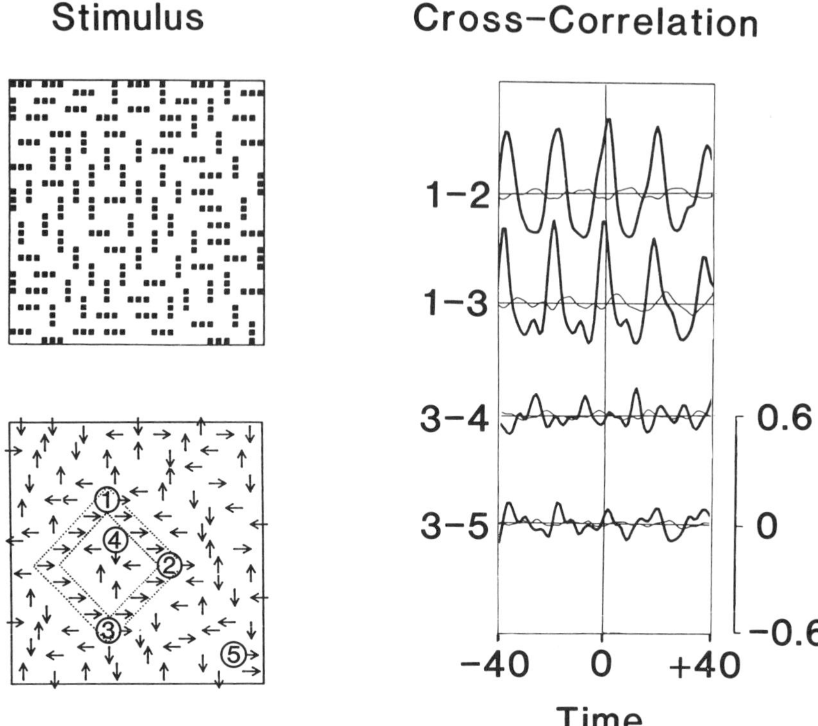

Figure 4. An example of grouping and segmentation in the model of Sporns et al., 1991b. **Left**: Stimulus presented to the model, consisting of 100 vertically and horizontally oriented light bars moving right, left, up, and down. In the top panel the light bars are shown at their starting positions; the bottom panel shows their corresponding directions of movement indicated by arrows. Encircled numbers with arrows in the bottom panel refer to the locations of recorded neuronal activity, corresponding cross-correlations are displayed on the right. "Electrodes" 1–3 recorded from neurons responding to the figure; "electrodes" 4 and 5 from neurons responding to the ground. **Right**: Cross-correlograms of neuronal responses to the stimulus shown on the left. Cross-correlograms are computed over a 100-ms sample period and subsequently averaged over 10 trials. Numbers refer to the locations of neuronal groups within the direction-selective repertoires (*see left*). Four correlograms are shown (figure-figure: 1–2, 1–3; figure-ground: 3–4, 3–5), computed between ms 201 and 300 after stimulus onset. The correlograms are scaled and shift-predictors (*thin lines*, averaged over nine shifts; Perkel et al., 1967b) are displayed for comparison. Reprinted from Sporns et al., 1991b, with permission of National Academy of Science, USA.

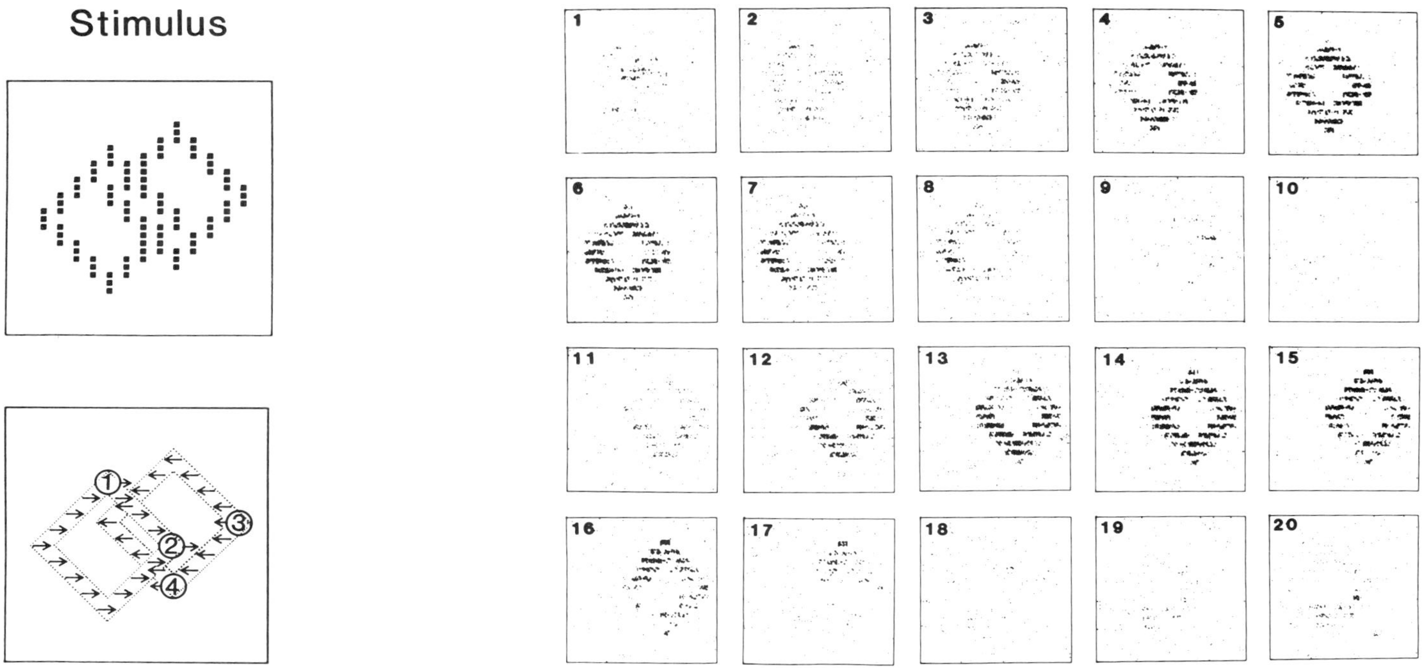

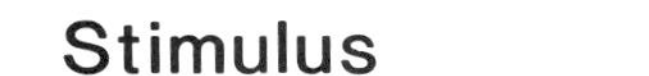

Figure 5. Frames taken from a movie (*right*) showing the responses of direction-selective groups in the model of figure-ground segregation (Sporns et al., 1991b) to a stimulus (*left*) containing two identical and overlapping, but differently moving figures. The frames show a continuous period of 20 ms (20 iterations) recorded about 150 ms after stimulus onset. Each frame displays the entire array of neuronal groups (16×16) selective for motion to the right and to the left, and arranged in an interleaved fashion (this accounts for the striped pattern). Each small dot within the array is an active neuron. For the first 10 ms (frames 1–10) mostly groups responding to the figure moving right are active; subsequently these groups are silent and groups responsive to the other figure become active (frames 11–20). The array of groups has been segregated into two cohorts oscillating independently from each other (in this movie segment they happen to be 180° out of phase). Notice that neuronal activity is strongly correlated both locally (in neighborhoods corresponding to groups) as well as over the entire extent of the figure. (left: modified from Sporns et al., 1991b). Reproduced with permission of National Academy of Sciences, USA.

The previous model of perceptual grouping and figure-ground segregation is clearly an instance where the anatomical connectivity has a predominant influence. In accord with experimental data, it incorporates preferential connections between groups that have similar orientation and direction specificity, and that are topographically neighboring. As a result, since objects tend to consist of similar features arranged more or less contiguously in space, whenever a coherent object is presented, the system readily produces a pattern of correlations that groups together the features corresponding to the object and segregates them from the background. In general, it may be assumed that the anatomical connectivity selected for during evolution and stabilized during individual experience has incorporated such useful principles. This is probably also the case with the relative segregation in the pattern of connectivity among different areas (e.g., different visual areas), among subsystems within and across areas (e.g., parvocellular and magnocellular streams), and among domains within an area (e.g., ocular dominance and orientation columns).

In other cases, the pattern of correlations may be determined chiefly by the fine temporal organization of neuronal activity. The most obvious example of this kind involves some clear-cut temporal structure in the input, as in the model of auditory segmentation by von der Malsburg and Schneider (1986). The amplitude of the different frequency components of a single sound will often be synchronously modulated. The synchronous wave of activity in the input fibers will induce synchronous activation in the set of neurons responding to the corresponding frequencies. Their correlated firing will express the grouping of the different frequency components into a single auditory event. Another sound will evoke synchronous activity in another set of neurons. Although all the neurons may be active and connected, the temporal structure of the input can dynamically segregate them into two independent cohorts (as discussed by Sporns et al., 1989, a cohort may be defined as an ensemble of groups that are strongly correlated among themselves).

Irrespective of the relative role of the connectivity and of the fine temporal structure of neuronal activity, it is extremely important to rely on further mechanisms in order to amplify and preserve the ensuing correlations in a feedforward way. As we have seen, one important mechanism, which has been employed in different contexts and formulations by Sporns et al. (1991b) as well as by von der Malsburg and Schneider (1986), may involve short-term changes in synaptic efficacy.

Temporal constraints on integration

As mentioned before, any mechanism accounting for perceptual integration must be fast, on the order of a few hundreds of milliseconds. This is apparent from a variety of psychophysical results, although the precise duration of perceptual processes is difficult to assess, due to disagreements about definitions, assumptions, and experimental approaches (cf. Richet, 1898; Boring, 1933; Blumenthal, 1977; Uttal, 1981). For instance, in visual perception, the minimum duration of an experience has been variously estimated to require about 60 ms (Serviere et al., 1977), 100 ms (Stroud, 1955), 125 ms (Lichtenstein, 1961), 130 ms (Efron, 1970), and 140 ms (Allport, 1968). At any rate, it seems safe to assume that processes such as perceptual grouping, texture segmentation, and figure-ground discrimination require less than 200 ms (e.g., Bergen and Julesz, 1983). Short stimulus presentations are often sufficient even for the perception of a complex visual scene: for instance, Biederman et al. (1982) conclude that "semantic relations, defined by the specific ways in which objects typically interact in the visual world, are accessed from a 150-ms presentation of a picture of a novel scene." Data coming from other modalities (e.g., Libet, 1978) as well as from several cognitive tasks (cf. Pöppel, 1985) also point to values somewhere between 50 and 500 ms. Thus, if the establishment of short-term correlations is indeed involved in perceptual integration, it should be consistent with temporal constraints of about this magnitude.

Interestingly, Gray et al. (1991) have shown that the onset of synchrony among neurons responding to different parts of coherent stimuli may take as little as a few tens of milliseconds. Furthermore, the duration of synchrony is highly variable, lasting from 40 to 430 ms, and within a response to a stimulus multiple episodes of coherent firing, varying in duration, amplitude, and phase, may alternate with episodes of asynchrony. Correspondingly, in our model of perceptual grouping and figure-ground segregation, synchronization after stimulus onset is rapid, usually within 100 to 200 ms (if one iteration is taken to correspond to 1 ms) (Sporns et al., 1991b). Multiple coherent episodes of various length may occur at different times in different trials. Furthermore, synchrony is transient (between 100 and 500 ms), and its offset is fast, as would be clearly required by the fact that the visual scene continuously changes due to eye movements. This is also consistent with well known perceptual phenomena (cf. Uttal, 1981), such as reversals of grouping, figure-ground (Rubin illusion), and depth (Necker cube). It should be mentioned that in the model episodes of correlated activity coincide with transient enhancement of reentrant connectivity due to short-term changes in synaptic efficacy, implying that the temporal characteristics of correlations are strongly influenced by ongoing short-term synaptic plasticity.

The question of effectiveness

Despite the considerable interest aroused by the discovery that neuronal groups display correlated activity for fractions of a second when responding to coherent stimuli, there is still some skepticism concerning the actual significance of these coherent oscillations. The question has been asked whether they should be considered as an "epiphenomenon" (Stryker, 1989).

To answer this question, it is important to distinguish between oscillations and correlations. With regard to oscillations *per se*, it is certainly possible that the presence of rhythmic activity at particular frequency ranges may give rise to "resonance" phenomena, which could produce significant effects in vast, reentrantly interconnected networks. In addition, the oscillatory properties of neuronal groups may interact in a variety of ways with biochemical or cellular processes involving synaptic modification (Levy and Steward, 1983) and different transmitter systems ("transmitter logic," see Edelman, 1987, Chapter 7). Finally, the spatiotemporal pattern of oscillations might play a critical role in guiding early morphogenetic events in the brain.

Although any or all of these mechanisms may be shown to exist, the main concern of this chapter is the problem of functional integration in the nervous system. In this regard, our proposal is that what really matters is the establishment of temporal correlations among neuronal groups, whether their firing pattern is oscillatory or not.

There is some indication that the appearance of short-term correlations, rather than of an increased firing rate, or of oscillatory activity, can be associated with the execution of behavioral tasks (Vaadia et al., 1991b). Recordings from the prefrontal cortex during behavioral sequences in which this part of the brain is definitely involved show that single neurons do not usually change their mean firing rate significantly (in strong contrast to neurons in primary sensory or motor cortices). Furthermore, there is so far no sign of fast oscillatory activity at the single cell level in this part of the cortex. As discussed by Abeles (Abeles et al., 1990), these findings are at least puzzling for advocates of "cell assemblies" as the basis for representation, if an assembly is characterized by the increased mean firing rate of its constituent cells. What is most intriguing, however, is that during a behavioral response, whereas mean activity levels for a given pair of neurons do not change their normalized cross-correlation does (Vaadia et al., 1991). The cross-correlograms are flat at the beginning; then, with the start of the behavioral response, they suddenly rise and stay elevated for about 250 ms before declining again.

Thus, at least in this case, a behavior coincides with a rise in the cross-correlation between neurons, but not with an increased, or rhythmic, firing rate. Of course, such a coincidence only suggests, but does not by itself demonstrate, that short-term correlations play a functional role in the execution of the task. The question remains whether correlations may be effective *per se*. Therefore, it is important to show that the presence of correlateo *vs* uncorrelated activity should make a substantial difference to the funaioning of the brain. There is a fundamental argument that illustrates this fact. Typically, several thousand synapses converge on a single cortical neuron. If these synapses are activated asynchronously, the summation of hundreds of excitatory postsynaptic potentials (EPSPs) is required in order to influence the target cell's probability of discharge. By contrast, as few as 10 EPSPs may be sufficient if they happen to be synchronous (Abeles, 1982). Thus, separate inputs cooperate optimally when they are strongly correlated. Interestingly enough, the width of the peak of the cross-correlograms obtained by Gray and Singer (1989) and Eckhorn et al. (1988) is generally around 6 to 8 ms, a value that closely matches the membrane time constant of cortical neurons (Lux and Pollen, 1966; Bindman et al., 1988).

A minimal model of effective integration. The argument that correlated activity *per se* can have a significant effect can be illustrated, in a simplified form, in a computer model. So far, our computer simulations have provided some insight into how neuronal activity can be integrated at various functional levels: within a local group of neurons and also within and between visual maps. None of the models has shown, however, how integration can become effective, for example, on behavior. In this section, we discuss a computer simulation that makes use of short-term correlations to integrate the activity of neuronal groups and produce a simple behavior. The model, a simplified version of the grouping and segmentation model, is a minimal one but it has some implications for the problem of effective integration in general.

As in the previous model, all groups discharge in an oscillatory fashion, and the efficacy of the reentrant connectivity changes on a short time scale. Instead of simulating full neuronal groups, we have substituted them with repertoires of 32 × 32 idealized groups, composed each of an excitatory and an inhibitory unit. This makes the model less realistic and more rigid, but is required in order to reduce the length of the simulations in real time. In addition, we have introduced a single group, called the effector, which is connected uniformly to all groups within the direction-selective repertoires. Such an arrangement is obviously unrealistic, since in a real nervous system several mapped and nonmapped regions would be involved in any behavioral response; nonetheless, the assumption of an effector is sufficient in order to illustrate the principle.

The model is supposed to respond only when it is presented with a single coherent object moving in a certain oblique direction (e.g. right-up). First, the system was trained to respond only to a square of a certain size moving right-up, irrespective of where it appeared in the visual field (see, e.g., Fig. 6A). The training sequence consisted of a number of squares presented at different positions in the visual field one at a time, moving in one of the four oblique directions. A value system similar to the ones used in the construction of the selective recognition automaton Darwin III (Reeke et al., 1990) was used to modify the probability of changing the strength of the connections from the direction-selective repertoire to the effector and thus to condition the system. As a result of this, the connections to the effector coming from the repertoires selective for movement to the left and down were weakened, whereas those coming from the repertoires selective for movement to the right and up were strengthened. At this point, the model was able to discriminate accuractely between squares moving in different directions (Fig. 6B).

Further training enabled the system to respond only to coherent squares, and not to separate line segments. The set of stimuli now consisted of either a coherent square moving right–up (the "positive" stimulus) or a collection of two vertical bars moving right plus two horizontal bars moving up (the "negative" stimulus, see Fig. 6C). (The individual bars had exactly the same length as the sides of the square.) During training, the system adjusted the strength of the connections coming from the "right" and "up" repertoires so that only the

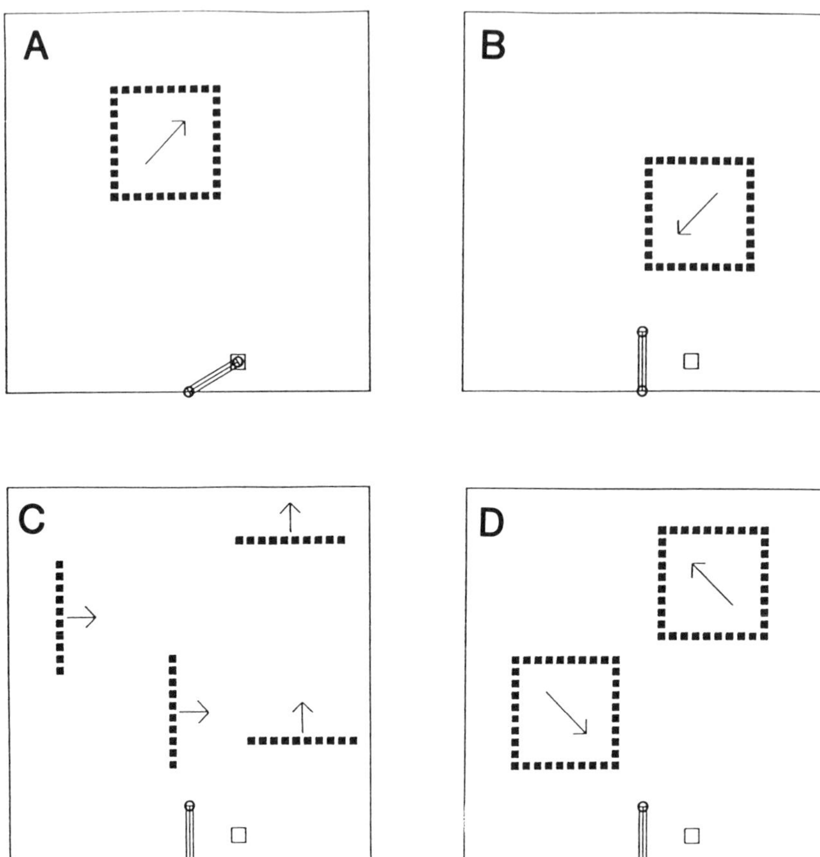

Figure 6. Examples of stimuli and "behavioral" responses of the minimal model of effective integration (see also Table 1). All four panels show the environment (input array) containing a visual stimulus (arrows indicating its direction of motion) and, at the bottom, a one-jointed effector. This effector can be in one of two positions: extended upward (resting position, "no response") or pointing to the right ("response"). When pointing to the right, the effector touches a lever (small square displayed near the bottom of the environment). This constitutes a "positive" behavioral response to the stimulus. All examples in panels A to D are after the completion of training. **A**: The model responds when presented with a coherent square moving right-up. No response occurs with a coherent square moving left-down (**B**), with a collection of separated bars moving right and up (**C**), or with simultaneously presented squares moving right-down and left-up (**D**).

Table 1. Response frequency for the minimal model of effective integration

Case fig. 6	Total	Number of trials response	No response
A	100	95	5
B	100	0	100
C	100	3	97
D	77	5	72

Note: The different cases (A) to (D) correspond to those displayed in Fig. 6. The sample period (length of a trial) was 260 ms starting with stimulus onset.

almost synchronous activation of units responding to the four sides of the square was able to excite the effector above threshold. After training was completed, the model responded only when presented with a coherent stimulus moving right–up (Fig. 6A), but not with a collection of separate line segments (Fig. 6C, see also Table 1). This is because groups responding to separate bars would not, in most cases, be activated synchronously. Thus, the model shows in an elementary way how short-term correlations among neuronal groups may be used to integrate the relevant characteristics of the stimulus and to respond appropriately.

The model was also tested with a potentially ambiguous stimulus, consisting of two coherent squares, one moving right–down, the other one moving left–up (Fig. 6D). As in the case of the stimulus shown in Figure 6C, all components of a square moving right–up were present. However, in this case they were not separated but constituted integral parts of two coherent objects (squares), which were simultaneously present in the visual field. Nonetheless, the system was not fooled by this arrangement, and the effector did not respond. This last case is particularly interesting in a comparison with an "assembly" model based on mean activity levels (see Fig. 3, middle). The latter could perhaps deal with the case depicted in Figure 6C, if the system were carefully designed so that, due to cooperative interactions, the mean activity level of units would be higher when they respond to a coherent long bar than when they respond to shorter isolated segments, but lower than when they respond to a whole coherent square. The connections between sensory and effector groups could be adjusted as in our model. However, an "assembly" model would fail in the case of Figure 6D. To the effector, the mean activity level of the groups responding to the two squares moving right–down and left–up would be indistinguishable from that of the groups responding to the square moving right–up, and erroneous responses would result.

It is of interest to compare some results obtained from the simulations presented above with data coming from experimental psychology. Studying the distribution of choice-reaction times of human subjects in sensory discrimination tasks, Pöppel has reported multimodal histograms with peaks regularly spaced by about 30 ms (Pöppel, 1970; see also Pöppel and

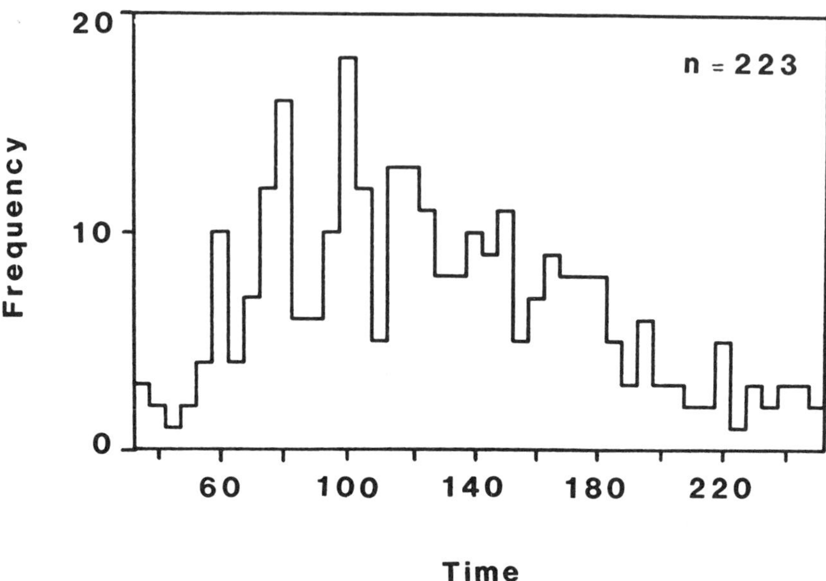

Figure 7. Histogram of time intervals between stimulus onset and onset of behavior recorded from 223 trials. The simulation was identical to the one shown in Fig. 6A, with a square moving right-up presented at different locations in the input array. The distribution shows multiple peaks at 60, 80, 100, and 120 ms after stimulus onset. Each trial lasted 260 ms, the bin-width is 5 ms. This histogram should be compared to a similar one in Pöppel (1970; see his Fig. 1).

Logothethis, 1986). According to Pöppel, the multimodality of the distributions indicates the presence of oscillatory neuronal activity in parts of the brain contributing to the response and, in particular, of a stimulus-locked component. This interpretation is entirely consistent with the results obtained from the present model. Figure 7 shows a histogram of the time intervals between presentation of the stimulus (a square moving right–up, as in Fig. 6A) and the response of the effector for 223 trials. The histogram reveals a multimodal distribution of response times with peaks spaced by about 20 ms (1 ms = 1 iteration); this corresponds to the period of the oscillatory activity in the direction-selective repertoires.

The hypothesis that the presence of correlated neuronal activity may affect behavior, as suggested by the previous computer simulation, may be amenable to experimental test. Such an experiment could involve an animal that has been conditioned to respond positively (e.g., by pressing a key) when presented with a particular coherent stimulus (e.g., a square moving right–up). While the animal is responding to a stimulus, neuronal responses could be recorded from appropriate locations in the cerebral cortex. One prediction is that coherency between different parts of the stimulus would appear only when the stimulus itself is coherent (as in Fig. 6A). Most importantly, a correlation should be found between the presence of coherent activity and a positive behavioral response. Conversely, if the animal makes an error, that is, the positive behavioral response fails to occur in the presence of the positive stimulus, coherent activity should be weak or absent. This should also be the case when the same bars composing the stimulus are moved independently (as in Fig. 6C). Furthermore, a correlation should be found between the onset of coherent neuronal activity (which is inherently variable) and that of the behavioral response.

Global Mappings and the Unity of Consciousness

As suggested before, the problem of integration, which is first encountered with linking and binding, culminates with the integration or unity of consciousness. According to William James, being "an integral thing not made of parts" (James, 1890, p. 177) is indeed a key property of consciousness. On the other hand, it has been argued that the emergence of even the most basic or primary form of consciousness requires complex brain systems dealing with perceptual categorization, memory, learning, biological self–nonself distinction, conceptual categorization, a memory of past value-category associations, and a reentrant pathway by which this memory can discriminate current perceptual categorizations (Edelman, 1989). This prompts the question of how the functions of all these brain systems may be effectively integrated. We propose that, even in the case of consciousness itself, the establishment through reentry of cooperative interactions resulting in temporal correlations may be the key to integration. In particular, reentry would take place simultaneously across several brain regions, within arrangements that have been called "global mappings." A global mapping has been defined as:

> ... a dynamic structure which contains multiple reentrant local maps, both motor and sensory, which interact with non-mapped regions to form a spatiotemporally continuous representation of objects and events. Through motor activity, a global mapping alters the sampling of the environment by sensory sheets. Each repertoire within the local maps of a global mapping disjunctively samples various aspects or features of the environment. Connection of these local maps in a global mapping serves to link these samples by reentry so that the various representations of features are correlated in space and time. (Edelman, *Neural Darwinism*, 1987, pp. 209–210)

In this respect, the fact that the oscillatory activity of distant neuronal groups can lock in with near-zero phase lag should be considered as an important indication of the presence and the effects of reentry. It should also be stressed that structures like the thalamus, the basal ganglia, the claustrum, and the hippocampus may be particularly important in linking parts of global mappings despite the long distances among brain areas. Because of their strategic position, they may facilitate the fast interaction among remote brain regions by establishing more direct synaptic routes between them, and allow the locking-in of distributed brain systems involved in the emergence of consciousness.

Conclusion

This chapter has examined some aspects of a fundamental problem of neural and mental function, that of neural integration at various levels. We have shown that computer models, based on the notions of neuronal groups and reentry and inspired by some recent findings about fast induced rhythms in the visual cortex, can address some simple instances of integration, such as linking and binding. We have also suggested a possible neural basis for perceptual grouping and figure-ground segregation, as well as for some of the Gestalt laws. In addition, we have presented a minimal model that indicates that having synchronous oscillations among neuronal groups may be functionally effective by giving rise to an elementary behavior, and we have proposed possible ways of experimentally confirming these ideas.

A main suggestion emerging from this analysis is that short-term correlations and reentry among neuronal groups may be one major key to the solution of the problem of integration at several levels, even up to those necessary for consciousness. Unfortunately, little is known about the existence, nature, and characteristics of short-term correlations outside the few visual areas explored until now. However, a reexamination of the available experimental results in view of these considerations seems to support this suggestion, since: 1) correlations are more easily observed among groups rather than single neurons, 2) correlations are found over long distances within an area, between different areas, and across the corpus callosum, 3) correlations have the right duration, that is, they last for 50 to 500 ms, and are highly dynamic, 4) the few examples at hand indicate that when parts of a stimulus should be "seen by the brain" as coherent or integrated, correlations have a near-zero phase lag, 5) in general, the width of the peak of the cross-correlograms is such as to be strongly effective on target neurons, 6) finally, recent experiments suggest that some behavioral tasks are associated with changes in short-term correlations among neurons, and not necessarily in neuronal activity. Accordingly, it would be particularly valuable if the renewed attention directed at induced rhythms in the cerebral cortex were accompanied by an increased interest in the study of patterns of short-term correlations in the nervous system.

Acknowledgments. This work was carried out as part of the Institute Fellows in Theoretical Neurobiology program at The Neurosciences Institute, which is supported by the Neurosciences Research Foundation. OS is a Charles and Mildred Schnurmacher Fellow. We are grateful to FIDIA, S.p.A., and to the National Science Foundation for a grant in support of computer resources.

References

Abeles M (1982): *Local Cortical Circuits.* Berlin: Springer–Verlag

Abeles M, Vaadia E, Bergman H (1990): Firing patterns of single units in the prefrontal cortex and neural network models. *Network* 1:13–25

Allport DA (1968): Phenomenal simultaneity and the perceptual moment hypothesis. *Br J Psychol* 59:395–406

Alonso A, Llinás RR (1989): Subthreshold Na^{+}-dependent theta-like rhythmicity in stellate cells of entorhinal cortex layer II. *Nature* 342:175–177

Ashby, WR (1956): *An Introduction to Cybernetics.* New York: Wiley

Barlow HB (1981): Critical limit factors in the design of the eye and visual cortex. *Proc R Soc Lond B* 212:1–34

Basar E (1980): *EEG–Brain Dynamics.* Amsterdam: Elsevier

Bauer RH, Jones CN (1976): Feedback training of 36–44 EEG activity in visual cortex and hippocampus of cats: evidence for sensory and motor involvement. *Physiol Behav* 17:885–890

Bergen JR, Julesz B (1983): Parallel versus serial processing in rapid pattern discrimination. *Nature* 303:696–698

Biederman I, Mezzanotte RJ, Rabinowitz JC (1982): Scene perception: detecting and judging objects undergoing relational violations. *Cogn Psychol* 14:143–177

Bindman LJ, Meyer T, Prince CA (1988): Comparison of the electrical properties of neocortical neurons in slices in vitro and in the anesthetised rat. *Exp Brain Res* 69:489–496

Blumenthal, AL (1977): *The process of cognition.* Englewood Cliffs, N.J.: Prentice Hall

Boring EG (1933): *The Physical Dimensions of Consciousness.* New York: Dover (reprinted 1963)

Bouyer JJ, Montaron MF, Rougeul A (1981): Fast fronto-parietal rhythms during combined focused attentive behavior and immobility in cat: cortical and thalamic localizations. *Electroencephalogr Clin Neurophysiol* 51:244–252

Bouyer JJ, Montaron MF, Vahnée JM, Albert MP, Rougeul A (1987): Anatomical localization of cortical beta rhythms in cat. *Neuroscience* 22:863–869

Bressler SL (1990): The gamma wave: a cortical information carrier? *Trends Neurosci* 13:161–162

Bullock TH, McClune MC (1989): Lateral coherence of the electrocorticogram: a new measure of brain synchrony. *Electroencphalogr Clin Neurophysiol* 73:479–498

Bush PC, Douglas RJ (1991): Synchronization of bursting action potential discharge in a model network of neocortical neurons. *Neur Comput* 3:19–30

Caelli T (1985): Three processing characteristics of visual texture segmentation. *Spatial Vision* 1:19–30

Chagnac-Amitai Y, Connors BW (1989): Synchronized excitation and inhibition driven by intrinsically bursting neurons in neocortex. *J Neurophysiol* 62:1149–1162

Damasio AR (1989): Time-locked multiregional retroactivation: a systems-level proposal for the neural substrates of recall and recognition. *Cognition* 33:25–62

Eckhorn R, Bauer R, Jordan W, Brosch M, Kruse W, Munk M, Reitboeck HJ (1988): Coherent oscillations: a mechanism of feature linking in the visual cortex? Multiple electrode and correlation analyses in the cat. *Biol Cybern* 60:121–130

Eckhorn R, Reitboeck HJ, Arndt M, Dicke P (1989): A neural network for feature linking via synchronous activity: results from cat visual cortex and from simulations. In: *Models of Brain Function*, Cotterill RMJ, ed. Cambridge, UK: Cambridge University Press, pp 255–272

Edelman GM (1978): Group selection and phasic re-entrant signalling: a theory of higher brain function. In: *The Mindful Brain*, Edelman GM, Mountcastle VB, eds. Cambridge, MA: MIT Press, pp 51–100

Edelman GM (1987): *Neural Darwinism. The Theory of Neuronal Group Selection.* New York: Basic Books

Edelman GM (1989): *The Remembered Present. A Biological Theory of Consciousness.* New York: Basic Books

Efron R (1970): The minimum duration of a perception. *Neuropsychologia* 8:57–63

Engel AK, König P, Gray CM, Singer W (1990): Stimulus-dependent neuronal oscillations in cat visual cortex: II. Inter-columnar interaction as determined by cross-correlation analysis. *Eur J Neurosci* 2:588–606

Engel AK, König P, Kreiter A, Gray CM, Singer W (1991): Temporal coding by coherent oscillations as a potential solution to the binding problem: physiological evidence. In: *Nonlinear Dynamics and Neuronal Networks*, Schuster HG, ed. Weinheim, FRG: VCH, pp 3–25

Finkel LH, Edelman GM (1989): The integration of distributed cortical systems by reentry: a computer simulation of interactive functionally segregated visual areas. *J Neurosci* 9:3188–3208

Freeman WJ, Skarda CA (1985): Spatial EEG patterns, non-linear dynamics and perception: the neo-Sherringtonian view. *Brain Res Rev* 10:147–175

Freeman WJ, van Dijk BW (1987): Spatial patterns of visual cortical fast EEG during conditioned reflex in a rhesus monkey. *Brain Res* 422:267–276

Galambos R, Makeig S, Talmachoff PJ (1981): A 40-Hz auditory potential recorded from the human scalp. *Proc Natl Acad Sci USA* 78:2643–2647

Gerstein G (1970): Functional associations of neurons: detection and interpretation. In: *The Neurosciences. Second Study Program*, Schmitt FO, ed. New York: The Rockefeller University Press, pp 648–671

Gilbert CD, Wiesel TN (1989): Columnar specificity of intrinsic horizontal and corticocortical connections in cat visual cortex. *J Neurosci* 9:2432–2442

Gray CM, Engel AK, König P, Singer W (1990a): Stimulus-dependent neuronal oscillations in cat visual cortex: I. Receptive field properties and feature dependence. *Eur J Neurosci* 2:607–619

Gray CM, Engel AK, König P, Singer W (1991): Temporal properties of synchronous oscillatory neuronal interactions in cat striate cortex. In: *Nonlinear Dynamics and Neuronal Networks*, Schuster HG, ed. Weinheim, FRG: VCH, pp 27–55

Gray CM, König P, Engel AK, Singer W (1989): Oscillatory responses in cat visual cortex exhibit inter-columnar synchronization which reflects global stimulus properties. *Nature* 338:334–337

Gray CM, König P, Engel AK, Singer W (1990b): Synchronization of oscillatory responses in visual cortex: a plausible mechanism for scene segmentation. In: *Synergetics of Cognition*, Haken H, ed. Berlin: Springer, pp 82–98

Gray CM, Singer W (1987): Stimulus-specific neuronal oscillations in the cat visual cortex: a cortical functional unit. *Soc Neurosci Abst* 13:1449

Gray CM, Singer W (1989): Stimulus-specific neuronal oscillations in orientation columns of cat visual cortex. *Proc Natl Acad Sci USA* 86:1698–1702

Grossberg S, Mingolla E (1985): Neural dynamics of perceptual grouping: textures, boundaries, and emergent segmentations. *Percept Psychophy* 38:141–171

Henle M (1971): *The Selected Papers of Wolfgang Köhler*. New York: Liveright.

James W (1890): *The Principles of Psychology*. New York: Dover (reprinted 1950)

Jones EG, Powell TPS (1970): An antomical study of converging sensory pathways within the cerebral cortex of the monkey. *Brain* 93:793–820

Kammen DM, Holmes PJ, Koch C (1989): Cortical architecture and oscillations in neuronal networks: feedback versus local coupling. In: *Models of Brain Function*, Cotterill RMJ, ed. Cambridge, UK: Cambridge University Press, pp 273–284

Kienker PK, Sejnowski TJ, Hinton GE, Schumacher LE (1986): Separating figure from ground with a parallel network. *Perception* 15:197–216

Koffka K (1935): *Principles of Gestalt Psychology*. New York: Harcourt

Köhler W (1947): *Gestalt Psychology*. New York: Liveright

Levy WB, Steward O (1983): Temporal contiguity requirements for long-term associative potentiation/depression in the hippocampus. *Neuroscience* 8:791–797

Libet B (1978): Neuronal vs. subjective timing for a conscious sensory experience. In: *Cerebral Correlates of Conscious Experience*, Buser PA, Rougeul-Buser A, eds. Amsterdam: North-Holland, pp 69–82

Lichtenstein M (1961): Phenomenal simultaneity with irregular timing of components of the visual stimulus. *Percept Motor Skills* 12:47–60

Livingstone MS, Hubel DH (1987): Psychophysical evidence for separate channels for the perception of form, color, movement and depth. *J Neurosci* 7:3416–3468

Llinás RR (1990): Intrinsic electrical properties of mammalian neurons and CNS function. In: *Fidia Research Foundation Neuroscience Award Lectures, vol 4*. Raven Press: New York, pp 175–194

Luhmann HJ, Greuel JM, Singer W (1990a): Horizontal interactions in cat striate cortex: I: Anatomical substrate and postnatal development. *Eur J Neurosci* 2:344–357

Lux HD, Pollen DA (1966): Electrical constants of neurons in the motor cortex of the cat. *J Neurophysiol* 29:207–220

Melssen WJ, Epping WJM (1987): Detection and estimation of neural connectivity based on crosscorrelation analysis. *Biol Cybern* 57:403–414

Moore GP, Segundo JP, Perkel DH, Levitan H (1970): Statistical signs of synaptic interaction in neurons. *Biophys* J 10:876–900

Nakayama K, Silverman GH (1986): Serial and parallel processing of visual feature conjunctions. *Nature* 320:264–265

Palm G, Aertsen AMHJ, Gerstein GL (1988): On the significance of correlations among neuronal spike trains. *Biol Cybern* 59:1–11

Pearson JC, Finkel LH, Edelman GM (1987): Plasticity in the organization of adult cortical maps: a computer model based on neuronal group selection. *J Neurosci* 7:4209–4223

Perkel DH, Gerstein GL, Moore GP (1967a): Neuronal spike trains and stochastic point processes. I. The single spike train. *Biophys J* 7:391–418

Perkel DH, Gerstein GL, Moore GP (1967b): Neuronal spike trains and stochastic point processes. II. Simultaneous spike trains. *Biophys J* 7:419–440

Pöppel E (1985): *Grenzen des Bewusstseins. Über Wirklichkeit und Welterfahrung*. Stuttgart, FRG: Deutsche Verlags Anstalt, English edition (1988): *Mindworks. Time and Conscious Experience*. Orlando, FL: Academic Press

Pöppel E (1970): Excitability cycles in central intermittency. *Psychol Forschung*, 34: 1–9

Pöppel E, Logothetis N (1986): Neuronal oscillations in the human brain. *Naturwissenschaften* 73:267–268

Reeke G Jr, Finkel LH, Sporns O, Edelman GM (1990): Synthetic neural modeling: a multilevel approach to the analysis of brain complexity. In: *Signal and Sense: Local and Global Order in Perceptual Maps*, Edelman GM, Gall WE, Cowan WM, eds. New York: Wiley, pp 607–707

Richet C (1898): Forme et duree de la vibration nerveuse et l' unité psychologique de temps. *Revue Philosophique de la France et de l' Etranger* 45:337–350

Schillen TB, König P (1990): Coherency detection by coupled oscillatory responses—synchronizing connections in neural oscillator layers. In: *Parallel Processing in Neural Systems and Computers*, Eckmiller G, Hartmann R, Hauske G, eds. Amsterdam: Elsevier, pp 139–142

Schrödinger E (1958): *Mind and Matter*. Cambridge, UK: Cambridge University Press

Serviere J, Miceli D, Galifret Y (1977): A psychophysical study of the visual perception of "instantaneous" and "durable." *Vision Res* 17:57–63

Sheer DE (1970): Electrophysiological correlates of memory consolidation. In: *Molecular Mechanisms in Memory and Learning*, Ungar G ed. New York: Plenum Press, pp 177–211

Sheer DE (1976): Focused arousal and 40-Hz EEG. In: *The Neuropsychology of Learning Disorders*, Knight RM, Bakker DJ, eds. Baltimore: University Park Press, pp 71–87

Sheer DE, Grandstaff N (1970): Computer-analysis of electrical activity in the brain and its relation to behavior. In: *Current Research in Neurosciences: Topical Problems in Psychiatry and Neurology, vol 10*, Wycis HT, ed. Basel: Karger, pp 160–172

Sherrington C (1906, 1947): *The Integrative Action of the Nervous System*, 1st and 2nd eds. New Haven: Yale University Press

Singer W (1985): Activity-dependent self-organization of the mammalian visual cortex. In: *Models of the Visual Cortex*, Rose D, Dobson VG, eds. London: Wiley, pp 123–136

Sompolinsky H, Golomb D, Kleinfeld D (1990): Global processing of visual stimuli in a network of coupled oscillators. *Proc Natl Acad Sci USA* 87:7200–7204

Sporns O, Gally JA, Reeke GN Jr, Edelman GM (1989): Reentrant signaling among simulated neuronal groups leads to coherency in their oscillatory activity. *Proc Natl Acad Sci USA* 86:7265–7269

Sporns O, Tononi G, Edelman GM (1990): Coherent oscillations in a population-based model: their role in visual perception. *Soc Neurosci Abst* 16:961

Sporns O, Tononi G, Edelman GM (1991a): Dynamic interactions of neuronal groups and cortical integration. In: *Nonlinear Dynamics and Neuronal Networks*, Schuster HG, ed Weinheim, FRG: VCH, pp 205–240

Sporns O, Tononi G, Edelman GM (1991b): Modeling perceptual grouping and figure-ground segregation by means of active reentrant connections. *Proc Natl Acad Sci USA* 88:129–133

Spydell JD, Pattee G, Golde WD (1985): The 40 Hz event-related potential: normal values and effects of lesions. *Elearoencephalogr Clin Neurophysiol* 62:193–202

Stroud JM (1955): The fine structure of psychological time. In: *Information Theory in Psychology*, Quastler H, ed. Glencoe, IL: Free Press

Stryker MP (1989): Is grandmother an oscillation? *Nature* 338:297–298

Symonds LL, Rosenquist AC (1984): Laminar origins of visual corticocortical connections in the cat. *J Comp Neurol* 229:39–47

Treisman A (1988): Features and objects: the fourteenth Bartlett Memorial Lecture. *Q J Exp Psychol* 40A:201–237

Treisman A, Gelade G (1980): A feature-integration theory of attention. *Cogn Neuropsychol* 12:97–136

Uttal WR (1981): *A Taxonomy of Visual Processes.* Hillsdale, NJ: Lawrence Erlbaum

Van Essen DC (1985): Functional organization of primate visual cortex. In: *Cerebral Cortex, Vol.* 3, *Visual Cortex*, Peters A, Jones EG, eds. New York: Plenum Press, pp 259–329

Van Essen DC, Maunsell JHR (1983): Hierarchical organization and functional streams in the visual cortex. *Trends Neurosci* 6:370–375

von der Malsburg C, Schneider W (1986): A neural cocktail-party processor. *Biol Cybern* 54:29–40

Vaadia E, Ahissar E, Bergman H, Lavner Y (1991): Correlated activity of neurons: a neural code for higher brain functions? In: *Neuronal Cooperativity* Krüger J, ed. Berlin: Springer pp 249–279

Wertheimer M (1923): Untersuchungen zur Lehre von der Gestalt II. *Psychol Forsch* 4:301–350

Zeki S (1969): Representation of central visual fields in prestriate cortex of monkey. *Brain Res* 14:271–291

Zeki S (1978): Functional specialization in the visual cortex of the rhesus monkey. *Nature* 274:423–428

Zeki S, Shipp S (1988): The functional logic of cortical connections. *Nature* 335:311–317

Flexible Linking of Visual Features by Stimulus-Related Synchronizations of Model Neurons

Reinhard Eckhorn, Peter Dicke, Martin Arndt
and Herbert Reitboeck

Introduction

Our models of visual information processing are based on the hypothesis that synchronized activities of sensory neurons serve to define perceptual relations: the features represented by the synchronized neurons are assumed to be linked and, thus, integrated into a perceptual entity. Recently, we found stimulus-related synchronizations in cat visual cortex that could play such role. These results are presented in chapter 2, together with discussions of the following questions: 1. What are the visual situations where stimulus-related activities in the visual cortex do become synchronized? 2. Where and by which neural mechanisms are synchronizations generated? 3. What possible roles do the synchronizations play in visual processing?

In this chapter we present neural network models that are able to link features flexibly via stimulus specific synchronizations. The models were developed by us originally in order to explain the neuronal mechanisms of stimulus-induced oscillatory synchronizations in cat visual cortex (Eckhorn et al., 1989a, 1989b, 1990a, 1990b).

Model Characteristics

Single model neuron

Our model neuron has dynamic "*synapses*" that are represented by (one or two parallel) *leaky integrators* (Fig. 1A) (Eckhorn et al., 1989a, 1990b). During a synaptic input pulse the integrator is charged and its output amplitude rises steeply. This is followed by an exponential decay, determined by the leakage time constant. The decaying signal does permit prolonged "post-synaptic" interactions, such as temporal and spatial integration and amplitude modulation.

The *spike encoders'* adaptive properties are also realized by (one or two parallel) leaky integrators, in combination with a differential amplitude discriminator and spike former. The stabilizing effect of the negative feedback threshold mechanism is explained and discussed here.

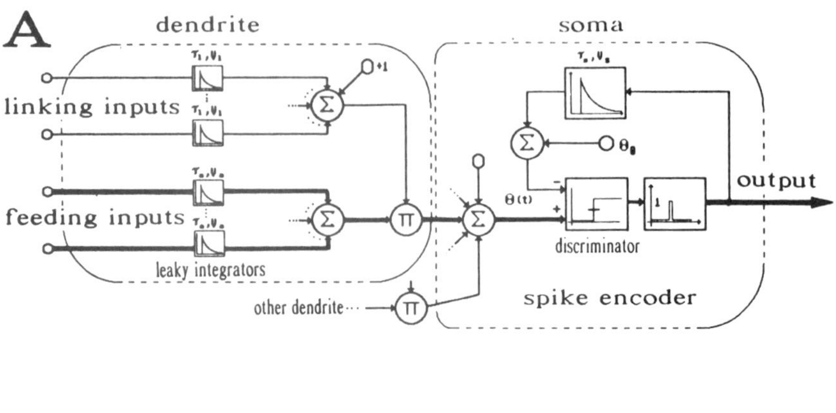

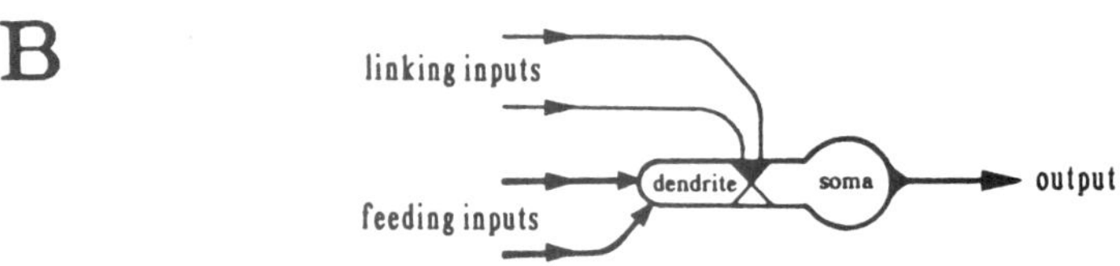

Figure 1. The model neuron. **A:** Circuit diagram. Linking and feeding inputs with leaky integrators on a single "dendrite" interact multiplicatively. Signals from different "dendrites" are summed and fed to the "spike encoder" in the "soma." **B:** Symbol for neuron in A. Reprinted with permission of Cambridge University Press from Eckhorn R, et al. (1989): A neural network for feature linking via synchronous activity: results from cat visual cortex and from simulations. In: *Model of Brain Function*, RMJ Cotterhill, ed. Cambridge University Press.

Two types of synaptic connections

Our model neuron has an important characteristic that provides for fast coupling between neurons without major degradation of the feature-encoding properties of the individual neuron. This characteristic is the result of the modulatory action the *linking inputs* exert on the feeding inputs (Fig. 1): The integrated signals from the linking inputs, together with a constant offset term (+1), interact multiplicatively with the integrated signals from the feeding inputs. Without linking input signals, the output of the "neural multiplier" is identical to the (integrated) feeding signals (multiplication by +1). This interaction assures fast and relatively unaffected signal transfer from the feeding synapses, which is an important requirement for fast "stimulus-locked synchronizations" and for the preservation of the "receptive field (RF) properties." With nonzero activity at the linking inputs, the integrated signal from the feeding inputs is modulated via the multiplier, and the threshold discriminator will now switch at different times, thereby shifting the phase of the output pulses. In network models of other groups that also use synchronization for feature linking, possible degradations of a model neuron's local coding properties by certain types of coupling networks, as far as we know, have not been considered yet (Baird, 1986; Freeman, 1987; Kammen et al., 1989; Kuramoto 1991; Schillen and König, 1990; but Sompolinsky et al., 1991).

In our models, feeding synapses are strong; they can include short and long time constants for the decay of synaptic potentials, and their overall number is small compared to the linking synapses. Linking synapses are weak, and they also can have fast and slow transfer properties (Eckhorn et al., 1991b).

The modulatory linking synapses used in our model neuron are neurophysiologically plausible: Modulation in real neurons might be achieved by changes in the dendritic membrane potential due to specific types of synapses that act locally (or, via electrotonic spread, also distantly) on voltage-dependent subsynaptic channels, thereby modulating the postsynaptic efficacies. In neocortical circuitry, it seems probable that mainly a subgroup of special "bursting neurons", (Llinás, 1988) is coupled via linking connections and such a network has been modeled only by us.

Simplified wiring principles for models of sensory systems

We modeled visual cortical areas in a simplified way as a network of coupled feature maps (Eckhorn et al., 1989a, 1989b, 1990a, 1990b). Special types of connections are necessary for this: 1) the models have to obey the constraints of sensory systems, where single neurons represent stimulus features via their RF properties, 2) these features shall be linked flexibly by forming synchronized assemblies with those neurons that represent a coherent stimulus region (Eckhorn et al., 1988, 1991a; Gray et al., 1989). In the visual system RF properties of individual neurons at a certain level are probably generated by convergent summation of signals from a preceding level that leads to a superposition of the input RF properties (Eckhorn et al., 1988, 1991a, 1991b). In our models, accordingly, topographically corresponding positions in any two successive layers of model neurons (feature maps) (Kohonen, 1982) are connected in forward direction (with respect to the input) via *feeding synapses*. It is assumed that relevant feature combinations, that almost always occur in combination, are represented as features of single neurons. These feature combinations are not separable at the respective level of a feature map.

Flexible synchronization between model neurons is generally mediated via linking connections and they can project in forward, lateral, or backward directions (well outside the topographic ranges of feature representations by individual model neurons). Some of these "simplifying assumptions" of connections in sensory systems (for a two-layer network with three neurons) are schematically illustrated in Figure 2. We use such networks for our simulations of stimulus-related synchronizations.

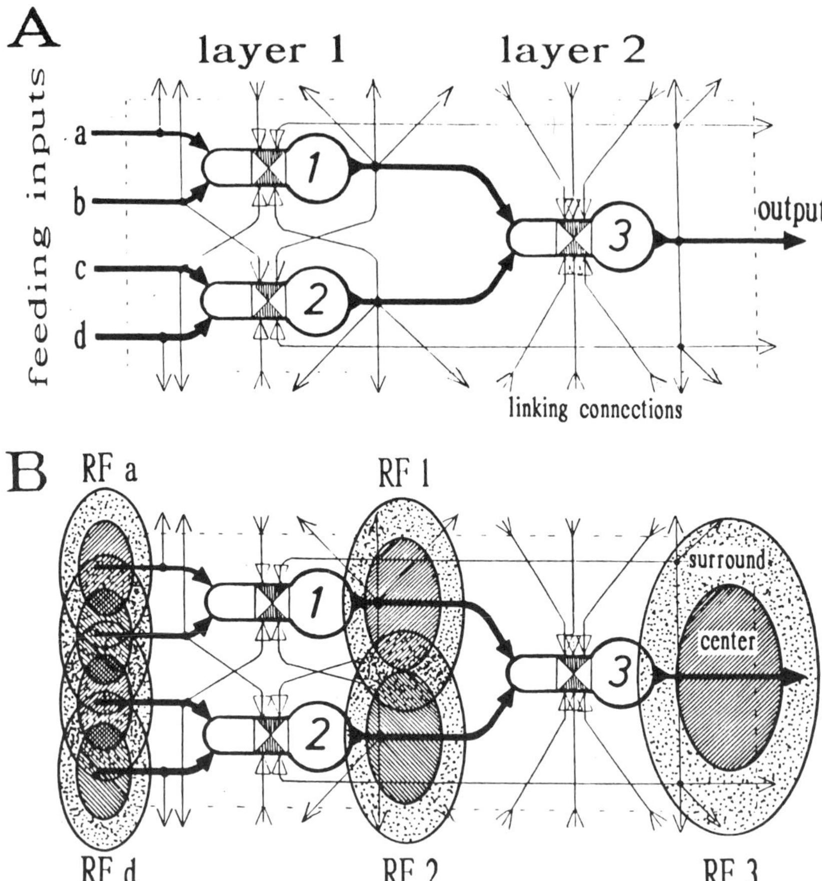

Figure 2. Schema of feeding and linking connections in sensory systems. **A:** Three schematic neurons are arranged in two layers with feeding (thick lines) and linking connections (thin lines). Feeding connections from lower level model neurons converge on feeding synapses at higher level neurons. They can activate the target neurons while their linking inputs (thin lines) are not activated. The stimulus features that are represented by an individual model neuron are determined by superposition of the feeding input's features (corresponding to receptive fields of real sensory neurons (RFa—RF3, with center and surround, shown in B). Linking connections project in forward, lateral, and backward directions and they are more numerous than feeding connections in order to provide a large number of different possible assemblies of model neurons that can synchronize their activities. Reprinted with permission of VCN–Verlag from Eckhorn R, et al. (in press): Stimulus-related facilitation and synchronization among visual cortical areas: experiments and models. In: *Nonlinear Dynamics and Neuronal Networks*, Schuster HG, Singer W, eds. Stuttgart: VCN–Verlag.

Dynamic Properties of Layered Networks

One-layer network shows basic behavior of stimulus-related synchronizations

To ascertain the special properties of our model neurons with respect to stimulus-related synchronizations, we began with a single linear array of coupled neurons (Fig. 3A). This network was interconnected according to the "simplified wiring principles" described above (Eckhorn et al., 1988b, 1991b). In the present simulations, the features represented by individual neurons are assumed to be identical except for the spatial positions of the features that were chosen to be equidistantly aligned. Each model neuron is connected to four neighbors at each side. The (positive) coupling strength of the linking synapses declines linearly with lateral distance. A further simplification is that each neuron has only one feeding input to which the "visual" input is fed as an analog signal. Before the simulations of dynamic network interactions the amplitudes of these signals are derived from stimulus intensity distributions by application of local filters with appropriate spatiotemporal features. Noise was added to the feeding signals in order to mimic irregularities due to the superposition of spike inputs to many similar feeding synapses and to simulate internal stochastic processes.

Figure 3B shows a simulation of region linking where the input "intensity function" is switched on and then moves at constant velocity across the feeding inputs of the model neurons. Such "stimulus situation" may represent a patch of light that moves across the retinotopically arranged "RFs" of the model neurons.

Two-layer network simulates synchronizations between two cortical areas

Two one-dimensional layers with mutual feedback already show basic properties of stimulus-related synchronizations similar to those observed between neural assemblies in cat visual cortex (Fig. 4) (Eckhorn et al., 1990a, 1990b, 1991b, 1991c). The layers have the same intralayer connections as the one-dimensional layer Figure 3. Stimulus features represented in layer 2 are (here) determined by the convergence of feeding inputs from (four) neighboring layer 1 neurons. Convergence causes enlarged "feature areas" due to the superposition of features from layer 1 neurons [corresponding to RF enlargements in visual neurons on which cells with smaller RFs converge].

The dynamic response of two-layer networks (Figs. 4A, D) is shown in the simulation results Figure 4B, E. Two stimulus regions (patches) of enhanced intensity are applied to the feeding inputs of layer 1. In order to demonstrate the model's robustness in generating stimulus-induced synchrony we introduced two impediments: 1) the stimulus amplitudes at the patches differed by a factor of two, which causes the burst rates of the driven neurons to differ appreciably, and 2) the stimuli were not switched on simultaneously, but in

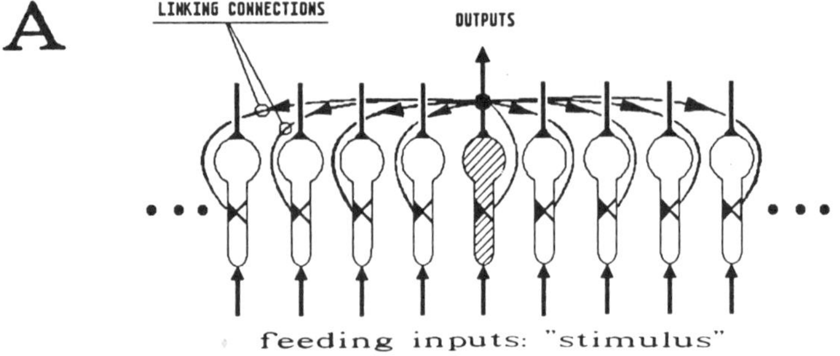

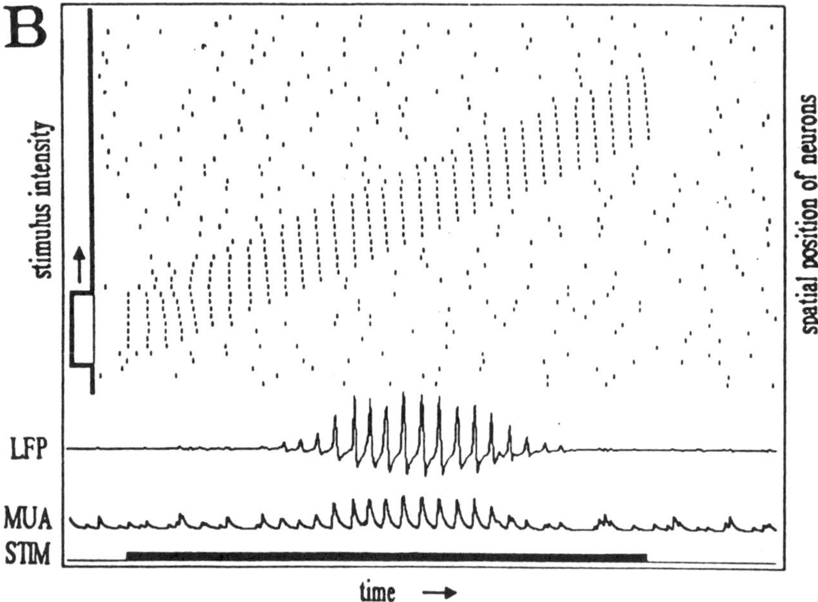

Figure 3. Stimulus-induced oscillations are synchronized via lateral linking connections in a single-layer network. **A:** Network of single layer of 50 model neurons with lateral linking connections (shown for one neuron). *Thick lines*: feeding connections; *thin lines*: linking connections. Weights of linking connections decline linearly with lateral distance from projecting neuron. **B:** Simulation result. *Abscissa*: time; *Ordinate*: position of model neuron (and its "receptive field") in the one-dimensional feature map. Dashes indicate occurrence times of output impulses of the 50 model neurons. The random maintained activity is due to analog noise that was continuously added to each feeding input. The black horizontal bar indicates the on-duration of enhanced "stimulus intensity" that moved with constant velocity across the array of feeding inputs, beginning at the lowermost 10 and ending at the 10 uppermost neurons. (In the visual system this would correspond to a moving patch of light activating a retinotopically organized cortical area at a constant speed.) Note the highly synchronized impulses inside the moving "stimulated" region and the stochastic activities elsewhere. LFP: Time course of local "slow wave field potential" calculated as average of the "membrane potentials" U_m of 10 model neurons in the middle of the array. MUA: Time course of low-pass filtered impulse responses of the same 10 model neurons. Modified from Eckhorn R, et al. (1988).

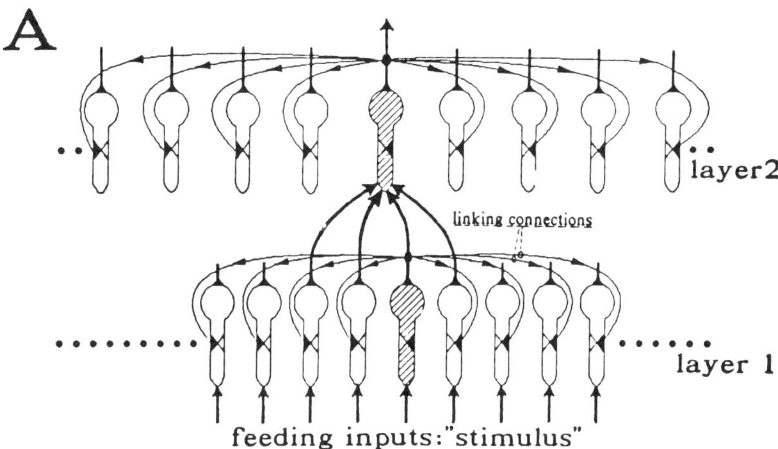

Figure 4. Stimulus-induced oscillations in spatially separate assemblies of model neurons are synchronized via feedback linking connections from a second layer. **A:** Network with two layers. *Layer 1*: 50, *layer 2*: 23 neurons; weights of lateral linking connections as for Fig. 3. The only connections between the layers are of the feeding type and they project from layer 1 to layer 2. Full output connectivity is shown for only one layer 1 and one layer 2 neuron (*hatched symbols*). **B:** Simulation result with network A. *Abscissa*: time; *Ordinate*: positions of neurons (and their "receptive fields"; neurons at corresponding positions of the ordinates of layer 1 and 2 panels have overlapping receptive fields). Dashes indicate occurrence times of output impulses of the model neurons in layer 1 and layer 2. Black horizontal bars indicate on-durations of two input stimulus subregions with enhanced amplitudes (a and b, respectively); the spatial distribution of stimulus intensities (*left side*) is drawn to scale with the positions of the the layer 1 neurons that are stimulated by the respective amplitudes at their feeding inputs. Note the synchronizations of rhythmic impulse bursts of neurons within each stimulus subregion a and b in layer 1 (dense aggregations of dots), and the independence of the burst occurrences in the two stimulus subregions. This is quantified in **C:** Auto- and cross-correlograms of the impulse activities in the centers of the stimulus subregions a and b (positions indicated by dashed horizontal lines in Fig. 4B), derived from simulation runs that were 20 times longer than the shown duration. The flat cross-correlogram indicates independence of the two rhythmic burst activities. **D:** Network with added backward linking connections from layer 2 to layer 1. **E:** Simulation result including backward linking connections. Note the synchronization between impulse bursts occurring in layer 1 neurons at the positions of enhanced stimulus intensities (a and b) in layer 1, and the precise spatial separation of the two synchronized subregions by a "gap" of "spontaneously" active neurons. Layer 2 activities at the corresponding "receptive field" positions indicate that the synchronization across the activity gap in layer 1 is mediated via the horizontal linking connections in layer two and their feedback linking connections to layer 1. This network supports the formation of a common synchronized state in both layers while preserving the spatial details of the input stimulus distribution. The two vertical dashed lines indicate the duration of a cycle of the rhythmic burst activities. They are in phase in layer 1 of E and out of phase in B. **F:** Correlograms of activities (sig. a and sig. b, E) from simulation E with active backward linking connections. Oscillatory cross-correlogram indicates synchronization among bursts in stimulus subregions a and b. Modified from Eckhorn, et al. (1990b).

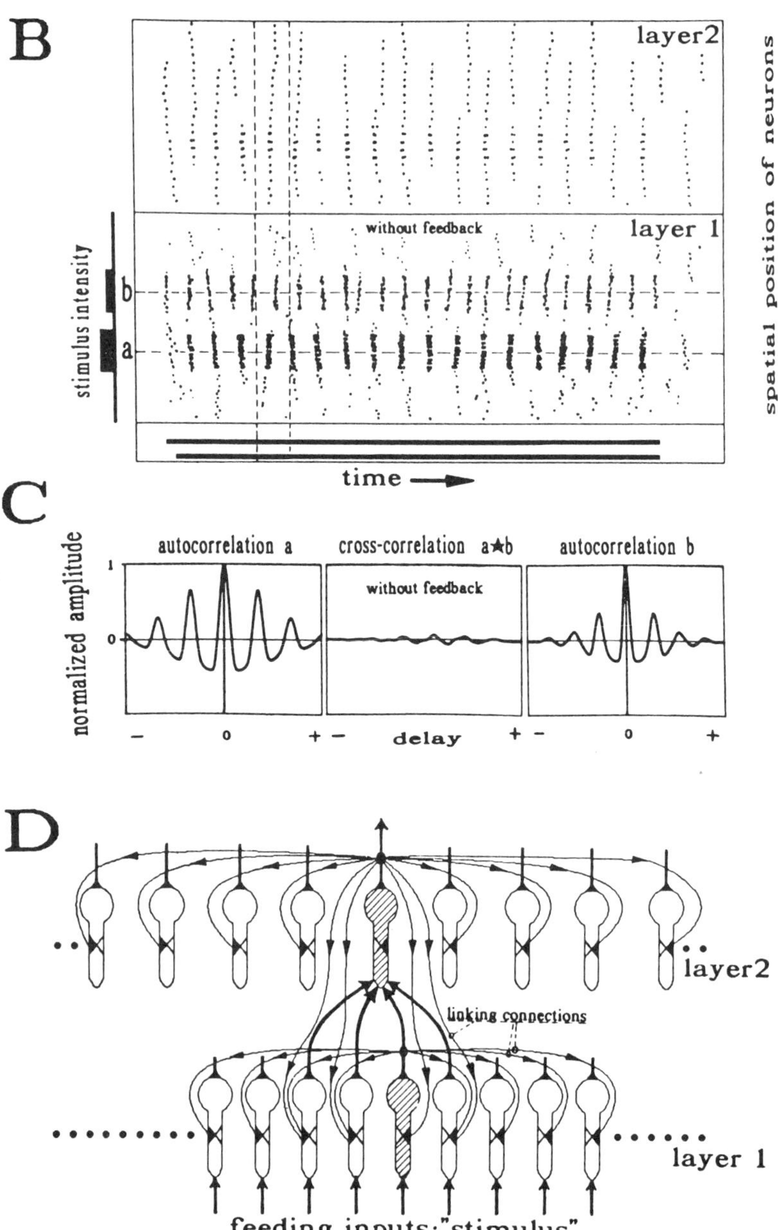

Figure 4 (*Continued*)

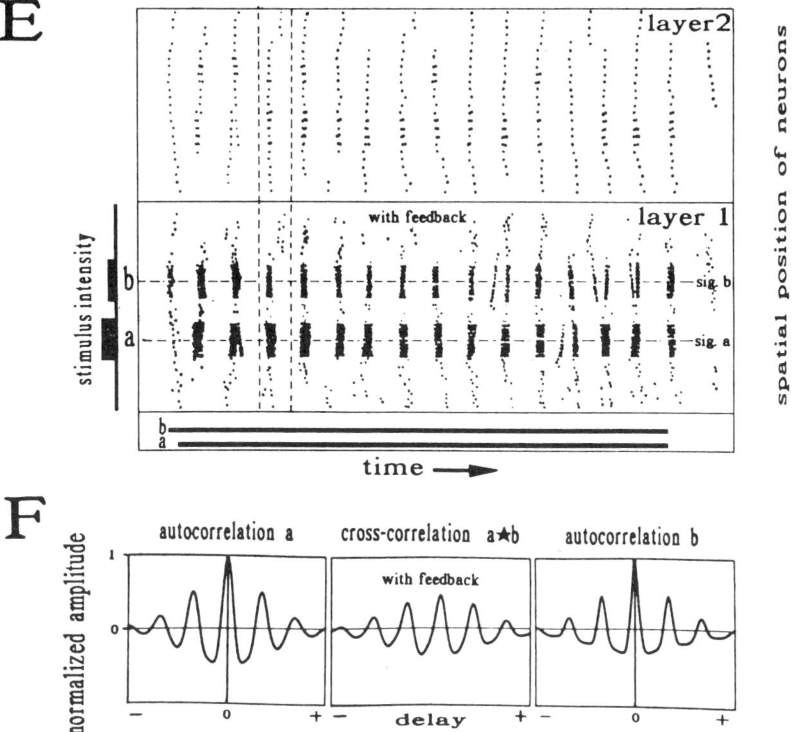

Figure 4 (*Continued*)

temporal succession. Stimulus-locked synchronizations due to on-transients were thus prevented. In the simulations Figure 4A through C there are only feedforward connections (from layer 1 to 2). Rhythmic bursts that are synchronized within each stimulus patch region are generated in both layers but the burst frequencies at the two stimulus patch positions differ markedly. We obtained quantitative measures of correlation between the activities at the centers of the stimulus patches (sig. a and b in Figs. 4B, E) by calculating the cross-correlations between the respective output activities of the model neurons. Figure 4C (center) shows a flat correlogram, indicating uncorrelated activities between stimulus patch regions and the action of forward feeding connections only. Synchronization, however, quickly develops if the layer 2 to 1 feedback linking connections are added. The degree of synchronization between the burst activities induced by the two spatially separate "stimulus patches" is quantified in the cross-correlogram Figure 4F (for more details see legend). "Interpatch" synchronization occurs mainly because layer 2 neurons are influenced by and affect large regions in layer 1: layer 2 neurons receive convergent inputs from four layer 1 neurons, they have interlayer connections to four neighbors at each side, and they project back to four layer 1 neurons.

Layer 2 neurons can thus span (fill in) the gap of nonstimulated neurons in layer 1.

The synchronization between layer 1 and layer 2 activities at corresponding positions (of stimulus representations) parallels our observations in cat visual cortex: simultaneous recordings from A17 and A18 showed that assemblies in A17 and A18 could be synchronized if they had overlapping RFs and if they were activated by the same stimulus (Eckhorn et al., 1988, 1991a).

Stimulus-Locked (Nonrhythmic) and Stimulus-Induced (Rhythmic) Synchronizations are Supported by the Same Feeding–Linking Network

We proposed that two different types of synchronization support perceptual feature linking in visual cortex: stimulus-locked and stimulus-induced synchronizations (Eckhorn et al., 1989b, 1990a, 1990b).

Stimulus-locked synchronizations are directly driven by fast and sufficiently strong stimulus transients, that is they are generally not oscillatory, but follow the time course of the stimulus transients. In recent neural network simulations of our group we showed that "near neural synchrony," initially generated by a stimulus transient that was applied to several neighboring feeding inputs in parallel, is enhanced via the same lateral and/or feedback linking connections that mediates correlated stimulus-induced rhythmic activities (Eckhorn et al., 1990b; Pabst et al., 1989; Reitboeck, 1989).

A demonstration of an interesting effect in our model networks with stimulus-locked responses is given in the simulations in Figure 5A: synchronization of the activities in two separate stimulus patches is forced mainly by applying two strong input impulses simultaneously. Shortly after the initial stimulation, a second impulse is given at patch 1 position only. Synchronized activity appears, however, also at patch 2. This effect of "filling-in" across spatial and temporal gaps is due to the facilitatory action of signals supplied via the lateral and feedback linking connections, interacting with the temporal "response tails" of the feeding inputs' leaky integrators. Such simulations mimic psychophysically observed mechanisms of "preattentive" perceptual facilitation and integration of spatially and temporally dispersed stimuli (e.g., Altmann et al., 1986; Snowden and Braddick, 1990; Wilson and Singer, 1981).

The stimulus-induced rhythmic synchronizations that were discovered in cat visual cortex are assumed to be produced internally via a self-organizing process among stimulus-driven local "oscillating units" that are mutually interconnected (Eckhorn et al., 1988, 1991a; Gray et al., 1989; Schillen and König, 1990; Schuster and Wagner, 1990; Snowden and Braddick, 1990; Sporns et al., 1989). The results of our simulations support this assumption. Feeding signals with moderate transients cause our model neurons to respond initially with rather irregular repetitive discharges, uncorrelated among different neurons, but subsequently the neurons mutually synchronize

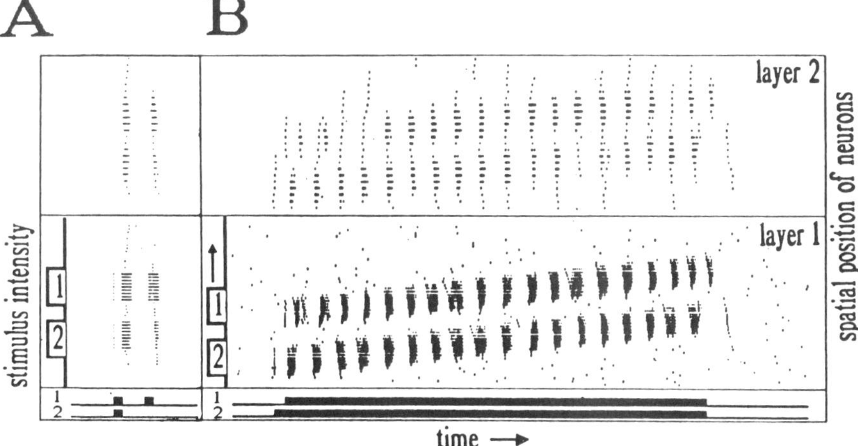

Figure 5. Stimulus-locked activities and stimulus-induced oscillatory activities are facilitated and synchronized via the same feeding-linking networks. The network Fig. 4D was used. **A:** Two stimulus impulses were presented in short succession at layer 1 feeding inputs in the positions of "patch 1," while a single impulse only was given at "patch 2" inputs. Note the synchronized bursts of spikes in both layers at the former "patch 2" position although the second stimulus was applied at "patch 1" position only. This effect of spatiotemporal "filling-in" is due to the facilitatory action of signals supplied via the lateral and feedback linking connections on the "response tails" at the feeding inputs' leaky integrators. **B:** Phase-lock among synchronized bursts of spikes in two subregions activated by a pair of moving "stimulus" subfields. Note the "filling-in" across the "stimulus gap" via layer 2 neurons. *Modified from* Eckhorn R, et al. (1990): Feature linking among distributed assemblies: simulations and results from cat visual cortex. *Neur Comput* 2:293–306.

their activities via the linking connections (Eckhorn et al., 1989a, 1989b, 1990a, 1990b, 1991b, 1991c). In our simulations, the same linking network supports phase-locking of both stimulus-locked and gamma-spindle synchronizations (Eckhorn et al., 1990b; Pabst et al., 1989). It is therefore reasonable to assume that this is likely to be the case also in visual cortex.

The simulation in Figure 5B demonstrates "rhythmic linking" among separate regions when the stimulus patches move in parallel. Again, synchronization of activities in the activated subregions is achieved via lateral and feedback linking connections of layer 2. Although a high level of noise was continuously applied to the feeding inputs of all model neurons in both layers, the synchronized moving "activity patches" maintain almost constant extent and clear separation. In such dynamic spatiotemporal input situations, neurons at the region boundaries must either join or leave the synchronized assembly. Region linking is thus accomplished by our model, even though the synchronized "patches" are moving and are separated by a gap of spontaneously active neurons.

Such synchronization from a higher to a lower level might also be responsible for the stimulus-induced synchronizations we observed in cat visual cortex. Stimulation with coarse gratings not only induced synchronized oscillations within the stimulated region of a single stripe in area 17, but it also induced synchronized activities among A17 positions that were stimulated by other, neighboring stripes (Eckhorn et al., 1988, 1991a).

Multiple-Level Feedback Ensures Sensitive and Stable Performance of Real and Simulated Neural Networks

Visual processing is stable and effective over a broad range of variations in input parameters and internal states, although excitatory synaptic connections in the neocortex outnumber the inhibitory ones by a factor of more than five (Braitenberg, 1986). In most neural network models it is, however, a formidable problem to achieve stable and sensitive behavior over a wide dynamic range. It is particularly difficult and time-consuming to choose parameters and "working ranges" in models with nonlinear properties and many parameters, if sufficiently distributed stabilizing mechanisms were not included. It seems worthwile, therefore, to ask how real neural networks achieve stable behavior and how neural stabilizing mechanisms can be included in model networks in order to keep them stable within a suitable working range.

In the brain, stability of performance includes states of "maintained" and evoked activities of rhythmic and nonrhythmic time courses. In our network simulations comparable states are present, and we discuss the influence of the different components and connections of the network with respect to their actions on stabilization, sensitization, and general information-processing properties.

At the level of single model neurons, the *negative feedback action of the spike encoders* is one of the most powerful factors for stabilization and for the generation of temporal structures (e.g., rhythms) because its influence is evenly distributed over the network. It functions in the following way: the spike encoder with its adaptive properties is realized via a leaky integrator, in combination with a differential amplitude discriminator and spike former (Eckhorn et al., 1989a, 1989b, 1990a, 1990b). The amplitude discriminator triggers the spike former when its input, the "membrane voltage" $U_m(t)$, exceeds the variable threshold $\theta(t)$. An output spike of the neuron immediately charges the leaky integrator to such high value of $\theta(t)$ that $U_m(t)$ cannot exceed $\theta(t)$ during and immediately after the generation of an output spike. This transitory elevation of $\theta(t)$ produces absolute and relative "refractory periods" in the spike generation. The spike encoder responds to a positive jump of U_m with a sudden increase in its discharge rate. After the first burst of spikes, subsequent spikes appear at increasingly longer intervals, since the burst charged the threshold integrator to a high value of $\theta(t)$. A negative jump of U_m, especially after a burst of spikes, leads to an abrupt pause in the discharge, until the output of the threshold integrator went down to the low value of U_m.

For the present simulations this "temporal contrast enhancement" is a desirable property of the spike encoder because it supports the formation of "isolated bursts." Such bursts are efficient temporal "markers" for fast and strong synchronizations among connected neurons. The formation of single and repetitive bursts is, in addition, supported in special types of sensory neurons by specific nonlinear feedback characteristics of dendritic and somatic membranes that can, for example, generate subthreshold oscillations that influence spike probability (for an overview see Llinás, 1988). In conclusion, single (model) neurons are already capable of controlling their level of activation and of generating single or repetitive transient outputs in response to sustained inputs.

At the level of locally coupled model neurons, *inhibitory feedback via interneurons* is probably an essential local circuit component in real neural networks. Fast-acting inhibitory loops via interneurons can serve to "chop" sustained activations of excitatory neurons into repetitive bursts by rhythmic suppression (in the γ range, see Chapter 2). In circuits where inhibitory interneurons receive their inputs from several excitatory neurons and project back onto the same group, they would force synchronization of the chopped activities with zero mean phase differences within the group of similar neurons and with phase differences of up to 180° between excitatory and inhibitory neurons. Sustained inhibitory reactions by local interneurons, however, suppress prolonged activations after a single short burst in excitatory neurons; that is, it mainly reduces the overall activity of a network. We did not yet include such local inhibitory feedback in our models because it was not essential for the effects studied by us so far.

Local facilitatory feedback coupling is provided in our models through excitatory linking connections from neighboring neurons of the same layer. The excitatory linking can transiently enhance the sensitivity of feeding inputs. This may result in an activating influence of the linking connections onto the overall state of the network that could drive it out of its working range. Such an "overdrive" is counteracted at the local level mainly by the negative feedback in the spike encoders. Mutual facilitation via linking synapses, on the other hand, is a desirable property in our models because it helps to synchronize the model neurons. Rhythmic activities are synchronized with zero phase differences if the local linking connections are symmetric and if the cells' activations are similar.

In the network simulations in Figures 6 and 7 loops with excitatory and inhibitory feeding and linking synapses have been used to interconnect distributed assemblies (in different layers). For this broadly diverging interlayer, feedback loops with slow inhibitory synapses were added to the fast excitatory and more narrowly diverging linking feedback used in the two-layer simulations above. In these simulations the excitatory linking connections support fast, phase-locked synchronizations with zero phase shift in neuron groups that are activated by a common input ("stimulus"). The slow decay of the activations in these circuits support prolonged mutual facilitations. The slowly acting inhibitory loops, on the other hand, "desensitize" the neurons of

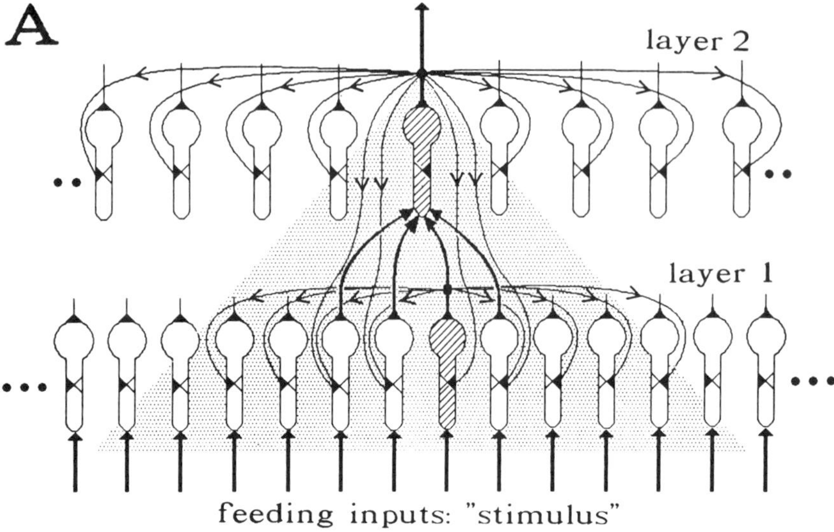

Figure 6. Additional negative feedback keeps two-layer-network in appropriate working range for high contrast region definitions. **A:** Network used for the simulation B. It has, in addition to the network in Fig. 4D, slowly acting ($\tau = 30$ ms), broadly diverging negative feedback projections, indicated for a single layer 2 neuron by the shaded pyramid. The weights of the negative feedback connections decline laterally according to a Gaussian function. Layer 1: 50 neurons, layer 2: 23 neurons. **B:** Simulation results with two-layer network of A. The left panels show the spike trains of all layer 1 and layer 2 model neurons over a short period of time. Note the highly synchronized activities in the subarea of enhanced stimulus intensity (indicated by *black square* at left side of layer 1) and the synchronized activities at the corresponding region in layer 2, due to the fast acting intra- and interlayer linking connections. Note also the lack of stochastic "spontaneous" activities in and around the "stimulated subregions" due to the slowly acting negative feedback of stimulus-activated layer 2 neurons on those of layer 1. The right panel of **B** shows a superimposogram of spatial correlation profiles of layer 1 neurons ($n = 50$). A single correlation profile was obtained by calculating the correlation coefficients between the spike trains of one "reference neuron" and all other neurons and plotting them over space (position of neurons, simulating receptive field positions). Each layer 1 neuron was taken as reference. The correlation profiles indicate the high degree of correlation between neurons of the stimulated center region and near zero correlation with neurons in the direct neighborhood. **C:** Simulation results without negative feedback from layer 2 onto layer 1; the remaining interconnections and simulation parameters are identical to network A and simulation B. Note in C (*left panel*) in both layers the higher average rates of stochastic activities and the less precise restriction of rhythmically synchronized activities to the "stimulus subregions," compared with B. The corresponding superimposogram of the spatial correlation profiles (C, *right panel*) directly shows the lower signal-to-noise ratios between the stimulated region and the surround.

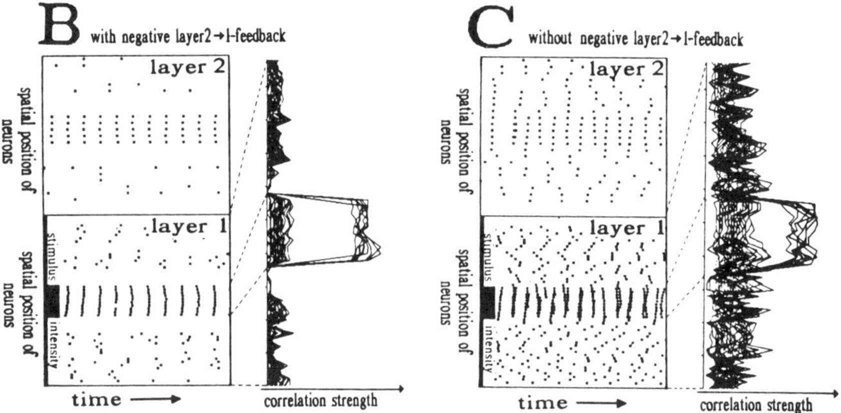

Figure 6 (*Continued*)

the input layer in an activated region and its surround by a slight negative shift of their membrane potentials. Such feedback control of the input layer sensitivities results in highly enhanced spatiotemporal contrasts: the activities in regions of stimulus-induced activition (with synchronized bursts of impulses) are enhanced, whereas the spontaneous activities in the surrounding regions are suppressed (Figs. 6 and 7).

The network in Figure 6A was also used for the simulation of focal attention by activating selected groups of neighboring neurons in the second layer via "top down" connections. In these simulations even exclusively stochastic (spontaneous) input signals caused the network to generate synchronized high frequency rhythms in a focal region while activities in a surround belt were inhibited. Such model results parallel those of investigations of focal attention in humans and animals where focal attention was found to induce 40-Hz rhythms in cortical parts of that sensory modality to which a subject had shifted its attention (for a review, see Sheer, 1989).

Additional "nonspecific" control inputs in every model neuron can act to shift the network's general "working range" to more sensitive or insensitive states corresponding to shifts of alertness in the brain. In our simulations we used offsets in the neuron's membrane potentials (Fig. 7) generated via feeding inputs (or a common threshold offset) in order to model such a "shift of alertness."

In conclusion, if negative feedback is present at several levels of organization and if it is distributed extensively over the network, as in the present simulations, model parameters including time constants, coupling strengths, and the degree of convergence and divergence of the connections can be varied over a broad range without changing the overall basic processing capabilities of the network. Even the addition of spike propagation delays (proportional to distance) does not crucially deteriorate phase-linking as long as the delays (in the region of cells to be linked) are shorter than the time constant of the feeding synapses.

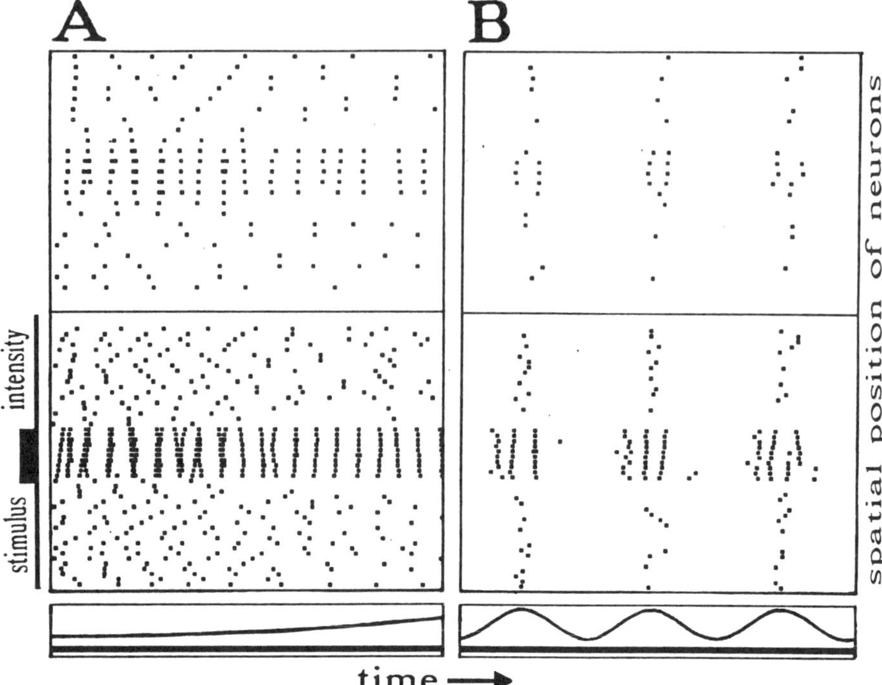

Figure 7. Changes of working range in two-layer network including fast facilitatory and slow inhibitory feedback connections. The same network from Fig. 6A was used. **A:** Simulation results with shift of the networks working range by continuous increase in the action of the slow negative feedback (as indicated in the lowermost frame). Note the reduction of impulse rates specifically in and around the stimulus-activated region and the improving "spatial correlation contrast" with increasing negative feedback. **B:** Rhythmic shifts in the working range of the two-layer network by low frequency feeding input on the "membrane potentials" U_m of all model neurons while the negative feedback has a strength according to the right portion of A. Such a low frequency rhythm induces rhythmic spatial activation profiles with synchronized activities according to the stimulus intensity distribution. Note again the clear separation of the stimulated center region from its "silent" surround.

High and Low Frequency Rhythms

Two main rhythms of different mean frequency can be generated by our model networks if two parallel leaky integrators with short and long time constants are used in synapses and in threshold mechanisms, and when the slowly acting interlayer inhibition (Fig. 6A) is included. The short time constants in the spike encoders support the generation of high impulse rates and those in the "synapses" ensure the transmission of temporal details of the spike patterns. The formation of common high frequency synchronized states among stimulus-driven neurons is dominated by these fast system components (range, 35–80 Hz). The generation of low frequency rhythms (range, 7–16 Hz), on the other hand, is dominated in our model networks by the influence of the diffusely projecting (slow) inhibitory feedback connections from higher to lower order layers (e.g., Fig. 6A). In order to model feature linking by stimulus-related synchronizations in the visual cortex with our networks, it is essential that the high frequency rhythms are in phase in the same and in different layers of the model network. The low frequency rhythms are supported by the slow negative feedback connections and they are generally out of phase in different layers of the model. The negative feedback transiently reduces the activities at and around the positions of stimulus-related activations; evoked activities ("signals") are slightly reduced in their amplitudes whereas "spontaneous" activities ("noise") are suppressed below threshold. Synchronized "signals" and uncorrelated "noise" are thus affected differently. Whereas stimulus-induced "signals" are mainly facilitated by the fast mechanisms, "noise" is suppressed. Such suppressive action has also been observed in the visual cortex (see chapter 2 in this book).

In the visual cortex as well as in our models, ongoing fast and slow rhythms can be interrupted by strong transient inputs. The formation of common synchronized oscillatory states is transiently suppressed, as we have argued before (Eckhorn et al., 1991a), because neurons initially respond to the same common stimulus with different spike patterns. Rhythmic states that are due to "self-organization" processes, including α and γ electroencephalogram (EEG) rhythms, are therefore restricted to more sustained input conditions.

Initially, short time constants (about 6 ms) were chosen in our simulations in order to obtain a system that can react rapidly to transient inputs (stimulus-locked synchronizations) and that can generate fast rhythms in the 50-Hz range (Eckhorn et al., 1989a, 1989b, 1990a). More recently, we introduced leaky integrators with longer time constants (about 30 ms) in order to generate medium duration "memory effects." Short aperiodic or fast rhythmic signals are thus integrated, resulting in a prolonged facilitatory action, for example, on rhythmic bursts at linking inputs (Fig. 5) or in prolonged inhibition of the diffusely projecting feedback connections from layer 2 to 1 (Figs. 6 and 7). The facilitation of sustained synchronizations is especially desirable in the models in order to increase the momentary activity differences between neurons that represent, for example, the features of an object and those of a background.

The generation of fast and slow rhythms in groups of coupled model neurons is due both to properties of the single neuron (time constants of leaky integrators) and to their specific feedback connections. In networks of real neurons, spike transmission times (delays) and/or postsynaptic signal bandpass properties of membranes can greatly influence the generation of rhythms in different frequency bands (e.g., Başar, 1979; Llinás, 1988). More detailed physiological investigations and modelings are necessary in order to test the hypothesis that the above-mentioned mechanisms in our models might play a significant role in the generation of high and low frequency rhythms in the brain.

Summary and Conclusions

For explanations of our physiological results (Chapter 2) we introduced special model neurons that are interconnected via feeding and linking "synapses". The model neurons are topographically arranged in "visual feature maps" (feature maps, in our models, correspond to retinotopically arranged cortical areas). *Feeding connections* simulating, for example, thalamocortical inputs project in forward directions. They mainly determine the features individual model neurons are responding to, thus, simulating neurons of the visual cortex and their receptive field (RF) properties. Linking connections, simulating intrinsic and cortico-cortical association fibers, project broadly within the same and between different feature maps. Signals at linking inputs modulate those at feeding inputs. Stimulus-activated neurons that are coupled via linking connections can thus mutually influence their activity patterns, producing a common synchronized state at high frequencies (35–80 Hz). Two one-dimensional layers of model neurons with mutual feedback linking connections, already, show basic properties of stimulus related synchronizations, similar to those observed by us in cat visual cortex. In our models we can identify different mechanisms and feedback loops for high frequency ("γ-like") and for lower frequency ("α-like") rhythms. Generation of low frequency rhythms is supported by inhibitory feedback connections with relatively long time constants. Furthermore, we could show that two types of stimulus-related synchronizations, stimulus-locked (non-rhythmic) and stimulus-induced (rhythmic) synchronizations, are supported by the same feeding-linking network. In our model networks, stimulus-locked responses can suppress ongoing or stimulus-induced oscillatory activities, similar to our observations in cat visual cortex. Our simulation results corroborate the assumption that multiple level feedback ensures sensitive and stable performance for the flexible linking of visual features in real as well as simulated neural networks.

Acknowledgments. The authors acknowledge the helpful comments on a previous version of the manuscript by Prof. T.H. Bullock. This project was sponsored by Deutsche Forschungsgemeinschaft Re 547/2-1, and Ec 53/4-1 and by Stiftung Volkswagenwerk I/64605.

References

Altmann L, Eckhorn R, Singer W (1986): Temporal integration in the visual system: influence of temporal dispersion on figure-ground discrimination. *Vision Res* 26: 1949–1957

Baird B (1986): Nonlinear dynamics of pattern formation and pattern recognition in the rabbit olfactory bulb. *Physica* 22D: 150–175

Başar E (1979): Combined dynamics of EEG and evoked potentials I. and II. *Biol Cybern* 34: 1–19, 21–30

Braitenberg V (1986): Two views of the cerebral cortex. In: *Brain Theory*, Palm G, Aertsen A, eds. Heidelberg–New York: Springer-Verlag, pp 81–96

Eckhorn R, Bauer R, Jordan W, Brosch M, Kruse W, Munk M, Reitboeck HJ (1988): Coherent oscillations: A mechanism of feature linking in the visual cortex? Multiple electrode and correlation analysis in the cat. *Biol Cybern* 60: 121–130

Eckhorn R, Dicke P, Kruse W, Reitboeck HJ (1991b): Stimulus-related facilitation and synchronization among visual cortical areas: experiments and models. In: *Nonlinear Dynamics and Neuronal Networks*, Schuster HG, Singer W, eds. Stuttgart: VCN-Verlag

Eckhorn R, Reitboeck HJ, Arndt M, Dicke P (1989a): Feature linking via stimulus-evoked oscillations: experimental results from cat visual cortex and functional implications from a network model. *Proceed Int Joint Conf Neural Networks, Washington. IEEE TAB Neural Network Comm*, San Diego, I: 723–730

Eckhorn R, Reitboeck HJ, Arndt M, Dicke P (1989b): A neural network for feature linking via synchronous activity: results from cat visual cortex and from simulations. In: *Models of Brain Function*, Cotterill RMJ, ed. Cambridge University Press Cambridge (UK), pp 255–272

Eckhorn R, Reitboeck HJ, Arndt M, Dicke P (1990b): Feature linking among distributed assemblies: simulations and results from cat visual cortex. *Neur Comput* 2: 293–306

Eckhorn R, Reitboeck HJ, Dicke P, Arndt M, Kruse W (1990a): Feature linking across cortical maps via synchronization. In: *Parallel Processing in Neural Systems and Computers*, Eckmiller R, Hartmann G, Hauske G, eds. Amsterdam New York North-Holland, pp 101–104

Eckhorn R, Schanze T, Brosch M, Salem W, Bauer R (1991a): Stimulus-specific synchronizations in cat visual cortex: multiple microelectrode and correlation studies from several cortical areas. In: *Induced Rhythms in the Brain*, Başar E, Bullock TH, eds. Boston: Birkhäuser Boston Inc. pp 47–80

Eckhorn R, Schanze T, Reitboeck HJ (1991c): Neural mechanisms of flexible feature linking in the visual system. In: *Mathematical Approaches to Brain Functioning Diagnostics*, Dvorak I, Holden AV, eds. Proceedings in Nonlinear Science Manchester New York: Manchester University Press pp 407–428

Freeman WJ (1987): Simulation of chaotic EEG patterns with a dynamic model of the olfactory system. *Biol Cybern* 56: 139–150

Gray CM, König P, Engel AK, Singer W (1989): Oscillatory responses in cat visual cortex exhibit inter-columnar synchronization which reflects global stimulus properties. *Nature (Lond)* 338: 334–337

Kammen DM, Holmes PJ, Koch C (1989): Cortical architecture and oscillations in neuronal networks: feedback versus local coupling. In: *Models of Brain Function*, Cotterill RMJ, ed. Cambridge–New York–Melbourne: Cambridge University Press, pp 273–284

Kohonen T (1982): Self-organized formation of topologically correct feature maps. *Biol Cybern* 43: 59–69

Kuramoto Y (1991): Collective synchronization of pulse-coupled oscillators and excitable units. *Physica D* (in press)

Llinás RR (1988): The intrinsic electrophysiological properties of mammalian neurons: insights into central nervous system function. *Science* 242:1654–1664

Pabst M, Reitboeck HJ, Eckhorn R (1989): A model of pre-attentive region definition in visual patterns. In: *Models of Brain Function*, Cotterill RMJ ed. Cambridge–New York–Melbourne: Cambridge University Press, pp 137–150

Reitboeck HJ (1989): Neuronal mechanisms of pattern recognition. In: *Sensory Processing in the Mammalian Brain*, Lund JS, ed. New York: Oxford University Press, pp 307–330

Reitboeck HJ, Eckhorn R, Arndt M, Dicke P, Stoecker M (1991): In Neural network models for the simulation of basic visual information processing tasks. In: *Mathematical Approaches to Brain Functioning Diagnostics*, Holden AV, *Proceedings in Nonlinear Science Series*, Manchester: Manchester University Press pp 257–270

Reitboeck HJ, Eckhorn R, Pabst M (1987): A model for figure/ground separation based on correlated neural activity in the visual system. In: *Computational Systems–Natural and Artificial*, Haken H, ed. Berlin–Heidelberg–New York: Springer-Verlag, pp 44–54

Reitboeck HJ, Pabst M, Eckhorn R (1988): Texture description in the time domain. In: *Computer Simulation in Brain Science*, Cotterill RMJ, ed. Cambridge (UK): Cambridge University Press, pp 479–494

Schillen TB, König P (1990): Coherency detection by coupled oscillatory responses synchronizing connections in neural oscillator layers. In: *Parallel Processing in Neural Systems and Computers*, Eckmiller R, Hartmann G, Hauske G, eds. Amsterdam Elsevier, North-Holland, pp 139–142

Schuster HG, Wagner P (1990): A model for neuronal oscillations in the visual cortex (Part I + II). *Biol Cybern* 64:77–85

Sheer DE (1989): Sensory and cognitive 40-Hz event-related potentials: behavioral correlates, brain function, and clinical application. In: *Springer Series in Brain Dynamics 2*, Başar E, Bullock TH, eds. Berlin–Heidelberg: Springer–Verlag, pp 339–374

Snowden RJ, Braddick OJ (1990): Differences in the processing of short-range apparent motion at small and large displacements. *Vision Res* 30:1211–1222

Sompolinsky H, Golomb D, Kleinfeld D (1991): Global processing of visual stimuli in a neural network of coupled oscillators. *Proc Nat Acad Sci USA* (in press)

Sporns O, Gally JA, Reeke GN, Edelman GM (1989): Reentrant signaling among simulated neuronal groups leads to coherency in their oscillatory activity. *Proc Natl Acad Sci USA* 86:7265–7269

Synergetics of the Brain: An Outline of Some Basic Ideas

H. HAKEN

Synergetics as a Conceptual Tool in Brain Research

The interdisciplinary field of synergetics (Haken, 1983, 1987) studies the behavior of complex systems, that is, systems composed of very many elements, or parts, or subsystems. It focuses its attention on those systems that can develop spatial, temporal, or functional structures on macroscopic scales. Examples are provided in physics by fluids that can form specific patterns (e.g., honeycomb patterns or oscillations), laser physics and nonlinear optics, where a great variety of oscillations and wave propagation phenomena occur, chemistry with a formation of macroscopic spiral or ring wave patterns, models in biology of population dynamics, morphogenesis, evolutional processes, and a variety of other fields. Over the past two decades it could be shown that self-organization is governed by general principles that can be summarized as follows: When specific control parameters, which may be the energy input into a system or a specific signal flow, change, the former state of the system becomes unstable and new kinds of structures may emerge. Despite the fact that the system is originally described in general by an enormous number of variables, close to the instability point the dynamics and structure formation are governed by rather few variables, the so-called order parameters. The behavior of the individual elements or parts is governed, or in technical terms, enslaved, by the order parameters. Because of the broad validity of these general principles, profound analogies in the behavior of quite different systems show up so that one complex system can be modeled by another system, which at least close to instability points can be much simpler than the complex system under consideration.

In the following I wish to discuss some phenomena occurring in the brain in light of these findings. In particular I shall focus my attention on electric activity as shown in electroencephalograms (EEGs) but also in intracellular electric activity.

The Brain as a Physical System

In this section I wish to discuss what kind of phenomena we know of the brain that can be produced by physical systems. Among the most prominent processes we wish to consider are oscillations. Oscillations can be found in many physical systems. They may be the oscillations of a pendulum, of springs, of coupled springs, as well as of electronic or electrical circuits, or the specific light oscillations in lasers. Whereas physicists generally aim at building oscillators with stable frequencies, it is well known that in reality a continuous frequency drift fluctuation occurs that is caused by a variety of parameter changes. Thus, the difference between an oscillation in a physical system and a biological rhythm is of a quantitative and not a qualitative nature. Note that these temporal changes need not be noise but can occur quite coherently, for instance when in a laser the distance between the mirrors is changed by thermal expansion. A pendulum or a weight fixed at a vertical spring can perform oscillations, but because of damping these oscillations die out. Oscillations that last forever can be produced in these systems only by external periodic forces so that the question arises how in turn their periodic motion was produced. With respect to biological applications, the class of self-sustained oscillators is of much more relevance. In this case the capability of performing oscillations is an internal property and not imposed on the system from the outside. An example that has proven to be very fruitful in the field of synergetics is the light source laser (Haken, 1984, 1985). In a somewhat oversimplified picture, the laser process can be described as follows: In the gas laser an ensemble of gas atoms is enclosed in a cylindrical tube. The atoms may be excited from the outside by an electric current, whereby the individual electrons of the atoms can be brought to an upper state. From there they can go over to the so-called ground state by the emission of a light wave track. This can be compared to throwing pebbles into water; a wildly excited water surface emerges. In this sense each lamp produces chaotic light that is a superposition of uncorrelated, or in other words, incoherent light wave tracks. On the other hand, when the laser is energetically excited more and more, suddenly a new phenomena occur, where the individual emission processes become correlated and a well ordered macroscopic light wave emerges. The light field has become coherent. As it transpires, a laser may serve as an analogue for the coherent firing of many neurones so as to produce macroscopic electric activities. It is worthwhile to mention a number of phenomena that may be produced by lasers. Namely, a laser can either oscillate at one specific frequency and in this way may suppress the existence of all other oscillations. In other situations the coexistence of oscillations at several frequencies becomes possible when the frequencies are independent of each other.

If differences of combinations of frequencies become smaller than some critical value, such frequencies can become locked, that is, instead of different frequencies, which were formerly present, only one is present, which represents the so-called frequency locked state. In lasers, by frequency-locking, pulses can be formed that run back and forth within the laser. At a still higher energy input and under specific circumstances, a new phenomenon may set in. The macroscopic oscillations may enter the regime of deterministic chaos. These chaotic motions can be described by a few degrees of freedom, that is, by a so-called low-dimensional attractor. (Applications of chaos theory to brain theory may be found in Başar, 1990.) When a laser is coupled to a nonlinear device, such as specific crystals, the frequency of its oscillation can be changed into so-called subharmonics (i.e., frequencies that are only half or a fraction of the former frequency) or to higher harmonics, in which case the frequency is an integer multiple of the laser frequency. Whereas the individual atoms may be considered as small antennas that produce light at a more or less well defined frequency and give rise to the laser light oscillation at a related frequency, oscillations can be produced also by systems whose parts do not show oscillations at all. Examples are provided by fluids. When a fluid layer is heated from below, it may first form specific spatial patterns, such as rolls. But at a higher energy input these rolls begin to oscillate. The oscillation frequency is determined by quantities like dimensions, viscosity, and so forth, but not by any oscillation frequency of the individual molecules of which the fluid is composed. Similar remarks can be made with respect to chemical reactions, where under a steady influx of chemical reactants and a steady outflux of the end-products, oscillations can be sustained indefinitely. These oscillations are not forced on the system from the outside, nor do the individual parts of the chemical reaction show any oscillations. Only by the interplay of several chemical reactions going on do these oscillations arise and manifest themselves in a periodic change of color. These oscillations may be periodic with one frequency or with several frequencies (quasiperiodic) or they may become chaotic (i.e., quite irregular), but still being governed by few degrees of freedoms (order parameters).

In conclusion, we may state that macroscopic oscillations may be produced by the coupling of oscillators with the same or closely related frequencies, or by coupling of otherwise nonoscillating elements. A simple example for the latter is also provided by strings of violins. A further general observation may be made that was alluded to before, namely, when we change a single control parameter, such as the power input into a system, the system may run through a hierarchy of so-called instabilities, and at each instability point a new kind of structure is formed. For instance, in a laser we may find the range from incoherent emission over to a coherent wave over to laser light pulses to laser light chaos. In the book of Kandel (Kandel, 1979) on *Aplysia*, a diagram of four different cells is shown that exhibit precisely the behavior just described. This may have an important biological consequence, namely, different kinds of behavior may be produced by exactly the same type of cell but just with one control parameter changed, which may for instance be the number of ionic channels. Generalizing from physics to the whole class of self-organizing systems studied by synergetics, we may make a number of important general remarks. There is no one-to-one correspondence between a nonlinear system and its performance. More precisely, one individual system may show qualitatively different states of operation or spatiotemporal patterns. On the other hand, one specific kind of operation can be realized by quite different systems. This means in general that a specific operation of a system can be modeled by a variety of other systems. How can we decide between different models? Or in other words, what further criteria can we apply to distinguish between them? In general, such differentiation will become possible when we look at a more microscopic level. As it appears for the moment, at least some features of macro-EEG data from the scalp with widely spaced electrodes could be imitated to a larger or smaller extent by physical systems. However, an important issue remains, namely, the relation between these physical processes and mental tasks, such as cognition, motor control, or introspection. In this author's opinion a main task will be to establish correlations between this latter kind of process and physical processes that are observed in the brain.

Significance of Oscillations

One may speculate why the mammalian brain prefers to use oscillations for the transmission and processing of information rather than steady state signals. There are a number of reasons for this:

With respect to steady fields it is difficult to fix a zero. Fields may build up in a way that cannot be easily controlled. In oscillating fields the zero line is set automatically. Oscillations contain much more information that any steady state, namely, they possess both an amplitude and a frequency. This allows the system either to let signals pass at different frequencies (the multiplex concept), or to frequency-lock them so that logical functions can be performed. By coupling modes together at different frequencies, qualitatively new phenomena may occur, such as pulses. In this respect, the recent experimental findings by Gray et al. (1990), Eckhorn and Reitböck (1990), and others are of utmost interest. They show that different neurones can mode-lock. What is the meaning of frequency-locking? It may serve for a discrimination between background and foreground. A recent mathematical model of mine (Haken, 1990) shows that in this way moving objects can be identified and recognized against the background. This discrimination between different objects is even simpler than in the case when the objects do not move. As was suggested by Singer and others, frequency-locking may be a general principle of correlating features to form patterns. Besides movement, common features include color and so forth. Quite clearly, more experimental results are needed to get a clearer picture of the meaning of frequency-locking. As just mentioned, though, models of recognition processes are promising. A further promising field for the application of the general concepts of synergetics is EEG analysis. Here we used data by Lehmann (Zürich) (1971, 1972) on α-rhythms and on epileptic seizures. We could show that in epileptic seizures the dynamics are determined by a few order parameters and their detailed dynamics in the frame of attractors could be determined. We have also analyzed multielectrode derivations taken by Lehmann in the case of α-rhythms. Because α-rhythms may easily break down, for instance when eyes are opened, we tentatively assume that these rhythms are close to an "instability point." According to our experience in synergetics, close to instability points spatial patterns can be considered as a superposition of a few basic simple patterns. In the case of the α-rhythms we were able to show that the spatial EEG pattern can be simulated by five elementary modes. The mode amplitudes undergo a low dimensional dynamics, but here a typical difficulty occurs that is caused by the nonstationarity of the data. For instance, in order to perform a dimensional analysis of the attractor in the sense of chaos theory, a sufficient number of measuring points is needed. If these points are chosen too closely to each other, the analysis exhibits coherence effects that are spurious. On the other hand, in order to avoid this difficulty, one has to take data points over an extended period. Here it turns out that the system is not stationary, which is shown as follows: We are able to determine the attractor of the order parameters for a short while, but then the system can no longer be described by this dynamic but undergoes a different one. It is as if the order parameters are hopping between several attracting states.

Acknowledgment. I wish to thank Prof. Ted Bullock for several very helpful comments.

References

Başar E (1990): *Chaos in Brain Function.* Berlin, New York: Springer

Ditzinger T, Haken H (1989): Oscillations in the perception of ambiguous patterns. *Biol Cybern* 61:279–287

Eckhorn R, Reitböck HJ (1990): Stimulus-specific synchronization in cat visual cortex and its possible role in visual pattern recognition. In: *Synergetics of Cognition*, Haken H, ed. Springer

Friedrich R, Fuchs A, Haken H (1991): Synergetic analysis of spatio-temporal EEG-patterns. In *Nonlinear wave process in excitable media*, Holden AV, Markus M, and Othmer HG, eds. New York: Plenum Press

Gray C, König P, Engel A, Singer W (1990): Synchronization of oscillatory responses in visual cortex: A plausible mechanism for scene segmentation. In: *Synergetics of Cognition*, Haken H, ed. Berlin, New York: Springer

Haken H (1983): *Synergetics, An Introduction*, 3rd ed. Berlin New York Springer

Haken H (1984): Laser Theory. In: *Encyclopedia of Physics*, Vol. XXV/2c. Fluegge S, ed. Berlin, New York: Springer

Haken H (1985): *Laser Light Dynamics.* Amsterdam: North Holland

Haken H (1987): *Advanced Synergetics, Instability Hierarchies of Self-Organizing Systems and Devices*, Berlin, New York: Springer

Haken H (1990): *Synergetic Computers and Cognition.* Berlin, New York: Springer

Kandel ER (1979): *Behavioral Biology of Aplysia.* San Francisco: Freeman

Lehmann D (1971): Multichannel topography of human alpha EEG fields. *Electroencephalogr Clin Neurophysiol* 31:439–449

Lehmann D (1972): Human scalp EEG fields: Evoked, alpha, sleep, and spike-wave patterns. In: *Synchronization of EEG Activity in Epilepsies*, Petsche H, Brazier MAB, eds. Berlin, New York: Springer

Epilogue

Brain Natural Frequencies are Causal Factors for Resonances and Induced Rhythms

Erol Başar*

The rationale of writing this epilogue is to help my own thinking about the results and discussions presented in the foregoing chapters. I do not aim to give a comprehensive account of all the chapters presented and all the ideas included in this book. Bullock has written most relevant introductory remarks, and I refer to his chapter for opening comment, chronology, and remarks about the chapters of the present volume.

One way of dealing with the problems at hand is to subdivide them according to the frequency bands, for example, "around 4 Hz," "around 10 Hz," "around 40 Hz," and then treat the theoretical implications and models. I will attempt this plan and try to distill my thought on induced rhythmicities and their connections with brain dynamics, including the chaotic approach.

Summary

I distinguish three topics concerning integrative aspects of brain signaling as points of entry into the problems of induced rhythms:

1) Can a single principle underlying high order neural processing be isolated? Or are there instead of a fundamental common principle multiple principles, some of them observable and some others beyond our scope? Or is the number of principles too high to permit generalizing the observations?

2) Are there common transfer functions in neural tissues of the brain? That is, can the transfer functions we compute have a common basis or meaning?

3) A general principle of high order neural processing may include analogies to the emergence of regular patterns from uniform matter: what is the role of dynamic pattern building? Concerning this topic, both tools of chaotic dynamics and concepts of Katchalsky's on dynamic pattern building have gained importance during the past few years.

Having in mind the idea that induced rhythmicities may be part of a general principle, our review distinguished four categories of rhythmicities em-

---

* With editorial assistance by Martin Schürmann

bracing both induced and spontaneous:

1) Rhythmicities around 10 Hz designated the alpha band;
2) those around 40 Hz, often designated the gamma band;
3) those in the 4–10 Hz band, called theta rhythms;
4) those in the 2 Hz band, often called delta waves.

If induced rhytbmicities really play an important role in brain signaling, how does the brain integrate oscillatory activity of its single neurons? Is reacting to internal or external events by the brain a transition from chaos to rhythmicity? And what principles underly the excitability of the brain? To deal with these questions, the epilogue contains remarks on synchrony and coherence of EEG activity, on oscillation and resonance and on the "chaotic approach" to the spontaneous EEG.

1) Conceptual aspects of EEG activity expressed in terms of synchrony and coherence may be important in integrating oscillatory neural activity.

1.1) As an example, the synchrony of alpha activity is discussed. It may be a sign of cooperative phenomena whose mechanisms are still to be uncovered. Coherence is a frequency-specific measure which can be equally high when the two time series are in phase or out of phase, that is, synchronized with any fixed phase lag between them. Its distribution and natural history are just beginning to be investigated.

1.2) Another example is the micro-EEG revealing spatio-temporal aspects of EEG synchrony.

2) Oscillation and resonance in neural tissues are variables with certain degree of independence from each other and from the foregoing, synchrony and coherence.

2.1) The cellular basis is an active experimental front. The example is cited of thalamic neurons behaving as oscillators and resonators.

2.2) Oscillation and resonance are a possible conceptual approach to link spontaneous and induced rhythmicities as will be outlined below in an "excitability rule".

2.3) An analysis of this relationship between spontaneous and induced rhythms contributes to the understanding of the differences between adults' and childrens' evoked potentials.

2.4) As an analogy to the excitability of neural tissues, dissipative structures —probably one of the simplest physical mechanisms of communication—and excitability in biological and biochemical systems are considered.

2.5) Biochemical oscillators even permit us to model multiple modes of neural oscillations. This is an important correlate to different modes of oscillation in thalamic neurons.

2.6) Another aspect of integration concerns the connections between and within cortical maps. It was hypothesized that responses are linked by reentry in interconnected networks.

3) Is external stimulation a prerequisite for exciting the brain? Internal events exciting neural tissues can be discovered using special paradigms. Even without such paradigms it is possible to demonstrate that the EEG is not merely "noise": this is achieved by methods of chaotic dynamics.

3.1) The existence of alpha and theta attractors by such methods is an interesting supplementary finding to the induced rhythmicities observed in the same frequency ranges.

3.2) High frequency attractors in cerebellum and brain stem have been demonstrated as well and should merit more attention.

It is concluded that induced rhythmicities and resonance phenomena are fingerprints of common transfer functions within the brain. Induced rhythmicities probably reflect most important functional activities. They are proposed as the base of a common language for investigators interested in field potentials, EEG and magnetoencephalography.

Some Integrative Aspects of Brain Signaling

One of the main topics of chapters of this book is the function of the brain's electromagnetic oscillatory activity and its possible roles in the coding of behaviorally relevant information in the central nervous system.

The higher order neural processing that leads to thinking, consciousness, and preparation for future acts has not been satisfactorily described in terms of neural oscillatory phenomena and the electroencephalogram (EEG) activity related to brain function. There are also no standard methods for clearly describing the functional and behavioral components of the brain's electrical activity.

Is there a "single principle" underlying high order neural processing?

It is usually assumed that there is no uniform code for behaviorally relevant information in the neuronal networks that constitute the central nervous systems. Edelman (1978) has raised the important question: "Does the brain operate according to a single principle in carrying out its higher order cognitive functions? That is, despite the manifold differences in brain subsystems and particularities of their connections, can one discern a general mechanism or principle that is required for the realization of cognitive functions? If so, at what level does the mechanism operate, cells, molecules, or circuits of cells?" In other words, has the brain, independent of its various special functions, some global strategies by means of which the internal communication and coordination among various neuronal networks is optimized?

To clarify these questions, in most of the chapters of this volume two important aspects of "induced rhythmicities" were discussed:

1. the neural origin of oscillatory phenomena
2. the relation of oscillatory phenomena to brain functions.

Are there common transfer functions in the neural tissues of the brain?

At this point I find it most pertinent to quote Fessard (1961), who tried to emphasize the role of neuronal networks in the brain:

> The brain, even when studied from the restricted point of view of sensory communications, must not be considered simply as a juxtaposition of private lines, leading to a mosaic of independent cortical territories, one for each sense modality, with internal subdivisions corresponding to topical differentiations.... The track of a single-unit message is doomed to be rapidly lost when one tries to follow it through a neuronal field endowed with network properties, within which the elementary message readily interacts with many others.... Unfortunately, we still lack principles that would help us describe and master such operations in which heterosensory communications are involved. These principles may gradually emerge in the future from an extensive use of multiple microelectrode recordings, together with a systematic treatment of data by modern electronic computers, so that pattern-to-pattern transformation matrices can be established and possibly generalized.... For the time being, it seems that we should do better to try to clear up such principles as seem to govern the most general transformations—or transfer functions—of multiunit homogeneous messages during their progressions through neuronal networks.

The definition of the transfer function, as commonly used in systems theory, is given in Chapter 8 of this book. This function presents the ensemble of amplitude and phase frequency characteristics of a system responding to excitation. In several chapters of the present volume the expressions network–resonance or brain resonance were used. In turn, resonant properties of a network are reflected in its transfer function. Accordingly, Fessard's aim can be possibly extended or interpreted in the sense of general systems theory as in the following paragraphs.

The brain has natural frequencies that are seemingly common in several neural populations. For example, induced gamma, theta, or alpha rhythmicities were reported in cortex, hippocampus, thalamus, and brain stem according to the experiments reported in most of the chapters of this volume. Freeman (1988) used the expression "common modes" for the existence of similar frequency channels in various networks of the brain. Further, the transfer function measures the ability of a network (here, neural networks of the brain) to increase (facilitate) or impede (inhibit) transmission of signals in given frequency channels. The existence of general transfer functions would then be interpreted as the existence of networks distributed in the brain that show similar frequency characteristics or facilitate or even increase the signal transmission in common frequency channels. In an electric system optimal transmission of signals is often reached when distributed subsystems of the system are tuned to the same frequency range. Does the brain have such subsystems tuned in similar frequency ranges, or do there exist common frequency modes in the brain?

Together the chapters of this book might provide a possible approach to this question. How to obtain the transfer function (or frequency characteristics) is described in many articles and books (Spekreijse and Van der Tweel, 1972; Başar, 1983a, Başar et al., Chapter 8 of this volume).

The broader question, "what are the neuronal correlates of the EEG and of EPs?," has been treated by several authors (see, e.g., Creutzfeldt et al., 1966, 1969; Verzeano, 1973; Freeman, 1975; Ramos et al., 1976; and for reviews see Başar 1980, 1983a, 1983b; Petsche et al., 1984; Steriade et al., 1990). Every model that tries to describe the EEG and field potentials offers a new window on the problem, as discussed elegantly by Bullock (this volume). Some of the chapters in this volume are examples of such "new windows."

Concepts of "dynamic pattern building," "synchrony" and "coherence"

In the present book several approaches extend the usefulness of analysis of dynamic patterns in brain signaling (Haken, Goldbeter, Sejnowski, this volume). The analysis of dynamic patterns with tools of the chaotic approach provides new important steps.

According to the discussion brought out by Katchalsky et al. (1974), the central question about building of dynamic patterns is: How does uniform matter, obeying physical principles, that is, laws of conservation of momentum, matter and energy, spontaneously develop regular patterns? In other words, how is it that a set of isotropic causes can give rise to anisotropic dynamic effects? This appears to be the root problem of morphogenesis; growing from it are more widely encountered problems of how preexisting static structures influence dynamic patterns.

In the book by Katchalsky et al. (1974) some dynamic patterns observed in geology, meteorology, and astrophysics were also described; for example, dynamic patterns on a large scale in clouds and the solar coronasphere.

The branch of mathematics that applies to dynamic systems is called the "dynamic system theory." Katchalsky et al. give examples of mathematical analysis of dynamic systems. There are the Lotka–Volterra scheme, relaxation oscillators (Van der Pol equation), and chemodiffusional systems. Each of these is a model or a tool that might reveal how dynamic patterns in brain activity are built.

Processes of synchrony of neural generators and coherency between neural populations are directly involved in the dynamic pattern building in brain's electrical activity. Therefore, the concepts of synchrony and coherence were treated by several authors trying to find correlations between EEG patterns and brain function (e.g., Bullock and McClune 1989, Bullock, this volume; Buzsáki; this volume; Lopes da Silva, this volume; Petsche and Rappelsberger, this volume). These concepts, which are also essential to understand the induced rhythmicities, will be treated later.

Freeman (1990) states: "In the view of neurobiologists, the function of our brains that we experience subjectively as remembering and recognizing are dynamic operations. These operations work on patterns of neural activity and transform them into other patterns of activity in our brains." Neuroscientists went a long but fruitful way since the suggestion of Katchalsky to observe the Zhabotinsky reaction as an example to see parallelisms in understanding pattern formation of the EEG. The approach with chaotic dynamics provides one of the routes to understand complex oscillations and nonlinear pattern formation. Accordingly, this epilogue has an appendix to present briefly the idea behind this approach and make somewhat easier the reading of a later section and of chapters and related work of authors such as Haken, Goldbeter, Lopes da Silva, Saermark, and Freeman. (For suggested reading see references of Tables 2 and 3 of the appendix.)

Induced and Spontaneous Rhythmicities: Examples of Observations from the 2-Hz Range to the 40-Hz Range

I will begin the discussion of questions raised in previous sections with examples of the several frequency bands "around 10 Hz," "around 40 Hz," "around 4 Hz," and so on.

Around 10 Hz

Andersen and Andersson (1968) published an interesting review on 10-Hz rhythms. In the following some of their features will be restated.

> "A particular feature of the thalamic relay nuclei is their ability to convert a single afferent volley to a series of rhythmic discharges along the thalamocortical fibers. [For a detailed account of thalamocortical circuits the reader is referred to Steriade et al., 1990b.]
>
> Several theories have been advanced to explain these rhythmic discharges. Adrian (1941) reported that rhythmic 10/sec activity following a single afferent volley could be recorded within or at the dorsal surface of the thalamus, even if the appropriate cortical area was removed. In other words, the thalamic nuclei contain a mechanism for the transfer of a single volley to a rhythmic 10/sec sequence without the presence of that cortical area to which the thalamocortical fibers project.
>
> Similar rhythmic activity was found by Bremer and Bonnet (1950) in the medial geniculate nucleus in response to a click. All these authors noted that the frequency of the evoked activity was around 10/sec, i.e., similar to that of the spontaneous rhythmic cortical waves. Adrian (1941) maintained that the after-discharges consisted of bursts of spikes separated by slow waves. A peripheral stimulus elicited a series of 3 to 7 such cycles. By recording from the white matter below the cortex, Adrian showed that the rhythmic discharge occurred in the thalamocortical fibers, indicating a thalamic origin of the after-discharges. Due to this rhythmic discharge in response to a single afferent volley, a series

> of waves are initiated in the cortex, appearing at a frequency of about 10/sec (Bartley and Bishop, 1933; Bishop, 1933; Jarcho, 1949; Bishop et al., 1953). In 1951 Chang advanced the hypothesis that a corticothalamic reverberating circuit should be the basis for the evoked rhythmic activity. The arguments for this explanation were the presence of a similar rhythmic activity in the thalamus and cortex, and the difficulty of recording thalamic rhythmic activity after removal of the appropriate cortical projection area. However, this theory is contradicted not only by the early reports of Adrian (1941) and Bremer and Bonnet (1950) but also by more recent observations by Adrian (1951), who critically tested the corticothalamic reverberating hypothesis, and by Galambos et al. (1952). Full support for the statement of Adrian and Bremer was given by Andersen, Brooks and Eccles (1964) and Andersen, Brooks, Eccles and Sears (1964)." (Andersen and Andersson, 1968)

Başar et al. (1976b; Başar 1980) reviewed and classified the field potential responses in the 10-Hz frequency range (the evoked alpha) starting with the alpha selectivity observed by Spekreijse and Van der Tweel. I now shorten this classification as follows:

1. alpha response at human occipital electrode upon sine modulated light stimulation (Van der Tweel and Verduyn Lunel, 1965; Regan, 1966; Spekreijse, 1966; Van der Tweel and Spekreijse, 1969)
2. enhanced alpha component with 500–600 ms latency (following alpha-blocking) at human scalp electrodes (Barlow and Estrin, 1971; Lansing and Barlow, 1972; Nogawa et al., 1976)
3. time-locking with 500–600 msec latency at scalp electrodes of human subjects with closed eyes upon auditory stimulation as tone bursts (Başar et al., 1976b)

4a. strong alpha resonance in the alpha channel in the auditory cortex, thalamus, reticular formation, inferior colliculus, hippocampus, and cerebellar cortex of the cat upon acoustic stimulation (tone bursts) (Başar et al., 1975a, 1975b, 1975c, 1976a)

4b. strong resonant alpha responses upon light stimulation in the visual pathway, reticular formation, and hippocampus of the cat. The stimulation was a light step function (Başar 1980)

5. enhancement and time-locked alpha response with 50–150 ms latency at scalp electrodes of human subjects sitting in a dimly illuminated room upon photic stimulation in form of a a step function (Başar et al., 1976b)

One of the most important publications on alpha activity is that by Pfurtscheller et al. (1988), in which the authors describe the alpha band rhythm and its event-related desynchronization. Emphasis is given to comparing the lower (6–10 Hz) and upper (9–13 Hz) alpha bands, this is, to the variety of rhythmicities in the frequency scale (see also Chapter by Pfurtscheller et al., this volume).

In this volume there is one more report that showed functionally related 10-Hz rhythmicities. Mangun (this volume) describes the P1-N1-P2-N2 sequence of the visual event-related potential in humans. This sequence of waves in the event-related potential has a characteristic frequency of 10 Hz. However, Mangun states that these responses are stimulus-induced and are to be distinguished from spontaneous or stimulus driven rhythms.

An important remark by Walter (1964), who is known as the discoverer of the contingent negative variation, is as follows:

> We've managed to check the alpha band rhythm with intracerebral electrodes in the occipital-parietal cortex; in regions which are practically adjacent and almost congruent one finds a variety of alpha rhythms, some of which are blocked by opening and closing the eyes, some are not, some are driven by flicker, some are not, some respond in some way to mental activity, some do not. What one sees on the scalp is a spatial average of a large number of components, and whether you see an alpha rhythm of a particular type or not depends upon which component happens to be the most highly synchronized process over the largest superficial area; there are complex rhythms in everybody.

My coworkers and I tentatively propose that activities of 1 to 4, 4 to 7, and 8 to 13 Hz serve as "operators" in the selective filtering of expected target stimuli. We suggested that Freeman's concept, as outlined below, can be generalized to various sensory systems and to other EEG frequencies such as 2, 5 to 6, and 8 to 13 Hz. Freeman (1975; Freeman and Skarda, 1985) has shown that the EEG of the olfactory bulb and cortex in awake, motivated rabbits and cats shows a characteristic temporal pattern consisting of bursts of 40- to 80-Hz oscillations, superimposed on a surface-negative baseline potential shift synchronized to each inspiration. Freeman has interpreted this finding as follows:

> The neural activity which is induced by an odor during a period of learning provides the specification for a neural template of strength connections between the neurons made active by that odor. Subsequently when the animal is placed in the appropriate setting, the template may be activated in order to serve as a selective filter for search and detection of the expected odor. (Freeman, 1979)

We used the expression "operative states" for degrees of brain synchronization in defined frequency channels (Başar et al, 1989). According to Lopes da Silva (1987), alpha networks with similar designs are distributed in various structures of the brain. Başar (1980) also takes the same viewpoint according to experimental results of field potentials in the cat brain.

In magnetoencephalography Saermark et al. (this volume) describe how it is possible to distinguish induced alpha and theta rhythmicities that can be recorded as more distinct 10-Hz or 5-Hz rhythmicities according to location of the detectors. Narici et al. (1990) presented results of a neuromagnetic study on the spatial structure of brain rhythms enhanced by photic and somatosensory stimulation. In the visual modality the synchronization was characterized by a potentiation of the subjects alpha. In the somatosensory modality two different activities were observed: one probably related to the rolandic mu rhythm, the second suggesting the presence of two widely separated and time correlated sources possibly driven by a unique deep clock. These authors conclude that the single frequency resonance elicited by visual stimulation may be located in a region close to the calcarine fissure. The experimental steps undertaken in the study of Narici et al. (1990) are promising for localization of rhythmicities and for their functional differentiation by means of magnetoencephalography.

Around 40 Hz

In the present volume, several fundamental chapters discuss the 40-Hz rhythmicities (Gray et al., Eckhorn, Tononi et al., Freeman, Galambos). With the recent discoveries of Gray and Singer (1987, 1989; Gray et al. 1989) at the cellular level and coherence studies of Eckhorn et al. (1988), a new important area has been opened and several important questions have emerged concerning the origin and functional significance of the 40-Hz activity (see also the chapter by Galambos in this volume). Besides the findings of Gray et al. and Eckhorn et al., I want to mention here another work of Llinás and Graves (1990), who have shown that in intracellular recordings from brain slices of guinea pig frontal cortex sustained subthreshold oscillatory activity around 40 Hz could be measured either spontaneously or upon direct depolarization. This form of activity was observed in the smooth or sparsely multipolar neurons of layer 4. Steriade et al. (1990) state that these last results suggest that the well defined 40-Hz rhythm observed in the cerebral cortex is driven by the intrinsic properties of neurons located in the same cerebral cortical layer that receives specific thalamocortical afferents (see also Llinás, this volume).

Gray and Singer (1987, 1989; Gray et al., 1989) have reported that neurons in the cat visual cortex exhibit oscillatory responses in the range of 40 to 60 Hz. These oscillations occur in synchrony for cells located within a functional column and are tightly correlated with local oscillatory field potentials. This led Gray and Singer to the working hypothesis that the synchronization of oscillatory responses of spatially distributed, feature-selective cells might be a way to establish relations between features in different parts of the visual field. Later, Gray and Singer (1989) provided evidence that neurons in spatially separate columns synchronize their oscillatory responses provided they are stimulated by one moving bar but not when they are stimulated by two bars moving similarly but not congruently. This synchronization occurs on the average with no phase difference and depends on the spatial separation and orientation preference of the cells.

The discovery made by Singer's group was later confirmed by Eckhorn et al. (1988, 1989a, 1988b), who raised the important question of whether coherent oscillations reflect a mechanism of "feature linking" in the visual cortex. They also found stimulus-evoked resonances of 35 to 85 Hz throughout the visual cortex when the primary coding channels were activated by their specific preferred stimuli (e.g., bars moving in the right orientation).

The results of the highly relevant experiments by the groups of Singer and later Eckhorn and their interpretations were commented upon by Stryker (1989): "Is Grandmother an oscillation? Is it possible that the neurons in visual cortex activated by the same object in the world tend to discharge rhythmically and in unison? Such a one-note neural harmony could, in principle at least, provide the neurons at higher cortical levels with stronger inputs so that they associate the activities of lower-order neurons with another." Stryker further notes, "Exploring the rhythms of the brain, revered by the pioneers of Electroencephalography but now mostly dismissed as irrelevant to neural information processing, may even come back into fashion."

As mentioned by Galambos and Makeig (1981), 40-Hz activity can be measured by scalp recordings. Galambos (this volume), one of the pioneers describing human 40-Hz evoked rhythmicities, provides an interesting classification of brain rhythm generators. He classifies "spontaneous," "induced," "evoked," and "emitted" 40-Hz rhythmicities (gamma band). Furthermore, the 10-Hz rhythmicities are classified with a similar strong schema, which can be, in turn, useful in search of functional correlates. Emitted rhythmicities to omitted stimuli in the fish brain, recently discovered by Bullock, are also illustrated in this relevant discussion by Galambos.

I also want to emphasize here an important review by Sheer (1989) who, based on his pioneering work on 40-Hz activity, summarizes a most important functional relationship of 40 Hz concerning focused attention as results of his own group and of other scientists working in this area.

In my opinion a word of caution in the study of 40-Hz oscillations should be pronounced. In the new trends there is an insistent search for 40-Hz potentials in cortex. However, we know from the literature that hippocampus has also rhythmic activity in this higher frequency range (for a review see Buszáki, this volume).

In Chapter 8 of this volume (Başar et al., this volume) we state that 40-Hz responsiveness is also an important component of the hippocampal evoked potentials: 40-Hz components of single epochs of hippocampal responses may reach magnitudes up to 200 μV upon sensory stimulation (Başar, 1980). Since 1972 we have published several studies showing that 40-Hz spontaneous and evoked activities do not only occur in cat hippocampus, but also 40-Hz activity or responsiveness can be triggered by several modalities of stimulation (see Başar, 1980, 1983). Accordingly, I enclose one of the tables published years ago (Başar, 1980) in which phase-locked 40-Hz enhancements were recorded not only in cat hippocampus but also in the brain stem (Table 1).

We see here that the auditory hippocampal 40-Hz response has a mean amplitude of 80 μV. The auditory cortex has the same response amplitude and thus the responsiveness to acoustical stimuli is comparable (for 40-Hz auditory response see also Başar et al., this volume). As in the case of alpha activity networks, I tend to assume that 40-Hz networks are distributed throughout the brain and that it is not possible to attribute to 40-Hz bursts only one or two types of function, but that this 40-Hz oscillatory activity

Table 1. Mean values of rms EEG and Evoked potentials from various intracranial structures of the cat brain during the waking state.

Center frequency	3 Hz		13 Hz		25 Hz		37 Hz		66 Hz		113 Hz	
Band limits	1–7 Hz		8–16 Hz		15–35 Hz		25–49 Hz		46–86 Hz		82–144 Hz	
	Mean	s.d.	Mean	s.d.	Mean	s.d.	Mean	s.d.	Mean	s.d.	Mean	s.d.
EEG (μV) (rms values)												
GEA	195	27	100	26	52	17	40	18	22	6	13	6
MG	261	68	112	16	59	13	41	6	22	7	15	7
IC	125	33	56	3	29	12	15	4	10	5	8	
RF	129	67	66	15	32	7	21	5	16	6	18	6
HI	194	57	81	29	51	14	43	16	28	14	16	14
EP (μV) (maximal values)												
GEA	339	129	234	73	210	72	104	54	54	22	49	20
MG	332	77	249	47	137	47	76	12	50	16	35	7
IC	210	112	102	21	61	23	32	10	29	20	22	2
RF	217	113	156	29	77	28	51	14	48	23	54	41
HI	338	146	160	30	100	22	82	23	52	19	33	22
X (enhancement factors)												
GEA	1.9	0.5	2.4	0.5	3.2	1.4	2.7	0.7	2.4	0.5	3.7	1.3
MG	1.5	0.5	2.3	0.4	2.4	0.4	2.0	0.6	2.3	0.4	2.5	0.3
IC	1.7	0.5	2.0	0.3	2.3	0.3	2.6	0.7	2.6	0.7	2.5	0.5
RF	1.6	0.5	2.5	0.6	2.4	0.8	2.5	0.5	2.9	0.6	2.8	0.6
HI	2.2	0.7	2.0	0.7	2.3	0.9	2.0	0.6	2.0	0.4	2.1	0.4

The EEG and evoked potentials were pass-band filtered as shown. The frequency channels are specified by their band limits and center frequencies at the top.
The filtered EP components were time-locked components in various bands. These are mean values of results from 11 experiments on 11 cats. For the method, explanation of experiments and definition of the enhancement factor the reader is referred to Başar et al., 1979a and to Başar, 1980. This is a modified version of tables published in those works.
GEA, auditory cortex, Gyrus ectosylvianus anterior; MG, medial geniculate nucleus; IC, inferior colliculus; RF, reticular formation; HI, hippocampus.

might occur in several structures during several sensory and cognitive tasks and showing several types of delays. As Freeman (1975) showed, 40-Hz bursts can occur before odor targets. They can appear accompanying slow P300 activity in the cat hippocampus (Başar-Eroglu and Başar, 1991; Başar et al., this volume). They can appear in expectancy states before arrival of a target (Başar et al., 1989). For the functional significance of 40-Hz activity in the cat brain one should also cite Rougeul et al. (1979).

Around theta

The rhythmic slow activity (RSA or theta rhythm) may be considered as the "fingerprint" of all limbic structures, although it is most prominent in the hippocampal formation. Lopes da Silva (this volume Lopes da Silva et al. 1990b) discusses the possible functional significance of RSA as follows:

1. RSA may serve a "gating function" on the flow of information through the hippocampus.
2. RSA may facilitate the "matching" of the "resonance" between the hippocampal formation outputs and the circuits of target structures.
3. RSA can have a facilitating role in the induction/enhancement of long-term potentiation in the circuits of the hippocampus and of target structures.

Hippocampal theta activity has been extensively analyzed since the pioneering work of Grastyán et al. (1959) and Adey et al. (1960). There is evidence that this activity can be induced during various physiological and behavioral conditions. In Table 2 there are a few examples of cat experiments during exploration and searching behavior, and during motor behavior and special displacement. Also during sensory stimulation in the cat brain 5-Hz induced activity was observed. This table has examples of only the cat hippocampus. An extended review on functionally related theta activity is given by O'Keefe and Nadel (1978).

The examples shown in the tables should make clear that it is usually not possible to relate spontaneous and induced rhythmicities only to a single function. There are at least 20 papers indicating that hippocampal theta activity can be controlled in various brain stem nuclei (Vertes, 1982). Accordingly, a concept of distributed networks in the brain and multifunctional theta activity should be considered for global approaches to understand brain-induced rhythmicities in general.

Lopes da Silva (this volume) put forward the hypothesis that oscillatory states in neuronal networks may constitute a mechanism used by the nervous system to regulate changes of state in these networks.

I also draw attention here to a review by Swanson (1983), in which it is concluded that hippocampal formation may be thought of as a class of complex "supramodal association cortex" that receives and integrates information from each of the sensory modalities, and that it projects back to complex polymodal and other supramodal association areas, to visceromotor control

Table 2. Hippocampal EEG during exploration, orientation reflex, and searching behavior, cat

	Theta frequency (Hz)
Grastyán et al., 1959	5
Adey et al., 1960	4.0–7.5
Bennett et al., 1973	4.7
Grastyán and Vereczkei, 1974	4–5

Hippocampal EEG during motor behaviors: spatial displacement

	Behavior and theta frequency (Hz)
Adey et al., 1960	5–6
Holmes and Adey, 1960	5–6
Elazar and Adey, 1967	5–6
Whishaw and Vanderwolf, 1973	5
Grastyán and Vereczkei, 1974	6–7

Hippocampal EEG during sensory stimulation

	Theta frequency (Hz)
Green and Arduini, 1954	5
Grastyán et al., 1959	5

systems (particularly in the hypothalamus) and to striatum. The conclusion of Swanson is based on several physiological and anatomical investigations (e.g., Jones and Powell, 1970; Mesulam et al., 1977). Besides theta resonances in hippocampus (see Table 2), 40-Hz resonances to acoustical stimuli and the delayed P300-40 Hz complex during cognitive tasks in cat (see Başar et al., this volume) should be also mentioned. Andersen (1975) showed rhythmic potentials or resonances about 10 Hz. The hippocampus, as a supramodal association structure, is involved in several spontaneous and induced rhythmicities. An early work by Horowitz et al. (1973) already reported hippocampal 40-Hz activity.

Pioneering experiments of Adey on induced theta ryhthmicities. Adey and co-workers started early pioneering work on theta rhythms in the limbic system of the cat brain during conditioning by using spectral techniques and the coherence concept (see Adey et al., 1960, Elazar and Adey, 1967; see also Table 2).

These workers published several experiments in which the field potentials of the cat brain could be functionally related by using, for the first time, the coherence function to compare EEG activity between various nuclei of the brain, although the common view was that the EEG is an epiphenomenon [see commentary of Adey (1989) and Table 2]. The induced theta rythmicities in the limbic system of the cat brain and the concept that emerged of "task relevant coherency and rhythmicity changes of theta activity" belong to landmarks in the EEG research and have to be considered as relevant readings in the research area of this book.

Around 2 Hz

Steriade et al. (1990a, this volume) point out that until recently, delta waves (0.5–4 Hz) were commonly thought to be exclusively generated in the cerebral cortex. However, earlier data pointed out that rhythmic slow waves (1–2 Hz) were focally recorded in the ventrolateral thalamic nucleus and were suppressed by midbrain stimulation. Further, these authors emphasize two sets of recent data indicating that delta-type oscillations can be triggered in thalamic cells. The recent publication by Steriade et al. (1990) is also important for summarizing in detail the role of thalamocortical neurons and brain stem neurons as possible generators of delta activity.

Analysis of slow waves during cognitive processes gained importance in the last 10 years: Rockstroh et al. (1984) reviewed the literature. With the benefit of a long period of their own empirical research they compared the relationships of slow cortical potentials of the human EEG with various phyiological functions such as attention, arousal, preparation, and expectancy. Such studies merit considerable attention since these authors included in their integrative approach processes of alpha feedback and contingent negative variation (CNV) not included in this book. We also showed induced rhythmicities around 2 to 4 Hz during decision-making processes at the hearing threshold (Başar et al., this volume).

Accordingly, induced delta activity might gain importance in the coming years from the functional viewpoint. This frequency range should not be considered only as a sign of sleep stages or pathological conditions.

How Does the Brain Integrate Oscillatory Activity of Neurons? Exciting the Brain: A Transition From Chaos to Rhythmicity

After dealing with the topics of synchrony and coherence in EEG research, I shall try to discuss the principles possibly underlying induced rhythmicities: *oscillation*, *resonance*, and *excitability* in neural tissues. Afterward, the impact of chaotic dynamics on EEG research will be sketched.

Synchrony and coherence of neural activity

Synchrony of brain electrical activity as well as coherence are important aspects of brain electrical activity that should be discussed before every attempt to relate the observed rhythmicities to brain function. Is synchrony of EEG necessarily a sign of cooperative activity and synergy within the brain?

Synchrony of generators and the concept of coherence. According to Elul (1972), a synchronized group of neurons as well as a randomly related population of generators are potentially capable of producing activity resembling the EEG, and summed activities from these two systems may well appear closely similar, as long as we do not know what amplitudes to expect in the extracellular fields.

To understand the cause of the similarity we have to consider the sum of two sinusoidal potentials of the same frequency, say, 10 Hz, leaving aside consideration of amplitudes. Unless these waves are exactly opposed in phase, they will sum to form a sinusoid at the same frequency of 10 Hz. If we add a third sinusoid at 10 Hz to the summed waveform, again the output will be at 10 Hz, and so on for any number of independent sinusoids. Although cortical neurons do not necessarily produce pure sinusoidal waves, the same principle applies to the summation of EEG rhythms, by Fourier's principle, that each complex waveform can be broken down to a number of pure sinusoids. These sinusoids, taken one frequency at a time, can be combined from the respective generators in like manner, yielding a summed output with the same frequency content as the component complex wave forms.

Elul states:

> With a synchronized population, a tenfold change in EEG amplitude also may ensue from reduction in activity in all cortical neurons involved. However, an additional alternate mechanism for reduction in amplitude exists in this situation. This mechanism involves desynchronization. It is quite obvious that the maximal output from a group of generators is attained when they are all in synchrony; even if the output from each generator is not decreased, the summed output will diminish when the generators lose synchrony.

Elul indicates that the magnitude of the change in output from a group of synchronized generators due to desynchronization is often neglected. From the systems theory we know that if the output from a single generator is V, then given a large population of N generators that are synchronized, the summed output will be NV. When the generators lose synchrony among themselves, the output may decrease to $\sqrt{NV}$. For any number of generators N, which is realistic in terms of cortical nerve cell populations, the changes in amplitude involved in desynchronization can be quite staggering. To give an example, Elul considers a population of one million generators (10^6) (if we consider the cells as generators, then we have to consider about 20 mm^3 of cortex). The summed output from this population would decrease in amplitude 1000 times in the transition from synchrony to randomness. Smaller changes (e.g., tenfold) would require only very minimal divergence from total synchrony; that is, only a small fraction of the total cell population need be synchronized to produce the gross EEG.

In this context it is also useful to mention analyses by Cooper et al. (1965), who showed that cortical areas of several cm^2 have to be involved in the same wave pattern to become visible at all on the scalp since the bone and its underlying tissues act as low-pass filters.

According to the consideration of Elul, the increase in the amplitude of 10-Hz activity, which is often called "synchronized alpha" by EEG scientists, cannot be necessarily considered as a sign of cooperative activity and synergy between individual generators. (This assumption excludes the possibility that individual generators increase their voltage.) However, the 10-Hz enhancement induced by sensory stimulation seemingly forces the individual generators to act in synergy (for the "rule of excitement states" see below; for an analogy with the reordering of elementary magnets, see Başar et al., this volume).

Bullock and McClune (1989) proposed that the significant definition of synchrony for neural activity is any level of congruence above that of coincidence in a fraction of the neighboring generators or a volume of tissue, in a defined frequency band. Furthermore, they explained the coherence as follows: "Coherence might mean 1) that both loci have a component of the energy at that frequency following a common driver, or 2) it might mean one of the loci drives the other, or 3) they reciprocally cooperate, or 4) it might result from current spread." The discussion of these authors leaves open a host of questions such as whether true oscillations are a general or a special case, the possibility of resonance, whether evoked potentials arise from the same fraction of the population as the ongoing EEG or recruit largely new generators. The mentioned paper is a significant description of concepts of synchrony, coherence, and varied degrees of synchrony and is most useful for the reader interested in the topics of the present epilogue.

We have a new and complementary approach to the conclusion that EEG generally involves some synergy. This is the approach with chaotic dynamics, which has partially demonstrated that activities in "alpha," "theta," and "delta" bands cannot be considered as simple noise and that activities in these frequency channels do not arise from indeterminate, stochastic, and independent processes. (see below and the Appendix).

Spatiotemporal aspects of EEG synchrony. The chapter by Petsche and Rappelsberger (this volume) analyzes carefully the EEG topography, emphasizing the spatiotemporal aspects of the EEG as a useful description. To give equal consideration to both temporal and spatial aspects, Petsche and Rappelsberger have developed a micro-EEG method. With this method they aimed to record from a small cortical volume with a number of electrodes the continuous cortical electrical behavior. In the application of this method the computation of coherence turned out to be useful. The estimation of coherence in human studies offers the possibility of a number of functional descriptors of the ongoing EEG. The degrees of coherence at each frequency between various neural populations and the changes of coherence even in scalp-recorded EEG provide important candidates for future applications in cognitive human neurophysiology. To me, the most important message coming from Petsche's laboratory is the fact that "the ensemble of EEG activities" covering alpha, beta, and theta bands is useful to describe the brain during various functional states, and not single frequency bands.

Oscillation and resonance

Oscillation and resonance in neural tissues belong to the core topics of this book. These phenomena have been investigated both at the cellular level and at the level of field potentials. Analogies from the field of simple cell culture are given as well.

An oscillation in our context is a periodic or quasiperiodic series. By extension, it is sometimes applied to a series of very few cycles. It need not be quite sinusoidal but is not generally applied to intermittent point processes themselves. Resonance here means the system acts as though it stores and releases energy at a characteristic frequency when stimulated aperiodically.

The cellular basis: thalamic neurons behaving as oscillators and resonators. In a highly important recent review, Llinás (1988) discussed the relevance of 8- and 10-Hz oscillations in the central neurons system. Llinás asks the following question: "How do the oscillatory properties of central neurons relate to the information-carrying properties of the brain as a whole?" Llinás (1988) describes the thalamic nervous oscillating at two distinct rhythms: if the cell is depolarized, it may oscillate at 10 Hz and if the cell is hyperpolarized, it tends to oscillate at 6 Hz. Llinás concludes that oscillation and resonance allow single elements in the central neurons system to be woven into functional states capable of representing and embedding external reference frames into neural connectivity. In addition to these embedding properties, oscillation and resonance generate global states such as sleep–wakefulness rhythms and probably emotional and attentive states. This conclusion, which was reached by using results of the resonance concept at the neuronal level, has parallels to my conclusion that various cognitive tasks or sensory communications result in a specific combination of various "resonant modes," and that the ensemble of resonant modes could achieve an important function in the sensory communication of the brain (Başar 1980, 1988b; see also Pfurtscheller et al., 1988).

Excitability of physiological systems and neural populations. Sato and coworkers introduced the expression "excitable physiological system." They studied the relation of visual evoked potentials to EEG by comparing the power spectra of the spontaneous activity with the rhythmic driven activity of the brain (Sato, 1963; Sato et al., 1971, 1977).

According to their experiments, the occipital recording of a relaxed human subject shows some spontaneous activity before photic flicker stimulation: Regarding its shape and the frequency positions of the power maxima the power spectrum of this activity is similar to the frequency characteristics obtained by the application of visual stimuli. According to these authors, the excitability of a physiological system is considered to be one of the most important factors that control the basic transfer function of the system.

In 1980 I derived a rule about excitability of neural populations according to the results of our own experiments on the relation between EEG and frequency characteristics of evoked potentials. Although this idea was inspired from publications of Sato and coworkers, the excitability rule of brain networks was more general, including several EEG frequency channels and intracranial recordings. Now I tend to call this rule the rule of "excitement states" of neural populations in order to avoid the interference with the rules of excitability of single neurons. This rule is summarized below (see also Başar, 1980; Başar, 1983a, 1983b);

> If a neural population is able to show spontaneous activity in a given frequency range, then this structure can be brought to a state of excitement in the same frequency range to sensory stimuli. According to my own measurements I can state that networks or neurons capable to give rise to spontaneous or excited 40 Hz field potentials are existent in various parts of the brain. These neural populations might react to given stimuli with different latencies or with different magnitude. There are several excitement states in theta, alpha and higher frequency ranges.

The question that would arise is the following: Why should the brain respond with a 40-Hz burst to various sensory stimulations in different parts of the brain? My viewpoint is that the brain is organized in such a way that the internal communication occurs in various defined frequency bands in order to accelerate and convey messages from one part of the brain to another in a resonant way. If a structure "A" is excitable in the 40-Hz frequency range and another structure "B" is also excitable in the same frequency range, then the communication between A and B is facilitated. I have written about this view in a speculative paper (Başar, 1988b).

In other words, the rule of excitement states of neural populations included "multiple oscillatory responses" of a given brain structure. In the following are examples of excitability in biological systems in which a similar rule seems to exist: excitability is related to spontaneity.

Oscillatory response susceptibility is related to spontaneous activity of neural populations activity: children's EEG/EP versus adult EEG/EP. According to statements of the previous section and of the next section, if a neural population does not have spontaneous oscillatory behavior in a given frequency range, then this population could not show excitement states or enhanced oscillatory response in the same frequency range. Children up to the age of 6 years usually do not have alpha activity. According to the rule of excitement states, children's evoked potentials should not show alpha response when they do not have spontaneous alpha activity. We performed experiments with 12 children 3 years of age.

Figure 1 shows a typical filtered evoked potential of a 3-year-old child and

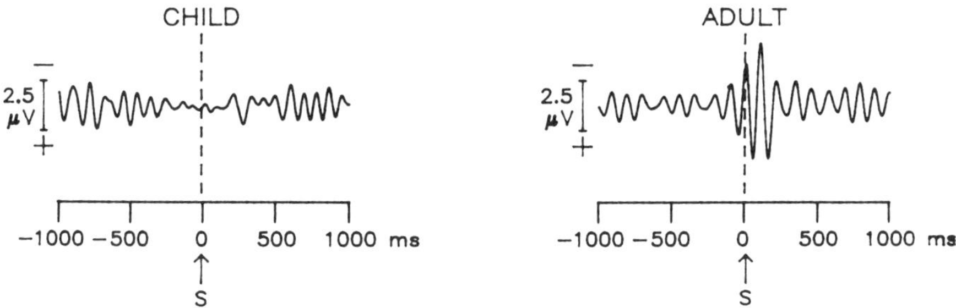

Figure 1. Alpha components of auditory EPs (filter limits: 8–13 Hz) recorded from a 3-year-old child and from an adult, respectively. Cz, vertex.

of an adult to a tone burst of 2000 Hz and 80 dB (Başar-Eroglu and Başar, unpublished results). Eleven of 12 children showed this behavior. Although filtered evoked potentials of adults show large alpha resonances (or what we have called "alpha enhancement"), children without alpha activity do not show this behavior. These results are an analogy to Goldbeter's view and the excitability rule described later. Children's brains without spontaneous alpha do not create alpha resonance upon sensory stimulation.

An analogy: dissipative structures and excitability in biological and chemical systems. In Prigoginian terms, all systems contain subsystems, which are continually fluctuating (Prigogine and Stengers, 1984). At times, a single fluctuation or a combination of them become so powerful, as a result of positive feedback, that it shatters the preexisting organization. At this revolutionary moment, a singular moment or a bifurcation point, it is inherently impossible to determine in advance in which direction change will take place: whether the system will disintegrate into randomness or leap to a now higher level of "order" or organization, which Prigogine called a "dissipative structure." (Such physical or chemical structures are termed "dissipative" because, compared with the simpler structures they replace, they require more energy to sustain them. Prigogine insists that order and organization can actually arise "spontaneously" out of disorder and chaos through a process of "self-organization.")

Let us here repeat a Gedankenexperiment described by Prigogine and Stengers (1984): "Suppose we have two kinds of molecules, 'red' and 'blue.' Because of the random motion of the molecules we would expect that at a given moment we would have more red molecules, say, in the left part of a vessel. Then a bit later more blue molecules would appear, and so on. The vessel would appear to us as 'violet,' with occasional irregular flashes of red or blue. However, this is not what happens with, for example, a chemical clock; here the system is all blue, then it abruptly changes its color to red, then again to blue. Because all these changes occur at regular time intervals, we have a coherent process."

Such a degree of order stemming from the activity of billions of molecules seems incredible, and indeed, if chemical clocks had not been observed, no one would believe that such a process is possible. To change color all at once, molecules must have a way to "communicate." The system has to act as a whole. Dissipative structures introduce probably one of the simplest physical examples for communication.

Goldbeter (1980) analyzed the behavior of two biological systems in which experimental evidence exists for excitable and/or oscillatory behavior. The first system is that of glycolytic oscillations; the second is the adenosine 3′, 5′-cyclic monophosphate (cAMP) signaling system, which controls periodic aggregation in the cellular slime mold *Dictyostelium discoideum.* Goldbeter and Caplan (1976) stated that sustained oscillations and excitability are closely associated in chemical systems. In other words, if a biological enzyme system demonstrates occasional or sustained oscillations, then this system is also excitable in the frequencies of the sustained oscillations. Later, Goldbeter and Segal (1980) described the ability to relay signals as an example of what in more general contexts is called excitability, that is, the ability of a system to amplify a small perturbation in a pulsatory manner. Support for their contention that in slime molds a single mechanism underlies both excitability and oscillating ability is the fact that both phenomena occur under closely related conditions in chemical systems such as the Belousov–Zhabotinsky reaction and in models for the nerve membrane and for an autocatalytic pH-controlled enzyme reaction. The statement of Goldbeter presents an excellent analogy to the findings or statements concerning the state of excitements of various brain structures in various frequency ranges discussed earlier.

As explained above, a brain structure is susceptible to go to a state of excitation with enhanced oscillations if it shows sustained oscillations in a given frequency channel. This is one of the striking examples of the usefulness of the study of dissipative structures in understanding the brain's excitement states with oscillatory behavior.

Modeling multiple modes of neuronal oscillations. Goldbeter and Moran (1988) analyzed the behavior of a two-variable cellular model in conditions where the model has multiple oscillatory domains in parameter space. This model (which is also explained by Goldbeter, this volume) represents an autocatalytic enzyme reaction with input of a substrate both from a constant source and from nonlinear-recycling of product into substrate. When two distinct oscillatory domains obtain as a function of the substrate injection rate, the system is capable of exhibiting two markedly different modes of oscillations for slightly different values of this control parameter. Phase plane analysis shows how the multiplicity of oscillatory domains depends on the parameters that govern the underlying biochemical mechanism of product recycling. Goldbeter and Moran analyzed the response of the model to various kinds of transient perturbations and to periodic changes in the substrate input that bring the system through the two ranges of oscillatory behavior. The results provided a qualitative explanation for experimental observations of two different modes of oscillations in thalamic neurons (Jahnsen and Llinás, 1984). The reader is also referred to the chapter by Goldbeter in this volume and to Llinás (1988).

Neural integration by correlation: the concept of reentry. The chapter by Tononi and coworkers (this volume) pays special attention to an orientation into the general problem of neural integration and includes several early as well as some new concepts on rhythmicities, Gestalt theory, mapping between neural groups, and the theory of group selection, proposed first in 1978 by Edelman (Edelman, 1978, 1987).

According to Edelman, the integration within and between cortical maps, allowing "a spatiotemporally continuous representation of objects or events" (Edelman, 1989, p. 56), is achieved through the establishment of temporal correlations (Edelman, 1978, 1987). Further, according to this worker these correlations are the result of a fundamental process called "reentry," which has been defined as the temporally ongoing parallel signaling between separate maps along ordered anatomical connections. "Reentry" is dynamic and can take place via multiple parallel and reciprocal connections between maps. "Reentry" takes place between populations of neurons rather than between single units. Such populations of neurons, called neuronal groups, form as the result of competitive and selective processes within cortical maps (Pearson et al., 1987). Neurons within a group tend to be strongly connected. At a higher level, the integration of perceptual and conceptual components is required to categorize objects. With regard to oscillations per se, it is certainly possible that the presence of rhythmic activity at particular frequency ranges may give rise to "resonance" phenomena, which could produce significant effects in vast networks interconnected by reentry . Correlations last for 50 to 500 ms and are highly dynamic (Sporns et al., 1989).

Tononi et al. (this volume) and Sporns et al. (1989) have developed a model consistent with the idea that reentry between neuronal groups links responses in distributed cortical systems and thus causes coherent firing. As demonstrated in this network model, coherent oscillations can be found among distinct neuronal groups that are responding to a single stimulus: Oscillations could act to isolate or sharpen coherent responses to a particular stimulus. While a neuronal group is engaged in cooperative discharges, other inputs to that group arriving out of phase or at a different frequency would be less efficient in exciting the group or would be suppressed altogether.

Haken's concept of synergetics (Haken, 1977; Haken, this volume) is based on coherent states of laser light. It should be noted that laser light is a much better means of communication than ordinary diffuse light. Laser is a sharpened light from coherent oscillation. Efficiency of the coherent laser light for communication and efficiency of cooperative discharges in a neural group are based on a similar principle. The reentry principle and its utility in brain function are, accordingly, reflected in several chapters of this book in which phase-locking of neural generators and transition to coherent oscillatory activity are discussed (see Bullock, Petsche, Lopes da Silva, Başar et al., this volume). Resonance phenomena reflect also a tuning effect or frequency sharpening effect; and these phenomena are discussed in most of the chapters of this volume.

Sporns et al. (1989) further predict that similar oscillations and phase coherencies will be found in other regions of the visual cortex, in areas devoted to other sensory modalities, and in motor areas—all of which contain strongly reentrant connections. This is a relevant theory that needs more experimental extension and that may also open new avenues of investigations at the cellular level.

The concept of coherent firing and the phase correlation between groups are types of descriptions about distributed resonance phenomena from which several experimental findings were already established with field potentials as well as zero-phase relation between brain structures (Başar, 1980; Eckhorn, 1988).

Chaotic activity in the "spontaneous" EEG

Some aspects of evoked electrical activity of the brain are discussed above. In a number of recent studies, "spontaneous" EEG was analyzed with concepts of chaotic dynamics. Some results will be sketched in the following sections and in the Appendix.

Attractors and synchrony: alpha and theta attractors. The concept of the strange attractor and of the correlation dimension D_2 will be explained in the Appendix. There are also several publications concerning this new approach, also cited in the Appendix. If a nonlinear signal has a finite correlation dimension then this signal may be considered as an almost deterministic signal as several investigators have shown for the case of human 10-Hz activity.

Figure 2 illustrates a comparative study of power spectra of a human subject. As is well known in the literature, the most ample alpha activity is registered in human occipital derivations, whereas the alpha activity in frontal regions is somewhat poorer. The correlation dimension computed for 3-min segments is also shown. Before computation of the correlation dimension the EEG activity was pass-band filtered between 5 and 15 Hz. It is important to note that in cases of desynchronization of alpha activity (manifested by missing alpha peaks in power spectra), the correlation dimension D_2 is not finite. Usually D_2 fluctuates between 5 and 8, demonstrating that the 10-Hz activity manifests deterministic chaos and not a pure noise behavior in the sense of general systems theory. There are several descriptions of the noise in neuronal

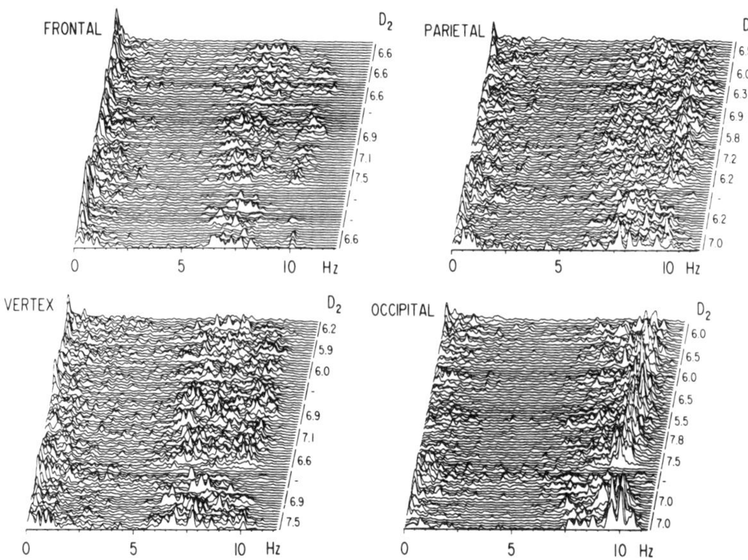

Figure 2. A comparative presentation of power spectra (compressed spectral arrays) and the correlation dimension D_2. Each D_2 value and the adjacent spectra were calculated from the same EEG segments. Simultaneous recordings from the same subject in frontal, central, parietal and occipital locations. Reprinted with permission of Springer-Verlag from Başar et al., 1990.

systems. The relevant definition of neurophysiological noise by Bullock is explained in the Appendix. The fact that all parts of the human brain do not manifest deterministic chaos over all times and in all brain locations is illustrated better in Figure 3, in which the frontal 10-Hz activity is small or disappeared over most of the time and where the correlation dimension D_2 does not show the behavior of a strange attractor. This may happen, for one reason, when the ratio of stochastic power to deterministic power falls when EEG power is low.

The parallelism between presumed synchrony of field potentials and the existence of a finite dimension D_2 could also be shown in the case of hippocampal theta activity. Röschke and Başar (1989) showed that during synchronized theta activity in the hippocampus of the cat, finite values of D_2 between 3.5 and 5 could be obtained. Figure 4 shows an example with the dimension about 4. If the hippocampus does not show regular theta activity, no finite dimension can be obtained. Lopes da Silva et al. (1990a) reported also that the hippocampus does not always show the behavior of deterministic chaos. The difficulty in describing the values of dimension in transition stages is described by Röschke and Başar (1989). The results outlined above manifest the parallelism between strange attractor behavior and the "state of synchrony" or the prominence of a band of activity in brain field potentials. Röschke and

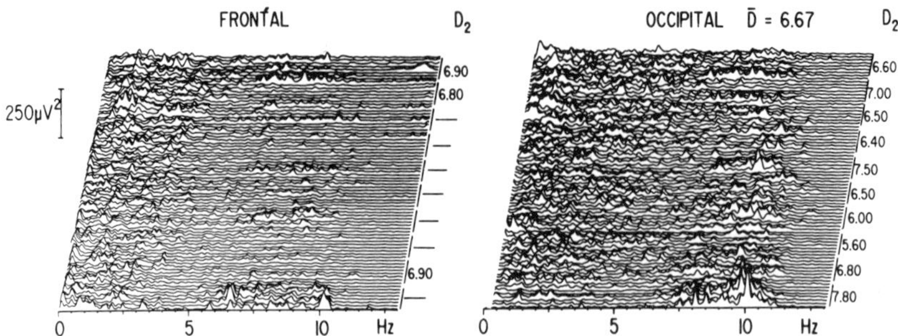

Figure 3. A comparative presentation of power spectra and D_2 for frontal and occipital locations. Another subject than in Fig. 2. Reprinted with permission of Springer-Verlag from Başar et al., 1990.

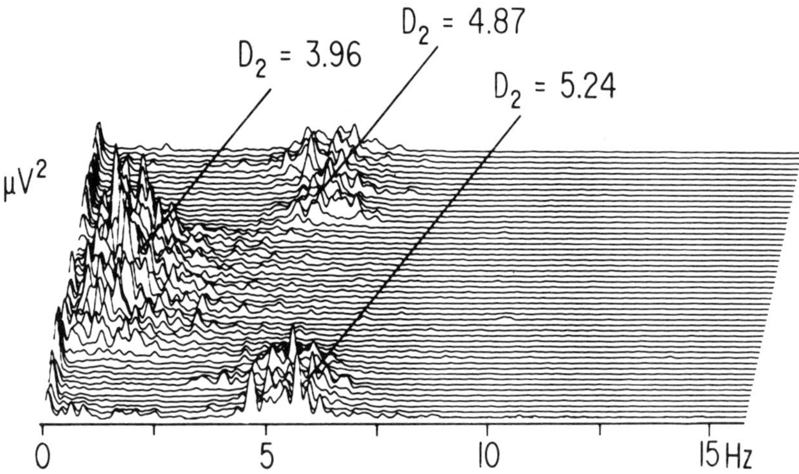

Figure 4. Power spectra (5-s epochs) of the hippocampus (cat "Jenny") and correlation dimension D_2 (for 40-s epochs) during theta activity (waking stage) and slow-wave sleep

Aldenhoff (1990, 1991) recently described also a parallelism between the number of resonance maxima in human evoked potentials and the dimensionality during various sleep stages: the dimensionality of EEG is higher in stages where the transfer function, computed from evoked potentials, shows multiple resonances.

High frequency attractors in cerebellum and brain stem. Although the spontaneous electrical activity of the brain, which we call EEG, has its most ample components in a frequency region between 1 and 50 Hz, it is well known that a number of higher frequency components can sometimes be observed in the field potentials of the brain. Since the days of Adrian and Yamagiwa (1935), it has been well known that the cerebellum sometimes depicts a high frequency component between 180 and 300 Hz. Röschke and Başar (1989) registered dominant spectral peaks in the frequency range between 200 Hz and 1000 Hz in four cats. Moreover, dimensionality of field potentials of four freely moving cats with chronically implanted electrodes in the cerebellar cortex and in the inferior colliculus were investigated. In the frequency range between 100 Hz and 1000 Hz for the cerebellum, a mean value of the correlation dimension of about $D_2 = 7$ and for the inferior colliculus a mean value of $D_2 = 6{,}7$ was obtained. However, finite dimensions were obtained only in approximately 25% of the studied data. In other words, in 75% of the investigated time periods the EEG signal cannot be distinguished from a random process. Only in 25% of the recordings can it be concluded that the high frequency activity was due to deterministic chaos. Simultaneous measurements in cortical electrodes did not show finite dimensions. Therefore, these authors excluded the possibility of extraneous sources at this low voltage level.

The same study (Röschke and Başar, 1989) showed that during slow-wave sleep (synchronous delta activity in all brain structures) nearly 75% of the sample recordings is due to a deterministic process.

Why is it important to mention here these results in the highest frequency range between 100 and 1000 Hz? For four decades the emphasis of neuroscientists has been concentrated on 4-Hz, 10-Hz, and 20-Hz activities of the brain. Only in the last decade analysis of 40-Hz activity gained some importance. If the cerebellar spontaneous activity around 100 to 300 Hz is not to be considered as largely noise, in the future this high frequency activity should merit more emphasis. Maybe this can turn out to be an important electrical activity to investigate also at the cellular level, just as the 40-Hz range has proved to be so interesting.

Conclusion: Induced Rhythmicities and Resonance Phenomena—Fingerprints of Common Transfer Functions Within the Brain

At the beginning of this Epilogue the quotation from Fessard referred to the search for general transfer functions of the brain. Broadening his use of the term, I tried to point out, in several chapters, that transfer functions of a dynamic system are often related to resonance phenomena. In this book we have several chapters describing the resonance phenomena in the brain as processes probably strongly related to function. Llinás (1988) emphasized the functional importance of cognitive- and movement-related functions of 5-Hz and 10-Hz resonances. Llinás (this volume) proposes that neuronal oscillations serve as elements 1) in a timing or pacemaker circuit, or 2) allowing synchronization of neuronal activity leading to coherence.

Freeman (1975) emphasizes the functional significance of 40-Hz resonances in the cortex (olfactory and visual). Gray et al. (1989) and Eckhorn et al. (1988)

describe conceptual models of the role of 40-Hz activity in sensory and cognitive processes of the cortex. Steriade et al. (1990a) and Buszákil (this volume) emphasize the role of thalamic oscillations in several processes ranging from sleep to tremor. Galambos emphasizes the role of 40-Hz activity during hearing and cognitive processes. Başar et al. (1991, this volume) point out resonances in 5-Hz, 10-Hz, and 40-Hz frequency ranges to sensory stimulation. These authors also mention the existence of emitted 40-Hz activity in the cat hippocampus (i.e., appearing after an omitted stimulus was due), and time-locked emitted 10-Hz activity in scalp records from human subjects during attentive behavior or during focussed attention. Başar and coworkers further assume that the evoked potential reflects ensembles of induced ryhthmicities in 4-, 10-, and 40-Hz frequency ranges.

Although according to the speculations of all these investigators several functions might be attributed to several ryhthms, and although there are often discrepancies in the description of functional relationships, one point is common in all these studies: The observed oscillatory phenomena showed in most of the cases some latency and some degree of "frequency locking," "phase coherence," and "time-locking" to a cognitive or sensory input. Sometimes there is a weak time-locking and sometimes a strong time-locking, but it is often existent (see also comparative analysis of Galambos in this volume). Further, it is important to emphasize that frequency and phase-locking in a neural population usually can be described as a resonant response of oscillators that can be coupled with internal or external signals applied to the central nervous system. It is possible that intrinsic oscillatory behavior of several neurons in the 10-Hz frequency range (as shown by Llinás) could be brought to synchrony and accordingly to produce huge potentials with homogeneous frequency upon stimulation. As we have shown recently (Başar, 1988a), bifurcation of 5-Hz or 10-Hz rhythmicities can be observed in single evoked potentials on the human scalp. It is a wonder that phenomena observed at the membrane level can be observed as population responses from human scalp recordings!

In this chapter Roy John's concept of hyperneurons is to be mentioned. He proposes that "afferent input via classical sensory pathways comes to a variety of primary receiving ensembles in multiple regions, via discrete pathways. These inputs activate a significant proportion of cells in many ensembles. These cells recruit other cells by local current flow comparable to or greater than that which we impose in our direct brain stimulation. A resonance is rapidly established between these ensembles, which are oscillating in a common mode." Comparing a group of neurons to a coupled resonating field, he states that "none of the single neuronal elements can be informed about the whole field. I suggest the name of 'hyperneuron' for this overall field, to indicate explicitly that it transcends the neurons from which it emerges. The individual neuron is important only insofar as it contributes negative entropy to the region" (John, 1989). I find this consideration useful, since the hyperneuron concept may be used as a representative picture of a neural population performing a hypothetical function.

My view is that if one had the desire to write equations to show or to demonstrate the most general transfer functions of the brain, then these equations should include nonlinear resonances in 2-Hz, 5-Hz, 10-Hz, 20-Hz, and 40-Hz frequencies. These frequencies should be considered as common modes and/or eigenvalues in several brain structures. Again, it is to be emphasized that for the time being it is difficult to predict all functional relationships. However, it could be assumed that similar resonators in various parts of the brain would facilitate the parallel processing in the brain, although this is a difficult idea to test.

Based on experimental observations ranging from the cellular level to the field potential level, I suggest that the induced rhythmicities in the brain (which have also the same frequency range as the spontaneous rhythms called EEG), reflect most important functional activities. The analysis of dynamic patterns as described at the beginning of this Epilogue and as it has been described by Haken (1977, 1983, and this volume) will certainly induce new ways of thinking in search of brain function.

I hope that the chapters presented in this volume will encourage the reader to plan experiments by taking into account frequencies of oscillations, to create new hypotheses, and to learn more about integrative functions of the brain. This viewpoint should also help to bring together neuroscientists working at the cellular level and at the level of field potentials both by EEG and MEG recording. I think a common language will emerge. This might well be the language of induced rhythmicities and EEG frequencies locked to a cognitive event or sensory stimulus.

Acknowledgment. Supported by Grant Nr. Ba 831/5-1 of DFG (Deutsche Forschungsgemeinschaft).

References

Adey WR, Dunlop CW, Hendrix CE (1960): Hippocampal slow waves: distribution and phase relations in the course of approach learning. *Arch Neurol* 3:74–90

Adey WR (1989): Do EEG-like Processes Influence Brain Function at a Physiological Level? In: *Dynamics of Sensory and Cognitive Processing by the Brain*, Başar E, ed. Berlin–Heidelberg: Springer–Verlag, pp 362–367

Adrian ED (1941): Afferent discharges to the cerebral cortex from peripheral sense organs. *J Physiol* 100:159–191

Adrian ED (1951): Rhythmic discharges from the thalamus. *J Physiol* 113:9–10P

Adrian ED, Yamagiwa K (1935): The origin of Berger rhythm. *Brain* 58:323–351

Andersen P (1975): Organization of hippocampal neurons and their interconnections. In: *The Hippocampus*, vol 1, Isaacson RL, Pribam KH, eds. New York: Plenum Press

Andersen P, Andersson SA (1968): *Physiological Basis of the Alpha Rhythm*. New York: Appleton-Century-Crofts

Andersen P, Brooks C McC, Eccles JC (1964): Electrical responses of the ventro-basal nucleus of the thalamus. *Prog Brain Res* 5: 100–113

Andersen P, Brooks CMcC, Eccles JC, Sears TA (1964): The ventro-basal nucleus of the thalamus: potential fields, synaptic transmission and excitability of both presynaptic and postsynaptic components. *J Physiol* 174: 348–369

Barlow JS, Estrin T (1971): Comparative phase characteristics of induced and intrinsic alpha activity. *Electroencephalogr Clin Neurophysiol* 30: 1–9

Bartley SH, Bishop GH (1933): The cortical response to stimulation of the optic nerve in the rabbit. *Am J Physiol* 103: 159–172

Başar E (1980): *EEG Brain Dynamics. Relation between EEG and Brain Evoked Potentials*. Amsterdam: Elsevier

Başar E (1983a): Toward a physical approach to integrative physiology. I. Brain dynamics and physical causality. *Am J Physiol* 14: R510–533

Başar E (1983b): Synergetics of Neuronal Populations. A Survey on Experiments. In: *Synergetics of the Brain*, Başar E, Flohr H, Haken H, Mandell AJ, eds. Berlin–Heidelberg: Springer–Verlag, pp 183–198

Başar E (1988a): EEG-Dynamics and Evoked Potentials in Sensory and Cognitive Processing by the Brain. In: *Dynamics of Sensory and Cognitive Processing by the Brain*, Başar E, ed. Berlin–Heidelberg: Springer–Verlag, pp 30–55

Başar E (1988b): Thoughts on Brain's Internal Codes. In: *Dynamics of Sensory and Cognitive Processing by the Brain*, Başar E, ed. Berlin–Heidelberg: Springer–Verlag, pp 381–384

Başar E, Başar-Eroglu C, Rahn E, Schürmann M (1991): Sensory and Cognitive Components of Brain Resonance Responses: an analysis of responsiveness in human and cat brain upon visual and auditory stimulation. *Acta Otolaryngol (Stockh)* (in press)

Başar E, Başar-Eroglu C, Röschke J, Schütt A (1989): The EEG is a quasi-deterministic signal anticipating sensory-cognitive tasks. In: *Brain Dynamics*, Başar E, Bullock TH, eds. Berlin–Heidelberg: Springer–Verlag, pp 43–71

Başar E, Gönder A, Özesmi C, Ungan P (1975a): Dynamics of brain rhythmic and evoked potentials. I. Some computational methods for the analysis of electrical signals from the brain. *Biol Cybern* 20: 137–143

Başar E, Gönder A, Özesmi C, Ungan P (1975b): Dynamics of brain rhythmic and evoked potentials. II. Studies in the auditory pathway, reticular formation and hippocampus during the waking stage. *Biol Cybern* 20: 145–160

Başar E, Gönder A, Özesmi C, Ungan P (1975c): Dynamics of brain rhythmic and evoked potentials. III. Studies in the auditory pathway, reticular formation and hippocampus during sleep. *Biol Cybern* 20: 161–169

Başar E, Gönder A, Ungan P (1976a): Important relation between EEG and brain evoked potentials. I. Resonance phenomena in subdural structures of the cat brain. *Biol Cybern* 25: 27–40

Başar E, Gönder A, Ungan P (1976b): Important relation between EEG and brain evoked potentials. II. A systems analysis of electrical signals from the human brain. *Biol Cybern* 25: 41–48

Başar-Eroglu C, Başar E (1991): Am Compound P300-40 Hz Response of the cat hippocampus. *Int J Neurophysiol* 60: 227–237

Bennett TL, Herbert PN, Moss DE (1973): Hippocampal theta activity and the attention component of discrimination learning. *Behav Biol* 8: 173–181

Bishop GH (1933): Cyclic changes in excitability of the optic pathway of the rabbit. *Am J Physiol* 103:213–224

Bishop GH, Jeremy D, McLeod JG (1953): Phenomenon of repetitive firing in lateral geniculate of cat. *J Neurophysiol* 16:437–447

Bremer F, Bonnet V (1950): Interprétation des réactions rhythmiques prolongées des aires sensorielles de l'écorce cérébrale. *EEG Clin Neurophysiol* 2:389–400

Bullock TH, McClune MC (1989): Lateral coherence of the electrocorticogram: a new measure of brain synchrony. *Electroencephalogr and Clin Neurophysiol* 73:479–498

Buzsáki G (1985): Theta rhythm: biophysical model of generation in the hippocampus. In: *Electrical Activity of the Archicortex*, Buzsáki G, Vanderwolf CH, eds. Budapest: Akadémiai Kiadó

Chang HT (1951): Dendritic potential of cortical neurons produced by direct electrical stimulation of the cerebral cortex. *J Neurophysiol* 14:1–21

Cooper R, Winter AL, Crow HJ, Walter WG (1965): Comparison of subcortical, cortical and scalp activity using chronically indwelling electrodes in man. *Electroencephalogr Clin Neurophysiol* 18:217–228

Creutzfeldt OD, Watanabe S, Lux HD (1966): Relations between EEG-phenomena and potentials of single cortical cells. I. Evoked responses after thalamic and epicortical stimulation. *Electroencephalogr Clin Neurophysiol* 20:1–18

Creutzfeldt OD, Rosina A, Ito M, Probst W (1969): Visual evoked response of single cells and of EEG in primary visual area of the cat. *J Neurophysiol* 32:127–139

Eckhorn R, Bauer R, Jordan W, Brosch M, Kruse W, Munk M, Reitboeck HJ (1988): Coherent oscillations: a mechanism of feature linking in the visual cortex? *Biol Cybern* 60:121–130

Eckhorn R, Bauer R, Reitboeck HJ (1989b): Discontinuities in visual cortex and possible functional implications: relating cortical structure and function with multielectrode/correlation techniques. In: *Brain dynamics*, Başar E, Bullock TH, eds. Berlin–Heidelberg: Springer–Verlag, pp 267–278

Eckhorn R, Reitboeck HJ, Arndt M, Dicke P (1989a): Feature linking via stimulus—evoked oscillations: experimental results from cat visual cortex and functional implications from a network model. IEEE and INNS on Neural Networks, Washington, June 18–22, 1989

Edelman GM (1978): Group selection and phasic re-entrant signalling: a Theory of higher brain function. In: *The Mindful Brain*, Edelman GM, Mountcastle VB, eds. Cambridge: MIT Press

Edelman GM (1987): *Neural Darwinism. The Theory of Neuronal Group Selection.* New York: Basic Books

Edelman GM (1989): *The Remembered Present. A Biological Theory of Consciousness.* New York: Basic Books

Elazar Z, Adey WR (1967): Spectral analysis of low frequency components in the electrical activity of the hippocampus during learning. *Electroencephalogr Clin Neurophysiol* 23:225–240

Elul R (1972): Randomness and synchrony in the generation of the electroencephalogram. In: *Synchronization of EEG Activity in Epilepsies*, Petsche H, Brazier MAB, eds. Wien–New York: Springer–Verlag

Fessard A (1961): The role of neuronal networks in communication within the brain. In: *Sensory Communication*, Rosenblith WA, ed. Cambridge: MIT Press, pp 585–606

Freeman WJ (1975): *Mass Action in the Nervous System.* New York: Academic Press
Freeman WJ (1979): Nonlinear gain mediating cortical stimulus-response relations. *Biol Cybern* 33:237–247
Freeman WJ (1988). Nonlinear neural dynamics in olfaction as a model for cognition. In: *Dynamics of Sensory and Cognitive Processing by the Brain*, Başar E, ed. Berlin Heidelberg New York: Springer-Verlag, pp 19–28
Freeman WJ (1990): Searching for signal and noise in the chaos of brain waves. In: *The Ubiquity of Chaos*, Knasner S, ed. American Association for the Advancement of Science, Washington
Freeman WJ, Skarda CA (1985): Spatial EEG patterns, non-linear dynamics and perception: the neo-Sheerringtonian view. *Brain Res Rev* 10:147–175
Galambos R, Makeig S (1981): Dynamic changes in steady-state responses. In: *Dynamics of sensory and cognitive processing of the brain*, Başar E, ed. Heidelberg: Springer–Verlag, pp 103–122
Galambos R, Rose JE, Bromiley RB, Hughes JR (1952): Microelectrode studies on medial geniculate body of cat. II. Response to clicks . *J Neurophysiol* 15:359–380
Goldbeter A (1980): Models for oscillations and excitability in biochemical systems. *Mathematical Models in Molecular and Cellular Biology*, Segel LA, ed. Cambridge: Cambridge University Press
Goldbeter A, Caplan SR (1976): Oscillatory enzymes. *Annu Rev Biophys Bioeng* 5: 449–476
Goldbeter A, Moran F (1988): Dynamics of a biochemical system with multiple oscillatory domains as a clue for multiple modes of neuronal oscillations. *Eur Biophys J* 15:277–287
Goldbeter A, Segal A (1980): Control of developmental transitions in the cyclic AMP signalling system of Dictyostelium discoideum. *Differentiation* 17:127–135
Grastyán E, Lissak K, Madarasz I, Donhoffer H (1959): Hippocampal electrical activity during the development of conditioned reflexes. *Electroencephalogr Clin Neurophysiol* 11:409–430
Grastyán E, Vereczkei L (1974): Effects of spatial separation of the conditioned signal from the reinforcement: a demonstration of the conditioned character of the orienting response or the orientational character of conditioning. *Behav Biol* 10:121–146
Gray CM, König P, Engel AK, Singer W (1989): Oscillatory responses in cat visual cortex exhibit inter-columnar synchronization which reflect global stimulus properties. Nature 338:334–337
Gray CM, Singer W (1987): Stimulus-specific neuronal oscillations in the cat visual cortex: a cortical function unit. *Soc Neurosci* 404:3
Gray CM, Singer W (1989): Stimulus-specific neuronal oscillations in orientation columns of cat visual cortex. *Proc Natl Acad Sci* 86:1698–1702
Green JD, Arduini A (1954): Hippocampal electrical activity in arousal. *J Neurophysiol* 17:533–557
Haken H (1977): *Synergetics. An Introduction.* Berlin: Springer
Haken H (1983): Synopsis and introduction. In: *Synergetics of the brain*, Başar E, Flohr H, Haken H, Mandell AJ, eds. Berlin–Heidelberg: Springer–Verlag, pp 3–27
Holmes JE, Adey WR (1960): Electrical activity of the entorhinal cortex during conditioned behaviour. *Am J Physiol* 199:741–744
Horowitz JM, Freeman WJ, Stoll PJ (1973): A neural network with a background level of excitation in the cat hippocampus. *Int J Neurosci* 5:113–123

Jahnsen H, Llinás R (1984): Ionic basis for the electroresponsiveness and oscillatory properties of guinea-pig thalamic neurones in vitro. *J Physiol* 349:229–247

Jarcho LW (1949): Excitability of cortical afferent systems during barbiturate anesthesia. *J Neurophysiol* 12:447–457

John ER (1989): Resonating fields in the brain and the hyperneuron. In: *Dynamics of Sensory and Cognitive Processing by the Brain*, Başar E, ed. Berlin–Heidelberg: Springer–Verlag, pp 56–87

Jones EG, Powell TPS (1970): An anatomical study of converging sensory pathways within the cerebral cortex of the monkeys. *Brain* 93:773–820

Katchalsky AK, Rowland W, Blumenthal R (1974): *Dynamics Patterns of Brain Cell Assemblies*. Massachusetts: MIT Press

Lansing RW, Barlow JS (1972): Rhythmic after-activity to flashes in relation to the background alpha which precedes and follows the photic stimuli. *Electroencephalogr Clin Neurophysiol* 32:149–160

Llinás RR (1988): The intrinsic electrophysiological properties of mammalian neurons: insights into central nervous system function. *Science* 242:1654–1664

Llinás RR (1990): Intrinsic electrical properties of mammalian neurons and CNS function. In: *Fidia Research Foundation Neuroscience Award Lectures*, vol 4. New York: Raven Press

Llinás RR, Graves A (1990): Intrinsic 40-Hz oscillatory properties of layer IV neurons in guinea-pig cerebral cortex in vitro. *Soc Neurosci Abstr* (in press)

Lopes da Silva FH (1987): Dynamics of EEGs as signals of neuronal populations: models and theoretical considerations. In: *Electroencephalography: Basic Principles, Clinical Applications and Related Fields*, Niedermeyer E, Lopes da Silva FH, ed. Baltimore–Munich: Urban and Schwarzenberg, pp 15–28

Lopes da Silva FH, Kamphuis W, van Neerven JMAN, Pijn JPM (1990a). Cellular and Network Mechanisms in the Kindling Model of Epilepsy: The Role of GABAergic Inhibition and the Emergence of Strange Attractors. In: *Machinery of the Mind*, John ER, ed. Boston Basel Berlin: Birkhäuser, pp 115–139

Lopes da Silva FH, Witter MP, Boeijinga PH, Lohman AHM (1990b): Anatomic organization and physiology of the limbic cortex. *Physiol Rev* 70:453–511

Mesulam MM, Van Hoesen GW, Pandya DN, Geschwind N (1977): Limbic and sensory connections of the inferior parietal lobule (area PG) in the rhesus monkey: a study with a new method for horseradish peroxidase histochemistry. *Brain Res* 136:393–414

Narici L, Pizella V, Romani GL, Torrioli G, Traversa R, Rossini PM (1990): Evoked α and μ-rhythm in humans: a neuromagnetic study. *Brain Res* 520:222–231

Nogawa T, Katayama K, Tabata Y, Ohshio T, Kawahara T (1976): Changes in amplitude of the EEG induced by a photic stimulus. *Electroencephalogr Clin Neurophysiol* 40:78–88

O'Keefe J, Nadel L (1978): *The Hippocampus as a Cognitive Map*. Oxford: Clarendon Press

Pearson JC, Finkel LH, Edelman GM (1987): Plasticity in the organization of adult cortical maps: a computer model based on neuronal group selection. *J Neurosci* 7:4209–4223

Petsche H, Pockeberger H, Rappelsberger P (1984): On the search for the sources of the electroencephalogram. *Neuroscience* 11:1–27

Pfurtscheller G (1988): Mapping of event-related desynchronization and type of derivation. *Electroencephalogr Clin Neurophysiol* 70:190–193

Prigogine I, Stengers I (1984): *Order Out of Chaos*. New York: Bantam

Ramos A, Schwartz E, John ER (1976): Evoked potential-unit relationship in behaving cats. *Brain Res Bull* 1:69–75

Regan D (1966): An effect of stimulus color on average steady-state potentials evoked in man. *Nature* 210:1056

Rockstroh B, Elbert T, Lutzenberger W, Birbaumer N (1984): *Slow Brain Potentials and Behavior*. Baltimore: Urban and Schwarzenberg

Röschke J, Aldenhoff J (1991): The dimensionality of human's electro-encephalogram during sleep. *Biol Cybern* 64:307–313

Röschke J, Aldenhoff JB (1991): Excitability and Susceptibility of the Brain's Electrical Activity during Sleep: an Analysis of Late Components of AEPs and VEPs. *Int J Neurosci* 56:255–272

Röschke J, Başar E (1989): Correlation dimensions in various parts of cat and human brain. In: *Brain Dynamics. Progress and Perspectives*, Başar E, Bullock TH, eds. Berlin–Heidelberg: Springer–Verlag, pp 131–148

Rougeul A, Bouyer JJ, Dedet L, Debray O (1979): Fast somatoparietal rhythms during combined focal attention and immobility in baboon and squirrel monkey. *Electroencephalogr Clin Neurophysiol* 46:310–319

Sato K (1963): On the linear model of the brain activity in electroencephalographic potentials. *Folia Psychiatr Neurol Jap* 17:156–166

Sato K, Kitajima H, Mimura K, Hirota N, Tagawa Y, Ochi N (1971): Cerebral visual evoked potentials in relation to EEG. *Electroencephalogr Clin Neurophysiol* 30: 123–128

Sato K, Ono K, Chiba G, Fukuta K (1977): Component activities in the autogressive activity of physiological systems. *Int J Neurosci* 7:239–249

Sheer DE (1989): Sensory and cognitive 40-Hz event-related potentials: behavioral correlates, brain function, and clinical application. In: *Brain Dynamics: Progress and Perspectives*, Başar E, Bullock TH, eds. Heidelberg: Springer–Verlag, pp 339–374

Spekreijse H (1966): *Analysis of EEG Responses in Man Evoked by Sinewave Modulated Light*. The Hague: Thesis, University of Amsterdam, Junk

Spekreijse H, Van der Tweel LH (1972): Systems analysis of linear and nonlinear processes in electrophysiology of the visual system. *Proc Kon Ned Akad van Wetensch* C75:77–105

Sporns O, Gally JA, Reeke GN Jr, Edelman GM (1989): Reentrant signaling among simulated neuronal groups leads to coherency in their oscillatory activity. *Proc Natl Acad Sci* 86:7265–7269

Steriade M, Gloor P, Llinás RR, Lopes da Silva FH, Mesulam MM (1990a): Basic mechnisms of cerebral rhythmic activities. *Electroencephalogr Clin Neurophysiol* 76:481–508

Steriade M, Jones EG, Llinás RR (1990b): Thalamic oscillation and signaling. New York: John Wiley (The Neurosciences Institute publication series)

Stryker MP (1989): Is grandmother an oscillation? *Nature* 338:297–298

Swanson LW (1983): The Hippocampus and the Concept of the Limbic System. In: *Neurobiology of the Hippocampus*, Seifert W, ed. London New York Paris: Academic Press

Van der Tweel LH, Spekreijse H (1969): Signal transport and rectification in the human evoked response system. *Ann NY Acad Sci* 156:678–695

Van der Tweel LH, Verduyn Lunel HFE (1965): Human visual response to sinusoidally modulated light. *Electroencephalogr Clin Neurophysiol* 18:587–598

Vertes RP (1982): Brain stem generation of the hippocampal EEG. *Prog Neurobiol* 19:159–186
Verzeano M (1973): The study of neuronal networks in the mammalian brain. In: *Bioelectric Recording Techniques. Part A. Cellular Processes and Brain Potentials*, Thompson RF, Patterson MM, eds. New York: Academic Press
Walter WG (1964): The convergence and interaction of visual, auditory, and tactile responses in human nonspecific cortex. *Ann NY Acad Sci* 112:320–361
Whishaw IQ, Vanderwolf CH (1973): Hippocampal EEG and behaviour: changes in amplitude and frequency of RSA (theta rhythm) associated with spontaneous and learned movement patterns in rats and cats. *Behav Biol* 8:461–484

Appendix

Chaos Approach to Brain Rhythmicities: Search for Causal Signals

The Conceptual Bridge Between Coherent Neural Firing and Brain Chaotic Dynamics

This appendix is a shortened version of a recent survey on "Chaotic Dynamics and Resonance Phenomena in Brain Function" in which the need to search for functional relations and/or parallelisms in chaotic brain dynamics and brain evoked ryhthmicities was already emphasized (Başar, 1990).

It is a wonder that we are able to measure theta, alpha, or gamma rhythmicities from human scalp recordings and not only stochastic signals. This is probably due to coherent firing of a large number of neurons. The chaotic approach provides one of the possibilties to partly demonstrate this view. This is a mathematical support among results of other methods or evidences based on neurological concepts also described in this book. I hope that the use of new empirical findings on induced ryhthms together with the chaotic approach will bridge results of experiments with electroencephalogram (EEG) signaling and events on the cellular level.

Several authors of this book (for example Bullock, Petsche and Rappelsberger, Başar, Tononi et al., Lopes da Silva, Haken, Goldbeter, Llinás, Freeman) used the concept of coherent activity of neural populations and/or of coherent neural firing. Phase transition, phase locking, and frequency locking emerged as leitmotivs to describe brain activity relevant for several functions (see also later in this Appendix). If in a physical system (e.g., laser light or magnetizable substances; see Başar et al. in this volume), (Fig. 1) the subunits of the system show a coherent behavior of activity, then a dramatic reduction of degrees of freedom in the entire behavior of this system is observed. Does the brain also have such a behavior? If the brain goes to a state of coherence during an intensive cognitive activity or when the brain is intensively bombarded with external sensory stimuli, should we then have a possibility to show, despite the large number of neurons involved in function during such

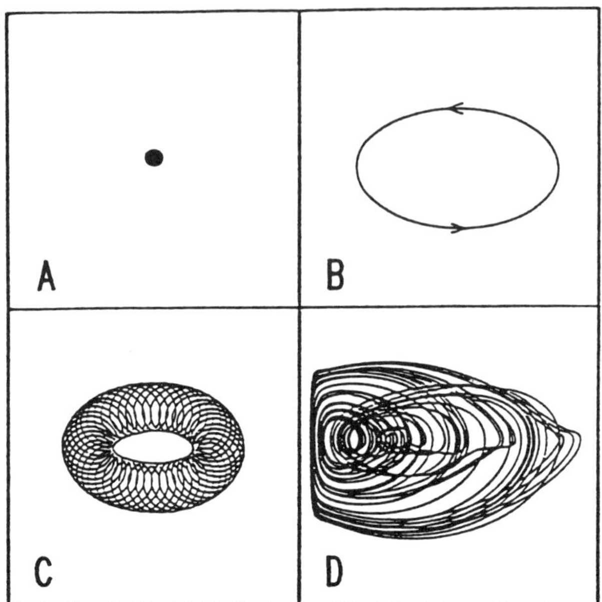

Figure 1. Types of attractors: **A**: fixed point; **B**: limit cycle; **C**: torus; **D**: projection of a strange attractor

a stage, a finite number of degrees of freedom? For about 8 years we have had the possibility of describing roughly the degrees of freedom of brain neural populations. This step is provided by computation of the correlation dimension of the EEG; this implies the chaotic approach to brain dynamics.

According to the reasoning above, I found it useful to append this methodological description on chaotic dynamics to the general treatise on brain-induced rhythmicities. Moreover, reading parts of the epilogue suggests the possibility that phenomena of synchrony, coherent states and transition to coherent states, and chaotic states are interwoven.

Chaos in Everyday Experience

A simple example of chaos in nature is described by Hooper (1983):

> Suppose you are sitting beside a waterfall watching a cascade of white water flow regularly over jagged rocks, when suddenly a jet of cold water splashes you in the face. The rocks have not moved, nothing has disrupted the water, and presumably no evil sprites inhibit the waterfall. So why does the water suddenly "decide" to splash you?

Physicists studying fluid turbulence have wondered about this kind of thing for several hundred years, and only recently have they arrived at some conclusions that seem to solve the problem at least in part: the waterfall's sudden random splashes do not come from some "imperceptible jiggle", but from the "inner dynamics" of the system itself. Behind the chaotic flow of turbulent fluids or the shifting cloud formations that shape the weather lies an abstract descriptor, which the physicists call a "strange attractor." What is an "attractor" and what makes it "strange"? We shall try to describe it again by using the simple explanation of Hooper (1983):

> Suppose one puts water in a pan, shakes it up, and then stops shaking it; after a time it will stop whirling and come to rest. The state of rest—the equilibrium state—can be described mathematically as a "fixed point," which is the simplest kind of attractor.

Let us now imagine the periodic movement of a metronome or a pendulum swinging from left to right and back again. From the viewpoint of geometry, this motion is said to remain within a fixed cycle forever. This is a second kind of attractor, the limit cycle. All of the various types of limit cycles share one important characteristic: regular, predictable motion. The third variety, the strange attractor, is irregular, unpredictable, or simply strange. For example, when a heated or moving fluid moves from a smooth, or laminar, flow to wild turbulence, it switches to a strange attractor.

Chaotic behavior in deterministic systems usually occurs through a transition from an orderly state when an external parameter is changed. In studies of these systems, particular attention has been devoted to the question of the route by which the chaotic state is approached. An increasing body of experimental evidence supports the belief that apparently random behavior observed in a wide variety of physical systems is caused by underlying deterministic dynamics of a low-dimensional chaotic (strange) attractor. The behavior exhibited by a system with chaotic attractor is predictable on short time scales and unpredictable (random) on long time scales.

Chaos is Between Strict Determination and Randomness

Chaos introduces an intermediate between strict determinism and randomness. A truly deterministic description of chaotic dynamics requires infinite precision in the choice of initial conditions and, thus, is a scientific chimera. Based on this evidence, Schuster (1988) considers that chaos introduces a fundamental uncertainty that is more general than Heisenberg's uncertainty in quantum mechanics.

The problem of nonlinear dynamics originates in planetary motions. Henri Poincaré was the first to investigate the complex behavior of simple mathematical systems. He analyzed topological structures in the phase space and discovered that the equation for the motion of planets could display an irregular or chaotic motion. In 1963 in a model of boundary layer convection Lorenz discovered that a system of three first-order nonlinear differential equations can exhibit a chaotic behavior. Poincaré's example was based on celestial dynamics; Lorenz discovered deterministic chaos in dissipative systems.

Lorenz Attractor

The differential equations of the Lorenz attractor are:

$$\dot{x} = \sigma(y - x),$$

$$\dot{y} = x(r - z) - y,$$

$$\dot{z} = xy - bz$$

where σ, b, r are constant parameters.

Although this model was derived for the convection instability in fluid dynamics, the single mode laser is also described by equations equivalent to the Lorenz equations (Haken, 1983).

The essential results derived from the Lorenz equations were

1. oscillations with a pseudorandom time behavior (or chaotic behavior)
2. trajectories that oscillate chaotically for a long time before they run into a static or periodic stable stationary state (preturbulence)
3. some trajectories alternate between chaotic and stable periodic oscillations (intermittency)
4. for certain parameter values trajectories appear chaotic although they stay in the neighborhood of an unstable periodic oscillation (noisy periodicity).

The phenomenon of deterministic chaos as clearly described by Lorenz's system is abundant in nature and technical systems and has important functional consequences. In Table 1 some nonlinear systems that display deter-

Table 1. Partial List of Systems found to be Chaotic*

Forced pendulum
Fluids near the onset of turbulence
Lasers
Nonlinear optical devices
Josephson junctions
Chemical reactions
Classical many-body systems (three-body problem)
Particle accelerators
Plasmas with interacting nonlinear waves
Biological models for population dynamics
Stimulated heart cells

It is understood that some examples of each class have been studied, and that no statement can be made as to the generality of chaos in each class.
*(From Schuster 1988)

ministic chaos are presented. The list is far from being complete, but it gives a good idea how different are the functions such systems can have.

EEG and Chaotic Dynamics

Does the EEG come from some "inperceptible jiggle" from the inner dynamics of the system itself?

In the decades following the first measurement of human EEG by Hans Berger and important developments by Lord Adrian and later Grey Walter, the pure EEG research remained somewhat in the shadow of new discoveries based on single neuron recordings. From the beginning of the 1960s the use of signal averagers enabled the EEG research scientists to extract the evoked potentials from the so-called "random-noise EEG." In this context, the event-related potentials that highly contributed to the understanding of cognitive functions and to clinical diagnostics have been considered as deterministic signals, whereas the EEG has been considered to be pure noise.

One of the most important developments in the field of chaotic dynamics was the discovery by Babloyantz et al. (1985), who pioneered by showing the strange attractor behavior of the EEG during slow-wave sleep stage by using the correlation dimension. In the same year some others had been able to show similar results from intracranial structures of the cat brain (Röschke and Başar, 1985; see references for tables 2 and 3).

In this short report we will mainly treat the description of the correlation dimension by reviewing existing studies.

Definitions and New Types of Expressions

For the neuroscientist who is not familiar with the jargon, some explanations will be given here. This step is useful although almost all the descriptions given are contained in various books (e.g., Schuster, 1988; Başar, 1990). However, we give in the following some important definitions to orient the reader.

Attractor

Attractor is defined as the property of a dynamic system that is manifested by the tendency under various but delimited conditions to go to a reproducible active state and stay there. The trajectory is a mathematical description of the sequence of values taken by a state variable in going from an initial or starting condition to an attractor, or through a sequence of attractors (Abraham and Shaw, 1983). *Transition* from one attractor to another is called a *state change* or *bifurcation*. Attractors can be periodic, quasiperiodic, or chaotic; the last are called strange attractors.

Fixed point

Simplest stable state solution. With increasing time, all trajectories tend to terminate in this point. *Stable fixed points* are static attractors (see Fig. 1A). A standard example is a pendulum that has come to rest after some time of oscillation, due to friction.

Limit cycle

Closed and recurrent trajectory in phase space. All trajectories tend to terminate in this cycle; no other closed cycle lies in its neighborhood. Without external drive, the limit cycle corresponds to a *Periodic stable* position of the nonlinear system, whose amplitude and frequency are determined by internal parameters of self sustained oscillations. Stable limit cycles act *as periodic attractors* (see Fig. 1B). The standard example is the attractor of a van der Pol oscillator. Limit cycles regularly occur with driven oscillators (Başar, 1980).

Torus

The systems trajectories move on a two-dimensional toroidal surface. Two frequencies are present, oscillations around the torus and along the torus (oscillations with two incommensurable frequencies). The trajectory never closes or covers the whole torus (see Fig. 1C). The trajectory on the torus is a quasiperiodic motion.

Strange attractor

The manifestation of a strange attractor is its activity, which appears to be random, but which is deterministic and reproducible if the input and initial conditions can be replicated (e.g., Lorenz Attractor, Rössler Attractor) (Fig. 1D). Since they cannot in practice be replicated, the manifestation is usually that after many trajectories, the phase plane is not evenly filled as it would be for a random time series, but is occupied by a quasipatterned line, never exactly repeated but clearly constrained.

Noise

Bullock describes noise in the general neurophysiology to mean "unwanted action" that interfers with desired signals (see Başar, 1990). This author further state:

> We should recognize the sharp difference between this dictionary usage and another current usage that refers to a stochastic sequence ("whiteness"). In the first meaning, noise is determined by the state of the receiver (sleep, attention) and depends on the usefulness, regardless of the charater; any unwanted sequence is regarded as noise whether it is a hiss, a whistle, or a voice. In the second meaning, noise is determined by the state of the sender (filter settings) and depends on the statistical character regardless of the use; any quasirandom

sequence is regarded as noise whether it is unwanted interference or a high resolution signal. The first meaning overlooks the difficulty of knowing what may be of value to a receiver; the second overlooks the difficulty of avoiding the common English sense, as in "signal-to-noise ratio."

According to the view of Bullock we should not use the term "noise" unless we are prepared to claim we know the codes and functions of the system and can recognize its signals. In the language of chaotic dynamics noise could be defined as "a signal showing irregular motion and that does not have a finite dimension." In other words, an irregular signal whose D_2 does not show saturation.

Correlation Dimension

The correlation dimension has become the most widely used measure to describe chaotic behavior. A valuable first step in the study of dynamical behavior, particularly when chaos is present, is measuring its dimensions and investigating how the dimensionality can change under different operational circumstances. A rigorous review of dimensions is given in several papers (see Tables 2 and 3). Less rigorously stated, it can be that the correlation dimension of a system's behavior is the minimum number of dimensions of a space that can contain the trajectories generated by the system. As Rapp et al. (see Tables 2 and 3) express it, the dimension of a system is its number of degrees of freedom. This definition is restricted but simple and useful. It is important to compare systems only by referring to the same quantity, usually the correlation dimension (D_2).

A system is periodic if its D_2 is a whole number (e.g., 2.0, 3.0, 4.0), and chaotic if D_2 is "fractal" (e.g., 2.1, 3.9., 4.5).

The values of correlation dimension in well studied chaotic physical systems rarely exceed 3.9 and some authorities question the meaning of values reported in some biological systems that already exceeds 4. The computation of D_2 requires some steps with judgemental determination, for example, of sampling rate, filter limits, or some other parameters.

As mentioned by several authors, the correlation dimension is not an absolutely satisfactory measure of complexity since similar systems, differing only in the value of some exponent, can have different fractal dimensions and can be regarded as more complex than a system with the next higher whole number.

The EEG has a Strange Attractor; The EEG is not Always Stochastic or Limit Cycle Activity

A new trend in brain research was initiated by evaluation of the correlation dimension D_2 of the brain's EEG during slow-wave sleep by Babloyantz et al. (1985) and shortly after that by application of the same algorithm to some

Table 2. Human EEG/MEG Data

Reference	Parameters	Results
Babloyantz et al. (1985)	$\Delta t = 10$ ms $N = 4000$ $\tau = 20$ ms EEG	Sleep stage 2: $D_2 = 5.03$ Sleep stage 4: $D_2 = 4.0–4.4$ Awake, alpha activity: $D_2 = 6.1$ Beta: D_2—no saturation
Rapp et al. (1986)	$\Delta t = 2$ ms $N = 1000–4000$ $\tau = 10–20$ ms EEG	Eyes closed, relaxed: $D_2 = 2.4$ ($N = 1000$) $D_2 = 2.6$ ($N = 4000$) Eyes closed, counting: $D_2 = 3.0$ ($N = 4000$)
Layne et al. (1986)	$\Delta t = 2$ ms $N = 1000–15000$ $\tau = 20$ ms (occipital) $\tau = 40$ ms (vertex) EEG	Awake, occipital: $D_2 = 5.5–6.6$ Awake, vertex: $D_2 = 6.5–7.7$
Başar et al. (1989b; 1990; this volume)	$\Delta t = 30$ ms $N = 16384$ points (segments of 3 min) $\Delta f = 100$ Hz EEG	Eyes closed, occipital/vertex/parietal/frontal: $D_2 = 5.5–8$ (Finite dimension only when data prefiltered between 5 and 15 Hz)
Dvorak and Siska (1986)	$\Delta t = 5$ ms $N = 1000–12000$ $\tau = 40$ ms EEG	Eyes closed: $D_2 = 3.8–5.4$ ($N = 1000$) $D_2 = 8–10$ ($N = 12000$)
Van Erp et al. (1987)	$\Delta t = 5–10$ ms $N = 1000–10000$ $\tau = 15–75$ ms EEG	Alpha rhythm: $D_2 = 5–6$ ($N = 1000$) $D_2 = 7–8$ ($N = 10000$) Beta rhythm: D_2—no saturation
Babloyantz et al. (1986)	$\Delta t = 0.83$ ms $N = 6000$ $\tau = 16–60$ ms EEG	Creutzfeldt-Jakob disease: $D_2 = 3.7–5.4$ Epileptic attack: $D_2 = 2.05$
Saermark et al. (1989; personal communication)	$\Delta t = 10$ ms $N = 4000–8000$ $\tau = 100$ ms MEG	Healthy subject: $D_2 = 11$ Epilepsy (2 patients): $D_2 = 7$ Epilepsy (2 patients): D_2—no saturation

D_2, Correlation dimension, N, number of data points; τ, time shift; Δt, sampling time; SWS, slow-wave sleep stage; REM, rapid-eye movement sleep; MEG, Magnetoencephalography; Δf, sampling frequency.

Table 3. Intracranial EEG (Animal Experiments)

Reference	Results
Başar et al. (1988), Röschke and Başar (1985, 1988)	Cat, SWS, cortex (epidural): $D_2 = 5.0 \pm 0.1$ Cat, SWS, hippocampus: $D_2 = 4.0 \pm 0.07$ Cat, SWS, reticular formation (mesencephalon): $D_2 = 4.4 \pm 0.07$ (the most stable data)
Röschke and Başar (1989)	Cat, inferior colliculus: $D_2 = 6.7$ Cat, reticular formation (mesencephalon): $D_2 = 7.05$ (unstable attractor, waking state, attractor properties in only 25% of recording time, „high frequency attractor,“ data filtered between 100 and 1000 Hz
Röschke and Başar (1989)	Cat, waking state, hippocampus: $D_2 = 4.00$ (during synchronized hippocampal theta activity)
Lopes da Silva et al. (1990)	Rat, hippocampus: $D_2 = 2\text{–}3$ or higher (unstable depending on location and on existence of epileptic discharge)
Skinner et al. (1989; this volume)	Rabbit, olfactory bulb: $D_2 = 5\text{–}6$ (event-related shifting from 5 to 6 in evoked activities with odor targets)

D_2, correlation dimension; SWS, slow wave sleep stage

pathological cases. Following the most important pioneering work by Babloyantz and coworkers, Röschke and Başar (1985) published results on the strange attractors in several intracranial structures of the cat brain during SWS and confirmed in a general way the results of Babloyantz et al. Further, Rapp and coworkers (1985) interpreted the waking EEG as chaotic behavior (for these references see Tables 2 and 3).

Why is the Descriptor Correlation Dimension Important?

Are the trajectories of the EEG comparable with those of a metronome? Certainly not. Can the EEG trajectories be compared with those of more complex systems presented in Table 1? Certainly not yet. However, the use of the parameter dimension is a first important step in this sense.

The unpredictability and so the attractor's degree of chaos is effectively measured by the parameter "dimension." Dimension is important to dynamics because it provides a precise way of speaking of the number of independent variables inherent in a motion. For a dissipative dynamical system, trajectories that do not diverge to infinity approach an attractor.

In Tables 2 and 3 the values of correlation dimensions D_2, computed by several research groups under different experimental conditions, are listed together. The computation parameters are also included in the tables on human EEG. In Table 2 the results of measurements on humans are presented; in Table 3 the experiments with intracranial recording of cat brain, rat brain, and rabbit brain are shown.

Most of the studies outlined in Tables 2 and 3 showed that the electrical activity (field potentials) are not random or stochastic, and they are generally fractal. Since the EEG has often finite dimensionality and limited degrees of freedom, it is to be hoped that the higher dimensionalities in the brain can be compared, in the future, with complex models yet to be developed. Computations with hypothetically developed neural models could help us to understand neural implications of these higher dimensionalities in the EEG provided that such models would include functional relevances to justification of fractal dimensions and high correlation dimensions greater than 3. Words of caution for these types of analysis and limits of interpretation are described by Bullock (1990) and Başar (1990).

References

Abraham RH, Shaw CD (1983): *Dynamics. The Geometry of Behaviour*, vols 1–3. Santa Cruz: Aerial

Babloyantz A, Nicolis C, Salazar M (1985): Evidence of chaotic dynamics of brain activity during the sleep cycle . *Phys Lett (A)* 11 : 152–156

Başar E, ed. (1980): *EEG–Brain Dynamics. Relation between EEG and Brain Evoked Potentials.* Amsterdam: Elsevier/North-Holland

Başar E, ed. (1990): *Chaos in Brain Function.* Berlin–Heidelberg–New York: Springer

Bullock TH (1990): An agenda for research on chaotic dynamics. In: *Chaos in Brain Function,* Başar E, ed. Berlin–Heidelberg–New York: Springer, pp 31–41

Haken H, ed. (1983): *Advanced synergetics.* Berlin–Heidelberg–New York: Springer

References to Tables 2 and 3

Babloyantz A, Destexhe, A (1986): Low dimensional chaos in an instance of epilepsy. *Proc Natl Acad Sci USA* 83 : 3513

Babloyantz A, Nicolis C, Salazar M (1985): Evidence of chaotic dynamics of brain activity during the sleep cycle. *Phys Lett (A)* 111 : 152–156

Başar E, Başar-Eroglu C, Röschke J (1988): Do coherent patterns of the strange attractor EEG reflect deterministic sensory-cognitive states of the brain. In: *From Chemical to Biological Organization,* Markus M, Müller Sc, Nicolis G, eds. Berlin–Heidelberg–New York: Springer, pp 297–306

Başar E, Başar-Eroglu C, Röschke J, Schult J (1989b): Chaos- and alpha-preparation in brain function. In: *Models of Brain Function*, Cotteril R, ed. Cambridge University Press, pp 365–395

Başar E, Başar-Eroglu C, Röschke J, Schult J (1990): Strange attractor EEG as sign of cognitive function. In: *Machinery of the Mind*, John ER, Harmony T, Prichep L, Valdes-Sosa A, Valdes- Sosa P, eds. Boston: Birkhäuser, pp 91–114

Dvorak I, Siska J (1986): On some problems encountered in the estimation of the correlation dimension of the EEG. *Phys Lett A* 118:63–66

Hooper J (1983): What lurks behind the wild forces of nature? Ask the connoisseurs of chaos. *Omni* 5:85–92

Layne SP, Mayer-Kress G, Holzfuss J (1986): Problems associated with dimensional analysis of electroencephalogram data. In: *Dimensions and Entropies in Chaotic Systems*, Mayer-Kress G, ed. Berlin–Heidelberg–New York: Springer, p 246

Lopes da Silva FH, Kamphuis W, van Neerven JMAM, Pijn JPM (1990): Cellular and network mechanisms in the kindling model of epilepsy: the role of GABAergic inhibition and the emerge of strange attractors. In: *Machinery of the Mind*, John ER, Harmony T, Prichep L, Valdes-Sosa M, Valdes-Sosa P, eds. Boston: Birkhäuser, pp 115–139

Rapp PE, Albano AM, Guzman GC, Greenbaum NN, Bashore TR (1986): In: *Nonlinear Oscillations in biology and chemistry*, Othmer HG, ed. Berlin–Heidelberg–New York: Springer, p 175 (Lecture Notes in Biomathematics, vol 66)

Röschke J, Başar E (1985): Is EEG a simple noise or a "strange attractor"? *Pflügers Arch* 405:R45

Röschke J, Başar E (1988): The EEG is not a simple noise: strange attractors in intracranial structures. In: *Dynamics of Sensory and Cognitive Processing by the Brain*, Başar E, ed. Berlin–Heidelberg–New York: Springer, pp 203–216

Röschke J. Başar E (1989): Correlation dimensions in various parts of cat and human brain in different states. In: *Brain Dynamics*, Başar E, Bullock TH, eds. Berlin–Heidelberg–New York: Springer, pp 131–148

Saermark K, Lebech J, Bak CK, Sabers A (1989): Magnetoencephalography and attractor dimension: normal subjects and epileptic patients. In: *Brain Dynamics*, Başar E, Bullock TH, eds. Berlin–Heidelberg–New York: Springer, pp 149–157

Schuster HG (1988): *Deterministic Chaos*. Weinheim: VCH

Skinner JE, Martin JL, Landisman CE, Mommer MM, Fulton K, Mitra M, Burton WD, Saltzberg B (1989): Chaotic attractors in a model of neocortex: dimensionalitites of olfactory bulb surface potentials are spatially uniform and event related. In: *Brain Dynamics*, Başar E, Bullock TH, eds. Berlin–Heidelberg–New York: Springer, pp 158–173

Van Erp MG (1988): *On Epilepsy: Investigations on the Level of the Nerve Membrane and of the Brain*. Leiden: Proefschrift Rijksuniversiteit

Index